Chemical Reagents
for
Protein Modification

2nd Edition

Author

Roger L. Lundblad, Ph.D.
Professor of Pathology and Biochemistry
Dental Research Center
University of North Carolina
Chapel Hill, North Carolina

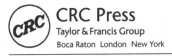

CRC Press
Taylor & Francis Group
Boca Raton London New York

CRC Press is an imprint of the
Taylor & Francis Group, an **informa** business

CRC Press
Taylor & Francis Group
6000 Broken Sound Parkway NW, Suite 300
Boca Raton, FL 33487-2742

Reissued 2019 by CRC Press

© 1991 by Taylor & Francis Group, LLC
CRC Press is an imprint of Taylor & Francis Group, an Informa business

No claim to original U.S. Government works

A Library of Congress record exists under LC control number:

Publisher's Note
The publisher has gone to great lengths to ensure the quality of this reprint but points out that some imperfections in the original copies may be apparent.

Disclaimer
The publisher has made every effort to trace copyright holders and welcomes correspondence from those they have been unable to contact.

ISBN 13: 978-0-367-26354-6 (hbk)
ISBN 13: 978-0-367-26355-3 (pbk)
ISBN 13: 978-0-429-29287-3 (ebk)

Visit the Taylor & Francis Web site at http://www.taylorandfrancis.com and the
CRC Press Web site at http://www.crcpress.com

PREFACE TO SECOND EDITION

It has been some seven years since the preparation of the first edition of this work. Although site-specific mutagenesis has proved to be a powerful technique for studying the relationship between structure and function in proteins, site-specific chemical modification continues to be a useful approach in this area. The revision has focused on some of the more popular techniques, including photoaffinity labeling and the modification of cysteine residues. Where possible, an attempt has been made to correlate the results from site-specific mutagenesis and site-specific chemical modification.

The author wishes to express his appreciation to Jarrod Jenzano for the preparation of many of the new chemical figures using the T^3 Scientific Word Processing Program (TCI Software Research Inc., Los Cruces, New Mexico). In addition, the support of colleagues at the University of North Carolina at Chapel Hill has been critical for the completion of this work. As with the first edition, the author acknowledges the continued intellectual support of the fifth floor of Flexner Hall at the Rockefeller University. In particular, the author expresses appreciation to Dr. Bryce Plapp of the University of Iowa and Dr. James Manning of the Rockefeller University.

The author's research programs are supported by Research Grants DE-06997 and DE-08671 from the National Institute of Dental Research.

Roger L. Lundblad

THE AUTHOR

Roger Lauren Lundblad, Ph.D. was Professor of Pathology and Biochemistry in the School of Medicine and Professor of Oral Biology in the Department of Periodontics in the School of Dentistry at the University of North Carolina at Chapel Hill. He is presently Director of Technology Development at Baxter Hyland Biotechnology in Hayward, California.

Dr. Lundblad received his undergraduate education at Pacific Lutheran University in Tacoma, Washington and the Ph.D. degree in biochemistry at the University of Washington in 1965. Prior to joining the faculty of the University of North Carolina in 1968, Dr. Lundblad was a Research Associate at the Rockefeller University.

Dr. Lundblad's research interests are in the use of solution chemistry techniques to study protein-protein interaction, with particular emphasis on the proteolytic enzymes involved in blood coagulation, salivary proteins, and the biochemistry of wound healing.

TABLE OF CONTENTS

Chapter 1
Site-Specific Chemical Modification of Proteins 1

Chapter 2
Amino Acid Analysis 21

Chapter 3
**Peptide Separation by Reverse-Phase High-Performance
Liquid Chromatography** 29

Chapter 4
Methods for Sequence Determination 37

Chapter 5
Chemical Cleavage of Peptide Bonds 49

Chapter 6
The Modification of Cysteine 59

Chapter 7
The Modification of Cysteine — Cleavage of Disulfide Bonds 95

Chapter 8
The Modification of Methionine 99

Chapter 9
The Modification of Histidine Residues 105

Chapter 10
The Modification of Lysine 129

Chapter 11
The Modification of Arginine 173

Chapter 12
Chemical Modification of Tryptophan 215

Chapter 13
The Modification of Tyrosine 239

Chapter 14
The Modification of Carboxyl Groups 267

Chapter 15
The Chemical Cross-Linking of Peptide Chains 287

Chapter 16
Affinity Labeling 305

Index 337

Chapter 1

SITE-SPECIFIC CHEMICAL MODIFICATION OF PROTEINS

The overall thrust of this book concerns the study of the solution chemistry of proteins using covalent modification of the various functional groups present in the protein. It is the purpose of this chapter to introduce the concept of the site-specific chemical modification of protein and how existence of site-specific chemical modification is established. Together with this subject, factors which influence the reactivity of the various functional groups in a protein will be considered.

We will define site-specific chemical modification as a chemical reaction which results in the *quantitative*, covalent derivatization of the functional group (i.e., primary amine, sulfydryl group, imidazole ring) of a *single, unique* amino acid residue in a protein without any demonstrable effect on either any other functional groups or the conformation of the molecule. This is an ideal pursuit which should be our foremost objective as organic chemists interested in the relationships between structure and function in a complex heteropolymer. There are several pragmatic considerations which tend to compromise our efforts in obtaining this ideal. First, few reagents are absolutely specific for a given type of functional group (i.e., sulfhydryl, phenolic hydroxyl, etc.) let alone for a specific residue within a functional group class. The status of analytical capabilities precludes unambiguous detection of loss less than 3 to 5% of an amino acid unless that modification is associated with the appearance of a unique derivative (i.e., *S*-carboxymethylcysteine, 3-nitrotyrosine) which can be easily identified. Second, it is unlikely that chemical modification of a single amino acid residue can be accomplished without *any* concomitant conformational change. Although this is a frequent criticism of chemical modification, it is, in general, *without significant merit* in the consideration of *specific chemical modification*. Admittedly, few investigators rigorously evaluate the extent of conformational change which occurs as a result of chemical modification but in such instances only minor change is seen.[1-5] However, this may well reflect the level of sophistication of conformational analysis since marked changes in protein stability can be observed.[5]

Establishment of the accomplishment of specific chemical modification is not a trivial process. There are a number of criteria to be fulfilled which are considered below.

Establishing the stoichiometry of modification is a relatively straightforward process. First, the molar quantity of modified residue is established by analysis. This could be spectrophotometric as, for example, with the trinitrophenylation of primary amino groups, the nitration of tyrosine with tetranitromethane (Figure 1), or the alkylation of tryptophan with 2-hydroxy-5-nitrobenzyl bromide or by amino acid analysis to determine either the loss of a residue as, for example, in photo-oxidation of histidine and the oxidation of the indole ring of tryptophan with *N*-bromosuccinimide or the appearance of a modified residue such as with *S*-carboxymethylcysteine or N^1- or N^3-carboxymethylhistidine. In the situation where spectral change or radiolabel incorporation is used to establish stoichiometry, analysis must be performed to determine that there is not a reaction with another amino acid. For example, the extent of oxidation of tryptophan by *N*-bromosuccinimide can be determined spectrophotometrically but amino acid analysis is *required* to determine if modification has also occurred with another amino acid such as histidine.

In case of the site-specific chemical modification of a protein, it must be established that the modification of one residue mole per mole of protein (or functional subunit) has occurred without modification of another amino acid (e.g., modification has only occurred with lysine and not with tyrosine). This must be established with each study. The reaction pattern of a given reagent with free amino acids or amino acid derivatives does not necessarily provide the basis for reaction with such amino acid residues in protein. Furthermore, the reaction

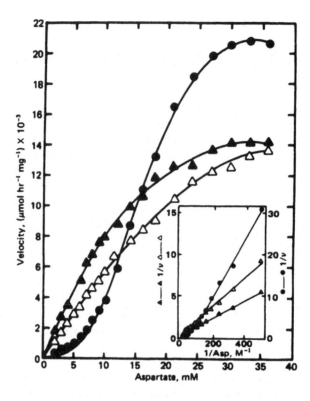

FIGURE 1.   The effect of nitration on the cooperative behavior of aspartate transcarbamylase. Shown is the effect of aspartate concentration on aspartate transcarbamylase activity with the reconstituted native enzyme (●) and with the enzyme reconstituted with the nitrated catalytic subunit in the presence (△) and absence (▲) of CTP. (From Landfear, S. M., Evans, D. R., and Lipscomb, W. N., *Proc. Natl. Acad. Sci. U.S.A.*, 75, 2654, 1978. With permission.)

pattern of a given reagent with one protein cannot necessarily be extrapolated to all proteins. It is of critical importance to appreciate that the results of a chemical modification can be markedly affected by reaction conditions (e.g., pH, temperature, solvent and/or buffer used, degree of illumination, etc.). Establishment of stoichiometry does not necessarily mean that this modification has occurred at a unique residue (unique in terms of position in the linear peptide chain — not necessarily unique with respect to reactivity). It is, of course, useful if there is a change in biological activity (catalysis, substrate binding, ion binding, etc.) which occurs concomitant with the chemical modification. Ideally, one would like to establish a direct relationship (i.e., 0.5 mol/mol of protein with 50% activity modification; 1.0 mol/mol of protein with 100% activity modification). This occurs frequently with affinity labels such as the peptide chloromethyl ketones[6,7] or with reaction at the active cysteinyl residues in sulfhydryl proteases.[8-10] More frequently, one might have the situation where there are several moles of a given amino acid modified.[11]

In some of these situations it is possible to fractionate the protein into uniquely modified species. The separation of carboxymethyl-HIS[12]-pancreatic ribonuclease from carboxymethyl-HIS[119]-pancreatic ribonuclease is a classic example of this type of a situation.[11] More recently, it has been possible to separate various derivatives of lysozyme obtained from the modification of carboxyl groups.[12] Frequently, however, while there is good evidence that multiple modified species are obtained as a result of the reaction, it is not possible to separate uniquely modified species. As an example, consider recent studies on the modification of thrombin by tetranitromethane.[13] In these studies, apparent stoichiometry of inactivation was obtained with equivalent modification of two separate tyrosine residues (Tyr 71 and Tyr 85 in the B chain) and it was not possible to separate these derivatives. As a result it was necessary to use techniques such as those described below to obtain an understanding of the inactivation reaction.

The approach advanced by Ray and Koshland[14] is based on establishing a relationship between the rate of the loss of biological activity and the rate of the modification of amino acid residues. This basically involves the comparison of the second-order rate constants for the modification of one or more amino acid residues and the loss of biological activity.

The statistical approach advanced by Tsou[15-17] is based on establishing a relationship between the number of residues modified and the change in biological activity. As noted by Tsou, this approach is quite valuable when it is difficult to accurately determine the rate of functional group modification as for example with N-bromosuccinimide or 2-hydroxy-5-nitrobenzyl bromide. With this approach it is necessary to determine the relationship between the number of residues (functional groups) modified and biological activity. In Tsou's least complicated example, the biologically essential groups are all of the same type and both essential and nonessential groups are modified at the same rate. Assuming that the modification of any essential group results in the loss of activity, the fraction of biologically active protein remaining will be equal to the fraction of activity remaining (denoted as a). In the situation where there is a single essential group, the fraction of essential groups remaining after any period of modification (denoted as x_c) will be equal to a. In the situation where the number of essential groups is i (by definition greater than 1) among all functional groups of type X, the fraction of each essential group remaining after a period of modification will be x_c. Only those proteins which have all their essential groups intact will retain full activity. Therefore:

$$a = x_c^i \qquad \text{or} \qquad a^{1/i} = x$$

When all groups of type X react at the same rate, then x_c will be equal to the fraction of the overall fraction of unmodified type X groups and

$$a^{1/i} = x$$

The use of this approach requires the plotting of log a vs. log x; the slope of the resulting line yields i. A number of investigators plot a (activity) vs. m (residues modified).

Horiike and McCormick[18] have explored the approach of relating changes in activity to extent of chemical modification. These investigators state that the original concepts which form the basis of this approach are sound[14,15] but that extrapolation from a plot of activity remaining vs. residues modified is not necessarily sound. Such extrapolation is only valid if the "nonessential" residues react much slower (rate at least 100 times slower). Given a situation where all residues within a given group are equally reactive toward the reagent in question, the number of essential residues obtained from such a plot is correct only when the total number of residues is equal to the number of essential residues which is, in turn, equal to 1.0. However it is important to emphasize that this approach is useful when there is a difference in the rate of reaction of an *essential* residue or residues and all other residues in that class as is the example in the modification of histidyl residues with diethyl pyrocarbonate in lactate dehydrogenase,[19,20] and pyridoxamine-5'-phosphate oxidase.[21] Some examples of the application of Tsou plots to specific chemical modification are presented in Figures 2 to 4.[21-23]

Unequivocal support for site-specific chemical modification can only be obtained from establishing that reaction occurred at a unique (in terms of position on the peptide chain)

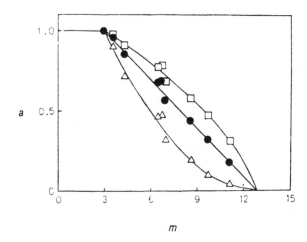

FIGURE 2. A Tsou plot for the modification of pepsin with trimethyloxonium fluoroborate. Shown is a plot of (a) vs. (m) where a is the
remaining catalytic activity and m is the number of methyl groups incorporated from reaction with trimethyloxonium fluoroborate. The line for
i = 2 (●) is the least-squares straight line for these points. The lines for
i = 1 (△) and i = 3 (□) are the theoretical curves based upon the
i = 2 line. (From Paterson, A. K. and Knowles, J. R., *Eur. J. Biochem.*,
31, 510, 1972. With permission.)

amino acid residue. This generally involves the isolation of a peptide fragment containing
the modified residue. A decade ago this was a very laborious task which required substantial
amounts of protein. Recent developments in the application of high-performance liquid
chromatography to the analysis of peptides (reviewed in Chapter 3) have greatly decreased
the amount of time and materials required for this analysis. It is of critical importance that
the investigator maintain very careful records of the yield of modified residue at each
fractionation step in order to be certain that the modified peptide is truly representative of
the stoichiometrically modified site on the protein.

The establishment of a definite, unambiguous relationship between a specific chemical
modification and a change in the catalytic activity, a change in the nature/magnitude of an
allosteric response, or a change in the characteristics of a specific binding site is, in general,
more difficult than one would expect considering the relatively large number of papers
purporting to have elucidated such a relationship. It is difficult to completely exclude the
argument that "activity" has been modified strictly secondary to the placement of steric
bulk "on" a functional group as opposed to a direct effect on the participation of the
functional group in the "activity". This argument was advanced to explain, in part, the
effect of the modification of the active site serine of chymotrypsin with diisopropylphosphorofluoridate. Subsequent work which showed that conversion to dehydroalanine also
resulted in the complete loss of enzyme activity obviated this particular argument.[24] Koshland
and Neet also described the formation of "thiol-subtilisin", a derivative of subtilisin where
the active-site serine has been converted to a cysteine residue.[25] Although a cysteinyl residue
functions at the active site of sulfhydryl proteases such as papain,[8] ficin,[10] and streptococcal
proteinase,[9] the analogous derivative of subtilisin, thiol-subtilisin, has, at best, 1% of the
enzymatic activity of subtilisin. It is of interest to note that conversion of the active-site
cysteine to a serine residue in papain resulted in a completely inactive enzyme.[26] In both of
the studies a "functionally conservative" *chemical* mutation resulted in the essentially complete loss of catalytic activity.

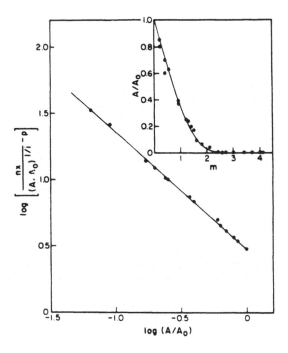

FIGURE 3. A Tsou plot for the modification of pyridoxamine phosphate oxidase by diethylpyrocarbonate. The data were plotted using the following equation:

$$\log \left[\frac{nx}{A/A_o^{1/i}} - p \right]$$
$$= \log(n - p) + \left(\frac{\alpha - 1}{i} \right) \log(A/A_o)$$

where A/A_o is the fraction of enzyme molecules retaining full activity, n is the number of modifiable residues of type X consisting of p residues, of which i are essential, react with the reagent at a pseudo-first-order rate constant k_1 and $n - p$ residues which are not essential reacting at a pseudo-first-order rate constant $k_2(-\alpha k_1)$, and x is the number of residues remaining after reaction with reagent. The data are plotted assuming that in the above equation $n = 4$ and $p = i = 1$. The inset describes the relationship between the number of histidyl residues modified per mole of enzyme (m) and A/A_o. (From Horiike, K., Tsuge, H., and McCormick, D. B., *J. Biol. Chem.*, 254, 6638, 1979. With permission.)

Increased insight into these data has been derived from recent studies on the site-specific mutagenesis of rat trypsin.[27,28] In the first of these studies,[27] a cysteinyl residue was introduced in place of the active-site serine residue by site-specific mutagenesis and the catalytic activity characterized with various substrates. While 'thiol-trypsin (trypsin S195C) was active, the value for k_{cat} for trypsin in S195C was reduced by a factor of 3.4×10^5 with respect to the native enzyme. In a subsequent crystallographic study of trypsin S195C, it was determined that there are likely steric considerations, such as blocking of the oxyanion hole by the sulfur atom, that contribute to the low levels of activity.

One of the better approaches to the problem of relating changes in "activity" to a specific chemical modification is being able to demonstrate that the reversal of modification (see Figures 5 and 6)[29,30] is directly associated with the reversal of the change(s) in biological

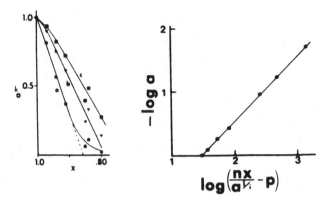

FIGURE 4.   The left figure is a Tsou plot for the modification of arginine residues in transketolase by phenylglyoxal. The abscissa is a ratio of unmodified arginine residues to the total number of arginine residues. The ordinate is a where a is the fraction of activity remaining and i is a small integer. A linear segment is generated in the case where p residues including i essential residues react at a rate k and n − p residues react with rate αk. The following equation adapted from Tsou:

$$nx = pa^{1/i} + (n - p)\, a^{\alpha/i}$$

reduces to

$$a^{1/i} = \frac{nx - (n - p)}{p}$$

when $\alpha \ll 1$. This gives a straight line with the x intercept equal to n − p/n. This is represented by the extrapolation of the linear portion of the curve to the x axis: a, i = 1, b, i = 2, c, i = 3. The best fit is provided by i − 1 and in this case p = 4 to 5 residues/active site. The right figure describes the determination of α (the constant relating the reaction rates of rapidly and slowly reacting residues). The following equation

$$nx = pa^{1/i} + (n - p)\, a^{\alpha/i}$$

adapted from Tsou can be rearranged as:

$$\log (nx/a^{1/i} - p) = \log (n - p) + [(\alpha - 1)/i]\, \log a,$$

where i and p are determined as described above. α is determined from the slope of the resulting line. In this situation, α = 0.023 implying that the rapidly reacting residues have a rate constant approximately 40-fold greater than the slowly reacting residues. (From Kremer, A. B., Egan, R. M., and Sable, H. Z., *J. Biol. Chem.*, 255, 2405, 1980. With permission.)

activity. Demonstrating that the ''effects'' of a specific chemical modification are reversible lends support *against* the argument that such ''effects'' are a result of irreversible and ''nonspecific'' conformation change.

A careful study of site-specific chemical modification can provide extensive information about the organic chemistry of this class of heteropolymers. The process of the elucidation of the differences in reactivities of various residues in a protein can provide considerable insight into the possible function of such residues. An excellent example of the information which can be obtained from a careful study is provided by Holbrook and Ingham.[19] This study used reaction with diethylpyrocarbonate to investigate the properties of a histidyl

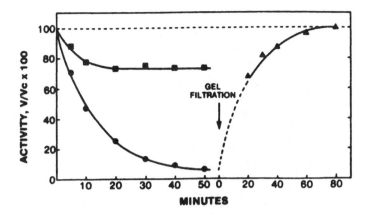

FIGURE 5.   The reversible modification of pyridoxamine-5′-phosphate oxidase by 2,3-butanedione. The enzyme (2.1 μM) was incubated with 10 mM 2,3-butanedione in the presence of 5 μM flavin mononucleotide (FMN) in either 50 mM potassium borate, pH 8.0 (●) or 50 mM potassium phosphate, pH 8.0 (■). The reaction mixture in borate was passed over a G-25 Sephadex column and assayed for enzyme activity (▲). The arrow indicates the time at which the reaction mixture in borate was applied to the gel filtration column. (From Choi, J.-D. and McCormick, D. B., *Biochemistry*, 20, 5722, 1981. With permission.)

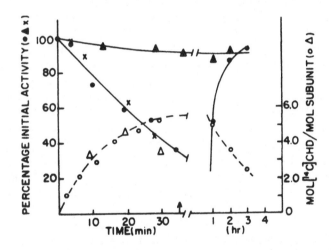

FIGURE 6.   The reversible modification of ADP-glucose synthetase by 1,2-cyclohexanedione (CHD). The enzyme was incubated with 10 mM [^{14}C] CHD in the presence (●,○) or absence (x, △) of 50 mM sodium tetraborate. The control (▲) was incubated in the absence of CHD. Portions were removed at the indicated times for the determination of incorporated radioactivity (open symbols) or fructose diphosphate-stimulated enzyme activity (closed symbols). The arrow indicated the time of addition of 0.2 M hydroxylamine. (From Carlson, C. A. and Preiss, J., *Biochemistry*, 21, 1929, 1982. With permission.)

residue suggested to be present at the active site of this enzyme. Both the essential histidine and N-acetylhistidine reacted optimally with diethylpyrocarbonate at pH 6.8. The rate for reaction of the active site histidine (216 M^{-1} s^{-1}) was approximately 10-fold greater than that for N-acetylhistidine (24 M^{-1} s^{-1}) implying enhanced reactivity of the essential histidine as a reflection of a unique microenvironment. Our laboratory[31] has also been able to use

Table 1
DISSOCIATION
CONSTANTS FOR
NUCLEOPHILES IN
PROTEINS

Potential nucleophile	pKa
Carboxyl	4.6
Imidazole	7.0
Sulfhydryl	7.0
Alpha-amino	7.8
Phenolic hydroxyl	9.6
Epsilon-amino	10.2

reaction with diethylpyrocarbonate as a measure of the change in the nucleophilicity of the active-site histidine associated with the conversion of bovine α-thrombin to β-thrombin.

To gain a thorough appreciation of the events involved in the specific chemical modification of proteins, it is necessary to understand some of the basic organic chemistry of the functional groups on the protein and the reagents which react with these functional groups.

Most of the reactions which will be described in the following pages are not actually a result of the reagent in question attacking the functional groups on the protein with the subsequent formation of a covalent bond but rather nucleophilic attack by the functional group on the protein on an electron-poor center such as the carbonyl carbon of an α-haloacid (e.g., iodoacetic acid).

Before going further it might be useful to define some terms that we will be using. When most of us think of acids we tend to think of substances such as hydrochloric acid, sulfuric acid, and acetic acid, substances which can donate protons in aqueous solution to form hydronium ions (H_3O^+). Likewise a base is most usually considered to be a substance (e.g., hydroxide ion — OH^-) which can accept protons. In other words, by this definition a base possesses an unshared electron pair with which it can attract and hold a proton. This is the classical Bronsted definition of acids and bases. Organic chemists find it more useful to use the Lewis definition of acids and bases. Using this definition, an acid is a substance that can form a covalent bond by accepting an electron pair and a base has an unshared electron pair. Taking this a step further then, Lewis acids are electrophilic while Lewis bases are nucleophilic.

As we have indicated above, the majority of the chemical reactions to be described later involve nucleophilic addition by a functional group on the protein molecule. Nucleophilic addition proceeds by either an S_N1 mechanism or an S_N2 mechanism.

Now we can go somewhat further and equate a nucleophilic species with an electron-rich center and an electrophilic species with an electron-deficient center. A list of the nucleophilic functional groups in proteins is given in Table 1. In general the most potent nucleophile in a protein is sulfur with nitrogen considerably less potent followed in potency by oxygen and carbon.

It is useful to consider some factors which influence the reactivity of nucleophilic centers in proteins. From a consideration of the three-dimensional structure of proteins the majority of polar amino acids (i.e., Lys, Arg, Gly, Asp) are located on the exterior surface of the molecule while the majority of the hydrophobic (nonpolar) residues are located in the interior of these molecules. Thus, a gradient of polarity (dielectric constant) will exist going from the surface of the protein into the interior. Such a gradient could also be considered to exist in "pocket-like" indentations on the protein surface. For example, the area immediately adjacent to the active site and substrate site S_1 in thrombin is definitely hydrophobic with respect to the surrounding environment and the aqueous solution. This is best demonstrated by the increase in the fluorescence of $N\alpha$-dansyl-L-arginine-N-(3-ethyl-1,5-pentanediyl) amide upon binding to the active-site region.[32]

It should follow from the above discussion that the surface of a globular protein is definitely not homogeneous with respect to electrical charge or, more critically for our consideration, with respect to dielectric constant. As a result of this lack of homogeneity, a variety of surface polarities will surround the various functional groups. The physical and chemical properties of any given functional group will be strongly influenced by the nature (e.g., polarity) of the local microenvironment. Changes in the polarity of the microenvironment can have a profound effect on the dissociation of acids. For example consider the effect of the addition of an organic solvent, ethyl alcohol, on the pKa of acetic acid. In 100% H_2O, acetic acid has a pKa of 4.70. The addition of 80% ethyl alcohol results in an increase of the pKa to 6.9. In 100% ethyl alcohol the pKa of acetic acid is 10.3. This is particularly important in considering the reactivity of nucleophilic groups such as amino groups, cysteine, carboxyl groups, and the phenolic hydroxyl group. In the case of the primary amines present in protein, these functional groups are not reactive except in the free base form. In other words the proton present at neutral pH must be removed from the ϵ-amino group of lysine before this functional group can function as an effective nucleophile. A listing of the "average" pKa values for the various functional groups present in protein is also given in Table 1.

Other factors which can influence the pKa of a functional group in a protein include hydrogen binding with an adjacent functional group, the direct electrostatic effect of the presence of a charged group in the immediate vicinity of a potential nucleophile and finally, direct steric effects on the availability of a given functional group.

There is another consideration which can in a sense be considered either a cause or consequence of microenvironmental polarity. This has to do with the functional groups/ environment immediately around the nucleophilic species in question. These are the "factors" that can cause a "selective" increase (or decrease) in reagent concentration in the vicinity of a potentially reactive species. The most clearly understood example of this is the process of affinity labeling. Another situation can be related to the differences in polarity of the microenvironment around a nucleophilic center. This is considered in Chapter 13 and is discussed by Myers and Glazer.[33] There is also the consideration that a charged reagent can be either attracted to or repelled from the vicinity of a nucleophilic center. This is easily demonstrated by the differences in the comparative rates of modification of the active-site cysteinyl residue by chloroacetic acid and chloroacetamide in papain.[34]

In the study of the effect of chemical modification on enzymes, it is of critical importance to differentiate between modifications which have an actual effect on catalysis (the *actual process* of bond-breaking and bond-making), modifications which have an effect on the microenvironment of enzymes and modifications which have a primary effect on the process of substrate recognition (the modification of the aspartic acid residue at S_1, see Figure 7, in trypsin[35] is an excellent example of such a modification).

Another major use of chemical modification has been in the determination of the primary structure of proteins. This includes reagents such as cyanogen bromide for the chemical cleavage of specific peptide bonds, citraconic anhydride for the reversible blocking of lysine residues to restrict tryptic cleavage to arginine residues, and the reversible blocking of arginine residues with 1,2-cyclohexanedione to restrict tryptic cleavage to lysine residues.

The detailed description of these techniques is given in Chapter 5. The ability to apply techniques such as cyanogen bromide cleavage directly to polyacryamide gel electrophoretograms or to protein blots has increased the usefulness of these techniques.

The use of protein sequence information derived from the sequence analysis of cDNA for a specific protein has largely supplanted direct sequence analysis of intact proteins by classical primary structure analysis.[36-38] This is not to say that the primary structure analysis of proteins

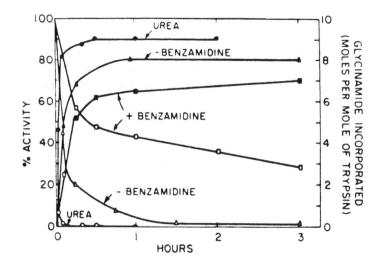

FIGURE 7.   The modification of β-trypsin with *N*-(3-dimethyl amino propyl)*N*-ethyl carbodiimide HCl (EDC) and glycinamide in the presence and absence of benzamidine and in the presence of urea as indicated in the figure. Modification of carboxyl groups was determined by the incorporation of radiolabeled glycinamide (■, ▲, ●) and catalytic activity (□, △, ○) was determined with benzoyl-arginine ethyl ester. (From Eyl, A. W., Jr. and Inagami, T., *J. Biol. Chem.*, 246, 738, 1971. With permission.)

is without value, but it is our feeling that the primary value of such analysis is to obtain information regarding the site of specific chemical modification (discussed above), the site of post-translational modification (such as the formation of γ-carboxyglutamic acid, ester-ification or *N*-methylation), the verification of "site-specific" mutagenesis, or to obtain sufficient primary structure information for the synthesis of a suitable cDNA probe which can be subsequently used for the isolation of specific messenger RNA.

The use of specific chemical modification to study changes in environment has been studied over the past 30 years. There is some consensus that the study of Kirtley and Koshland[39] provided the basis for the concept of using "reporter" groups to study changes in the microenvironment surrounding a site of modification. This study used 2-bromoace-tamido-4-nitrophenol to modify a limited number of sulfhydryl groups in glyceraldehyde-3-phosphate dehydrogenase. The modified protein has a λ_{max} at 390 nm ($\epsilon = 7100 \ M^{-1}$ cm^{-1}) between pH 7.0 and pH 7.6. The addition of the coenzyme, NAD, caused a marked change in the spectral properties (decrease in absorbance at approximately 375 nm and increase in absorbance at approximately 420 nm) of the modified enzyme which is consistent with a change in the microenvironment around the modified residue (increase in polarity of medium which results in increased formation of the nitrophenolate ion). The reaction of 2-hydroxy-5-nitrobenzyl bromide with tryptophanyl residues to yield the 2-hydroxy-5-nitro-benzyl derivative[40] (see Chapter 12) and the reaction of tetranitromethane with tyrosyl residues[41] to form these 3-nitrotyrosyl derivatives (see Chapter 13) were developed shortly after this study and have been extensively used to study microenvironmental changes in the modified proteins (Figures 8 to 10).

The use of spin-labeled reagents to determine the conformational environment at enzyme-active sites and other binding sites on proteins has been of considerable interest during the past decade. Berliner and co-workers have been particularly active in this area.[42] One early study used spin-labeled derivatives of diisopropylphosphorofluoridate to study the active site environment of trypsin[43] (Figures 11 to 13). Subsequent studies used various spin-label derivatives (piperidinyl nitroxide, pyrrolidinyl nitroxide and pyrrolinyl nitroxide substituent groups) of phenylmethylsulfonyl fluoride to compare microenvironments surrounding the active sites in α-chymotrypsin and trypsin.[44,45] These reagents have been more recently used

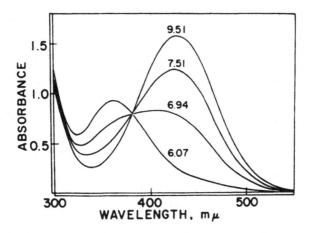

FIGURE 8. The absorption spectrum of *N*-acetyl-3-nitrotyrosine (0.25 m*M*) in 0.2 *M* Tris, 0.2 *M* acetate, 0.5 *M* NaCl at the pH indicated in the figure. (From Riordan, J. R., Sokolovsky, M., and Vallee, B. L., *Biochemistry,* 6, 358, 1967. With permission.)

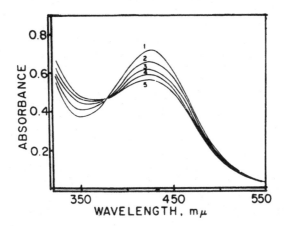

FIGURE 9. Changes in the absorption spectrum of nitrated carboxypeptidase in the presence of a competitive inhibitor, β-phenylpropionate. The spectra were determined in 0.2 *M* Tris, 0.2 *M* acetate, 0.5. NaCl, pH 8.0. The concentrations of β-phenylpropionate were 1 (none), 2 (0.01 *M*), 3 (0.025 *M*), 4 (0.05 *M*), and 5 (0.1 *M*). (From Riordan, J. R., Sokolovsky, M., and Vallee, B. L., *Biochemistry,* 6, 358, 1967. With permission.)

to study the active site of thrombin.[46,47] The preparation of spin-labeled pepsinogen has been reported.[48] This study used a *N*-hydroxy succinimide ester derivative, 3-[[(2,5-dioxo-1-pyrrolidiny)oxyl] carbonyl]-2,5,-dihydro-2,2,5,5,-tetramethyl-1H-pyrrolyl-1-oxy, to modify lysyl residues in pepsinogen. Coupling was accomplished at pH 7.0 (0.1 *M* sodium phosphate) for 7 h at 22°C resulting in the derivatization of approximately three amino groups. Figure 14 shows the change in the ESR spectrum of the modified protein upon activation (it is noted that the modified protein retained full potential peptic activity). Figure 15 shows this change in greater detail at pH 2.38 while Figure 16 shows an apparent lag phase when activation is performed at pH 2.77. It is clear that the change in the "signal" generated by the label is a measure of the rate of proenzyme to enzyme transformation as shown in Figure 17.

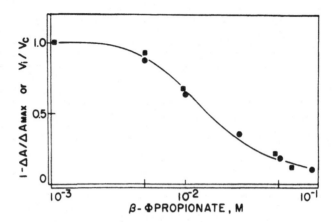

FIGURE 10. The effect of a competitive inhibitor, β-phenylpropionate on the esterase activity (■) and the absorbance at 428 nm (●) of nitro-carboxypeptidase. $\Delta A/\Delta A_{max}$ represents the fractional decrease in absorbance at 428 nm resulting from the indicated concentration of β-phenylpropionate. ΔA_{max} is the maximal decrease in absorbance at 428 nm obtained by extrapolation to infinite concentration of β-phenylpropionate. V/Vc is the ratio of catalytic activity in the presence (V) and absence (Vc) of β-phenylpropionate. (From Riordan, J. R., Sokolovsky, M., and Vallee, B. L., *Biochemistry*, 6, 358, 1967. With permission.)

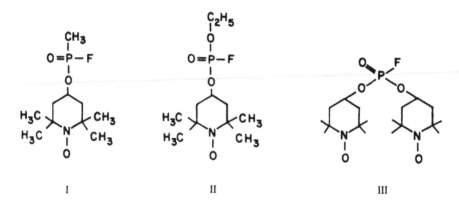

FIGURE 11. The structures of spin-labeled derivatives used to study the conformation of trypsin as shown in Figures 12 and 13. These are various derivatives of diisopropylphosphorofluoridate. Compound I is 1-oxyl-2,2,6,6-tetramethyl-4-piperidinylmethylphosporofluoridate. (From Berliner, L. J. and Wong, S. S., *J. Biol. Chem.*, 248, 1118, 1973. With permission.)

Fluorescent probes have been particularly useful in the study of protein structure. A rigorous review of this area is beyond the scope of the present work and only a limited number of examples will be considered. One exceptional study[49] in this area used a dansylpeptide chloromethyl ketone to label the active site of blood coagulation factor Xa and then subsequently used this derivative to study the stoichiometry of interaction with the other components of the prothrombin-activation enzyme complex (Figures 18 to 20). One of the major problems in the labeling of proteins to obtain fluorescent derivatives is the difficulty in achieving selective modification. One clever approach to this problem has been advanced by Jackson and co-workers.[50] These investigators used the observation that 3-aminotyrosyl residues (obtained by reaction with tetranitromethane followed by a reduction with sodium

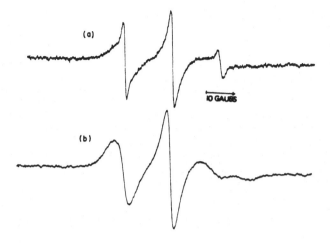

FIGURE 12. The electron spin resonance (ESR) spectra of trypsin labeled with compound I (see Figure 11). Spectrum (a) was obtained by modification at pH 5.5 for 10 to 20 h followed by gel filtration at pH 3.5. Spectrum (b) was obtained by labeling for 1 to 2 h at pH 7.7 followed by gel filtration, collodion bag concentration and dialysis at pH 3.5. (From Berliner, L. J. and Wong, S. S., *J. Biol. Chem.*, 248, 1118, 1973. With permission.)

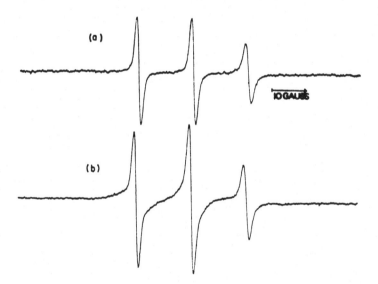

FIGURE 13. The ESR spectra of trypsin. Sample (a) was inert trypsin obtained from chromatographic fractionation of spin-labeled enzyme described in Figure 12. Sample (b) was obtained with α-β-trypsin labeled with compound I (see Figure 11) and then treated with added commercial trypsin. (From Berliner, L. J. and Wong, S. S., *J. Biol. Chem.*, 248, 1118, 1973. With permission.)

hydrosulfite) are more reactive than other primary amino functions in a protein to obtain a preparation of an apolipoprotein specifically modified (Figure 21) with 5-dimethylamino-naphthalene-1-sulfonyl chloride (dansyl chloride). These investigators were subsequently able to use the increase in the fluorescence associated with the binding of the dansyl-apolipoprotein to a phospholipid vesicle (Figure 22) to examine kinetics of association of phospholipid with apolipoprotein (Figure 23).

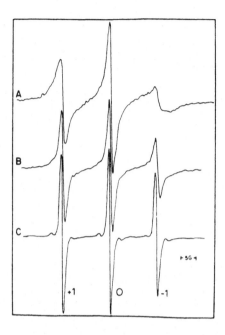

FIGURE 14.   The ESR spectrum of porcine pepsinogen and pepsin preparations. The protein derivatives have been labeled with 3-[[(2,5-dioxo-1-pyrrolidinyl)oxy]carbonyl]-2,5-dihydro-2,2,5,5-tetramethyl-1H-pyrrolyl-1-oxy. Spectrum A shows spin-labeled pepsinogen in 0.02 *M* sodium phosphate, pH 7,0; spectrum B with the same solution as A with a 2.0:1 molar ratio of pepstatin brought to pH 1.5 with HCl; spectrum C shows the spin-labeled pepsinogen solution taken to pH 1.3 for 300 min with HCl. (From Twining, S. S., Sealy, R. C., and Glick, D. M., *Biochemistry*, 20, 1267, 1981. With permission.)

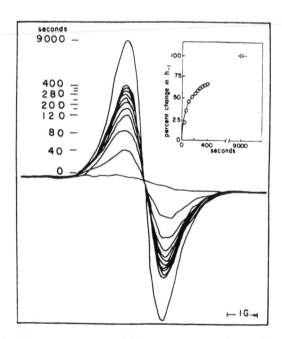

FIGURE 15.   Repeated scans of the downfield peak following activation of the spin-labeled pepsinogen preparation described in Figure 14. The ESR spectrum of the peak was scanned at 40-s intervals following the acidification of the spin-labeled pepsinogen preparation to pH 2.38 with HCl. The insert shows the peak height vs. time. (From Twining, S. S., Sealy, R. C., and Glick, D. M., *Biochemistry*, 20, 1267, 1981. With permission.)

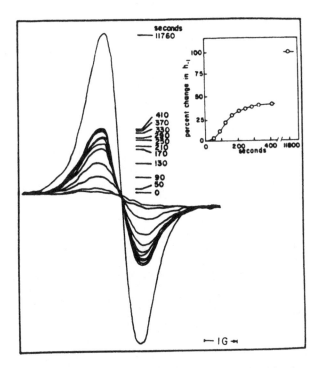

FIGURE 16. Conformational changes in pepsinogen occurring during the activation to pepsin. This figure shows repeated ESR spectra of the downfield peak following the activation of spin-labeled pepsinogen following acidification of a 32.3 μM solution to pH 2.77. The insert shows the peak height vs. time. (From Twining, S. S., Sealy, R. C., and Glick, D. M., *Biochemistry*, 20, 1267, 1981. With permission.)

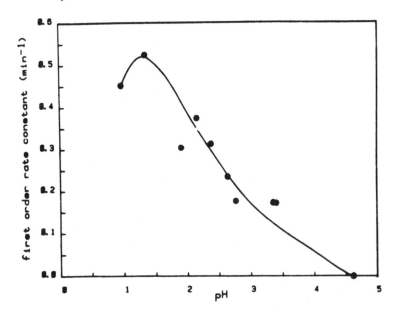

FIGURE 17. The study of the rate of ESR changes of spin-labeled pepsinogen as a function of pH. The acidified pepsinogen solutions were analyzed as described in Figure 21. The first-order rate constants were determined from the initial 20% of the total change in spectra. (From Twining, S. S., Sealy, R. C., and Glick, D. M., *Biochemistry*, 20, 1267, 1981. With permission.)

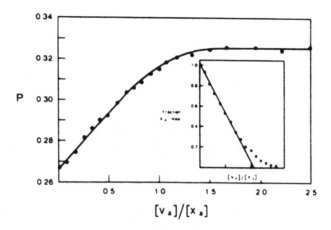

FIGURE 18.   The interaction of fluorescent factor Xa with factor Va
in the presence of phospholipid and calcium ions. The factor Xa had
been modified with Dansyl-Glu-Gly-Arg-chloromethyl ketone. The value
for fluorescence polarization (P) is plotted vs. the concentration of factor
Va added. The inset shows a plot of the factor Xa free (not in complex
formation as assessed by fluorescence polarization data) vs. the total
factor Xa added. Extrapolation of the data indicated in the insert suggests
a binding stoichiometry of 1:1 between factor Xa and factor Va in the
presence of calcium ions and phospholipid. (From Nesheim, M. E.,
Kettner, C., Shaw, E., and Mann, K. G., *J. Biol. Chem.*, 256, 6537,
1981. With permission.)

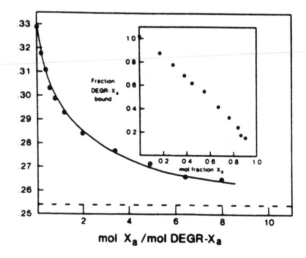

FIGURE 19.   The displacement of fluorescent factor Xa (see Figure 18)
from complex with factor Va in the presence of calcium ions and phospholipid by unlabeled factor Xa. Fluorescence polarization values (ordinate) are plotted vs. the ratio of unlabeled factor Xa to fluorescent factor
Xa (abscissa). The inset shows the fraction of fluorescent factor Xa bound
to factor Va, calculated from polarization values, vs. the mole fraction of
unlabeled factor Xa. (From Nesheim, M. E., Kettner, C., Shaw, E., and
Mann, K. G., *J. Biol. Chem.*, 256, 6537, 1981. With permission.)

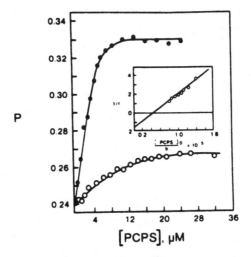

FIGURE 20. The binding of fluorescent factor Xa (see Figure 18) to phospholipid in the presence (closed circles) and absence (open circles) of factor Va. The degree of binding was assessed by the degree of fluorescence polarization (P). The inset shows a double reciprocal analysis of the binding isotherm for the factor Va-independent interaction of factor Xa with phospholipid. (From Nesheim, M. E., Kettner, C., Shaw, E., and Mann, K. G., *J. Biol. Chem.*, 256, 6537, 1981. With permission.)

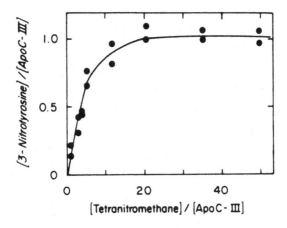

FIGURE 21. The modification of apolipoprotein C-III (apoC-III) with tetranitromethane. The extent of nitrotyrosine formation is plotted vs. the molar excess of tetranitromethane. (From Cardin, A. D., Jackson, R. L., and Johnson, J. D., *J. Biol. Chem.*, 257, 4987, 1982. With permission.)

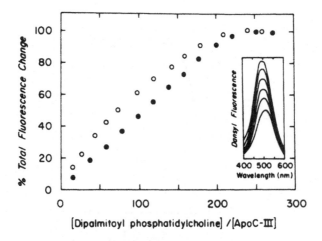

FIGURE 22.   The increase in fluorescence of labeled apoC-III (the nitrated apoC-III was reduced with dithionite and subsequently reacted with dansyl chloride to provide the fluorescent derivative) (open circles) and native apoC-III (closed circles) occurring on interaction with dipalmitoyl phosphatidyl choline unilamellar vesicles. Intrinsic fluorescence was utilized with the native apolipoprotein. The inset shows the increase and wavelength shift in dansyl fluorescence emission with dansyl-apoC-III after successive additions of dipalmitoyl phosphatidyl choline. (From Cardin, A. D., Jackson, R. L., and Johnson, J. D., *J. Biol. Chem.*, 257, 4987, 1982. With permission.)

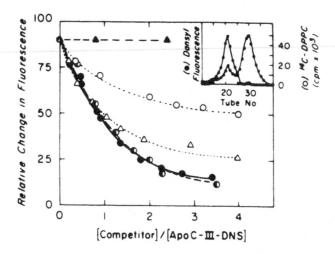

FIGURE 23.   The decrease in dansyl fluorescence intensity of labeled apoC-III (see Figure 28) occurring on the addition of bovine serum albumin (▲), apolipoprotein C-I (○), apolipoprotein C-II (△), apolipoprotein A-I (●, or apolipoprotein C-III (◖). (From Cardin, A. D., Jackson, R. L., and Johnson, J. D., *J. Biol. Chem.*, 257, 4987, 1982. With permission.)

REFERENCES

1. **Plapp, B. V., Zeppezauer, E., and Brändén, C. I.**, Crystallization of liver alcohol dehydrogenase activated by the modification of amino groups, *J. Mol. Biol.*, 119, 451, 1978.

2. **Zisapel, N., Mallul, Y., and Sokolovsky, M.**, Tyrosyl interactions at the active site of carboxypeptidase B, *Int. J. Peptide Protein Res.*, 19, 480, 1982.

3. **Kirschner, M. W. and Schachman, H. K.**, Conformational studies on the nitrated catalytic subunit of aspartate transcarbamylase, *Biochemistry*, 12, 2987, 1973.

4. **Landfear, S. M., Evans, D. R., and Lipscomb, W. N.**, Elimination of cooperativity in aspartate transcarbamylase by nitration of a single tyrosine residue, *Proc. Natl. Acad. Sci. U.S.A.*, 75, 2654, 1978.

4a. **Kumar, G. K., Beegen, N., and Wood, H. G.**, Involvement of tryptophans at the catalytic site and subunit-binding domains of transcarboxylase, *Biochemistry*, 27, 5972, 1988.

5. **Okajima, T., Kawata, Y., and Hamaguchi, K.**, Chemical modification of tryptophan residues and stability changes in proteins, *Biochemistry*, 29, 9168, 1990.

6. **Shaw, E., Mares-Guia, M., and Cohen, W.**, Evidence for an active-center histidine in trypsin through use of a specific reagent, 1-chloro-3-tosylamido-7-amino-2-heptanone, the chloromethyl ketone derived from N^α tosyl-L-lysine, *Biochemistry*, 4, 2219, 1965.

7. **Schoellmann, G. and Shaw, E.**, Direct evidence for the presence of histidine in the active center of chymotrypsin, *Biochemistry*, 2, 252, 1963.

8. **Glazer, A. N. and Smith, E. L.**, Papain and other plant sulfhydryl proteolytic enzymes, in *The Enzymes*, Vol. 3, Boyer, P. D., Ed., Academic Press, New York, 1971, 502.

9. **Gerwin, B. I.**, Properties of the single sulfhydryl group of streptococcal proteinase. A comparison of the rates of alkylation by chloroacetic acid and chloroacetamide, *J. Biol. Chem.*, 242, 451, 1967.

10. **Englund, P. T., King, T. P., Craig, L. C., and Walti, A.**, Studies on ficin. I. Its isolation and characterization, *Biochemistry*, 7, 163, 1968.

11. **Crestfield, A. M., Stein, W. H., and Moore, S.**, Alkylation and identification of the histidine residues at the active site of ribonuclease, *J. Biol. Chem.*, 238, 2418, 1963.

12. **Yamada, A., Imoto, T., Fujita, K., Okasaki, K., and Motomura, M.**, Selective modification of aspartic acid-101 in lysozyme by carbodiimide reaction, *Biochemistry*, 20, 4836, 1981.

13. **Lundblad, R. L., Noyes, C. M., Featherstone, G. L., Harrison, J. H., and Jenzano, J. W.**, The reaction of bovine alpha-thrombin with tetranitromethane. Characterization of the modified protein, *J. Biol. Chem.*, 263, 3729, 1988.

14. **Ray, W. J., Jr. and Koshland, D. E., Jr.**, A method for characterizing the type and numbers of groups involved in enzyme action, *J. Biol. Chem.*, 236, 1973, 1961.

15. **Tsou, C.-L.**, Relation between modification of functional groups of proteins and their biological activity. I. A graphical method for the determination of the number and type of essential groups, *Sci. Sinica*, 11, 1535, 1962.

16. **Tsou, C.-L.**, Kinetics of substrate reaction during irreversible modification of enzyme activity, *Adv. Enzymol.*, 61, 381, 1988.

17. **Zhou, J.-M., Liu, C., and Tsou, C.-L.**, Kinetics of trypsin inhibition by its specific inhibitors, *Biochemistry*, 28, 1070, 1989.

18. **Horiike, K. and McCormick, D. B.**, Correlations between biological activity and the number of functional groups chemically modified, *J. Theoret. Biol.*, 79, 403, 1979.

19. **Holbrook, J. J. and Ingram, V. A.**, Ionic properties of an essential histidine residue in pig heart lactate dehydrogenase, *Biochem. J.*, 131, 729, 1973.

20. **Bloxham, D. P.**, The chemical reactivity of the histidine-195 residue in lactate dehydrogenase thiomethylated at the cysteine-165 residue, *Biochem. J.*, 193, 93, 1981.

21. **Horiike, K., Tsuge, H., and McCormick, D. B.**, Evidence for an essential histidyl residue at the active site of pyridoxamine (pyridoxine)-5'-phosphate oxidase from rabbit liver, *J. Biol. Chem.*, 254, 6638, 1979.

22. **Paterson, A. K. and Knowles, J. R.**, The number of catalytically essential carboxyl groups in pepsin. Modification of the enzyme by trimethyloxonium fluoroborate, *Eur. J. Biochem.*, 31, 510, 1972.

23. **Kremer, A. B., Egan, R. M., and Sable, H. Z.**, The active site of transketolase. Two arginine residues are essential for activity, *J. Biol. Chem.*, 255, 2405, 1980.

24. **Strumeyer, D. H., White, W. N., and Koshland, D. E., Jr.**, Role of serine in chymotrypsin action. Conversion of the active serine to dehydroalanine, *Proc. Natl. Acad. Sci. U.S.A.*, 50, 931, 1963.

25. **Neet, K. E. and Koshland, D. E., Jr.**, The conversion of serine at the active site of subtilisin to cysteine: a "chemical mutation", *Proc. Natl. Acad. Sci. U.S.A.*, 56, 1606, 1966.

26. **Clark, P. I. and Lowe, G.**, Conversion of the active-site cysteine residue into a dehydroserine, a serine and a glycine residue, *Eur. J. Biochem.*, 84, 293, 1978.

27. **Higaki, J. N., Evnin, L. B., and Craik, C. S.**, Introduction of a cysteine protease active site into trypsin, *Biochemistry*, 28, 9256, 1989.

28. **McGrath, H. E., Wilke, M. E., Higaki, J. N., Craik, C. S., and Fletterick, R. J.,** Crystal structures of two engineered thiol trypsins, *Biochemistry,* 28, 9264, 1989.

29. **Choi, J.-D. and McCormick, D. B.,** Roles of arginyl residues in pyridoxamine-5'-phosphate oxidase from rabbit liver, *Biochemistry,* 20, 5722, 1981.

30. **Carlson, C. A. and Preiss, J.,** Involvement of arginine residues in the allosteric activation of *Escherichia coli* ADP-glucose synthetase, *Biochemistry,* 21, 1929, 1982.

31. **Lundblad, R. L., Nesheim, M. E., Straight, D. L., Sailor, S., Bowie, J., Jenzano, J. W., Roberts, J. D., and Mann, K. G.,** Bovine alpha- and beta-thrombin. Reduced fibrinogen-clotting activity of beta-thrombin is not a consequence of reduced affinity for fibrinogen, *J. Biol. Chem.,* 259, 6991, 1984.

32. **Nesheim, M. E., Prendergast, F. G., and Mann, K. G.,** Interactions of a fluorescent active-site-directed inhibitor of thrombin: dansylarginine *N*-(3-ethyl-1,5-pentanediyl) amide, *Biochemistry,* 18, 996, 1979.

33. **Myers, B., II and Glazer, A. N.,** Spectroscopic studies of the exposure of tyrosine residues in proteins with special reference to the subtilisins, *J. Biol. Chem.,* 246, 412, 1971.

34. **Chaiken, I. M. and Smith, E. L.,** Reaction of chloroacetamide with the sulfhydryl groups of papain, *J. Biol. Chem.,* 244, 5087, 1969.

35. **Eyl, A. W., Jr. and Inagami, T.,** Identification of essential carboxyl groups in the specific binding site of bovine trypsin by chemical modification, *J. Biol. Chem.,* 246, 738, 1971.

36. **Ambrose, B. J. and Pless, R. C.,** DNA sequencing: chemical methods, *Methods Enzymol.,* 152, 522, 1987.

37. **Barnes, W. M.,** Sequencing DNA with dideoxyribonucleotides as chain terminators: hints and strategies for big projects, *Methods Enzymol.,* 152, 538, 1987.

38. **Spoerel, N. A. and Kafatos, F. C.,** Identification of genomic sequences corresponding to cDNA clones, *Methods Enzymol.,* 152, 588, 1987.

39. **Kirtley, M. E. and Koshland, D. E., Jr.,** The introduction of a "reporter" group at the active site of glyceraldehyde-3-phosphate dehydrogenase, *Biochem. Biophys. Res. Commun.,* 23, 810, 1966.

40. **Loudon, G. M. and Koshland, D. E., Jr.,** The chemistry of a reporter group: 2-hydroxy-5-nitrobenzyl bromide, *J. Biol. Chem.,* 245, 2247, 1970.

41. **Riordan, J. R., Sokolovsky, M., and Vallee, B. L.,** Environmentally sensitive tyrosyl residues. Nitration with tetranitromethane, *Biochemistry,* 6, 358, 1967.

42. **Berliner, L. J., Ed.,** *Spin Labeling: Theory and Applications,* Academic Press, New York, 1975.

43. **Berliner, L. J. and Wong, S. S.,** Evidence against two "pH locked" conformations of phosphorylated trypsin, *J. Biol. Chem.,* 248, 1118, 1973.

44. **Berliner, L. J. and Wong, S. S.,** Spin-labeled sulfonyl fluorides as active site probes of protease structure. I. Comparison of the active site environments in α-chymotrypsin and trypsin, *J. Biol. Chem.,* 249, 1668, 1974.

45. **Wong, S. S., Quiggle, K., Triplett, C., and Berliner, L. J.,** Spin-labeled sulfonyl fluorides as active site probes of protease structure. II. Spin label synthese and enzyme inhibition, *J. Biol. Chem.,* 249, 1678, 1974.

46. **Berliner, L. J. and Shen, Y. Y.,** Probing active site structure by spin label (ESR) and fluorescence methods, in *Chemistry and Biology of Thrombin,* Lundblad, R. L., Fenton, J. W., II, and Mann, K. G., Eds., Ann Arbor Science, Ann Arbor, Mich., 1977, 197.

47. **Berliner, L. J., Bauer, R. S., Chang, T.-L., Fenton, J. W., II, and Shen, Y. Y. L.,** Active-site topography of human coagulant (α) and noncoagulant (γ) thrombins, *Biochemistry,* 20, 1831, 1981.

48. **Twining, S. S., Sealy, R. C., and Glick, D. M.,** Preparation and activation of spin-labelled pepsinogen, *Biochemistry,* 20, 1267, 1981.

49. **Nesheim, M. E., Kettner, C., Shaw, E., and Mann, K. G.,** Cofactor dependence of factor Xa incorporation into the prothrombinase complex, *J. Biol. Chem.,* 256, 6537, 1981.

50. **Cardin, A. D., Jackson, R. L., and Johnson, J. D.,** 5-Dimethylaminonaphthalene-1-sulfonyl-3-amino-tyrosyl apolipoprotein C-III. Preparation, characterization and interaction with phospholipid vesicles, *J. Biol. Chem.,* 257, 4987, 1982.

Chapter 2

AMINO ACID ANALYSIS

In the course of exploring some of the early literature on chemical modification, specifically the initial application of photo-oxidation to the study of proteins,[1,2] we had occasion to examine some papers from 1949 to 1952. We were mildly surprised to see that microbial growth assays and specific enzyme assays were still used to determine changes in the amino acid composition of proteins.[3,4] These studies required substantial quantities of protein and, as such, were limited to proteins such as chymotrypsin, lysozyme, and various albumins which could be readily obtained in such quantities. In addition to the limitations posed by the quantities of material required, the lack of accuracy inherent in these approaches led to the application[5] of chromatography to the problem of determining amino acid composition. This specific era of protein chemistry has been reviewed by Fruton.[6] The application of chromatography to the analysis of amino acid composition occurred in the laboratories of Stanford Moore and William H. Stein at The Rockefeller Institute for Medical Research (now The Rockefeller University). This led to the further development of the ninhydrin reaction for the detection of amino acids[7] and the earlier invention of the automatic fraction collector for use in the chromatographic fractionation. The introduction of ion-exchange resin in 1954[8] reduced the time required for the analysis of a single hydrolyzate from 10 days to 5 days. The introduction of the automated amino acid analyzer in 1958[9,10] reduced this time to 24 h and this in turn had been reduced to 6 h by 1966 using two-column methodology. The further development of ion-exchange resins made the use of single column analysis possible. This, together with other technical advances, reduced the time required for a single analysis to 2 to 4 h with sensitivity at the nmol level.[11] Of major importance in this increase in both speed and sensitivity was the development of narrow-bore or microbore columns.[12,13] The critical events in the development of the apparatus used today are also reviewed in several of the preceding references[12,13] and several more recent state-of-the-art reviews.[14-16]

The critical aspects of amino acid analysis at the present time are sample preparation, including hydrolysis and pre-column derivatization (does the method used to produce amino acids from the peptide or protein under study accurately represent the composition?), preparation of the solvents used for the chromatographic fractionation, and the reproducibility of the analytical system. Reproducibility of the analytical system includes reproducibility of the spectrophotometric analytical system, maintenance of an extremely reproducible flow rate, and the accuracy of the data analysis system. Implicit in this last area is the accuracy of the amino acid standard used for calibration of the system. With ninhydrin-based detection systems, consideration needs to be given to the possibility of reagent decomposition.

The preparation of the sample will first be discussed. The strategy is somewhat different depending upon the qualitative and quantitative demands on the information desired. If the objective is to rigorously determine the amino acid composition of newly isolated protein, it is essential to know the *chemical* purity of the preparation. Here it would be assumed that a single macromolecular component (protein) is present. In the absence of other analytical information regarding the nature of the protein preparation (i.e., carbohydrate content, nucleic acid content, etc.), it is of critical importance to know precisely how much material (mass) is present at the start so that the investigation can accurately determine what portion (percentage) of the sample is recovered as amino acid. The careful investigator would also know what portion of the sample is moisture or inorganic components detected as % ash. Impurities can also contribute to artifactual results other than inaccurate estimates of the amount of protein present. The presence of nucleic acid in a sample can result in the formation of artifactual amounts of glycine.[25] Inorganic constituents can pose a number of difficulties.

Ionic chromium can irreversibly bind to the ion-exchange columns used for amino acid analysis.[26] This effect can be prevented by addition of one or two extra buffers prior to the increase in pH to an alkaline value (i.e., pH 7.6) for the elution of basic amino acids in the single-column system. A similar effect of gold has been observed. A systematic study has explored the effect of cupric ions and ferric ions[27] on the recovery of amino acids after acid hydrolysis (6 N HCl, 20 to 22 h/110°C). The presence of these metal ions results in the conversion of cysteine/cystine to cysteic acid and methionine to methionine sulfoxide.

In general, adequate results for the amino acid composition of a protein (excluding tryptophan content) can be obtained from careful hydrolysis in 6 N HCl. Effective exclusion of oxygen during the hydrolysis is essential for the accurate determination of composition. This is easily achieved by the careful deaeration of the sample prior to placement in a hydrolysis oven or block.[28] Accurate values for serine, threonine, and tyrosine require samples hydrolyzed for several periods of time (i.e., 22 h, 48 h, 72 h) such that extrapolation back to zero time can be accomplished.

Hydrolysis in 6 N HCl precludes the determination of tryptophan since this amino acid is destroyed under these conditions. It was therefore necessary to rely on a spectrophotometric method,[29,30] or somewhat tedious and occasionally unreliable methods[31,32] for alkaline hydrolysis. The introduction of 2-hydroxy-5-nitrobenzyl bromide[33] provided a reliable spectral method but required an independent determination of protein concentration and composition and is only applicable to soluble proteins. Molner-Perl and Pinter-Sazaki[34] have developed a technique for the determination of tryptophan in intact proteins based on reaction with acid ninhydrin. Nozaki[35] recently revised the use of second-derivative spectroscopy for the determination of the tryptophan content of proteins. The work of Hugli and Moore[36] provided a reliable method for base hydrolysis and subsequent analysis. The conditions developed by these investigators result in the accurate determination of tryptophan, and the presence of carbohydrate does not interfere with the analysis. Although alkaline hydrolysis and spectroscopy are still of value (the use of base hydrolysis, for example, is now not essential for the determination of tryptophan but is essential for the determination of γ-carboxyglutamic acid[37,39]), the work of Liu and co-workers has largely supplanted their use in the quantitative determination of tryptophan in proteins which do not contain substantial carbohydrate. This group reported the development of the use of tosyl acid (*p*-toluenesulfonic acid) for the hydrolysis of proteins to determine tryptophan.[40] This procedure was effective despite having several disadvantages. The major problem is that tosyl acid is a solid which generally must be recrystallized from HCl prior to use and it is difficult to obtain completely free of HCl. The inclusion of indole or 3-(2-aminoethyl) indole was observed to improve the yield of tryptophan and, therefore, the reproducibility of analyses. The use of 4.0 N methanesulfonic acid as outlined in a subsequent publication from Liu's laboratory[41] has proved to be more effective than tosyl acid. The condition for the hydrolysis of proteins are 4.0 N methanesulfonic acid (containing 0.2% 3-[2-aminoethyl] indole) at 115°C for 22 h (it may be necessary to include other time periods of hydrolysis such as 48 h and 72 h for the reasons given above for 6 N HCl as well as to assure the cleavage of all peptide bonds). Sartin and co-workers[42] have reported that the inclusion of mercaptoacetic acid, phenol, and 3-(2-aminoethyl) indole in 6.0 N HCl (100-μl sample in H_2O, 100 μl concentrated HCl, 1 μl mercaptoacetic acid, 10 μl of 5% phenol, and 5 μl of 2% 3-(2-aminoethyl) indole) resulted in the effective recovery of tryptophan for subsequent analysis. Chiou and Wang[43] have modified this technique by using 4 M methanesulfonic acid at 160°C for 45 min. Complete recovery of cysteine and tryptophan is obtained under these conditions. The presence of carbohydrate (greater than 5%) results in the excessive loss of tryptophan using any of these procedures such that alkaline hydrolysis or some alternative analytical approach (i.e., 2-hydroxy-5-nitrobenzyl bromide, N-bromosuccinimide) may be preferable. There have been significant advances in hydrolysis technology. The use of a mixture of hydrochloric acid and trifluoroacetic acid (TFA) (HCl:TFA; 2:1) has been recommended for the hydrolysis of hydrophobic proteins.[44] The technique is rapid (25 min/166°C) and TFA is suggested to be necessary for the hydrolysis of peptide bonds involving hydrophobic amino acids. Tryptophan is destroyed under these conditions. Chiou and Wang[45] have described the use of microwave irradiation for the acid hydrolysis (6 N HCl) of peptides and proteins. Microwave irradiation (0.96 kW) for 8 min yielded hydrolyzates comparable to those obtained with 6 N HCl (24 h/110°C). Conditions for the acid hydrolysis of proteins blotted onto polyvinyl difluoride membranes have also been reported.[46,47] A gas-phase hydrolysis technique has been described by Metzer et al.,[48] which uses conventional HCl hydrolysis conditions (24 h/110°C). Although there is no time advantage with this technique, it does permit the simultaneous processing of a large number of samples.

Most analytical systems are based on the detection of the respective amino acids in the effluent from the analytical columns by reaction with ninhydrin.[7] The ninhydrin systems in use are based either on a methyl cellosolve solvent[7-9] or on dimethyl sulfoxide.[49] Our laboratories use the dimethyl sulfoxide-based system as we find this reagent more stable on storage, the dimethyl sulfoxide does not have the severe toxic properties of methyl cellosolve and the color yields for most amino acids are superior. The primary problem in the use of the ninhydrin system is concerned with reagent preparation. The source of ninhydrin is critical and we have found that only Pierce Chemical Company, Rockford, Ill., has continually provided material of excellence. We have, on occasion, used material from other sources which has had equivalent performance but there was extensive batch-to-batch variation.

Figure 1 shows the chromatographic separation of amino acids via conventional ion-exchange technology following by post-column detection with the ninhydrin reagent. This data was obtained using Beckman Instruments System Gold®. Figure 2 shows the analysis of physiological fluids using the same technology.

The use of fluorogenic reagents to detect amino acids has been increasing during the past decade. Fluorescamine (4-phenylspiro[furan-2-(3H), 1'-phthalan]-3,3'-dione) was introduced by Udenfriend and co-workers[50] for the detection of amino acids. At the time, the reagent provided greater sensitivity for most amino acids than did the ninhydrin reagent but did not detect amino acids such as proline or hydroxyproline. Felix and Turkelsen[51] reported the use of post-column derivatization of proline with N-chlorosuccinimide which permitted effective reaction with fluorescamine. Further studies[52] on the chemistry of the reaction of fluorescamine with amino acids have created a solid base for the use of this reagent for amino acid analysis using colorimetric rather than fluorescence detection. Further developments of note in the use of this reagent include the use of alkaline sodium hypochlorite for the post-column derivatization of amino acids. A recent review of this technique has appeared.[22]

Another fluorescence-based system based on the use of o-phthalaldehyde has been developed.[54,55] An excellent review[23] has recently appeared regarding the use of o-phthalaldehyde in amino acid analysis. Our laboratories do not have any practical experience with either fluorescamine or o-phthalaldehyde but it is our impression that o-phthalaldehyde has been more useful. It is water soluble which makes this compound somewhat easier to use from a technical viewpoint. Both reagents require the post-column derivatization of amino acids which requires a sometimes tedious plumbing arrangement. It is also our impression that solvent purity is a more critical factor with either of these reagents than with ninhydrin. The reader is directed to the review[23] cited above for a more critical comparison of the various detection systems.

Amino acid analysis by high-performance liquid chromatography (HPLC) following pre-column derivatization with either dansyl chloride[56] or phenylisothiocyanate[57] has proved to be extremely useful. Sensitivity can be easily achieved at the nmol level, using either

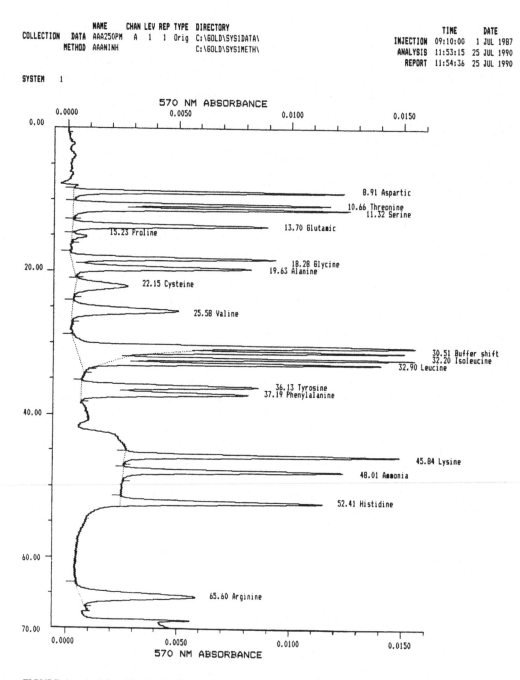

FIGURE 1.   Amino acid analysis of protein hydrolyzate with post-column derivatization with ninhydrin. Note buffer change artifacts at injection, 28 min, and 44 min. Response monitored at 570 and 440 nm (proline). Column temperature was 50°C and coil temperature was 30°C. Obtained using System Gold® technology. (Figure courtesy of Beckman Instruments.)

technique. The separation of PTC-amino acids using HPLC analysis on an ISCO Instruments system is shown in Figure 3.

In conclusion it is important to emphasize that reagent purity and a clean laboratory environment are both critical for the successful application of current technology in amino acid analysis. A thorough discussion of these factors is beyond the limited scope of this present writing and the reader is directed to several reviews[11,14,15,28] which consider these various factors in adequate detail.

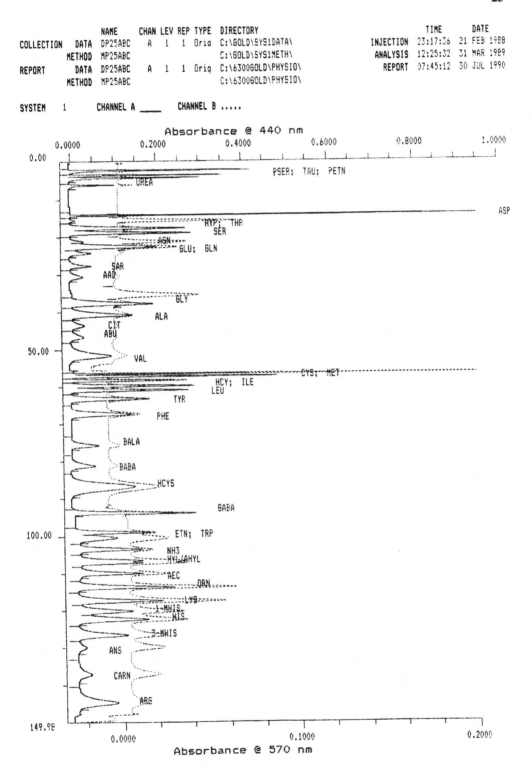

FIGURE 2. Amino acid analysis of physiological fluids with post-column derivatization with ninhydrin. Response monitored at both 570 and 440 nm. Column temperature was 50°C and coil temperature was 30°C. Obtained using System Gold® technology. (Figure courtesy of Beckman Instruments.)

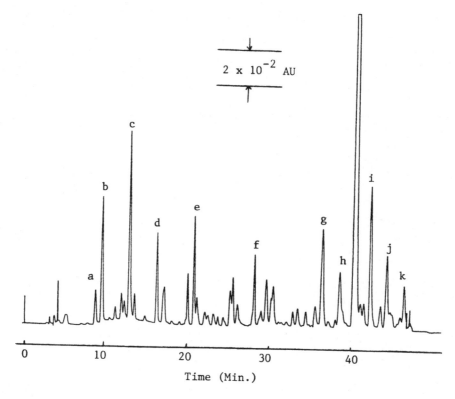

FIGURE 3. Amino acid analysis using pre-column derivatization with phenylisothiocyanate. The column was a C^{18}-reverse phase with 50 mM sodium acetate, pH 6.5 as the initial solvent. Elution was accomplished with an acetonitrile/methanol gradient. The effluent was monitored at 269 nm using an ISCO HPLC System. a, asx; b, glx; c, gly; d, his; e, ala; f, thr; g, tyr; h, val; i, leu; j, phe, k, lys. (Courtesy of ISCO Scientific.)

REFERENCES

1. **Weil, L. and Buchert, A. R.,** Photooxidation of crystalline β-lactoglobulin in the presence of methylene blue, *Arch. Biochem. Biophys.,* 34, 1, 1951.
2. **Weil, L., James, S., and Buchert, A. R.,** Photooxidation of crystalline chymotrypsin in the presence of methylene blue, *Arch. Biochem. Biophys.,* 46, 266, 1952.
3. **Snell, E. E.,** The microbiological assay of amino acids, *Adv. Protein Chem.,* 2, 85, 1945.
4. **Tristram, G. R.,** The amino acid composition of proteins, in *The Proteins,* Vol. 1, Part A, Neurath, H. and Bailey, K., Eds., Academic Press, New York, 1953, 185.
5. **Moore, S. and Stein, W. H.,** Partition chromatography of amino acids on starch, *Ann. N.Y. Acad. Sci.,* 49, 256, 1948.
6. **Fruton, J. S.,** *Molecules and Life; Historical Essays on the Interplay of Chemistry and Biology,* Wiley-Interscience, New York, 1972, 148.
7. **Moore, S. and Stein, W. H.,** A modified ninhydrin reagent for the photometric determination of amino acids and related compounds, *J. Biol. Chem.,* 211, 907, 1954.
8. **Moore, S. and Stein, W. H.,** Procedures for the chromatographic determination of amino acids on four per cent cross-linked sulfonated polystyrene resins, *J. Biol. Chem.,* 211, 893, 1954.
9. **Moore, S., Spackman, D. H., and Stein, W. H.,** Chromatography of amino acids on sulfonated polystyrene resins. An improved system, *Anal. Chem.,* 30, 1185, 1958.
10. **Spackman, D. H., Stein, W. H., and Moore, S.,** Automatic recording apparatus for use in the chromatography of amino acids, *Anal. Chem.,* 30, 1190, 1958.
11. **Moore, S.,** The precision and sensitivity of amino acid analysis, in *Chemistry and Biology of Peptides,* Meienhofer, J., Ed., Ann Arbor Sci., Ann Arbor, Mich., 1972, 629.

12. **Krejci, V. K. and Machleidt, W.**, Verbessere Methodik der Aminosäuren– analyse im Nanomol-Bereich, *Hoppe Seyler's Z. Physiol. Chem.*, 350, 981, 1969.
13. **Liao, T.-H., Robinson, G. W., and Salnikow, J.**, Use of narrow-bore columns in amino acid analysis, *Anal. Chem.*, 45, 2286, 1973.
14. **Hamilton, P. B.**, Micro and submicro determinations of amino acids by ion-exchange chromatography, *Meth. Enzymol.*, 11, 15, 1967.
15. **Hare, P. E.**, Subnanomole-range amino acid analysis, *Meth. Enzymol.*, 47, 3, 1977.
16. **Benson, J. R.**, Improved ion-exchange resins, *Meth. Enzymol.*, 47, 19, 1977.
17. **Hirs, C. H. W.**, A buffer system for amino acid analysis with automatic integrators, *Meth. Enzymol.*, 91, 3, 1983.
18. **Elzinga, M. and Alonzo, N.**, Analysis for methylated amino acids in proteins, *Meth. Enzymol.*, 91, 8, 1983.
19. **Bohlen, P.**, Analysis for imino acids with *o*-phthalaldehyde, *Meth. Enzymol.*, 91, 26, 1983.
20. **Inglis, A. S.**, Single hydrolysis method for all amino acids, including cysteine and tryptophan, *Meth. Enzymol.*, 91, 26, 1983.
21. **Chang, J.-Y., Knecht, R., and Braun, D. G.**, Amino acid analysis in the picomole range by precolumn derivatization and high-performance liquid chromatography, *Meth. Enzymol.*, 91, 41, 1983.
22. **Pan, Y.-C. E. and Stein, S.**, Amino acid analysis with postcolumn fluorescent derivatization, in *Methods of Protein Microcharacterization*, Shively, J. E., Ed., Humana Press, Clifton, NJ, 1986, 105.
23. **Jones, B. N.**, Amino acid analysis by *o*-phthalaldehyde precolumn derivatization and reverse-phase HPLC, in *Methods of Protein Microcharacterization*, Shively, J. E., Ed., Humana Press, Clifton, NJ, 1986, 121.
24. **Harris, E. L. V.**, Amino acid analysis by precolumn derivatization, in *Methods in Molecular Biology*, Vol. 3, Walker, J. M., Ed., Humana Press, Clifton, NJ, 33, 1988.
25. **Paddock, G. V., Wilson, G. B., and Wang, A.-C.**, Contribution of hydrolyzed nucleic acids and their constituents to the apparent amino acid composition of biological components, *Biochem. Biophys. Res. Commun.*, 87, 946, 1979.
26. **Bech-Anderson, S.**, Single-column analysis of amino acids in hydrolysates of samples containing chromic oxide, *J. Chromatogr.*, 179, 227, 1979.
27. **Brummel, M., Gerbeck, C. M., and Montgomery, R.**, Effects of metals on analytical procedures for amino acids and carbohydrates, *Anal. Biochem.*, 31, 331, 1969.
28. **Moore, S. and Stein, W. H.**, Chromatographic determination of amino acids by the use of automatic recording equipment, *Meth. Enzymol.*, 6, 819, 1963.
29. **Goodwin, T. W. and Morton, R. A.**, Spectrophotometric determinations of tyrosine and tryptophan in proteins, *Biochem. J.*, 40, 628, 1946.
30. **Edelhoch, H.**, Spectroscopic determination of tryptophan and tyrosine in proteins, *Biochemistry*, 6, 1948, 1967.
31. **Dreze, A.**, Le dosage du tryptophane dans les milieux naturels. II. La stabilité du tryptophane au cours de l'hydrolyse alcaline effectuée en présénce d'hydrates de carbone, *Bull. Soc. Chim. Biol.*, 42, 407, 1960.
32. **Noltmann, E. A., Mahowald, T. A., and Kuby, S. A.**, Studies on adenosine triphosphate transphorylases. II. Amino acid composition of adenosine triphosphate-creatine transphosphorylase, *J. Biol. Chem.*, 237, 1146, 1962.
33. **Barman, T. E. and Koshland, D. E., Jr.**, A colorimetric method for the quantitative determination of tryptophan residues in proteins, *J. Biol. Chem.*, 242, 5771, 1967.
34. **Molner-Perl, I. and Pinter-Szakacs, M.**, Spectrophotometric determination of tryptophan in intact proteins by the acid ninhydrin method, *Anal. Biochem.*, 177, 16, 1989.
35. **Nozaki, Y.**, Determination of tryptophan, tyrosine and phenylalanine by second derivative spectroscopy, *Arch. Biochem. Biophys.*, 277, 324, 1990.
36. **Hugli, T. E. and Moore, S.**, Determination of the tryptophan content of proteins by ion-exchange chromatography of alkaline hydrolysates, *J. Biol. Chem.*, 247, 2828, 1972.
37. **Hauschka, P. V.**, Quantitative determination of γ-carboxyglutamic acid in proteins, *Anal. Biochem.*, 80, 212, 1977.
38. **Kuwada, M. and Katayama, K.**, A high-performance liquid chromatographic method for the simultaneous determination of γ-carboxyglutamic acid and glutamic acid in proteins, bone, and urine, *Anal. Biochem.*, 117, 259, 1981.
39. **Price, P. A.**, Analysis for gamma-carboxyglutamic acid, *Meth. Enzymol.*, 91, 13, 1983.
40. **Liu, T.-Y. and Chang, W. H.**, Hydrolysis of proteins with *p*-toluenesulfonic acid. Determination of tryptophan, *J. Biol. Chem.*, 246, 2842, 1971.
41. **Simpson, R. J., Neuberger, M. R., and Liu, T.-Y.**, Complete amino acid analysis of proteins from a single hydrolysate, *J. Biol. Chem.*, 251, 1936, 1976.
42. **Sartin, J. L., Hugli, T. E., and Liao, T.-H.**, Reactivity of the tryptophan residues in bovine pancreatic deoxyribonuclease with *N*-bromosuccinimide, *J. Biol. Chem.*, 255, 8633, 1980.

43. **Chiou, S.-H. and Wang, K.-T.,** Simplified protein hydrolysis with methanesulfonic acid at elevated temperature for the complete amino acid analysis of proteins, *J. Chromatogr.,* 448, 404, 1988.
44. **Tsugita, A. and Scheffler, J.-J.,** A rapid method for acid hydrolysis of protein with a mixture of trifluoroacetic acid and hydrochloric acid, *Eur. J. Biochem.,* 124, 585, 1982.
45. **Chiou, S.-H. and Wang, K.-T.,** Peptide and protein hydrolysis by microwave irradiation, *J. Chromatogr.,* 491, 424, 1989.
46. **Tous, G. I., Fausnaugh, J. L., Akinyosoye, O., Lackland, H., Winter-Cash, P., Victorica, F. J., and Stein, S.,** Amino acid analysis on polyvinyl difluoride membranes, *Anal. Biochem.,* 179, 50, 1989.
47. **Nakagawa, S. and Fukuda, T.,** Direct amino acid analysis of proteins electroblotted onto polyvinylidene difluoride membrane from sodium dodecyl sulfate-polyacrylamide gel, *Anal. Biochem.,* 181, 75, 1989.
48. **Meltzer, N. M., Tous, G. I., Gruber, S. and Stein, S.,** Gas-phase hydrolysis of proteins and peptides, *Anal. Biochem.,* 160, 356, 1987.
49. **Moore, S.,** Amino acid analysis: aqueous dimethyl sulfoxide as solvent for the ninhydrin reaction, *J. Biol. Chem.,* 243, 6281, 1968.
50. **Udenfriend, S., Stein, S., Bohlen, P., and Dairman, W.,** A new fluorometric procedure for assay of amino acids, peptides and proteins in the picomole range, in *Chemistry and Biology of Peptides,* Meienhofer, J., Ed., Ann Arbor Sci., Ann Arbor, Mich., 1972, 655.
51. **Felix, A. M. and Turkelsen, G.,** Total fluorometric amino acid analysis using fluorescamine, *Arch. Biochem. Biophys.,* 157, 177, 1973.
52. **Felix, A. M., Toome, V., DeBernardo, S., and Weigele, M.,** Colorimetric amino acid analysis using fluorescamine, *Arch. Biochem. Biophys.,* 168, 601, 1975.
53. **Böhlen, P., and Mellet, M.,** Automated fluorometric amino acid analysis: the determination of proline and hydroxyproline, *Anal. Biochem.,* 94, 313, 1979.
54. **Cronin, J. R. and Hare, P. E.,** Chromatographic analysis of amino acids and primary amines with *o*-phthalaldehyde detection, *Anal. Biochem.,* 81, 151, 1977.
55. **Lund, E., Thomsen, J., and Brunfeldt, K.,** The use of *o*-phthalaldehyde for fluorescence detection in conventional amino acid analyzers. Sub-nanomole sensitivity in the analysis of phenylthiohydantoin-amino acids, *J. Chromatogr.,* 130, 51, 1977.
56. **Stocchi, V., Piccoli, G., Magnani, M., Palma, F., Biagiarelli, B., and Cucchiarini, L.,** Reversed-phase high-performance liquid chromatography separation of dimethylaminoazobenzene sulfonyl- and dimethylaminoazobenzene thiohydantoin-amino acid derivatives for amino acid analysis and microsequencing studies at the picomole level, *Anal. Biochem.,* 178, 107, 1989.
57. **Cohen, S. A. and Strydom, D. J.,** Amino acid analysis utilizing phenylisothiocyanate derivatives, *Anal. Biochem.,* 174, 1, 1988.

Chapter 3

PEPTIDE SEPARATION BY REVERSE-PHASE HIGH-PERFORMANCE LIQUID CHROMATOGRAPHY

The previous edition of this book included a brief discussion of more classical techniques for peptide purification such as two-dimensional electrophoresis and thin-layer chromatography. Although there is still some use of these techniques, almost all of the work since 1984 has focused on HPLC or specialized affinity approaches. It is not possible to discuss the current status of peptide purification in any depth, and the reader is directed toward several reference works for further detail.[1-11]

Reverse-phase high-performance liquid chromatography (HPLC) has developed recently into a useful method for analytical and preparative "mapping" of peptide mixtures, allowing peptides containing sites of chemical modification to be isolated for identification.

Improvement in chromatographic efficiency is achieved by decreasing the particle size of the stationary phase. The resulting decrease in sample bandspreading allows better resolution, faster separation, and higher detection sensitivity. The basis of the technique commonly known as HPLC is a stationary phase made of 10-μm diameter or smaller particles to yield High Performance. High Pressure is then required to make the liquid mobile phase flow through a column of this packing, and the necessary pump, sample injection valve, detector, and associated equipment lead to a High-Priced system. Snyder and Kirkland[12] provide a thorough discussion of the theory and practice of HPLC.

The original expectation in development of HPLC was that existing thin-layer and column chromatographic separation methods would be transferred to columns packed with small, uniform-sized, rigid particles. This implied a stationary phase of unmodified silica. However, the retention properties of a silica surface are very sensitive to moisture levels. Elution times may be difficult to reproduce, and long column equilibration times may be required following solvent changes. Attempts to improve reproducibility of retention properties by masking the surface silanol groups led to the development of packing materials having covalently bonded surface phases. The most successful of these have been the so-called C-18 or ODS (octadecylsilyl) packings, which have 18-carbon hydrocarbon chains bonded to the surface silanols. The use of these and other hydrophobic bonded-phase packings is known as "reverse-phase" chromatography because the stationary phase is nonpolar and the mobile phase polar, which happens to be the reverse of most older methods of partition liquid chromatography.

The bonded reverse-phase supports are versatile and provide reproducible retention, rapid equilibration to new solvent conditions, and good column life when used within the pH range of 2 to 7.5. Mobile phases are based on water or aqueous buffers; sample retention is controlled by the proportion of a water-miscible organic solvent, often acetonitrile or an alcohol, in the mobile phase. The higher the volume fraction of organic solvent, the "stronger" the mobile phase, that is, the more hydrophobic and better able it is to elute sample components from the nonpolar stationary phase. Simple mixtures of chemically similar small molecules can be adequately separated in a reasonable time with a single properly selected mobile phase composition ("isocratic" elution). More complex mixtures or those having a wider range of polarities require a solvent compositional gradient for efficient analysis. The retention of peptides and proteins on reverse-phase columns is highly dependent on solvent strength[13] and on their amino acid compositions; gradient elution is necessary for most polypeptide mixtures.

The application of reverse-phase HPLC to proteins and peptides lagged behind its use for smaller molecules. The size and chemical complexity of polypeptides cause their retention characteristics to be affected by a number of factors. These include the pH of the mobile phase, the buffer system used, the organic mobile phase component, the nature of the bonded

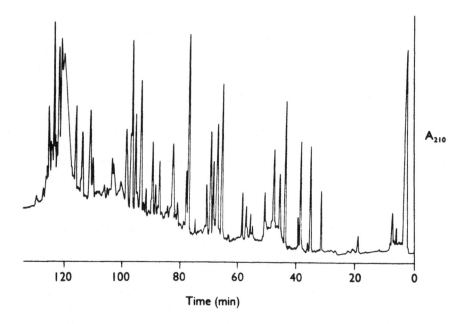

A_{210}

Time (min)

FIGURE 1.   Tryptic digest of reduced and carboxymethylated human blood coagulation Factor IX. Column, Ultrasphere-ODS, 0.46 × 25 cm; flow rate 1 ml/min; temperature 25°C. Solvent A = 0.05 M sodium phosphate, pH 2.95; solvent B = acetonitrile. Gradient program: 0 to 28% B in 114 min, then to 62% B in 30 min; both segments linear.

stationary phase surface, and the pore size of the stationary phase. Usable elution systems have now been worked out and high-resolution separations can be achieved, particularly of peptides up to about 2 dozen amino acids in length.

For small peptides such as most of those produced by tryptic digestion, ordinary C-18 columns can be used. We have obtained good results[14] with the system recommended by Schroeder and co-workers[15] for the mapping of hemoglobin tryptic peptides.[14,15] A Beckman Ultrasphere-ODS column, 0.46 × 25 cm, is eluted at 1 ml/min with a phosphate-acetonitrile gradient at ambient temperature. The aqueous component is approximately 50 mM phosphate, pH 2.95. The gradient rate is 0.25% increase in acetonitrile per minute up to 28% acetonitrile, followed by 1.1% increase per minute to a final acetonitrile concentration of 62%. A typical chromatogram of a tryptic digest is shown in Figure 1.

The phosphate-acetonitrile eluent gives good resolution of peptides and allows absorbance monitoring at 210 nm for high-sensitivity detection. Its main defect is a lack of volatility. This level of phosphate salt will interfere in sequence analysis. Schroeder et al.[15] recommend rechromatography of individual peaks using 10 mM ammonium acetate adjusted to pH 6.07 with dilute acetic acid as the aqueous component of the mobile phase. We have generally used 5 mM phosphate, pH 6.5, for rechromatography, still with an acetonitrile gradient. Up to 1 ml of this eluent can be used for sequence analysis without further desalting. In either case the change in pH causes changes in relative peptide mobility so that any peaks which coeluted initially are separated during rechromatography.

Larger peptides give broader peaks[16] and are more sensitive to the nature of both the column packing and the mobile phase. Schroeder et al.[15] note poor elution of hemoglobin "core" peptides in the phosphate-acetonitrile system; they form sharper peaks if oxidized, and also are eluted better from a Zorbax TMS (trimethylsilyl) column than from the Ul-trasphere-ODS. Similarly, the broad peak late in the chromatogram shown in Figure 1 is a 35-amino acid glycopeptide (the "activation peptide" of human blood coagulation factor IX).[14] To separate it from the phosphate and the coeluting peaks, we chromatographed it on a VydacTP C-8 column with a gradient from 0.1% trifluoroacetic acid (TFA) to

2-propanol at a flow rate of 1.0 ml/min, a gradient rate of 0.5%/min, and a temperature of 45°C.

The Vydac TP packing material has 330-Å diameter pores. Several laboratories have shown that supports having 300 to 500-Å pores give better results with large peptides and proteins than the more commonly used supports which have pores of about 100 Å diameter.[17-20]

Either 1-propanol or 2-propanol is a stronger solvent for polypeptides than acetonitrile[21,22] and may be required for elution of some samples not eluted by the latter. However, propanol systems have a higher viscosity than acetonitrile systems. This causes higher column backpressure and lower efficiency (broader peaks).[16]

Phosphate or phosphoric acid has been found to give particularly good results in HPLC of peptides.[14,23-26] It is presumed that ion-pairing between peptide $R\text{-}NH_3^+$ groups and the hydrophilic anion $H_2PO_4^-$ increase the polarity of the migrating species, thus decreasing their retention. Some workers add perchlorate as a chaotropic agent to phosphate mobile phases.[27-29] Trifluoroacetic acid also works well;[21] larger perfluoridated acids have been used to provide more hydrophobic counterions and thus increase retention of hydrophilic peptides.[18,30,31]

Other mobile phase buffers used in reverse-phase HPLC of polypeptides include triethylamine phosphate[13,32-36] and, as noted previously, ammonium acetate.[14,37-46] All the mobile phase systems mentioned to this point are used with absorbance detection of peptides at 205 to 230 nm (and at 254 or 280 nm or other wavelengths if desired). Winkler[47,48] has proposed using absorbance at 215 nm instead of 210 or 205 nm to detect effluent peptide material when using an acetonitrile gradient in TFA to avoid baseline problems concomitant with increasing acetonitrile concentrations. We have found this to be quite useful. Fluorescence detection following postcolumn derivatization of peptides[17,28] allows the use of pyridine formate or acetate buffers and is very sensitive but destructive of the portion of the sample diverted to the detector. Wilson and co-workers have compared absorbance and fluorescence detection,[28] finding them both sensitive down to the picomole level. The fluorescence detector produces some peak broadening from postcolumn mixing of reagents, although this affects only the recorded trace and not the actual resolution of peptides in the portion of the eluent not passed through the detector. They found ultraviolet (UV) absorbance detection more susceptible to impurity and baseline problems.

Chemically modified peptides may be detected by their change in mobility relative to peaks of an unmodified digest, by specific absorbance or fluorescence characteristics of the modifying group, and/or radiolabel incorporated with the modifying group.

Cyanopropyl columns are less retentive than C-18 or C-8 columns and therefore useful for more hydrophobic peptides.[34,41] Alkylphenyl columns have been used for peptide separation.[32,49,50] Newer types of packings include diphenyl and short-chain hydrocarbon bonded phases.

Column performance for polypeptide separations is not necessarily related to performance for separation of small molecules. In the latter situation the sample is considered to undergo a series of equilibration steps between the mobile and stationary phases as it passes through the column.[51] Retention and separation are thus dependent on the column length (number of "theoretical plates" or equilibration steps). With polypeptides this is not the case; 5-cm columns separate as well as 25-cm columns;[19,52] only loading capacity is affected. Pearson et al.[52] attribute this phenomenon to the operation of an adsorption-desorption mechanism instead of the multi-step partitioning which occurs with smaller molecules.

Several groups have determined sets of coefficients for predicting retention of a peptide from its amino acid composition.[16,22,31,53,54] Each set is valid only for a specific chromatographic system (mobile phase, stationary phase, pH, temperature, flow rate, gradient rate, etc.).

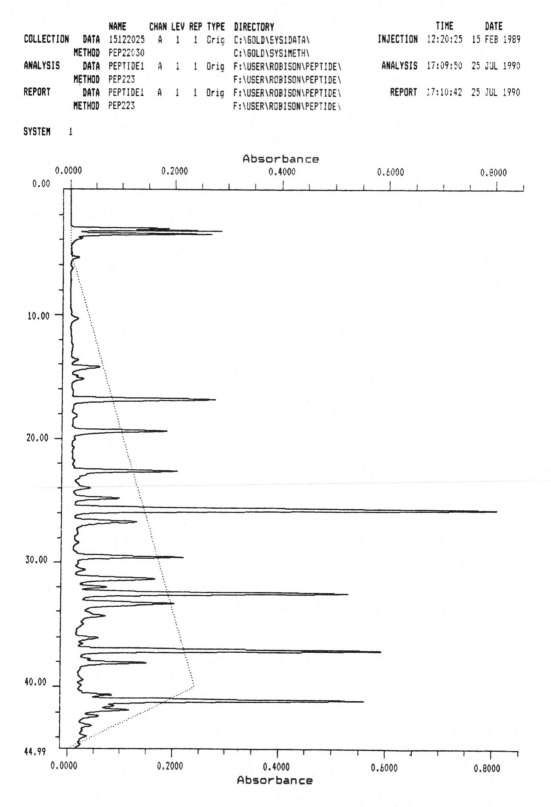

FIGURE 2.   HPLC separation of the tryptic digest of lysozyme on an Ultrasphere® C-18 Column. Initial solvent (solvent A) was 5% acetonitrile in 0.1% TFA, and solvent B is 75% acetonitrile in 0.1% TFA. A gradient from 0 to 30% B (shown by dotted line) at a flow rate of 1 ml/min. (This figure is courtesy of Beckman Instruments.)

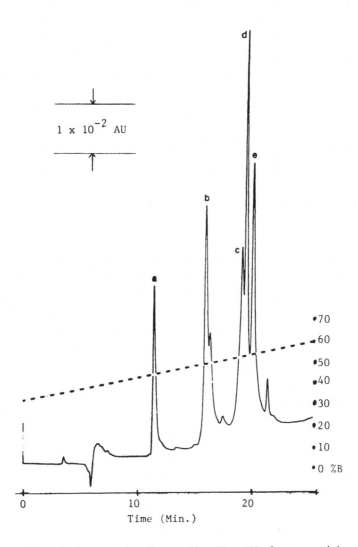

1×10^{-2} AU

d

b

e

c

a

•70
•60
•50
•40
•30
•20
•10
•0 %B

0   10   20

Time (Min.)

FIGURE 3.   The separation of cyanogen bromide peptides from sperm whale myoglobin on a C-4 Column. A gradient (dotted line) of acetonitrile in 0.1% TFA was used to develop the column. Effluent absorbance was monitored at 230 nm. (Courtesy of ISCO Scientific.)

Figure 2 shows the separation of the tryptic peptides from lysozyme on C-18-column, using a gradient of acetonitrile in TFA. Figure 3 depicts the separation of the cyanogen bromide peptides from sperm whale myoglobin using a C-4 column with an acetonitrile gradient in TFA. Figure 4 shows the separation of the tryptic peptides from sperm whale myglobin on a C-18 column using an acetonitrile gradient in TFA.

There have been some additional studies which are worth consideration. In virtually each of the individual chapters, there is some discussion of a unique approach to the purification of a peptide containing a modified amino acid. In addition, there have been recent studies directed toward the purification of hydrophobic peptides[56,57] as well as methodology for obtaining peptides from sodium dodecyl sulfate-solubilized proteins.[58] Finally, an interesting affinity approach based on the use of immobilized anhydrotrypsin has been developed for the purification of C-terminal peptides.[58]

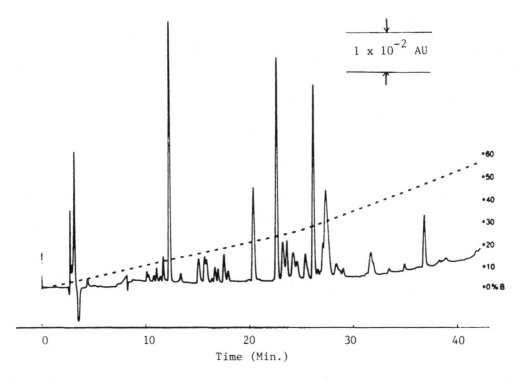

FIGURE 4.   The separation of tryptic peptides from sperm whale myoglobin on a C-18 Column. A gradient (dotted line) of acetonitrile in 0.1% TFA was used to develop the column. Effluent absorbance was monitored at 230 nm. (Courtesy of ISCO Scientific.)

REFERENCES

1. *CRC Handbook of HPLC for the Separation of Amino Acids, Peptides, and Proteins,* Hancock, W. S., Ed., CRC Press, Boca Raton, FL, 1984.
2. **Ito, Y.,** Countercurrent chromatography, *Meth. Enzymol.,* 91, 335, 1983.
3. **Hermodson, M. and Mahoney, W. C.,** Separation of peptides by reversed-phase high-performance liquid chromatography, *Meth. Enzymol.,* 91, 352, 1983.
4. **Nika, H. and Hultin, T.,** Analyzer for microscale peptide separation, *Meth. Enzymol.,* 91, 359, 1983.
5. **Croft, L. R.,** *Handbook of Protein Sequence Analysis,* John Wiley & Sons, Chichester, 1980.
6. **Petrides, P. E.,** Microisolation of biologically active polypeptides by reverse-phase liquid chromatography, in *Methods of Protein Microcharacterization,* Shively, J. E., Ed., Humana Press, Clifton, NJ, 1986, 3.
7. **Shively, J. E.,** Reverse-phase HPLC isolation and microsequence analysis, in *Methods of Protein Microcharacterization,* Shively, J. E., Ed., Humana Press, Clifton, NJ, 1986, 41.
8. **Mayes, E. L. V.,** Electrophoretic and chromatographic separation of peptides on paper, in *Methods in Molecular Biolology, Vol. 1,* Walker, J. M., Ed., Humana Press, Clifton, NJ, 1984, 21.
9. **Mayes, E. L. V.,** Peptide mapping by reverse-phase high pressure liquid chromatography, in *Methods in Molecular Biology, Vol. 1,* Walker, J. M., Ed., Humana Press, Clifton, NJ, 1984, 33.
10. **Simpson, R. J., Moritz, R. L., Begg, G. S., Rubira, M. R. and Nice, E. C.,** Micropreparative procedures for high sensitivity sequencing of peptides and proteins, *Anal. Biochem.,* 177, 221, 1989.
11. **Wilson, K. J.,** Micro-level protein and peptide separations, *TIBS,* 14, 252, 1989.
12. **Snyder, L. R. and Kirkland, J. J.,** *Introduction to Modern Liquid Chromatography,* 2nd ed., John Wiley & Sons, New York, 1979.
13. **Wehr, C. T., Correia, L., and Abbott, S. R.,** Evaluation of stationary and mobile phases for reversed-phase high performance liquid chromatography of peptides, *J. Chromatogr. Sci.,* 20, 114, 1982.
14. **Noyes, C. M. and Lundblad, R. L.,** unpublished data, 1981.

15. **Schroeder, W. A., Shelton, J. B., and Shelton, J. R.**, High performance liquid chromatography in the identification of human hemoglobin variants, in *Advances in Hemoglobin Analysis*, Hanash, S. M. and Brewer, G. J., Eds., Alan R. Liss, New York, 1981, 1.

16. **Meek, J. L. and Rossetti, Z. L.**, Factors affecting retention and resolution of peptides in high-performance liquid chromatography, *J. Chromatogr.*, 211, 15, 1981.

17. **Lewis, R. V., Fallon, A., Stein, S., Gibson, K. D., and Udenfriend, S.**, Supports for reverse-phase high-performance liquid chromatography of large proteins, *Anal. Biochem.*, 104, 153, 1980.

18. **van der Rest, M., Bennett, H. P. J., Solomon, S., and Glorieux, F. H.**, Separation of collagen cyanogen bromide-derived peptides by reversed-phase high-performance liquid chromatography, *Biochem. J.*, 191, 253, 1980.

19. **Pearson, J. D., Mahoney, W. C., Hermodson, M. A., and Regnier, F. E.**, Reversed-phase supports for the resolution of large denatured protein fragments, *J. Chromatogr.*, 207, 325, 1981.

20. **Wilson, K. J., Van Wieringen, E., Klauser, S., Berchtold, M. W., and Hughes, G. J.**, Comparison of the high-performance liquid chromatography of peptides and proteins on 100- and 300-Å reversed-phase suppots, *J. Chromatogr.*, 237, 407, 1982.

21. **Mahoney, W. C. and Hermodson, M. A.**, Separation of large denatured peptides by reverse phase high performance liquid chromatography. Trifluoroacetic acid as a peptide solvent, *J. Biol. Chem.*, 255, 11199, 1980.

22. **Wilson, K. J., Honegger, A., Stötzel, R. R., and Hughes, G. J.**, The behaviour of peptides on reverse-phase supports during high-pressure liquid chromatography, *Biochem. J.*, 199, 31, 1981.

23. **Hancock, W. S., Bishop, C. A., Prestidge, R. L., Harding, D. R. K., and Hearn, M. T. W.**, High-pressure liquid chromatography of peptides and proteins. II. The use of phosphoric acid in the analysis of underivatised peptides by reversed-phase high-pressure liquid chromatography, *J. Chromatogr.*, 153, 391, 1978.

24. **Fullmer, C. S. and Wasserman, R. H.**, Analytical peptide mapping by high performance liquid chromatography. Application to intestinal calcium-binding proteins, *J. Biol. Chem.*, 254, 7208, 1979.

25. **O'Hare, M. J. and Nice, E. C.**, Hydrophobic high-performance liquid chromatography of hormonal polypeptides and proteins on alkylsilane-bonded silica, *J. Chromatogr.*, 171, 209, 1979.

26. **Nice, E. C. and O'Hare, M. J.**, Simultaneous separation of β-lipotrophin, adrenocorticotropic hormone, endorphins and enkephalins by high-performance liquid chromatography, *J. Chromatogr.*, 162, 401, 1979.

27. **Meek, J. L.**, Prediction of peptide retention times in high-pressure liquid chromatography on the basis of amino acid composition, *Proc. Natl. Acad. Sci. U.S.A.*, 77, 1632, 1980.

28. **Wilson, K. J., Honegger, A., and Hughes, G. J.**, Comparison of buffers and detection systems for high-pressure liquid chromatography of peptide mixtures, *Biochem. J.*, 199, 43, 1981.

29. **Strydom, D. J. and Vallee, B. L.**, Characterization of human alcohol dehydrogenase isoenzymes by high-performance liquid chromatographic peptide mapping, *Anal. Biochem.*, 123, 422, 1982.

30. **Bennett, H. J. P., Browne, C. A., and Solomon, S.**, The use of perfluorinated carboxylic acids in the reversed-phase HPLC of peptides, *J. Liquid Chromatogr.*, 3, 1353, 1980.

31. **Browne, C. A., Bennett, H. J. P., and Solomon, S.**, The isolation of peptides by high-performance liquid chromatography using predicted elution positions, *Anal. Biochem.*, 124, 201, 1982.

32. **Rivier, J. E.**, Use of trialkyl ammonium phosphate (TAAP) buffers in reverse phase HPLC for high resolution and high recovery of peptides and proteins, *J. Liquid Chromatogr.*, 1, 343, 1978.

33. **Biedermann, K., Montali, U., Martin, B., Svendsen, I., and Ottesen, M.**, The amino acid sequence of proteinase A inhibitor 3 from baker's yeast, *Carlsberg Res. Commun.*, 45, 225, 1980.

34. **Chaiken, I. M. and Hough, C. J.**, Mapping and isolation of large peptide fragments from bovine neurophysins and biosynthetic neurophysin-containing species by high-performance liquid chromatography, *Anal. Biochem.*, 107, 11, 1980.

35. **Hancock, W. S., Capra, J. D., Bradley, W. A., and Sparrow, J. T.**, The use of reversed-phase high-performance liquid chromatography with radial compression for the analysis of peptide and protein mixtures, *J. Chromatogr.*, 206, 59, 1981.

36. **Hearn, M. T. W. and Grego, B.**, High-performance liquid chromatography of amino acids, peptides and proteins. XXXVI. Organic solvent modifier effects in the separation of unprotected peptides by reversed-phase liquid chromatography, *J. Chromatogr.*, 218, 497, 1981.

37. **Wilson, J. B., Lam, H., Pravatmuang, P., and Huisman, T. H. J.**, Separation of tryptic peptides of normal and abnormal α, β, γ, and δ hemoglobin chains by high-performance liquid chromatography, *J. Chromatogr.*, 179, 271, 1979.

38. **Hancock, W. S. and Sparrow, J. T.**, Use of mixed-mode, high-performance liquid chromatography for the separation of peptide and protein mixtures, *J. Chromatogr.*, 206, 71, 1981.

39. **Kehl, M. and Henschen, A.**, Characterization of the peptides released at the fibrinogen-fibrin conversion using high performance liquid chromatography, in *High Performance Chromatography in Protein and Peptide Chemistry*, Lottspeich, F., Henschen, A., and Hupe, K.-P., Eds., Walter de Gruyter, Berlin, 1981, 339.

40. **Kratzin, H. and Yang, C.-Y.**, Separation of enzymatic hydrolysates by reverse-phase HPLC, in *High Performance Chromatography in Protein and Peptide Chemistry*, Lottspeich, F., Henschen, A., and Hupe, K.-P., Eds., Walter de Gruyter, Berlin, 1981, 269.

41. **Ponstingl, H., Krauhs, E., Little, M., Kempf, T., Hofer-Warbinek, R., and Ade, W.**, Elucidation of tubulin amino acid sequence: preparative separation of peptides by reversed phase HPLC, in *High Performance Chromatography in Protein and Peptide Chemistry*, Lottspeich, F., Henschen, A., and Hupe, K.-P., Eds., Walter de Gruyter, Berlin, 1981, 325.

42. **Stüber, K., and Beyreuther, K.**, Preparative separation of peptides by high performance liquid chromatography. Use of volatile buffers transparent in the ultraviolet, in *High Performance Chromatography in Protein and Peptide Chemistry*, Lottspeich, F., Henschen, A., and Hupe, K.-P., Eds., Walter de Gruyter, Berlin, 1981, 205.

43. **Yang, C.-Y. and Kratzin, H.**, Chromatography and rechromatography of peptide mixtures by reverse-phase HPLC, in *High Performance Chromatography in Protein and Peptide Chemistry*, Lottspeich, F., Henschen, A., and Hupe, K.-P., Eds., Walter de Gruyter, Berlin, 1981, 283.

44. **Anderson, J. K. and Mole, J. E.**, Adaptation of reverse-phase high-performance liquid chromatography for the isolation and sequence analysis of peptides from plasma amyloid P-component, *Anal. Biochem.*, 123, 413, 1982.

45. **Lambert, D. T., Stachelek, C., Varga, J. M., and Lerner, A. B.**, Iodination of β-melanotropin, *J. Biol. Chem.*, 257, 8211, 1982.

46. **Oray, B., Jahani, M., and Gracy, R. W.**, High-sensitivity peptide mapping of triosephosphate isomerase: a comparison of high-performance liquid chromatography with two-dimensional thin-layer methods, *Anal. Biochem.*, 125, 131, 1982.

47. **Winkler, G., Wolshann, P., Briza, P., Heinz, F. X., and Kunz, C.**, Spectral properties of trifluoroacetic acid-acetonitrile gradient systems for spearation of picomole quantities of peptides by reversed-phase high-performance liquid chromatography, *J. Chromatogr.*, 34, 83, 1985.

48. **Winkler, G.**, Increasing the sensitivity of UV detection in protein and peptide separations when using TFA-acetonitrile gradients, *LC/GC*, 5, 1044, 1987.

49. **Hancock, W. S., Bishop, C. A., Meyer, L. J., Harding, D. R. K., and Hearn, M. T. W.**, High-pressure liquid chromatography of peptides and proteins. VI. Rapid analysis of peptides by high-pressure liquid chromatography with hydrophobic ion-pairing of amino groups, *J. Chromatogr.*, 161, 291, 1978.

50. **Hancock, W. S., Bishop, C. A., Battersby, J. E., Harding, D. R. K., and Hearn, M. T. W.**, High-pressure liquid chromatography of peptides and proteins. XI. The use of cationic reagents for the analysis of peptides by high-pressure liquid chromatography, *J. Chromatogr.*, 168, 377, 1979.

51. **Martin, A. J. P. and Synge, R. L. M.**, A new form of chromatogram employing two liquid phases. I. A theory of chromatography. II. Application to the micro-determination of the higher monoamino-acids in proteins, *Biochem. J.*, 35, 1358, 1941.

52. **Pearson, J. D., Lin, N. T., and Regnier, F. E.**, The importance of silica type for reverse-phase protein separations, *Anal. Biochem.*, 124, 217, 1982.

53. **Su, S.-J., Grego, B., Niven, B., and Hearn, M. T. W.**, Analysis of group retention contributions for peptides separated by reversed phase high performance liquid chromatography, *J. Liquid Chromatogr.*, 4, 1745, 1981.

54. **Sasagawa, T., Okuyama, T., and Teller, D. C.**, Prediction of peptide retention times in reversed-phase high-performance liquid chromatography during linear gradient elution, *J. Chromatogr.*, 240, 329, 1982.

55. **Arjomaa, P. and Hallman, M.**, Purification of a hydrophobic surfactant peptide using high-performance liquid chromatography, *Anal. Biochem.*, 171, 207, 1988.

56. **Feick, R. G. and Shiozawa, J. A.**, A high-yield method for the isolation of hydrophobic proteins and peptides from polyacrylamide gels for protein sequencing, *Anal. Biochem.*, 187, 205, 1990.

57. **Bosserhoff, A., Wallach, J., and Frank, R. W.**, Micropreparative separation of peptides derived from sodium dodecyl sulphate-solubilized proteins, *J. Chromatogr.*, 473, 71, 1989.

58. **Kumazaki, T., Terasawa, K., and Ishii, S.-I.**, Affinity chromatography on immobilized anhydrotrypsin: general utility for selective isolation of C-terminal peptides from protease digests of proteins, *J. Biochem.*, 102, 1539, 1987.

Chapter 4

METHODS FOR SEQUENCE DETERMINATION

I. INTRODUCTION

Determination of the amino acid sequence around a site of chemical modification provides unequivocal identification of its location in the proteins, providing the complete sequence of the protein is known. Although analysis of amino acid composition alone may allow identification of the peptide containing the modification, even a few cycles of sequence analysis serve to verify its purity and identity.

Most methods for the determination of amino acid sequence use the degradation scheme developed by Edman.[1,2] (The procedure was originally described as a micro-method requiring "only" 10 mg of amino acid per cycle.) Phenylisothiocyanate (PITC) reacts with the NH_2-terminal amino acid of a polypeptide at basic pH (see Scheme 1) to form a phenylthiocarbamyl derivative (Reaction 1). Acidification, generally with anhydrous acid, then cleaves off the first amino acid as its 2-anilino-5-thiazolinone derivative and exposes the amino group of the second amino acid (Reaction 2). The derivatized amino acid is removed by extraction, the remaining polypeptide is dried, and the cycle is repeated. The large difference in pH between coupling and cleavage allows the degradation to proceed by discrete steps, unlike exopeptidase digestions, which begin to release the second amino acid before all of the first has been removed.

Procedures for sequence analysis by the Edman degradation fall into two major categories differing in the type of method used for determination of the amino acid at each step. In so-called indirect Edman procedures, a portion of the sample is removed at the beginning and after each cycle and analyzed either quantitatively for total amino acid composition or qualitatively for the identity of the NH_2-terminal. In direct methods, the thiazolinone produced at each step is extracted, converted to the more stable thiohydantoin (Reaction 3), and identified. Manual procedures of both types are used; automated sequenators have generally used direct identification.

The following points apply to all Edman degradation techniques:

1. All procedures and identification methods should be practiced first on known peptides.
2. Ideally, known examples of derivatives from all amino acids from actual degradations should be observed in the identification system to be used.
3. Purity of reagents and solvents, particularly freedom from aldehydes and oxidants, is important.
4. Degradations are performed in an atmosphere of nitrogen or argon to exclude oxygen and air pollutants that can cause side reactions and block further degradation.[3,4] Manual degradation may be carried out in a glove box[5] or closed reaction vessel[6] to facilitate maintenance of an inert atmosphere.

II. INDIRECT EDMAN DEGRADATION

A. Subtractive

An aliquot of the peptide is removed after each cycle and subjected to hydrolysis and quantitative amino acid analysis. A typical procedure is outlined by Konigsberg:[7]

The medium for coupling can be (1) 50% aqueous pyridine containing 2% triethylamine, (2) N-ethylmorpholine per acetic acid per 95% ethanol per water (60:1.5:500:438), or (3) 50% pyridine containing 5% dimethylallylamine. The peptide is dissolved in coupling buffer and treated with a 50-fold excess of PITC at 37°C for 2 h. (Exclusion of oxygen and

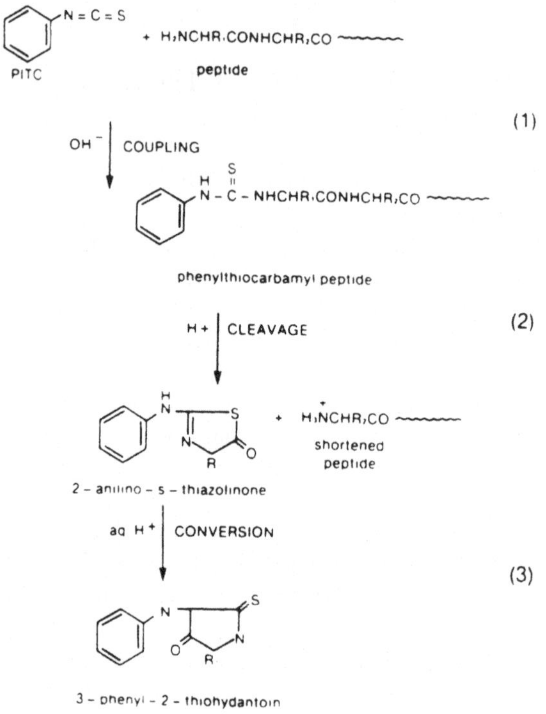

$$\text{PITC} \quad \text{N=C=S} \quad + \quad H_2NCHR_1CONHCHR_2CO \sim\sim\sim \quad \text{peptide}$$

(1)

$$OH^- \downarrow \text{COUPLING}$$

$$\text{phenylthiocarbamyl peptide} \quad \underset{H}{N}-\overset{\underset{\parallel}{S}}{C}-NHCHR_1CONHCHR_2CO \sim\sim\sim$$

(2)

$$H^+ \downarrow \text{CLEAVAGE}$$

$$\text{2 – anilino – 5 – thiazolinone} \quad + \quad H_2NCHR_2CO \sim\sim\sim \quad \text{shortened peptide}$$

$$aq \ H^+ \downarrow \text{CONVERSION}$$

(3)

$$\text{3 – phenyl – 2 – thiohydantoin}$$

SCHEME 1.

contaminants during coupling is particularly important in the subtractive method, since partial blockage of peptide will cause nonintegral loss of amino acid.)

After coupling, the sample is evaporated nearly to dryness and extracted three times with 1 to 2 ml benzene, then dried. Cleavage is carried out in anhydrous trifluoroacetic acid (TFA) at 25°C for 1 h or 40°C for 15 min. The TFA is evaporated; the residue is dissolved in 0.2 M acetic acid and heated at 40°C for 10 min. It is then extracted three times with benzene. An appropriate aliquot of the acetic acid solution is removed for hydrolysis and amino acid analysis (see Chapter 2). The remaining sample is dried and the cycle is repeated.

Subtractive degradation is applicable only to peptides small enough that loss of a single amino acid is clearly distinguishable in the amino acid analysis. The amount of peptide needed depends on the sensitivity of the analyzer and the number of Edman cycles to be carried out. Glu/Gln and Asp/Asn are not differentiated by the usual acid hydrolysis procedure, since Gln and Asn are deamidated.

B. Dansyl-Edman

Intensely fluorescent derivatives result from the reaction of 1-dimethylaminonaphthalene-5-sulfonyl (dansyl) chloride with free amino groups. Dansyl amino acid derivatives are stable to acid hydrolysis and exhibit yellow fluorescence.[8] The NH2-terminal of a peptide can therefore be identified by reacting it with dansyl chloride, hydrolyzing the peptide, and identifying the fluorescent derivative by electrophoresis or chromatography.[8-11] For sequence determination, an aliquot is removed at each cycle of degradation and analyzed in this way. Since 10 pmol of dansyl amino acid is readily detected,[11] the amount removed can be less than in subtractive Edman degradation. Also, the sample need only be washed after cleavage, so extractive losses of peptide may be less than with other procedures. The method requires no major equipment and is considered simple and easily learned.[12]

Instructions for dansyl-Edman degradation of about a nanomole of peptide are given by

Bruton and Hartley.[11] The sample is dissolved in 20 μl of water, a 10-pmol aliquot is removed for dansylation, and 20 μl of 5% (v/v) PITC in pyridine is added to the remainder. The tube is flushed with nitrogen and heated at 45°C for 1 h, then dried in a vacuum desiccator at 60°C for 30 min. TFA (20 μl) is added and the sample is incubated at 45°C for 30 min and dried *in vacuo* over NaOH. The residue is dissolved in 25 μl of water and extracted with four 150-μl portions of *n*-butyl acetate. The aqueous solution is dried *in vacuo* and redissolved in 20 μl of water. Another 10-pmol aliquot is removed for dansylation and the cycle repeated on the remainder.

The aliquots removed at each cycle are dried in a vacuum desiccator over P_2O_5. Two successive 2-μl portions of 0.1 *M* $NaHCO_3$ are added and dried to remove ammonia. Dansyl chloride solution (1 μl of a 1:1 mixture of water and a solution of 2.5 mg dansyl chloride per ml acetone) is added and the sample incubated at 37°C for 1 h. After drying, 5 μl of 6 *N* HCl is added. The tube is sealed and the peptide is hydrolyzed at 105°C for 16 h. The dansyl amino acids are identified by 2-dimensional thin-layer chromatography on 5 × 5 cm polyamide sheets.[10] A fine capillary is used for sample application to keep the spot as small as possible. A mixture of standards is run on the reverse side of the sheet. The solvent for the first dimension is 1.5% (v/v) formic acid. In the second dimension benzene/acetic acid 9:1 (or less toxic toluene/acetic acid 10:1) is run, followed in the same direction by ethyl acetate/methanol/acetic acid 20:1:1. The plate is dried and examined under UV light after each step. Resolution of certain spots may require a fourth solvent, 0.05 *M* trisodium phosphate/ethanol 3:1, also run in the second direction. As in the subtractive method, glutamine and asparagine are deamidated during hydrolysis. The thiazolinones may be recovered from the organic solvent, converted to the phenylthiohydantoins, and identified by one of the methods described later.

Gray and Smith developed a rapid dansyl-Edman procedure for five or six cycles on small peptides.[13] The sample is divided at the start into portions corresponding to the number of cycles to be carried out, and one tube is set aside before each cycle. The desired number of cycles is performed, with drying at 70°C *in vacuo* after each coupling and each cleavage, but with no solvent wash until the end. At that time all tubes are washed with water-saturated ethyl acetate to remove phenylthiourea and diphenylthiourea. Dansylation, hydrolysis, and identification are performed as described above.

Detailed instructions for a modified dansyl-Edman procedure suitable for analysis of proteins (which tend to become insoluble in the solvents used for peptides) are given by Weiner et al.[14]

III. DIRECT EDMAN DEGRADATION

A. Manual PITC

An extensive discussion of the factors affecting the Edman chemistry and of possible reagent, solvent, and temperature options for manual degradation is given by Tarr.[6] The manual Edman procedure described by Peterson et al.[15] has been widely used.

Levy recommends the following technique for 1 to 10 nmol of peptide.[16] Acid-washed polypropylene microcentrifuge tubes are used, and all manipulations of liquids are done with polypropylene micropipet tips. Argon is preferred for flushing since it is heavier than nitrogen and thus stays in the tubes better. The buffer for coupling consists of 15 ml pyridine, 1.18 ml dimethylallylamine, and 10 ml water; the pH is adjusted to 9.5 with TFA. Norleucine, 25 to 50 nmol, is added at the beginning of each cycle as a carrier and internal standard.

Coupling takes place with 40 μl buffer plus 3 μl PITC for 30 min at 50°C under argon. The sample is washed twice with heptane/ethyl acetate 10:1 and once with heptane/ethyl acetate 2:1, with vigorous mixing followed by centrifugation to separate the phases. The sample (aqueous phase) is dried under vacuum. Cleavage follows in 20 μl TFA for 20 min at 50°C. After vacuum drying the sample is dissolved in 40 μl of 30% pyridine, extracted with three 150-μl portions of benzene:ethyl acetate (1/2) and the cycle is repeated.

The benzene/ethyl acetate extract containing the thiazolinone is dried. Conversion to the phenylthiohydantoin is done in 40 μl 1 *N* HCl for 10 min at 80°C, followed by extraction with three 50-μl portions of ethyl acetate. All PTHs except PTH-Arg, -His, and -CysSO$_3$H are extracted by the ethyl acetate. The PTHs are identified by HPLC or one of the other methods described in Section IV of this chapter.

There have been significant advances in manual techniques for sequence analysis of peptides and proteins. Shively and co-workers[17,18] have developed an attractive apparatus for performing manual gas-phase Edman degradation reactions. Brandt and Frank[19] have also reported a manual technique for the gas-phase Edman degradation.

B. Manual DABITC/PITC

The Edman degradation can be carried out with the compound dimethylaminoazobenzene-4'-isothiocyanate (DABITC) in place of PITC.[20,21] The thiohydantoin amino acid derivatives (DABTHs) of this compound are red (ϵ_M, 436 nm $\cong$ 34,000), so they can be detected visually on thin layer sheets, with the further advantage that derivatives of non-amino acid impurities appear blue or are invisible. However, quantitative coupling with DABITC requires a temperature of 75°C. Consequently a double coupling is performed instead at 52°C; the second coupling is with PITC to drive the reaction to completion.

In the method developed by Chang et al.,[21] 2 to 8 nmol of peptide or protein are dried in an acid-washed tube and dissolved in 80 μl of 50% pyridine. Freshly prepared DABITC solution (2.82 mg/ml pyridine), 40 μl is added. The tube is flushed with nitrogen and heated at 52°C for 50 min. PITC, 10 μl, is added, followed by another 30-min incubation at 52°C. The mixture is extracted two or three times by 0.5-ml portions of heptane/ethyl acetate 2:1, with vortexing followed by centrifugation. The aqueous phase is dried under high vacuum. The sample is dissolved in 50 μl anhydrous TFA, flushed with nitrogen, sealed with a glass stopper, and heated at 52°C for 15 min. After drying in a vacuum desiccator, it is dissolved in 50 μl of water and extracted with 200 μl of butyl acetate. The sample is dried and the cycle repeated.

For conversion, the butyl acetate extract is evaporated; 20 μl of water and 40 μl of acetic acid saturated with HCl are added. Conversion is at 52°C for 50 min. The sample is dried, redissolved in ethanol, and applied to polyamide sheets for thin layer chromatography. Acetic acid/water, 1:2, is run in the first dimension and toluene/*n*-hexane/acetic acid, 2:1:1, in the second. DABTH-Leu and -Ile are resolved on silica gel plates in chloroform/ethanol, 100:3. The plates are dried and exposed to HCl vapor; DABTH spots are red. Sensitivity of detection is 5 to 25 pmol on polyamide, 25 to 50 pmol on silica.

Wilson, Hughes, and co-workers[22,23] have adapted the DABITC/PITC degradation scheme for use in automated sequenators. They prefer 1 *N* HCl or 20% TFA for the conversion step. DABITC is light-sensitive and not very stable in solution, so appropriate precautions must be taken. Fischer and Howden[24] have described a manual sequence technique for picomole quantities of peptide using the 4-*N*,*N'*-dimethylaminoazobenzene 4'-thiohydantoin derivatives.

C. Spinning-Cup Sequenator

In 1967 Edman and Begg[25] published a description of a machine for automatically performing the Edman degradation of proteins. Essentially a "robot chemist", the sequenator or sequencer carries out the coupling, wash, cleavage, and extraction steps of the cycle. Conversion of thiazolinones to thiohydantoins is still often performed manually, although automated converters have been devised.[26,27]

The heart of the sequenator is a spinning glass cup in a temperature-controlled reaction chamber. The protein or peptide sample is deposited in a thin film in the lower half of the cup. Reagents for coupling or cleavage are added to cover the film. Solvents for extraction are run into the cup for several minutes, so that the liquid flows up over the precipitated sample, out through a tube at the top of the cup, and is directed by a valve to waste or a fraction collector. The sample can be dried by a stream of nitrogen followed by progressive degrees of vacuum. An inert atmosphere is maintained in the reaction chamber.

In addition to the convenience of unattended operation, the sequenator gives better results than manual degradation in extended sequence analyses of intact proteins. These tend to become insoluble precipitates after a few cycles of manual degradation, with concomitant poor yields and out-of-phase results. The spinning cup of the sequenator keeps the sample spread out in a thin film, thus maintaining efficiency of reaction and extraction.

For small peptides, on the other hand, the sequenator does not have as clear a performance advantage over manual techniques. With these samples it is more difficult to achieve adequate extraction of reagents, by-products, and thiazolinones without also washing out the sample. Manual procedures offer more flexibility and better control. A great deal of effort has gone into improving sequenator retention of small peptides, including modifying them to decrease their solubility in organic solvents[28,29] and use of nondegradable or artificial carriers.[30,31] The most successful carrier has been the polymer 1,5-dimethyl-1,5-diazaundecamethylene polymethobromide, commonly known as Polybrene.[32,33] Addition of 1 to 3 mg of Polybrene to the cup with the sample allows complete sequence analysis of even subnanomolar amounts of many peptides. Le Caer and Rossier[34] have reported that polyethyleneimine is superior to Polybrene for sequencing peptides and proteins since the precycling used to condition Polybrene-coated glass fiber filters was no longer necessary. Extremely hydrophobic peptides may still require manual degradation, but in general, automated sequence analysis is now as feasible for peptides as for proteins.

As with all sequence analysis techniques, the amount of sample required for automated Edman degradation is determined by the sensitivity of the identification method used, the repetitive yield on successive cycles of degradation, and the number of cycles to be run. Identification depends on both absolute sensitivity and levels of background contaminants. Besides whatever background is obtained from reagent impurities and side reactions, an increasing level of amino acid background arises during a sequence analysis because of small amounts of nonspecific cleavage of peptide bonds.[25] This background is proportional to the size of the polypeptide, and runs on intact proteins, commonly limited in length by the decreasing signal-to-noise ratio arising from decreasing yield and increasing background from nonspecific cleavage and cycle-to-cycle overlap. Peptides up to a few dozen residues in length, on the other hand, produce very little cumulative background and can be followed to the limits imposed by the sensitivity of the detection method used and/or the background from the degradation procedure.

We are able to achieve 93% repetitive yield on 250 pmol starting yield of a peptide using an unmodified Beckman 890C sequenator, Polybrene carrier, and Beckman chemicals. Identification of PTHs by HPLC with this system is possible down to 10 to 50 pmol, so complete sequence analysis of small peptides is possible and at least 20 cycles on larger ones. The first amino acids to be unidentifiable tend to be serine and proline.

We use the 0.1 M Quadrol sequenator program of Brauer et al.[32] with the following modifications. After coupling, the buffer is flushed from the delivery line with a short delivery of ethyl acetate. Delivery of heptafluorobutyric acid (HFBA) for cleavage is modified to use a minimum amount of acid, to avoid blowing acid vapors through the effluent valve, and to provide thorough flushing of acid from the delivery line. HFBA is delivered for 3 seconds, followed by 20 seconds of restricted vacuum to draw it into the cup. After cleavage and a preliminary drying step, n-chlorobutane is delivered briefly through the same line and dried. Extraction with n-chlorobutane follows. Three mg of Polybrene is added to the cup and put through one complete cycle before adding the sample. (Some authors find more extensive precycling of Polybrene necessary,[33,35] so there may be lot-to-lot variations in its purity.)

Some laboratories have devised extensive modifications of the spinning-cup sequenator.[33,36,37] These changes in conjunction with meticulous purification reagents provide decreased background levels and improved repetitive yields, thus allowing extended degradation on subnanomolar quantities of sample. Applications related to the topic of this book should not generally require such measures.

Automated devices for the conversion of thiazolinones to PTHs have been described.[26,27] Although they increase convenience and possibly recovery levels of unstable derivatives, their use places more exacting demands on system cleanliness, reagent purity, and the resolution of the identification method, and may in turn necessitate the further sequenator and reagent improvements described below. With an automatic converter the conversion mixture is dried down in a single phase. Thus, all the PTHs must be distinguished from each other and from all by-products during identification, whereas manual conversion divides the products between an organic and an aqueous phase, which are analyzed separately.

D. Solid-Phase Sequenator

One approach to the problem of sample loss during washing is covalent attachment of the peptide to a solid support.[38] The support beads are then placed in a temperature-controlled column or reaction chamber, and reagents and solvents are passed through.

Methods of covalent attachment have been summarized by Laursen.[39] Peptides can be attached to appropriate supports through the COOH-terminal homoserine produced by cyanogen bromide digestion, through lysine ϵ-NH$_2$ groups, or through carboxyl groups. In the latter method, aspartic and glutamic acid side chains tend to become bound in addition to the COOH-terminal carboxyl, causing gaps at those points in the sequence. Support materials are derivatized glass or polystyrene beads.[38,40]

The necessary repertoire of materials and attachment methods is cumbersome but may be used to achieve separation of peptide mixtures by selective coupling and sequences of COOH-terminal portions of larger peptides by trypsin digestion of bound material.[39]

Commercially available equipment for automated solid-phase Edman degradation is less expensive than liquid-phase (spinning-cup) machines. It may be possible to use less expensive chemicals, since more extensive washing is possible. Disadvantages are the extra time and work required for sample attachment to the solid support and sample losses due to incomplete coupling.

Powers[41] describes solid-phase methods for spinning-cup sequenators. These include both placing beads with peptides attached in the sequenator cup (and hoping they won't wash out and plug the effluent valve) and attaching peptides directly to the glass wall of the cup. These techniques have been mostly superseded by the simpler use of Polybrene carrier, but may be useful for particular problems.

Chang[42] has performed manual sequence analysis by the DABITC/PITC procedure on peptides attached to glass beads. No advantage was found over the corresponding liquid-phase manual method except for small peptides where extractive loss would be a problem without attachment.

E. Gas-Liquid Solid-Phase Sequenator

The gas-phase automatic sequenator devised by Hewick et al.,[43] is now the instrument of choice for performing the Edman degradation. The reader is directed to excellent reviews by Shively,[44,45] Hunkapiller et al.,[46] and Allen[47] for a complete description of this technology. This technology has been quite useful in the direct sequence analysis of proteins blotting from polyacrylamide gel electrophoretograms.[48-50] Bhown et al.[51] have described a method for the conversion of a spinning-cup sequenator to a gas-phase instrument.

IV. IDENTIFICATION METHODS FOR DIRECT EDMAN DEGRADATION

A. High-Performance Liquid Chromatography

HPLC offers high resolution, quantitative analysis, and high sensitivity; it is currently the method of choice for identification of PTH amino acids in sequence analysis.

The methods most commonly used today are similar in general principle to that of Zimmerman et al.;[52] i.e., a 25-cm C-18 reverse-phase column is used, with isocratic or gradient elution by a mobile phase of buffered aqueous sodium acetate and acetonitrile at elevated temperature. Other bonded-phase column packings such as cyanopropyl[53] or phenylalkyl[54] types are also used, as are other solvents and buffer salts. Even C-18 columns from different manufacturers differ in retention characteristics, so experimental conditions optimized for one column may have to be adjusted if a column from another source is used.

The desired result is adequate separation of all PTH amino acids from each other and from any by-products of the Edman degradation. If the conversion procedure used includes extraction from an acidic aqueous phase by ethyl acetate, then PTH-Arg, -His and hydrophilic by-products remain in the aqueous phase and need only be separated from each other, which is not difficult. Retention of the PTHs extracted by ethyl acetate is adjusted by changing the temperature and the proportion of organic solvent in the mobile phase.

We find it helpful in establishing optimal conditions to measure the retention of the individual PTHs over a range of solvent strengths and temperatures. If retention times are plotted on a logarithmic scale as a function of solvent strength or temperature, separation between lines for the individual PTHs is essentially proportional to resolution.[55]

All the PTHs except PTH-dehydrothreonine (derived from PTH-Thr) are easily detected at 254 nm with the common mercury lamp absorbance monitor. PTH-dehydrothreonine is detectable at 313 or 323 nm. In the case of serine, little or no PTH-Ser is seen in samples from our sequencing system (manual conversion in 1 N HCl) nor is there any peak visible at 323 nm; the only peak seen elutes after all the other PTHs and absorbs at 254 nm. It may be a dehydrated and polymerized product, as described by Chang for the DABITC degradation.[56] Other laboratories do report detection of serine as PTH-dehydroserine absorbing at 313 to 323 nm and eluting at an intermediate position among the PTHs[37,57] or (in the presence of dithiothreitol) as a derivative eluting near PTH-Ala and absorbing at 254 nm.[33,58] It is, therefore, essential that elution and absorbance characteristics be determined for the product(s) of Edman degradation of known serine residues in the particular sequence determination procedure to be used.

Gradient elution is more rapid than isocratic but may not save time in repetitive analyses because of the time required for column re-equilibration. It also causes baseline fluctuations at high detector sensitivity. The principal advantage of gradient elution in PTH analysis may be increased sensitivity of detection for the late-eluting serine derivative mentioned above. Reproducibility and flexibility are important in a solvent gradient system for PTH analysis. We use a complex gradient profile which includes a nominal temporary drop in solvent strength at one point (although the actual change is damped by the mixing chamber and is more likely only a plateau, see Figure 1). Total analysis time including re-equilibration is under 35 min. A faster analysis is possible in which PTH-Lys elutes between PTH-Trp and -Phe, but background peaks (e.g., diphenylthiourea) from the sequenator then co-elute with PTH-Trp.

Detection of PTHs is possible at the picomole level with the UV monitor. As discussed earlier (Section III.C.), sensitivity in actual sequence analysis depends partly on levels of background from the sample and the degradation system.

B. Thin-Layer Chromatography

Thin-layer methods are inexpensive and have the particular advantage of speed, since

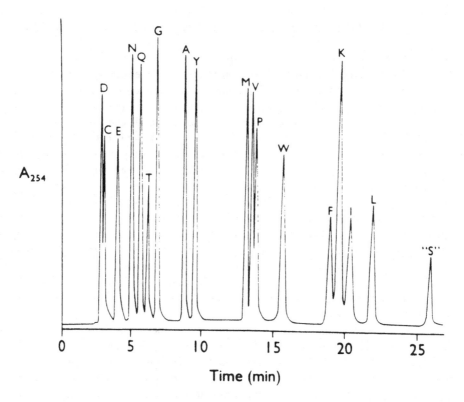

FIGURE 1.   Separation of PTH amino acids on Ultrasphere-ODS column, 0.46 × 25 cm. Flow rate 1 ml/min, temperature 55°C. Solvent A = 0.01 M sodium acetate, pH 4.9; solvent B = acetonitrile. Gradient program: percent B increased linearly from 27 to 46.9% in 11 min, then dropped immediately to 30% and held there 1 min, and finally increased to 49% in 10 min. PTHs: D, aspartic acid; C, carboxymethylcysteine; E, glutamic acid; N, asparagine; Q, glutamine; T, threonine; G, glycine; A, alanine; Y, tyrosine; M, methionine; V, valine; P, proline; W, tryptophan; F, phenylalanine; K, lysine; I, isoleucine; L, leucine; "S", serine product.

derivatives from a number of cycles of degradation can be processed simultaneously. Lack of quantitation is less of a problem in sequence analysis of pure samples of peptides, since they do not develop the degree of overlap and background from nonspecific cleavage that long runs on proteins produce. PTHs are detected under 254 nm UV light as dark spots on a fluorescent background.

PTH identification procedures using silica gel plates include those of Jeppsson and Sjöquist,[59] Solal and Bernard,[60] and Inagami and Murakami.[61] We have found that a change in the binder used in Eastman plates in the late 1970s made them incompatible with some of the organic solvents recommended in these papers. However, the solvent xylene/95% ethanol/acetic acid, 50:50:0.5, recommended by Inagami[62] for PTH-His and -Arg is compatible with the new binder, and the same mixture with twice the proportion of xylene works well for most of the other PTHs. Inagami and Murakami[61] recommend marking the positions of spots under UV light, then spraying the plate with 0.5% ninhydrin in n-butanol, drying, and heating at 95 to 110°C for 10 to 15 min. Many of the PTHs develop characteristic colors useful for their identification. Sensitivity is about 1 to 5 nmol.

Kulbe[63] recommends solvent systems for 1- and 2-dimensional TLC on polyamide sheets. Solvent I is toluene/n-pentane/acetic acid, 60:30:16, and Solvent II is 25% aqueous acetic acid. Solvent II is run at right angles to Solvent I for maximum resolution, or in the same direction if several sequence cycles are to be analyzed on one sheet. Sensitivity is 0.05 to 0.2 nmol.

C. Hydrolysis and Amino Acid Analysis

This procedure is slower than others, a disadvantage for its use as the primary means of identification in extended sequence analysis. However, it does provide quantitative results and is valuable as a supplementary or confirmatory means of identification.

Smithies et al.[64] recommend hydrolysis of the thiazolinones or PTHs in 57% hydriodic acid (HI) at 127°C for 20 h. PTH-alanine, -serine, -carboxymethylcysteine, or -cysteine all hydrolyze to alanine. Threonine is identified as α-aminobutyric acid. PTH-tryptophan gives glycine plus alanine, and methionine is destroyed. Alkaline hydrolysis in 0.2 M NaOH plus 0.1 M sodium dithionite allows recovery of methionine and tryptophan and differentiation of alanine from serine or cysteine.

Mendez and Lai[65] prefer hydrolysis in 5.7 N HCl containing 0.1% $SnCl_2$ for 4 h at 150°C.

V. COOH-TERMINAL DEGRADATION

Methods for sequential degradation from the carboxyl terminals of peptides have not yet achieved the efficiency of the NH_2-terminal methods just described. Most such procedures involve reaction with thiocyanate or thiocyanic acid to form the 2-thiohydantoin derivative of the COOH-terminal amino acid.[66] Meuth et al.[67] describe advances in technique, stating that repetitive yield is about 90%. Attachment of the sample to a derivatized glass support aids in separating peptide from reagents but seems to lower recoveries of some amino acid thiohydantoins. In 1987, Hawke et al.[68] reported a significant advance in the isothiocyanate-based chemistry for the stepwise degradation of peptides and proteins from the carboxyl terminus using trimethylsilylisothiocyanate. Bailey and Shively[69] have extended this study and by using aqueous triethylamine for cleavage, have developed a useful technique for the stepwise degradation of peptides from the carboxyl terminus.

REFERENCES

1. **Edman, P.,** A method for the determination of the amino acid sequence in peptides, *Arch. Biochem.,* 22, 475, 1949.
2. **Edman, P.,** Method for determination of the amino acid sequence in peptides, *Acta Chem. Scand.,* 4, 283, 1950.
3. **Ilse, D. and Edman, P.,** The formation of 3-phenyl-2-thiohydantoins from phenylthiohydantoin amino acids, *Aust. J. Chem.,* 16, 411, 1963.
4. **Schroeder, W. A.,** Degradation of peptides by the Edman method with direct identification of the PTH-amino acid, *Meth. Enzymol.,* 11, 445, 1967.
5. **Meagher, R. B.,** Rapid manual sequencing of multiple peptide samples in a nitrogen chamber, *Anal. Biochem.,* 67, 404, 1975.
6. **Tarr, G.,** Improved manual sequencing methods, *Meth. Enzymol.,* 47, 335, 1977.
7. **Konigsberg, W.,** Subtractive Edman degradation, *Meth. Enzymol.,* 11, 461, 1967.
8. **Gray, W. R. and Hartley, B. S.,** A fluorescent end-group reagent for proteins and peptides, *Biochem. J.,* 89, 59P, 1963.
9. **Gray, W. R.,** Sequential degradation plus dansylation, *Meth. Enzymol.,* 11, 469, 1967.
10. **Hartley, B. S.,** Strategy and tactics in protein chemistry, *Biochem. J.,* 119, 805, 1970.
11. **Bruton, C. J. and Hartley, B. S.,** Chemical studies on methionyl-tRNA synthetase from *Escherichia coli*, *J. Mol. Biol.,* 52, 165, 1970.
12. **Croft, L. R.,** *Introduction to Protein Sequence Analysis,* John Wiley & Sons, New York, 1980, 110.
13. **Gray, W. R. and Smith, J. R.,** Rapid sequence analysis of small peptides, *Anal. Biochem.,* 33, 36, 1970.
14. **Weiner, A. M., Platt, T., and Weber, K.,** Amino-terminal sequence analysis of proteins purified on a nanomole scale by gel electrophoresis, *J. Biol. Chem.,* 247, 3242, 1972.
15. **Peterson, J. D., Nehrlich, S., Oyer, P. E., and Steiner, D. F.,** Determination of the amino acid sequence of the monkey, sheep and dog pro-insulin C-peptides by a semi-micro Edman degradation procedure, *J. Biol. Chem.,* 247, 4866, 1972.

16. **Levy, W.,** Manual Edman sequencing techniques for proteins and peptides at the nanomole level, *Meth. Enzymol.,* 79, 27, 1981.
17. **Shively, J. E., Miller, P., and Ronk, M.,** Microsequence analysis of peptides and proteins. VI. A continuous flow reactor for sample concentration and sequence analysis, *Anal. Biochem.,* 163, 517, 1987.
18. **Haniu, M. and Shively, J. E.,** Microsequence analysis of peptides and proteins. IX. Manual gas-phase microsequencing of multiple samples, *Anal. Biochem.,* 173, 296, 1988.
19. **Brandt, W. F. and Frank, G.,** Manual gas-phase isothiocyanate degradation, *Anal. Biochem.,* 168, 314, 1988.
20. **Chang, J. Y., Creaser, E. H., and Bentley, K. W.,** 4-*N*,*N*-Dimethylamino-azobenzene 4'-isothiocyanate, a new chromophoric reagent for protein sequence analysis, *Biochem. J.,* 153, 607, 1976.
21. **Chang, J. Y., Brauer, D., and Wittmann-Liebold, B.,** Micro-sequence analysis of peptides and proteins using 4-*N*,*N*-dimethylaminoazobenzene 4'-isothiocyanate/phenylisothiocyanate double coupling method, *FEBS Lett.,* 93, 205, 1978.
22. **Hughes, G. J., Winterhalter, K. H., Lutz, H., and Wilson, K. J.,** Microsequence analysis. III. Automatic solid-phase sequencing using DABITC, *FEBS Lett.,* 108, 92, 1979.
23. **Wilson, K. J., Hunziker, P., and Hughes, G. J.,** Microsequence analysis. IV. Automatic liquid-phase sequencing using DABITC, *FEBS Lett.,* 108, 98, 1979.
24. **Fischer, P. M. and Howden, M. E. H.,** Analysis of 4-N,N'-dimethylaminoazobenzene 4-thiohydantoin amino acids at sub-picomole levels by high-performance liquid chromatography: simultaneous manual sequencing of picomole quantities of several polypeptides, *Anal. Biochem.,* 177, 46, 1989.
25. **Edman, P. and Begg, G.,** A protein sequenator, *Eur. J. Biochem.,* 1, 80, 1967.
26. **Wittmann-Liebold, B., Graffunder, H., and Kohls, H.,** A device coupled to a modified sequenator for the automated conversion of anilinothiazolinones into PTH amino acids, *Anal. Biochem.,* 75, 621, 1976.
27. **Horn, M. J. and Bonner, A. G.,** Automatic conversion, microsequencing and other advances in solid-phase sequence analysis, in *Solid Phase Methods in Protein Sequence Analysis,* Previero, A. and Coletti-Previero, M.-A., Eds., Elsevier/North Holland, Amsterdam, 1977, 163.
28. **Rochat, H., Bechis, G., Kopeyan, C., Gregoire, J., and Van Rietschoten, J.,** Use of parvalbumin as a protecting protein in the sequenator: an easy and efficient way for sequencing small amounts of peptides, *FEBS Lett.,* 64, 404, 1976.
29. **Silver, J. and Hood, L.,** Automated microsequence analysis in the presence of a synthetic carrier, *Anal. Biochem.,* 60, 285, 1974.
30. **Tarr, G. E., Beecher, J. F., Bell, M., and McKean, D. J.,** Polyquaternary amines prevent peptide loss from sequenators, *Anal. Biochem.,* 84, 622, 1978.
31. **Klapper, D. G., Wilde, C. E., III, and Capra, J. D.,** Automated amino sequence analysis of small peptides utilizing Polybrene, *Anal. Biochem.,* 85, 126, 1978.
32. **Brauer, A. W., Margolies, M. N., and Haber, E.,** The application of 0.1 *M* Quadrol to the microsequence of proteins and the sequence of tryptic peptides, *Biochemistry,* 14, 3029, 1975.
33. **Hunkapiller, M. W. and Hood, L. E.,** Direct microsequence analysis of polypeptides using an improved sequenator, a nonprotein carrier (Polybrene), and high pressure liquid chromatography, *Biochemistry,* 17, 2124, 1978.
34. **Le Caer, J. P. and Rossier, J.,** On the use of polyethyleneimine as a carrier for protein sequencing: comparison with Polybrene, *Anal. Biochem.,* 169, 246, 1988.
35. **Henschen-Edman, A. and Lottspeich, F.,** Aspects on automated and microscale sequencing, in *Methods in Peptide and Protein Sequence Analysis,* Birr, C., Ed., Elsevier/North-Holland, Amsterdam, 1980, 105.
36. **Wittmann-Liebold, B. and Lehmann, A.,** New approaches to sequencing by micro- and automatic solid phase technique, in *Methods in Peptide and Protein Sequence Analysis,* Birr, C., Ed., Elsevier/North Holland, Amsterdam, 1980, 49.
37. **Shiveley, J. E.,** Sequence determinations of proteins and peptides at the nanomole and subnanomole level with a modified spinning cup sequenator, *Meth. Enzymol.,* 79, 31, 1981.
38. **Laursen, R. A.,** Solid-phase Edman degradation. An automatic peptide sequencer, *Eur. J. Biochem.,* 20, 89, 1971.
39. **Laursen, R. A.,** Coupling techniques in solid-phase sequencing, *Meth. Enzymol.,* 47, 277, 1977.
40. **Machleidt, W. and Wachter, E.,** New supports in solid-phase sequencing, *Meth. Enzymol.,* 47, 263, 1977.
41. **Powers, D. A.,** Solid-phase sequencing in spinning-cup sequenators, *Meth. Enzymol.,* 47, 299, 1977.
42. **Chang, J. Y.,** Manual solid phase sequence analysis of polypeptides using 4-*N*,*N*-dimethylaminoazobenzene 4'-isothiocyanate, *Biochim. Biophys. Acta,* 578, 188, 1979.
43. **Hewick, R. M., Hunkapiller, M. W., Hood, L. E., and Dreyer, W. J.,** A gas-liquid solid phase peptide and protein sequenator, *J. Biol. Chem.,* 256, 7990, 1981.
44. **Shively, J. E.,** Comparison of the spinning cup and gas-phase instruments, in *Methods of Protein Microcharacterization,* Shively, J. E., Ed., Humana Press, Clifton, NJ, 1986, 195.

45. **Shively, J. E., Paxton, R. J., and Lee, T. D.,** Highlights of protein structural analysis, *Trends Biochem. Sci.,* 14, 246, 1989.

46. **Hunkapiller, M. W., Granlund-Moyer, K., and Whitely, N. W.,** Gas-phase protein/peptide sequencer, in *Methods of Protein Microcharacterization,* Shively, J. E., Ed., Humana Press, Clifton, NJ, 1986, 223.

47. **Allen, G.,** *Sequencing of Proteins and Peptides,* Elsevier, Amsterdam, 1989.

48. **Xu, Q.-Y. and Shively, J. E.,** Microsequencing analysis of peptides and proteins. VIII. Improved electroblotting of proteins onto membranes and derivatized glass-fiber sheets, *Anal. Biochem.,* 170, 19, 1988.

49. **Hseih, J.-C., Lin, E.-P., and Tam, M. F.,** Electroblotting onto glass-fiber filter from an analytical isoelectrofocusing gel: a preparative method for isolating proteins for N-terminal microsequencing, *Anal. Biochem.,* 170, 1, 1988.

50. **Yuen, S., Hunkapiller, M. W., Wilson, K. J., and Yuan, P. M.,** Applications of tandem microbore liquid chromatography and sodium dodecyl sulfate-polyacrylamide gel electrophoresis/electroblotting in microsequence analysis, *Anal. Biochem.,* 168, 5, 1987.

51. **Bhown, A. S., Wayland, J. L., Jr., Lynn, J. D., and Bennett, J. C.,** Conversion of the Beckman liquid phase sequencer to a gas-liquid phase sequencer, *Anal. Biochem.,* 175, 39, 1989.

52. **Zimmerman, C. L., Appella, E., and Pisano, J. J.,** Rapid analysis of amino acid phenylthiohydantoins by high-performance liquid chromatography, *Anal. Biochem.,* 77, 569, 1977.

53. **Johnson, N. D., Hunkapiller, M. W., and Hood, L. E.,** Analysis of phenylthiohydantoin amino acids by high-performance liquid chromatography on DuPont Zorbax cyanopropylsilane columns, *Anal. Biochem.,* 100, 335, 1979.

54. **Henderson, L. E., Copeland, T. D., and Oroszlan, S.,** Separation of amino acid phenylthiohydantoins by high-performance liquid chromatography on phenylalkyl support, *Anal. Biochem.,* 102, 1, 1980.

55. **Noyes, C. M.,** Optimization of complex separations in HPLC: application to phenylthiohydantoin amino acids, *J. Chromatogr.,* 226, 451, 1983.

56. **Chang, J. Y.,** The destruction of serine and threonine thiohydantoins during the sequence determination of peptides by 4-N,N-dimethylaminoazobenzene 4′-isothiocyanate, *Biochim. Biophys. Acta,* 578, 175, 1979.

57. **Wittmann-Liebold, B.,** Application of HPLC-techniques to the separation of PTH-amino acid derivatives and peptides, in *High Performance Chromatography in Protein and Peptide Chemistry,* Lottspeich, F., Henschen, A., and Hupe, K.-P., Eds., Walter de Gruyter, Berlin, 1981, 223.

58. **Shiveley, J. E., Hawke, D., and Jones, B. N.,** Microsequence analysis of peptides and proteins. III. Artifacts and the effects of impurities on analysis, *Anal. Biochem.,* 120, 312, 1982.

59. **Jeppsson, J.-O. and Sjöquist, J.,** Thin-layer chromatography of PTH amino acids, *Anal. Biochem.,* 18, 264, 1967.

60. **Solal, M. C. and Bernard, J. L.,** Miniature thin-layer chromatography of phenylthiohydantoin amino acids. Application of automatic Edman degradation, *J. Chromatogr.,* 80, 140, 1973.

61. **Inagami, T. and Murakami, K.,** Identification of phenylthiohydantoin amino acids by thin-layer chromatography on a plastic-backed silica-gel plate, *Anal. Biochem.,* 47, 501, 1972.

62. **Inagami, T.,** Simultaneous identification of PTH derivatives of histidine and arginine by thin-layer chromatography, *Anal. Biochem.,* 52, 318, 1973.

63. **Kulbe, K. D.,** Micropolyamide thin-layer chromatography of phenylthiohydantoin amino acids (PTH) at the subnanomolar level. A rapid microtechnique for simultaneous multisample identification after automated Edman degradation, *Anal. Biochem.,* 59, 564, 1974.

64. **Smithies, O., Gibson, D., Fanning, E. M., Goodfliesh, R. M., Gilman, J. G., and Ballantyne, D. L.,** Quantitative procedures for use with the Edman-Begg sequenator. Partial sequences of two unusual immunoglobulin light chains, Rzf and Sac, *Biochemistry,* 10, 4912, 1971.

65. **Mendez, E. and Lai, C. Y.,** Regeneration of amino acids from thiazolinones formed in the Edman degradation, *Anal. Biochem.,* 68, 47, 1975.

66. **Stark, G. S.,** Sequential degradation of peptides from their carboxyl termini with ammonium thiocyanate and acetic anhydride, *Biochemistry,* 7, 1796, 1968.

67. **Meuth, J. L., Harris, D. E., Dwulet, F. E., Crowl-Powers, M. L., and Gurd, F. R. N.,** Stepwise sequence determination from the carboxyl terminus of peptides, *Biochemistry,* 21, 3750, 1982.

68. **Hawke, D. H., Lahm, W.-H., Shively, J. E., and Todd, C. W.,** Microsequence analysis of peptides and proteins: trimethylsilylisothiocyanate as a reagent for COOH-terminal sequence analysis, *Anal. Biochem.,* 166, 298, 1987.

69. **Bailey, J. M. and Shively, J. E.,** Carboxy-terminal sequencing: formation and hydrolysis of C-terminal peptidylthiohydantoins, *Biochemistry,* 29, 3145, 1990.

Chapter 5

CHEMICAL CLEAVAGE OF PEPTIDE BONDS

The elucidation of the covalent structure of a protein requires the development of specific, reproducible methods for cleavage of the protein into fragments of a size amenable to structural analysis. Proteolytic enzymes such as trypsin, chymotrypsin, and pepsin have proved quite useful in the cleavage of specific peptide bonds in proteins. In addition to the use of specific proteases, the nature of certain amino acid residues has permitted the development of nonenzymatic chemical methods for the cleavage of certain peptide bonds. Site-specific chemical cleavage can also be used for the cleavage of fusion proteins[1] and *in situ* in polyacrylamide gels or on protein blots when the use of proteases is impractical.

Partial acid hydrolysis is the oldest of the various chemical approaches to the cleavage of specific peptide bonds. This was one of the principal approaches used by Sanger in his primary structure work on insulin.[2-4] Although there are problems with this approach reflecting the variability in the yields of specific fragments as well as danger of deamidation of certain asparagine and glutamine residues, the technique still has potential for use in the structural analysis of proteins. Schultz[5] has reviewed the recent work in this area. The general principle of partial acid hydrolysis is based on the use of dilute acid at a pH just adequate to maintain the β-carboxyl group of aspartic acid in the protonated form. Under these conditions, peptide bonds in which the carboxyl moiety is contributed by aspartic acid are cleaved 100-fold more rapidly than other peptide bonds. Specifically, the use of 0.03 N HCl *in vacuo* at 105°C for 20 h has been found to be satisfactory. This process has also been studied by Tsung and Fraenkel-Conrat.[6]

Cleavage of methionine-containing peptide bonds with cyanogen bromide[7] is certainly the most widely used method for specific chemical cleavage of peptide bonds (Figure 1). The reaction cleaves peptide bonds in which methionine contributes the carboxyl moiety. Methionine is converted into homoserine lactone during this process. There are several reasons for this high degree of popularity. First, the reaction is reasonably quantitative although, as indicated below, variable amounts of cyanogen bromide (CNBr) might be required. Second, the methionine content of most proteins is low[8] enough that a reasonably small number of fragments are obtained, providing a distinct advantage in primary structure analysis. Finally, the knowledge of the primary structure around methionine residues is of particular value in the design of primary DNA probes for the isolation and characterization of cDNA fragments in recombinant DNA research. The chemistry of this reaction is straightforward, involving the nucleophilic attack of the thioether sulfur on the carbon in cyanogen bromide followed by cyclization to form the iminolactone, which is hydrolyzed by water resulting in cleavage of the peptide bond. At acid pH this reaction does not generally, in and by itself, affect any other amino acid with the exception of cysteine, which is converted to cysteic acid. In this regard it is noted that one would rarely be working with a protein or peptide containing free sulfhydryl groups. The yield of cleavage is measured either by the loss of methionine or by the sum of homoserine and homoserine lactone after acid hydrolysis. This value is probably best determined by allowing complete conversion to homoserine with base at room temperature. Cleavage of peptide chains at methionine with cyanogen bromide proceeds best with a fully denatured protein in mild acid. Early work with this reaction used 0.1 M HCl as the solvent or 0.1 M HCl in 6 M guanidine hydrochloride. Most recent studies have used 70% formic acid, triflouroacetic acid,[10] or an equal mixture of formic acid and trifluoroacetic acid.[11] Use of formic acid has, on occasion, resulted in the blocking of amino-terminal residues via reaction with formaldehyde (present as a contaminant in the formic acid).[12] Acetic acid can also be used as solvent for this reaction. In general, the reaction proceeds effectively with a 20- to 100-fold molar excess of cyanogen bromide (added either as a solid

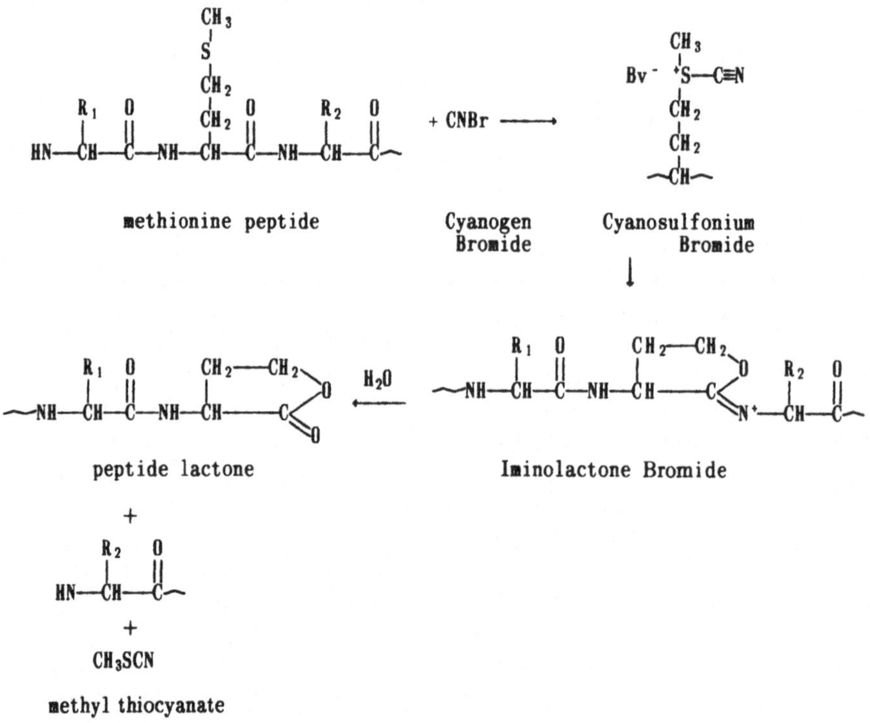

FIGURE 1.   A scheme for the cleavage of methionine-containing peptide bonds with cyanogen bromide.

to the protein or peptide dissolved in the solvent of choice). Solutions of acetic acid could also be used as solvent for the cyanogen bromide reaction. The molar ratio of cyanogen bromide to methionyl residues needs to be established for each peptide and protein under study. In the work on the structure of the pancreatic deoxyribonuclease it was necessary to use a 3000-fold molar excess to cleave a particular methionine-serine peptide bond.[13] In this regard it is of interest that methionine-123 in human serum albumin is converted to homoserine lactone by treatment with cyanogen bromide without concomitant peptide bond cleavage.[14] The conversion of methionine to methionine sulfoxide under conditions used for the cyanogen bromide cleavage has been reported.[15] With a tenfold molar excess of cyanogen bromide for 22 h at ambient temperature, 1% conversion to methionine sulfoxide was observed in 70% formic acid, 8% conversion in 0.1 M HCl, 64% conversion in 0.1 M citrate, pH 3.5, and 97% conversion in 0.1 M phosphate, pH 6.5.

There has been an increasing use of the cyanogen bromide reaction to determine the internal sequence of proteins which have been separated by polyacrylamide gel electrophoresis and subsequently transferred to a membrane via the process of protein blotting (western blotting). There are several reasons for pursuing this strategy with trace proteins. First, there is often difficulty in obtaining amino-terminal sequence from proteins on blots. Secondly, most of the interest in this procedure is directed toward obtaining primary structure information of sufficient quality to permit the development of suitable probes for cDNA preparation.

Simpson and Nice[16] developed a procedure for the *in situ* cyanogen bromide cleavage of proteins absorbed to the glass-fiber membranes developed for the gas-phase protein-peptide sequenator. The procedure was originally developed to determine internal sequence information from N-terminal blocked proteins. In the procedure described, satisfactory sequence information was obtained from 2.2 nmol (24 μg) cytochrome c. Cyanogen bromide (20 μl containing a 20-fold molar excess of reagent in 70% formic acid) was applied to the membrane. The membrane was then placed in a vacuum desiccator over CNBr/HCOOH for 16 h at ambient temperature. The membrane was air dried and taken to the sequenator.

Xu and Shively[17] have described improvements on the electroblotting of proteins. These investigators reported higher degrees of success with polyvinyldifluoride (PVDF) membranes. Transfer yields were markedly improved upon pretreatment of the membranes with Polybrene.

Scott et al.[18] described an additional approach to the cyanogen bromide cleavage of proteins on PDVF membranes followed by elution of the reaction products from the membranes with 2% sodium dodecyl sulfate/1% Triton X-100 in 50 mM Tris, pH 9.2. (Using bovine serum albumin as a model protein, these investigators obtained a 90% recovery of eluted peptides [10 μg protein applied to PVDF membrane].[19]) The heavy and light chains of antibody were separated by electrophoresis and transferred to a PVDF membrane. After staining with Ponceau Red, the bands were excised and placed in a 500-μl Eppendorf tube. Cyanogen bromide (150 μl; 150 μM in 70% formic acid) was added and the reaction allowed to proceed for 16 h at ambient temperature. The solvent was removed *in vacuo* and the peptides eluted (90 min/ambient temperature) with 75 μl of the Tris-detergent solvent described above. The peptides were separated by SDS-polyacrylamide gel electrophoresis and the bands subjected to gas-phase sequence analysis. Useful sequence information was obtained from 25 to 50 μg of parent immunoglobulin.

Sokolov et al.[20] describe a modified method for direct cyanogen bromide cleavage directly within the polyacrylamide gel. After identification of the proteins by either staining or autoradiography, the gel is sliced and dried. The dried gel is taken into 30 μl cyanogen bromide (200 mg/ml in 70% HCOOH). The reaction is allowed to proceed for 16 h at ambient temperature or 3 h at 37°C. The gel is then dried and the reaction products are separated by a second electrophoretic step. The drying of the gel prior to the cleavage step is critical to avoid protein loss during this procedure. An alternative approach has been developed by Jahnen et al.[21] These investigators isolated the fragments from the cyanogen bromide cleavage of proteins on polyacrylamide gel (the gel slices were dried by lyophilization prior to the cyanogen bromide cleavage step) by either a second electrophoretic step or by HPLC after elution. The electrophoretic step is recommended over the HPLC step.

The other methods for chemical cleavage of specific peptide bonds have been used somewhat infrequently. This is, in part, a reflection of the considerable success experienced with the cyanogen bromide reaction as well as the increased ability to determine more primary structure during a single run with the improved automated Edman degradation. There is, however, continued interest because of the possibility of peptide mapping as well as the ability to perform these reactions on a solid support such as a transfer membrane (i.e., nitrocellulose membranes, polyvinyldifluoride membranes).

A number of methods have been proposed for chemical cleavage at cysteine residues. One approach is based on the conversion of cysteine to dehydroalanine[22-24] and subsequent hydrolysis with either acid or base to release pyruvic acid and involves the conversion of cysteine to the dialkyl sulfonic salt with methyl bromide or methyl iodide at pH 6.0 and subsequent β-elimination in dilute bicarbonate with mild heating.[24] The use of 2,4-dinitrofluorobenzene for the modification of cysteine to form the *S*-dinitrophenyl derivatives at pH 5.6 has been reported.[24] The β-elimination of these derivatives was accomplished with sodium methoxide in methanol. Cleavage of the dehydroalanine-containing peptide bond was accomplished by heating (100°C) in dilute acid (0.01 M HCl) for 1 h. This reaction mixture was then lyophilized, treated with a volume of 0.1 M NaOH equivalent to the original volume of acid and one fifth volume of 30% hydrogen peroxide and then heated at 37°C for 30 min. The reaction mixture was then neutralized with acetic acid and excess peroxide removed with catalase. Alternatively, cleavage can be accomplished with bromide or performic acid.

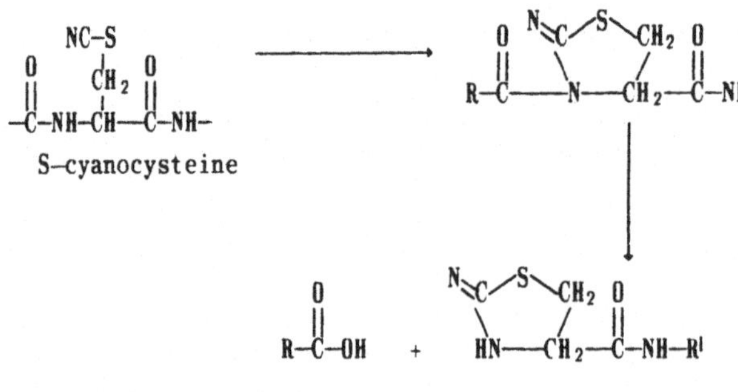

FIGURE 2.   A scheme for the cleavage of *S*-cyanocysteine-containing peptide bonds.

The cleavage of peptide bonds containing cystine (disulfide groups) has been examined in some detail.[25] In this reaction, cyanide reacts with cysteine to yield a sulfhydryl and a thiocyano group. The thiocyano-containing derivative at pH less than 8 will cyclize to form an acyliminothiazolidine ring which will then undergo hydrolysis to cleave the peptide bond (Figure 2). The formation of the iminothiazolidine can be followed by absorbance at 235 nm. An application of this approach has been advanced by Jacobson et al.[26] *S*-cyano-cysteine is obtained by reaction of cysteine or cystine with 2-nitro-5-thiocyano-benzoic acid. Cleavage of the *S*-cyanocysteine is achieved by incubation in 0.1 *M* sodium borate, 6 *M* guanidine, pH 9.0 at 37°C with the formation of 2-iminothiazolidine-4-carboxyl peptides. Virtually 100% cleavage was achieved for several proteins. This results in the formation of a free carboxyl group and a "blocked" amino terminal peptide (2-iminothiazolidine-4-carboxyl) derivative. This reaction has been recently used for the identification of reactive sulfydryl groups in phosphoglycerate kinase.[27] In this study, the two highly reactive cysteine residues (there are seven cysteine residues in the native protein) were modified with 5,5′-dithiobis (2-nitrobenzoate). An excess of KCN was added, resulting in the formation of *S*-cyanocysteine. The excess cyanide was removed by gel filtration. Incubation of the *S*-cyano protein in 6.0 *M* guanidine hydrochloride at pH 8.0 at 50°C resulted in peptide bond cleavage. Schaffer and Stark[28] have proposed a catalyst prepared from nickel chloride and sodium borohydride for the conversion of the 2-iminothiazolidine-4-carboxylate to alanine. These investigators also noted that cleavage could occur at phenylalanyl-seryl and phenylalanyl-threonyl peptide bonds. Lu and Gracy[29] have employed 2-nitro-5-thiocyanobenzoic acid to convert the cysteinyl residues in human placental glucosephosphate isomerase to *S*-cyanocysteine, followed by cleavage at the modified cysteine residues. Conversion to the *S*-cyanocysteinyl derivative was accomplished with a five- to tenfold molar excess of 2-nitro-5-thiocyanobenzoic acid in 0.2 *M* Tris-acetate, 6 *M* guanidinium chloride, pH 9.0 (protein previously incubated with adequate dithiothreitol — fourfold molar excess over sulfhydryls in the protein) for 5 h at 37°C. The modified protein was dialyzed extensively against 10% acetic acid and lyophilized. Cleavage of *S*-cyanylated protein was achieved by incubation in 0.2 *M* Tris-acetate, 6 *M* guanidium chloride, pH 9.0 at 37°C for 2 h. The average extent of cleavage obtained was approximately 80%.

Specific cleavage at tryptophanyl residues in peptides and proteins has been frequently used to obtain specific fragments. Cleavage of tryptophanyl peptide bonds with *N*-bromo-succinimide can occur as a side reaction of the *N*-bromosuccinimide oxidation of tryptophanyl residues (see Chapter 12) but generally requires a substantial molar excess of reagent with mild acid.[39] This reaction is generally accomplished in 70% acetic acid. Although cleavage is generally restricted to tryptophanyl residues, cleavage can also occur at tyrosyl and histidinyl residues. Cleavage at tryptophanyl residues under the above conditions generally occurs with an efficiency of 50 to 80% with peptides but is substantially less with proteins (10 to 50%).

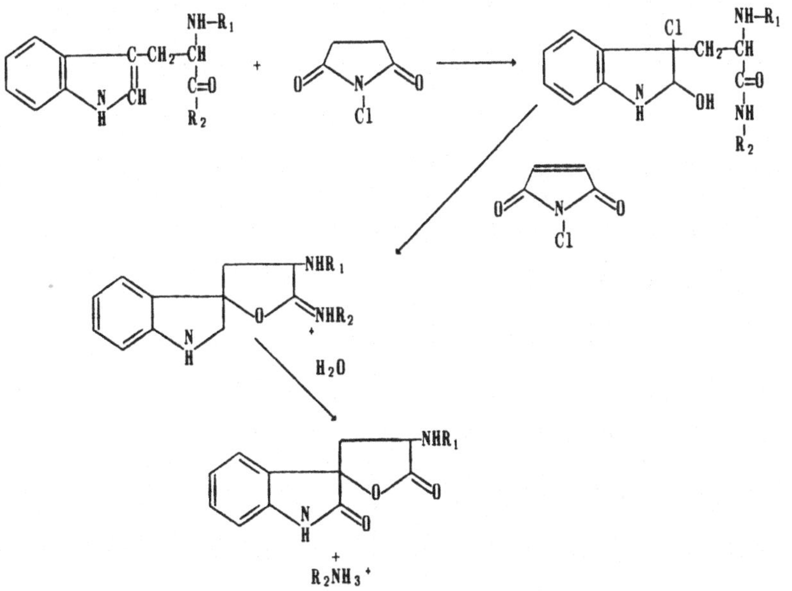

FIGURE 3. A scheme for the N-chlorosuccinimide cleavage of peptide bonds containing tryptophan.

BNPS-Skatole (2-(2-nitrophenylsulfenyl)-3-methyl-3-bromoindolenine) has been used for the cleavage of peptide bonds involving tryptophan.[31] The reaction conditions are similar to those utilized for N-bromosuccinimide, and the reaction mechanism is similar in terms of the production of an "active bromide". It is reported to be somewhat more selective than N-bromosuccinimide, but nonspecific cleavages do occur as does the conversion of methionine to methionine sulfoxide. The yield of peptide bond cleavage is similar to that reported with N-bromosuccinimide.

The specific cleavage of tryptophanyl peptide bonds with N-chlorosuccinimide[32] has been reported. The peptide bond cleavages (Figure 3) obtained with N-chlorosuccinimide (NCS) are much more specific than those achieved with either N-bromosuccinimide or BPNS-skatole. The cleavage of tryptophanyl peptide bonds requires a twofold excess of N-chlorosuccinimide in 50% acetic acid under ambient conditions. Cleavage of other peptide bonds was not detected under these conditions but methionine is converted to methionine sulfoxide, and cysteine to cystine. Model peptides were cleaved in approximately 40% yield while with several proteins yields from 19 to 50% were reported. Mechanistically, the reaction proceeds as described above for N-bromosuccinimide. The N-chlorosuccinimide should be recrystallized from ethyl acetate prior to use. Lischwe and Sung[33] examined the N-chloro-succinimide cleavage of proteins in some detail. Cytochrome c was used as the model protein. The protein was dissolved in water (1 nmol/ml) and the N-chlorosuccinimide dissolved in a buffer composed of 1.0 ml glacial acetic acid, 1 g urea, and 1 ml water. Four volumes of the protein solution were mixed with 10 volumes of the N-chlorosuccinimide in this buffer. The resulting solution in 4.68 M with respect to urea in 27.5% acetic acid. Approximately 50% of the tryptophanyl peptide bonds were cleaved after 30 min of reaction using a 10-fold molar excess of reagent. The oxidation of methionine (to methionine sulfoxide) and cysteine (to cysteic acid) occurs as a side reaction. More recently, the specific cleavage of tryptophanyl peptide bonds by N-chlorosuccinimide under these reaction conditions has been used to study epitope distribution in alpha-1-antiprotease inhibitor.[34] The use of 2,4,6-tribromo-4-methyl-cyclohexadione (TBC) for the cleavage of tryptophanyl peptide bonds in proteins has been advanced by Burstein and Patchornik.[35] The cleavage is

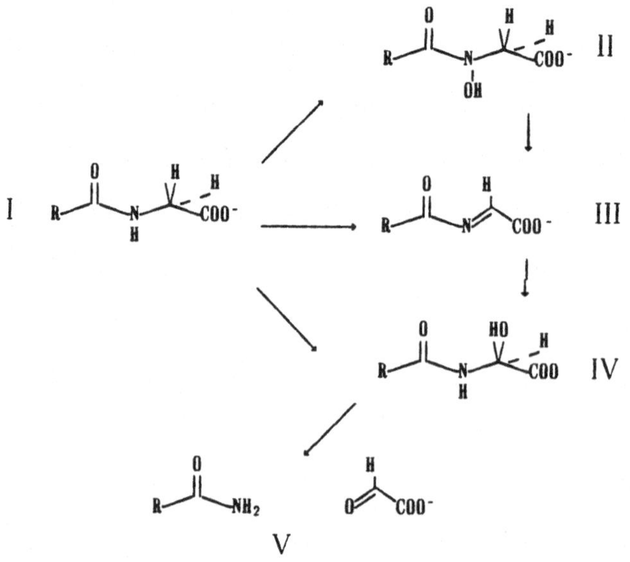

FIGURE 4.   A scheme for the oxidative cleavage of peptide bonds. (Adapted from Reference 39.)

fairly specific for tryptophanyl residues but modification of other amino acid residues was noted (tyrosine, methionine, cysteine, etc). Optimal conditions for the cleavage reaction were a threefold excess of reagent at pH 3.0 at ambient conditions for 15 min. Generally, 60 to 80% acetic acid is used as the solvent and the reaction is allowed to proceed in the dark. Approximately 50% cleavage of tryptophanyl-containing peptide bonds is obtained with synthetic peptides such as N-benzyloxy-carbonyl-tryptophanyl-glycine while 5 to 60% yields are reported with proteins such as lysozyme.

The cleavage of protein at asparaginyl-glycyl peptide bonds with hydroxylamine[36] has proved useful in selected circumstances. The reaction is generally performed in the presence of 6 M guanidium chloride at pH 9.0 with 2 M NH$_2$OH. The pH of the solution is maintained either with a pH-stat or with 0.2 M potassium carbonate. Generally, as with other means of peptide bond cleavage, optimal results are obtained with the reduced and alkylated protein. The reaction will yield a new amino-terminal amino acid and aspartyl hydroxyamate.

Cleavage at peptide bonds where the carboxyl group is contributed by tryptophan occurs upon reaction with o-iodosobenzoic acid. The reaction has been studied in detail by Hermodson and co-workers.[37,38] The reaction can be reasonably specific for tryptophan although some modification of methionine to form methionine sulfoxide is observed. The reaction is performed in 60 to 80% acetic acid in the presence of a denaturing agent such as guanidine. The occasional modification of tyrosyl residues seen with some preparations of o-iodosobenzoic acid has been shown to be a property of o-iodoxybenzoic acid contamination of certain o-iodosobenzoic acid preparations.[38] Pretreatment of the o-iodosobenzoic acid preparations with p-cresol obviates cleavage at tyrosyl peptide bonds. The site-specific oxidative cleavage of peptide bonds (Figure 4)[39] by either cupric ions or ferric ions is an exciting recent development in this area. Two research groups have reported elegant approaches to this problem.

Schepartz and Cuenoud[40] have reported the specific cleavage of calmodulin with a reagent based on the structure of trifluoroperazine (Figure 5). In these experiments, the trifluoroperazine-EDTA reagent (TFE), ferric ions and dithiothreitol were required for effective peptide bond cleavage in 10 mM Tris, pH 7.2. In a directly related approach, Hoyer et al.[41] attached ethylenediaminetetraacetic acid (EDTA) to biotin (Figure 6). The resulting derivative

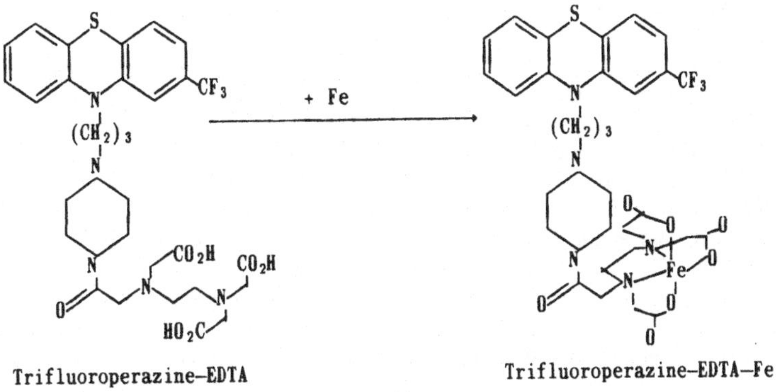

FIGURE 5. The structure of trifluoroperazine-EDTA.

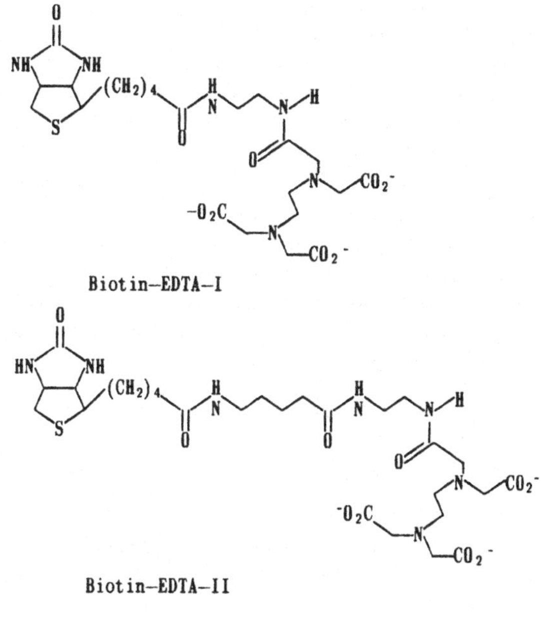

FIGURE 6. The structure of biotin-EDTA.

was used to place either a cupric ion or a ferric ion close to the biotin binding site on streptavididin. Relatively specific cleavage was obtained in solvent 50 mM borate, pH 7.5 containing 20 μM protein, 20 μM cupric chloride, and 20 μM biotin-EDTA.

The approach developed by these two groups has tremendous potential for both the study of protein structure, specific drug design, and specific cleavage of fusion proteins.

REFERENCES

1. **Forsberg, G., Baastrup, B., Brobjer, M., Lake, M., Jörnvall, H., and Hartmanis, M.,** Comparison of two chemical cleavage methods for preparation of a truncated form of recombinant human insulin-like growth factor I from a secreted fusion protein, *BioFactors,* 2, 105, 1989.
2. **Sanger, F.,** The terminal peptides of insulin, *Biochem. J.,* 45, 563, 1949.

3. **Sanger, F. and Tuppy, H.**, The amino-acid sequence in the phenylalanyl chain of insulin. I. The identification of lower peptides from partial hydrolysates, *Biochem. J.*, 49, 463, 1951.

4. **Sanger, F. and Thompson, E. O. P.**, The amino acid sequence in the glycyl chain of insulin. I. The identification of lower peptides from partial hydrolysates, *Biochem. J.*, 53, 353, 1953.

5. **Schultz, J.**, Cleavage at aspartic acid, *Meth. Enzymol.*, 11, 255, 1967.

6. **Tsung, C. M. and Fraenkel-Conrat, H.**, Preferential release of apartic acid by dilute acid treatment of tryptic peptides, *Biochemistry*, 4, 793, 1965.

7. **Gross, E.**, The cyanogen bromide reaction, *Meth. Enzymol.*, 11, 238, 1967.

8. **Tristram, G. R. and Smith, R. H.**, Amino acid composition of certain proteins, in *The Proteins*, 2nd ed., Neurath, H., Ed., Academic Press, New York, 1963, 45.

9. **Pan, Y.-C. and Stein, S.**, Amino acid analysis with postcolumn fluorescent derivatization, in *Methods of Protein Microcharacterization*, Shively, J. E., Ed., Humana Press, Clifton, NJ, 1986, 117.

10. **Morrison, J. R., Fidge, N. N., and Grego, H.**, Studies on the formation, separation, and characterization of cyanogen bromide fragments of human A1 apolipoprotein, *Anal. Biochem.*, 186, 145, 1990.

11. **Shively, J. E.**, Reverse-phase HPLC isolation and microsequence analysis, in *Methods of Protein Microcharacterization*, Shively, J. E., Ed., Humana Press, Clifton, NJ, 1986, 65.

12. **Shively, J. E., Hawke, D., and Jones, B. N.**, Microsequence analysis of peptides and proteins. III. Artifacts and the effects of impurities on analysis, *Anal. Biochem.*, 120, 312, 1982.

13. **Liao, T.-H., Salnikow, J., Moore, S., and Stein, W. H.**, Bovine pancreatic deoxyribonuclease A. Isolation of cyanogen bromide peptides; complete covalent structure of the polypeptide chain, *J. Biol. Chem.*, 248, 1489, 1973.

14. **Doyen, N. and LaPresle, C.**, Partial non-cleavage by cyanogen bromide of a methionine-cystine bond from human serum albumin and bovine α-lactalbumin, *Biochem. J.*, 177, 251, 1979.

15. **Joppich-Kuhn, R., Corkill, J. A., and Giese, R. W.**, Oxidation of methionine to methionine sulfoxide as a side reaction of cyanogen bromide cleavage, *Anal. Biochem.*, 119, 73, 1982.

16. **Simpson, R. J. and Nice, E. C.**, *In situ* cyanogen bromide cleavage of N-terminally blocked proteins in a gas-phase sequencer, *Biochem. Int.*, 8, 787, 1984.

17. **Xu, Q.-Y. and Shively, J. E.**, Microsequence analysis of peptides and proteins. VIII. Improved electroblotting of proteins onto membranes and derivatized glass-fiber sheets, *Anal. Biochem.*, 170, 19, 1988.

18. **Scott, M. G., Crimmins, D. L., McCourt, D. W., Tarrand, J. J., Eyerman, M. C., and Nahm, M. H.**, A simple *in situ* cyanogen bromide cleavage method to obtain internal amino acid sequence of proteins electroblotted to polyvinyldifluoride membranes, *Biochem. Biophys. Res. Commun.*, 155, 1353, 1988.

19. **Szewczyk, B. and Summers, D. F.**, Preparative elution of proteins blotted to immobilon membranes, *Anal. Biochem.*, 168, 48, 1988.

20. **Sokolov, B. P., Sher, B. M., and Kalinin, V. N.**, Modified method for peptide mapping of collagen chains using cyanogen bromide-cleavage of protein within polyacrylamide gels, *Anal. Biochem.*, 176, 365, 1989.

21. **Jahnen, W., Ward, L. D., Reid, G. E., Moritz, R. L. and Simpson, R. J.**, Internal amino acid sequencing of proteins by *in situ* cyanogen bromide cleavage in polyacrylamide gels, *Biochem. Biophys. Res. Commun.*, 166, 139, 1990.

22. **Witkop, B. and Ramachandran, L. K.**, Progress in non-enzymatic selective modification and cleavage of proteins, *Metabolism*, 13, 1016, 1964.

23. **Patchornik, A. and Sokolovsky, M.**, Nonenzymatic cleavages of peptide chains at the cysteine and serine residues through their conversion into dehydroalanine. I. Hydrolytic and oxidative cleavage of dehydroalanine residues, *J. Am. Chem. Soc.*, 86, 1206, 1964.

24. **Sokolovsky, M., Sadeh, T., and Patchornik, A.**, Nonenzymatic cleavages of peptide chains at the cysteine and serine residues though their conversion to dehydroalanine (DHAL). II. The specific chemical cleavage of cysteinyl peptides, *J. Am. Chem. Soc.*, 86, 1212, 1964.

25. **Catsimpoolas, N. and Wood, J. L.**, Specific cleavage of cystine peptides by cyanide, *J. Biol. Chem.*, 241, 1790, 1966.

26. **Jacobson, G. R., Schaffer, M. H., Stark, G. R., and Vanaman, T. C.**, Specific chemical cleavage in high yield at the amino peptide bonds of cysteine and cystine residues, *J. Biol. Chem.*, 248, 6583, 1973.

27. **Minard, P., Desmadril, M., Ballery, N., Perahia, D., Mouawad, L., Hall, L., and Yon, J. M.**, Study of the fast-reacting cysteines in phosphoglycerate kinase using chemical modification and site-directed mutagenesis, *Eur. J. Biochem.*, 185, 419, 1989.

28. **Schaffer, M. H. and Stark, G. R.**, Ring cleavage of 2-iminothiazolidine-4-carboxylates by catalytic reduction. A potential method for unblocking peptides formed by specific chemical cleavage at half-cystine residues, *Biochem. Biophys. Res. Commun.*, 71, 1040, 1976.

29. **Lu, H. S. and Gracy, R. W.**, Specific cleavage of glucosephosphate isomerase at cysteinyl residues using 2-nitro-5-thiocyanobenzoic acid: analyses of peptides eluted from polyacrylamide gels and localization of active site histidyl and lysyl residues, *Arch. Biochem. Biophys.*, 212, 347, 1981.

30. **Ramachandran, L. K. and Witkop, B.,** N-Bromosuccinimide cleavage of peptides, *Meth. Enzymol.,* 11, 283, 1967.

31. **Fontana, A.,** Modification of tryptophan with BNPS-skatole (2-(2-nitrophenylsulfenyl)-3-methyl-3-bromoindolenine), *Meth. Enzymol.,* 25, 419, 1972.

32. **Shechter, Y., Patchornik, A., and Burstein, Y.,** Selective chemical cleavage of tryptophanyl peptide bonds by oxidative chlorination with N-chlorosuccinimide, *Biochemistry,* 15, 5071, 1976.

33. **Lischwe, M. A. and Sung, M. T.,** Use of N-chlorosuccinimide/urea for selective cleavage of tryptophanyl peptide bonds in proteins, *J. Biol, Chem.,* 252, 4976, 1977.

34. **Zhu, X.-J. and Chan, S. K.,** The use of monoclonal antibodies to distinguish several chemically modified forms of human alpha-1-proteinase inhibitor, *Biochem. J.,* 246, 19, 1987.

35. **Burstein, Y. and Patchornik, A.,** Selective chemical cleavage of tryptophanyl peptide bonds in peptides and proteins, *Biochemistry,* 11, 4641, 1972.

36. **Bornstein, P. and Balian, G.,** Cleavage at Asn-Gly bonds with hydroxylamine, *Meth. Enzymol.,* 47, 132, 1977.

37. **Mahoney, W. C. and Hermodson, M. A.,** High yield cleavage of tryptophanyl peptide bonds by *o*-iodosobenzoic acid, *Biochemistry,* 18, 3810, 1979.

38. **Mahoney, W. C., Smith, P. K., and Hermodson, M. A.,** Fragmentation of proteins with *o*-iodosobenzoic acid: chemical mechanism and identification of *o*-iodoxybenzoic acid as a reactive contaminant that modifies tyrosyl residues, *Biochemistry,* 20, 443, 1981.

39. **Ramer, S. E., Cheng, H., Palcic, M. M., and Vederas, J. C.,** Fromation of peptide amides by peptideylglycine alpha-amidating monooxygenase: a new assay and stereochemistry of hydrogen loss, *J. Am. Chem. Soc.,* 112, 8526, 1988.

40. **Schepartz, A. and Cuenoud, B.,** Site-specific cleavage of the protein calmodulin using a trifluoroperazine-based affinity reagent, *J. Am. Chem. Soc.,* 112, 3247, 1990.

41. **Hoyer, D., Cho, H., and Schultz, P. G.,** A new strategy for selective protein cleavage, *J. Am. Chem. Soc.,* 112, 3249, 1990.

Chapter 6

THE MODIFICATION OF CYSTEINE

The sulfhydryl group of cysteine (Figure 1) is potentially the most reactive functional group in a protein. Cysteinyl residues are easily alkylated, acylated, arylated, and oxidized. The reactivity of cysteine is, as with most other functional groups in proteins, a reflection of the nucleophilic nature of the thiol groups. It is impossible to thoroughly discuss the reactions of protein sulfhydryl groups. The reader is directed to the excellent review by Liu[1] on the properties and reactions of sulfhydryl groups for a more extensive discussion of the chemistry of sulfur in proteins. In addition Kenyon and Bruice[2] review a collection of thiol reagents.

Cysteine is relatively sensitive to oxidation but there is little selectivity in these reactions. Mild oxidizing conditions can result in the formation of disulfide bonds with appropriately aligned cysteinyl residues. Formation of sulfenic acid is generally readily reversible unless stabilized by local conditions[3] and more highly oxidized forms such as cysteine-sulfonic acid are more frequently observed. More rigorous conditions such as treatment with performic acid result in the formation of cysteic acid.

Modification of cysteine with sodium tetrathionate (Figure 2)[4] is similar to oxidation. This reaction has the advantage of ready reversibility by mild reducing agents. Reaction with sodium tetrathionate has been used to study cysteine in chalcone isomerase.[5] The native enzyme was only slowly inactivated by sodium tetrathionate (pH 5.2 [50 mM MES], $k^2 <0.005$ M^{-1} min^{-1}; pH 7.5 [50 mM HEPES], $k^2 = 0.009$ M^{-1} min^{-1}; pH 9.4 [50 mM CHES], $k^2 = 0.093$ M^{-1} min^{-1}). In the presence of 6.0 M urea, the enzyme was rapidly inactivated (pH 7.5, $k^2 >690$ M^{-1} min^{-1}).

Methyl methanethiosulfonate was introduced by Smith et al.[6] as reagent for the reversible reaction of sulfydryl groups (Figure 3). This concept was extended by Bruice and Kenyon as a mechanism for introducing novel substituents[7] (see Figure 4) into proteins via modification of cysteine sulfydryl groups. These reagents have subsequently been used for the modification of site-specific mutants of carboxypeptidase Y.[8]

Cysteine is far more reactive as the thiolate anion. The pKa for the formation of the thiolate anion is 10.5 with free cysteine but is considerably reduced with the cysteinyl residue in peptide bond. For example, the pKa for the formation of the thiolate anion N-acetylcysteine ethyl ester is 8.5 while with N-formyl cysteine, it is 9.5. It is useful to compare these values with pKa values for other functional groups as is done in Table 1.

Haloacetates, the corresponding amides and derivatives have been extremely useful reagents for the specific modification of cysteinyl residues. These reagents react with cysteine via a S_N2 reaction mechanism to give the corresponding carboxymethyl or carboxamidomethyl derivatives (see Figure 5). When a rapid reaction is desired, the iodine-containing compounds are used. For example, the reaction of iodoacetate with cysteine is approximately twice as fast as the reaction of bromoacetate and 20 to 100 times as rapid as chloroacetate. There are situations in which fast reaction rates are not necessarily desirable, such as the studies of Gerwin on streptococcal proteinase.[9] This particular study was of considerable importance since it emphasized the importance of microenvironmental effects on the reaction of cysteine with α-halo acids and α-halo amides. Chloroacetic acid was far less effective than chloroacetamide. The sulfhydryl group at the active site of streptococcal proteinase has enhanced reactivity in that modification with iodoacetate readily occurred in the presence of 100- to 1000-fold excess of β-mercaptoethanol or cysteine. The enhanced reactivity of the active-site cysteine is also apparent from a comparison of the relative rates of modification of streptococcal proteinase and reduced glutathione. The rate of modification of streptococcal proteinase is 50 to 100 times more rapid than that of glutathione. The unique properties of

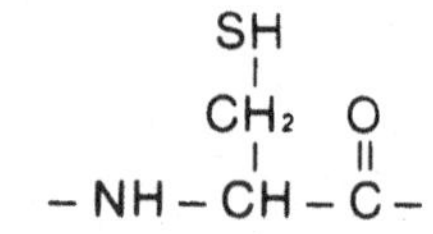

$$SH$$
$$|$$
$$CH_2 \quad O$$
$$| \quad \quad ||$$
$$-NH-CH-C-$$

FIGURE 1.   The chemical structure of covalently bound cysteine.

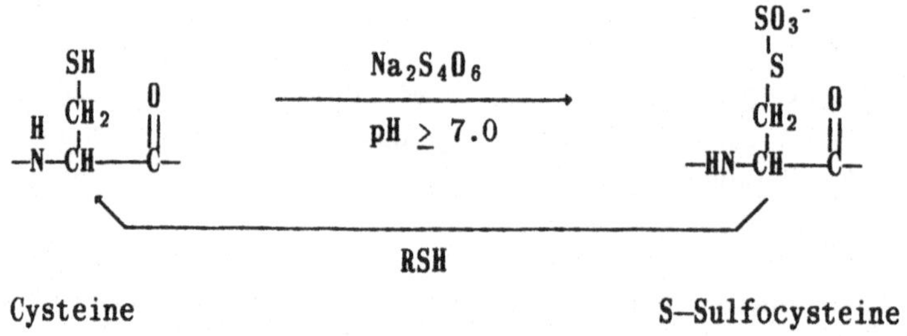

FIGURE 2.   Conversion of cysteine to *S*-sulfocysteine by reaction with sodium tetrathionate and reversal by exogenous thiols.

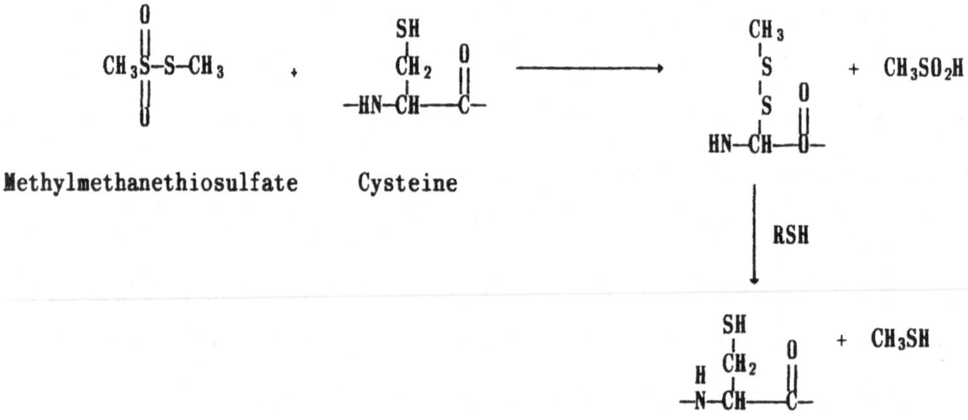

FIGURE 3.   The reaction of methyl methanethiosulfate with cysteine and reversal with exogenous thiols.

this cysteine residue can be explained in part by the presence of an adjacent histidyl residue which was demonstrated by an elegant series of studies by Liu.[10] Although histidine residues will react with α-halo acids and amides, the presence of an adjacent cysteine residue precluded the use of this class of reagents to demonstrate the presence of a histidyl residue at the active site of streptococcal proteinase. Liu took advantage of the reversible modification of cysteinyl residues with sodium tetrathionite to modify the active-site histidine.

The reaction of chloroacetic acid and chloroacetamide with papain has also yielded interesting results.[11,12] In studies with chloroacetamide, the active-site sulfhydryl group of papain reacts at a rate more than tenfold faster than free cysteine (5.78 M^{-1} s^{-1} vs. 0.429 M^{-1} s^{-1}).[11] As was the situation with streptococcal proteinase, there are dramatic differences in the rate of reaction of papain with chloroacetic acid and chloroacetamide. The reaction with chloroacetic acid has a pH optimum of approximately 7 while the optimum for reaction with chloroacetamide is at a pH greater than 9. A comparison of the effect of pH on the reaction of papain with chloroacetic acid and chloroacetamide is shown in Figure 6. This investigation

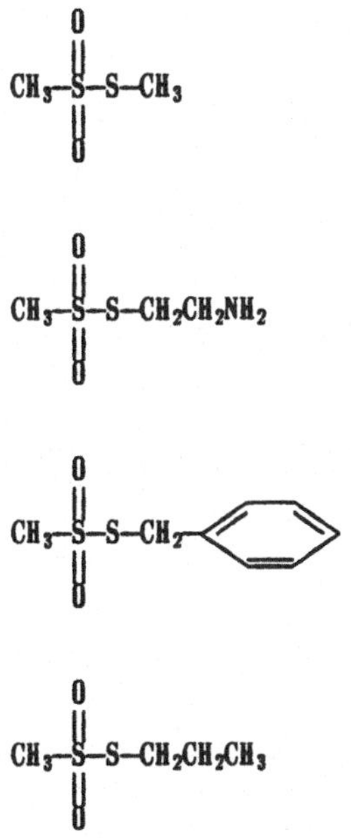

Methyl methanethiosulfonate

Aminoethyl methanethiosulfonate

Benzyl methanethiosulfonate

Propyl methanethiosulfonate

FIGURE 4. Structures of selected alkyl and aryl methanethiosulfates.

Table 1
ACID DISSOCIATION VALUES FOR FUNCTIONAL GROUPS IN PROTEINS

Functional Group	pKa
Carboxyl (Asp, Glu)	4.6
Imidazole (His)	7.0
Alpha-amino	7.8
Sulfhydryl (Cys)	8.5
Phenolic hydroxyl (Tyr)	9.6
Side-chain amino (Lys)	10.5

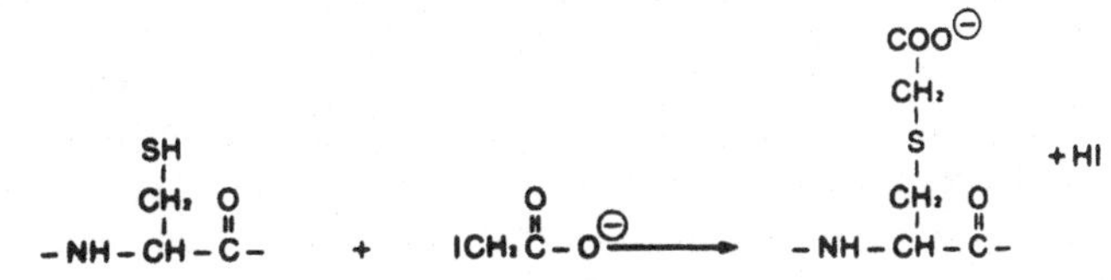

FIGURE 5. The modification of cysteine with iodoacetic acid to form *S*-carboxymethylcysteine.

notes the influence of the neighboring histidyl residue as has been discussed for streptococcal proteinase. These data further emphasize the importance of neighboring functional group effects on cysteinyl reactivity in proteins as well as the importance of rigorous evaluation of the effect of pH on the rate of the modification reaction.

The α-halo acids decompose in water, with the rate being far more rapid at alkaline pH. In the case of iodoacetic acid, the products are iodide and glycolic acid. We recrystallize the commercially obtained reagents and store over P_2O_5. The compounds are readily soluble

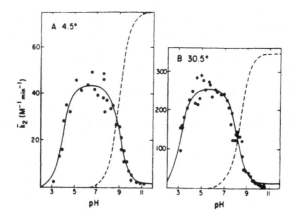

FIGURE 6.   The effect of pH on the second-order rate constant for the inactivation of papain by chloroacetic acid at low ionic strength (0.07). The broken lines are the theoretical curves for the reaction of papain with chloroacetamide under the same reaction conditions. (From Chaiken, I. M. and Smith, E. L., *J. Biol. Chem.*, 244, 5095, 1969. With permission.)

in water. In the case of the free acid, it is useful to dissolve the compound in base prior to addition to the reaction mixture. In the case of α-haloacetyl derivatives, the resultant *S*-carboxymethylcysteine is easily quantitated by amino acid analysis.

Jörnvall and co-workers[13] have used reaction with iodoacetate to probe differences in structure in wild-type β-galactosidase and various mutant forms of the enzyme. The modification reactions were performed in 0.1 M Tris, pH 8.1 under nitrogen in the dark. (This condition is of considerable importance since the α-halo acids are photolabile.) The reaction was terminated by the addition of excess β-mercaptoethanol. Kalimi and Love[14] have examined the reaction of the hepatic glucorticoid-receptor with iodoacetamide in 0.010 M Tris-0.25 M sucrose. Again, this reaction was performed in the dark. Kallis and Holmgren[15] have examined the differences in reactivity of two sulfhydryl groups present at the active site of thioredoxin. The pH dependence of the reaction with iodoacetate suggested that one group had a pKa value of 6.7 while the second was 9.0. Iodoacetamide showed the same pH dependence but the rate of reaction was approximately 20-fold greater than with iodoacetate. For example, at pH 7.2, the second-order rate constant for reaction with iodoacetate was 5.2 M^{-1} s^{-1} while it was 107.8 M^{-1} s^{-1} for iodoacetamide. The results from this study are shown in Figure 7. The low pK of one of the sulfhydryl groups was suggested to be a reflection of the presence of an adjacent lysine residue. Mikami and co-workers have examined the inactivation of soybean β-amylase with iodoacetamide and iodoacetate.[16] Inactivation with iodoacetamide occurred approximately 60 times more rapidly than with iodoacetate at pH 8.6. Hempel and Pietruszko[17] have shown that human liver alcohol dehydrogenase is inactivated by iodoacetamide but not by iodoacetic acid. These experiments were performed in 0.030 M sodium phosphate, pH 7.0 containing 0.001 M EDTA.

The reaction of sulfhydryl groups with iodoacetate[18] is still extensively used in the preparation of proteins for primary structure analysis, although pyridylethylation[19,20] is proving to be quite useful (Figure 8).

Dahl and McKinley-McKee[21] have made a rather detailed study of the reaction of alkyl halides with thiols. It is emphasized that reactivity of alkyl halides not only depends on the halogen but also on the nature of the alkyl groups. These investigators emphasized that the reactivity of an alkyl halide such as iodoacetate depends not only on the leaving potential of the halide substituent (I > Br >>> Cl; 130:90:1) but also on the nature of the alkyl group. The rate of reaction of 2-bromoethanol with the sulfydryl group of L-cysteine (pH 9.0)

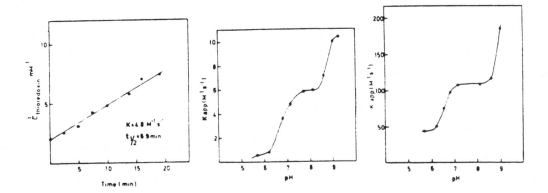

FIGURE 7. The left figure shows a time course for the reaction of thioredoxin and iodoacetic acid at pH 7.2. Analysis of this data yields a single second-order rate constant of 4.8 M^{-1} s^{-1} and a halftime of 6.9 min. The center figure shows the effect of pH on the second-order rate constant for the reaction between iodoacetic acid and thioredoxin. The figure on the right shows the effect of pH on the second-order rate constant for the reaction between iodoacetamide and thioredoxin. (From Kallis, G.-B. and Holmgren, A., *J. Biol. Chem.*, 255, 10261, 1980. With permission.)

ANALYSIS OF DISULFIDE BONDS

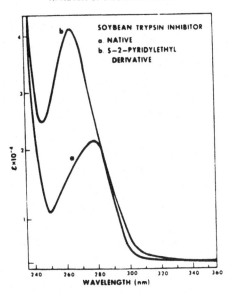

FIGURE 8. The UV absorption spectra of soybean trypsin inhibitor and the S-pyridylethylcysteinyl derivative of soybean trypsin inhibitor at a concentration of 0.5 mg/ml (23 μM) at pH 3.0 in 0.05 M glycine-HCl. (From Friedman, M., Krull, R. H., and Cavins, J. F., *J. Biol. Chem.*, 245, 3868, 1970. With permission.)

is approximately 1000 times less than that observed with bromoacetic acid. The reactions are extremely pH dependent, emphasizing the importance of the thiolate anion in the reaction.

While haloacetates and haloacetamides continue to be useful,[22-27] there has been far greater interest in the use of this chemistry as a mechanism for introducing a larger molecule which can serve as structural probe. Examples include 5-iodoacetamido-fluorescein[28] (Figure 9), 5-[2-((iodoacetyl)amino)ethyl]naphthalene-1-sulfonic acid (1,5-IAEDANS)[29-32] (Figure 10) and 4-(2-iodoacetamido)-TEMPO[24] (Figure 11). Iodoacetate has also been used for introducing a biotin probe (Figure 12) in proteins.[23]

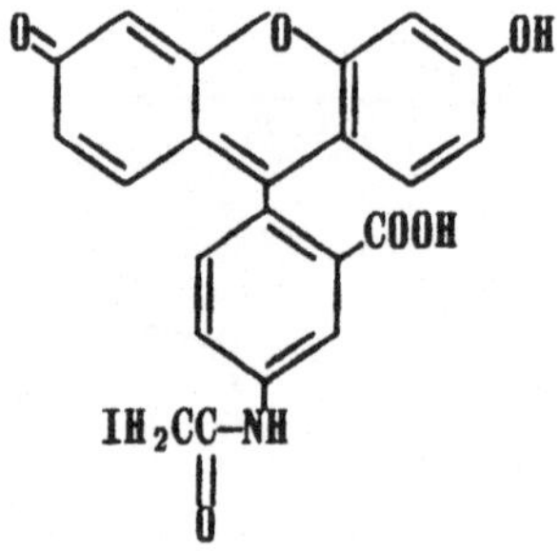

FIGURE 9. Structure of 5-iodoacetamidofluorescein.

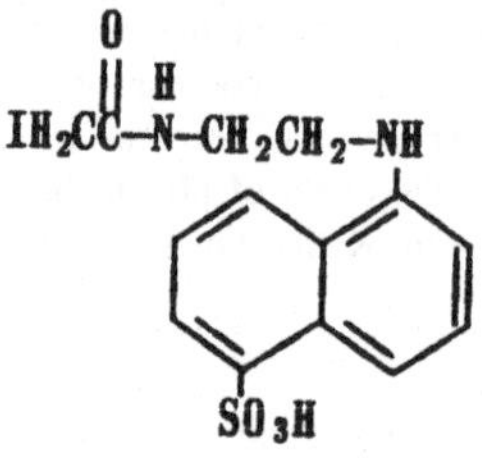

FIGURE 10. Structure of 5-[2-((iodoacetyl)amino-ethyl)amino]naphthalene-1-sulfonic acid (1,5-IAE-DANS).

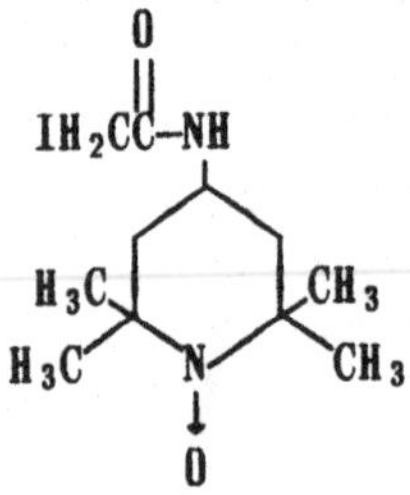

FIGURE 11. Structure of iodoacetamido-TEMPO.

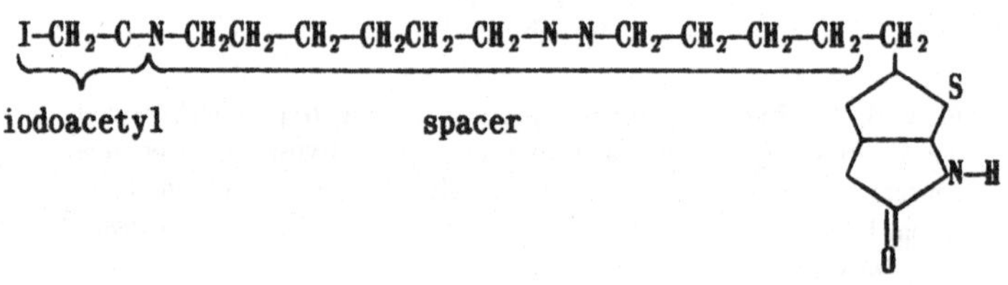

I—CH$_2$—C—N—CH$_2$CH$_2$—CH$_2$—CH$_2$CH$_2$—CH$_2$—N—N—CH$_2$—CH$_2$—CH$_2$—CH$_2$—CH$_2$

iodoacetyl   spacer

Biotin

FIGURE 12. Iodoacetyl derivative of biotin for coupling with protein sulfhydryl groups.

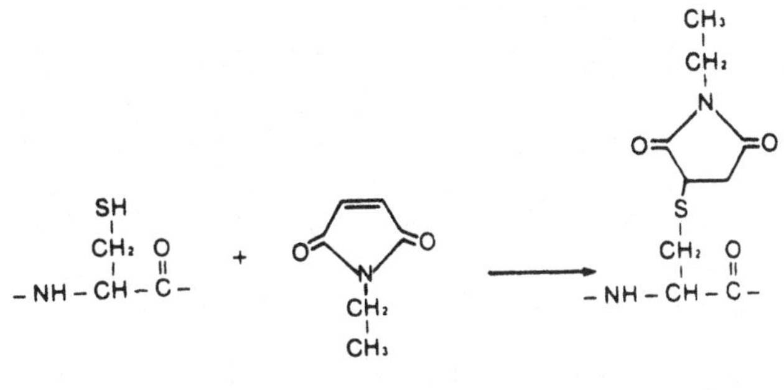

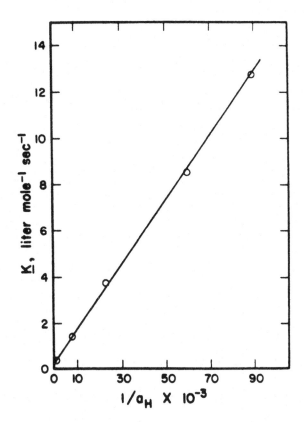

FIGURE 13.   The reaction of *N*-ethylmaleimide with cysteine.

FIGURE 14.   The pH dependence of the reaction of *N*-ethyl-maleimide with cysteine. (From Gorin, G., Martic, P. A., and Doughty, G., *Arch. Biochem. Biophys.*, 115, 593, 1966. With permission.)

N-Ethylmaleimide reacts with sulfhydryl groups (Figure 13) in proteins with considerable specificity.[33-35] The effect of pH on the reaction of free cysteine and *N*-ethylmaleimide is shown in Figure 14. These determinations were performed in the pH range of 3 to 5 and these investigators estimated that a rate constant of $1.53 \times 10^3 \, M^{-1} \, s^{-1}$ would be obtained at pH 7.0. This reaction can be followed spectrophotometrically by the decrease in absorbance at 300 nm, the absorbance maximum of *N*-ethylmaleimide. The extinction coefficient of *N*-ethylmaleimide is $620 \, M^{-1} \, cm^{-1}$ at 302 nm.[33] This reaction product yields *S*-succinyl cysteine on acid hydrolysis. Although the reagent is reasonably specific for cysteine, reaction with other nucleophiles must be considered.[36] The use of reaction with *N*-ethylmaleimide in the identification of selenocysteine has been proposed.[37] A "diagonal" procedure for the

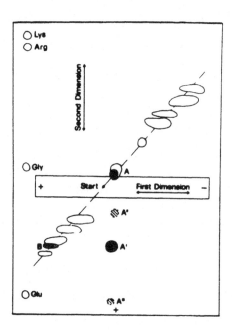

FIGURE 15. A "diagonal" method for the identification of cysteine peptides. A mixture of chymotryptic peptides containing a peptide with a cysteinyl residue alklylated with radiolabeled *N*-ethylmaleimide was subjected to diagonal electrophoresis with intervening exposure to ammonia for 5.5 h at 35°C. The treatment with ammonia results in the hydrolysis of the *N*-ethylsuccinimide to *N*-ethylsuccinamic acid thus generating a new negative charge permitting the resolution of the labeled peptides from the unlabeled peptides during the second electrophoresis. (From Gehring, H. and Christen, P., *Anal. Biochem.*, 107, 358, 1980. With permission.)

isolation of cysteine-containing peptides modified with *N*-ethylmaleimide has been reported (Figure 15).[38] This procedure is based on the hydrolysis of the reaction product of cysteine and *N*-ethylmaleimide to cysteine-*S*-*N*-ethyl succinamic acid generating a new negative charge.

There has been a considerable amount of interest recently in maleimide derivatives. For example, various derivatives of maleimide provide the basis for the design of cross-linking reagents (see Chapter 15). Brown and Matthews[39,40] have studied the reaction of lactose repressor protein with *N*-ethylmaleimide, two spin-label derivatives of *N*-ethylmaleimides and a fluorophore derivative. The investigators demonstrated that three sulfhydryl residues present in *Escherichia coli* lactose repressor protein monomer had distinctly different reaction characteristics. These data are presented in Figure 16. (The modification reactions were performed in 0.24 M potassium phosphate, pH 7.0 containing 5% (v/v) glycerol under nitrogen for 1 to 4 h.) The extent of reaction was determined by the reaction of the remaining free sulfhydryl groups with 2-chloromercuri-4-nitrophenol.[41,42] Modification at a specific cysteinyl residue was determined by reaction of the modified protein with 2-bromoacetamido-4-nitrophenol and quantitation of the three 5-(2-acetamido-4-nitrophenol)-cysteine-containing peptides following enzymatic digestion of the modified protein and gel filtration on G-50 Sephadex (0.1 M NH$_4$HCO$_3$ containing 2% (w/v) sodium dodecyl sulfate). The spin-labeled compounds showed the same pattern of reaction with the three cysteinyl residues as seen with *N*-ethylmaleimide. The fluorophore-derivative (*N*-(3-pyrene)maleimide) shows a slightly different reaction pattern. As is the situation for the α-halo acetyl derivatives, there has only been limited use of *N*-ethylmaleimide[29,43-46] during the past six years. However, the chemistry associated with the modification of sulfydryl groups with *N*-alkylmaleimides

67

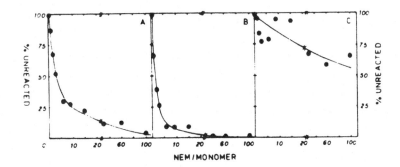

FIGURE 16. The reaction of *lac* repressor protein with *N*-ethylmaleimide at specific cysteine residues as function of *N*-ethylmaleimide concentration. Panel A shows reaction at cysteine-107, panel B shows reaction at cysteine-140, while panel C shows reaction at cysteine-281. (From Brown, R. D. and Matthews, K. S., *J. Biol. Chem.*, 254, 5128, 1979. With permission.)

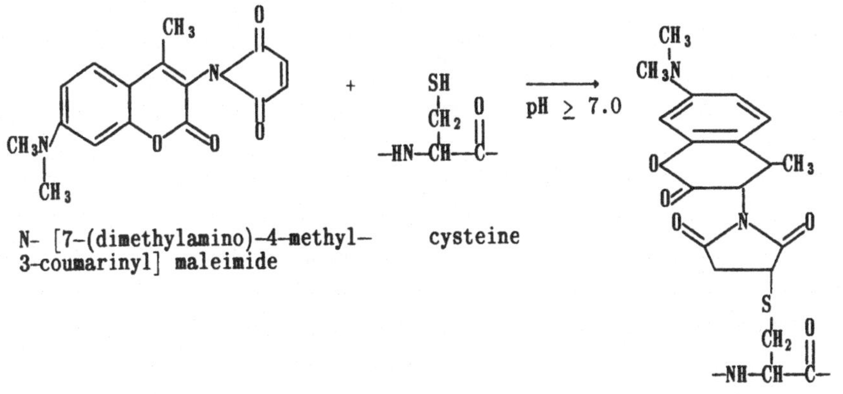

N- [7-(dimethylamino)-4-methyl-3-coumarinyl] maleimide   cysteine

FIGURE 17. Modification of a cysteinyl residue with a maleimido-fluorescent probe.

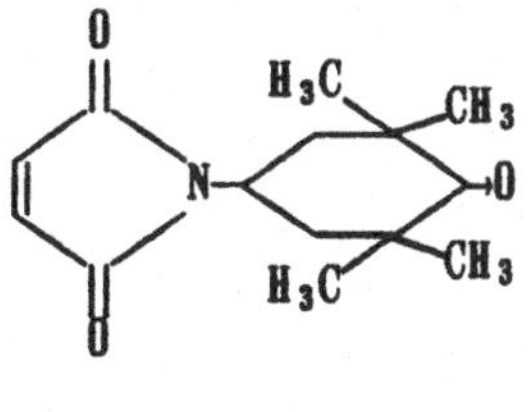

FIGURE 18. The structure of 4-maleimido-2,2,6,6,-tetramethyl-1-piperidinyloxy, a spin-label maleimide derivative.

has proved useful for introducing structural probes into proteins (Figure 17). Such probes include 4-maleimido-2,2,6,6-tetramethylpiperidine-1-oxyl[47] (Figure 18), maleimidotetramethylrhodamine,[30] *N*-(1-pyrenyl) maleimide[48] (Figure 19), 2,-(4-maleimidoanilino) napthalene-6-sulfonic acid,[49] 2,5-dimethoxy-4-stilbenylmaleimide,[49] rhodamine maleimide,[49] and eosin-5-maleimide[50] (Figure 20). Le-Quoc and colleagues have examined the effect of the nature of the *N*-substituent groups on the rate of sulfhydryl group modification in succinate dehydrogenase.[51] The derivatives used were *N*-ethylmaleimide, *N*-butylmaleimide, and *N*-benzylmaleimide. The most reactive thiol groups in succinate dehydrogenase are probably located in an apolar environment since the benzyl derivative reacted twice as fast as the

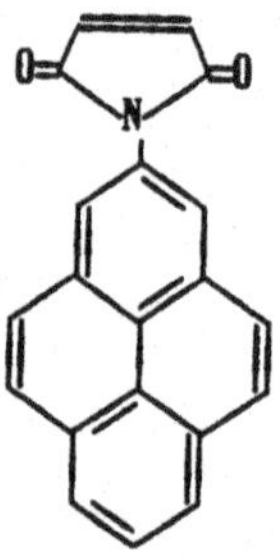

FIGURE 19.   The structure of *N*-(1-pyrenyl)male-
imide, a hydrophobic fluorescent maleimide-based
structural probe.

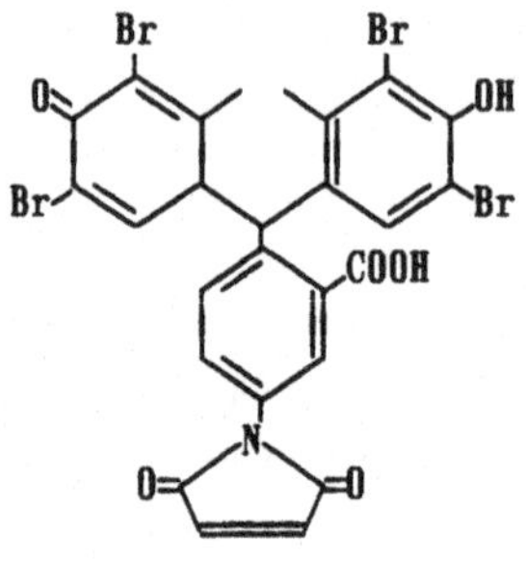

FIGURE 20.   The structure of eosin-5-maleimide.

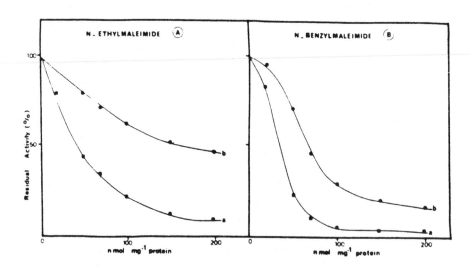

FIGURE 21.   The inactivation of succinate dehydrogenase with *N*-ethylmaleimide (panel A) or *N*-benzylmaleimide
(panel B) as a function of reagent concentration. Reaction a was performed with enzyme preparations preincubated
with 50 m*M* succinate, 3 m*M* thenoyltrifluoroacetone and 10 μg rotenone. Reaction b was performed with no
additions other than the maleimide derivatives, in 0.05 *M* sodium phosphate, pH 7.6. (From Le-Quoc, K., Le-
Quoc, D., and Guademer, Y., *Biochemistry,* 20, 1705, 1981. With permission.)

ethyl derivative, as shown in Figure 21 (these modification reactions were performed in
0.050 *M* sodium phosphate, pH 7.6, at 37°C).

A recent study has explored hydrophobic derivatives of *N*-ethylmaleimide (Figure 22) as
probes of the environment surrounding a sulfydryl group in membrane anion channels.[52]
Reaction with *N*-ethylmaleimide, *N*-benzylmaleimide, and *N,N'*-1,2-phenylenedimaleimide

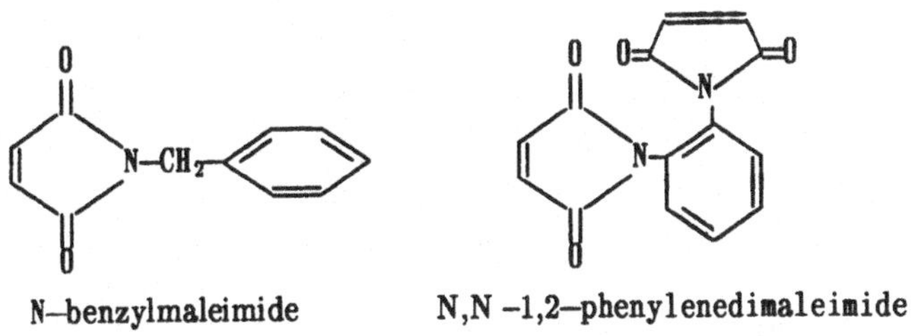

FIGURE 22. The structures of some hydrophobic *N*-alkylmaleimide derivatives, *N*-benzylmaleimide and *N*,*N*'-1,2,-diphenylenedimaleimide.

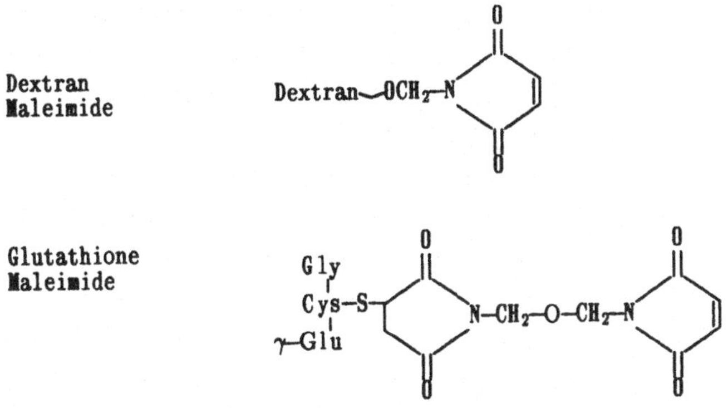

FIGURE 23. Some membrane-impermeant *N*-alkylmaleimide derivatives (from Reference 58).

was evaluated and the reaction rate increased with increasing hydrophobicity. *N*-Phenyl-maleimide has been used for the modification of a sulfydryl group in the acetylcholine receptor.[53,54] Detergent was required for the modification reaction (10 m*M* MOPS to 100 m*M* NaCl to 0.1 m*M* EDTA with 0.02% sodium azide and 1% cholate). These studies identified cysteine residues potentially important in membrane function. Subsequent studies using site-specific mutagenesis have supported the importance of these cysteinyl residues.[54]

Localization of sulfydryl groups within membranes has been achieved through the comparison of the reaction with membrane-permeant and membrane-impermeant derivatives (Figure 23).[44,46,55-57] The use of these reagents can be traced back to the original observations of Abbott and Schacter in 1976.[58] The basic concept is to provide either a polar derivative or a derivative with steric considerations which preclude passage through or into the membranes (c.f. dextran-maleimide in Figure 23). Maleimide derivatives of glucosamine have been synthesized as affinity labels for the human erythrocyte hexose transport protein.[59]

A particularly novel approach to this problem has been used by Koshland's laboratory to analyze aspartate receptor structure.[60] In this study, site-specific mutagenesis was used to place cysteinyl residues at six positions in the peptide chain. A new membrane-impermeant reagent (Figure 24) was used to study the reactivity of the individual sulfydryl residues. From these studies it was possible to ''map'' the domain structure of the receptor protein. Cysteinyl residues placed in the surface area could be modified by aqueous reagents while transmembrane areas could be excluded by lack of reaction with membrane-impermeant reagents. Finally, spatial proximity of multiple cysteinyl residues could be evaluated by disulfide bond formation.

4,4'-Diisothiocyanostilbene 2,2'-disulfonic acid (Figure 25) has been used to study the importance of specific sulfydryl groups in anion transport by membrane proteins.[61-63] Bimanes

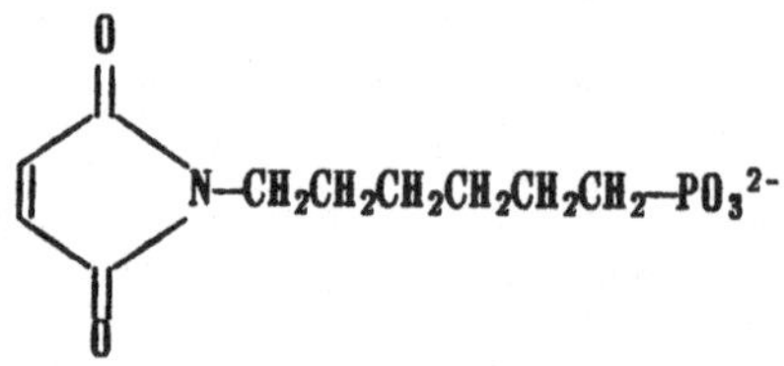

FIGURE 24. The structure of N-(6-phosphonyl)-n-hexyl)-maleimide (PHM), a membrane-impermeant N-alkylmaleimide. (From Falke, J. J., Dernburg, A. F., Sternberg, D. A., Zalkin, N., Milligan, D. L., and Koshland, D. E., Jr., Structure of a bacterial sensory receptor. A site-directed sulfhydryl study, *J. Biol. Chem.*, 263, 14,850, 1988. With permission.)

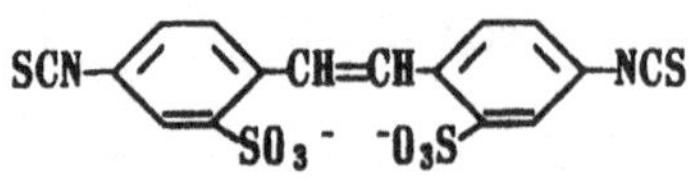

FIGURE 25. The structure of 4,4'-diisothiocyanostilbene-2,2'-disulfonic acid.

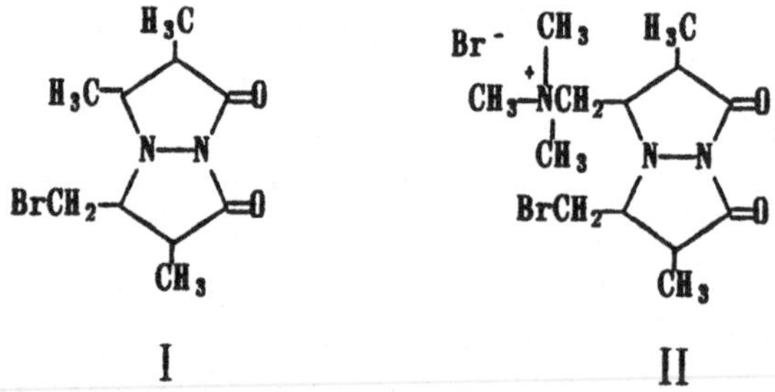

FIGURE 26. Structure of two bimane derivatives which have proved useful in the study of protein sulfydryl groups. (I) Monobromobimane, a relatively hydrophobic derivative; and (II) monobromotrimethylammonium bimane, a relatively hydrophilic derivative.

have proven to be useful structural probes for proteins. The structures of monobromobimane (I) and monobromotrimethylammonium bimane (II) are shown in Figure 26. These are two examples of various derivatives available with monobromobimane being considered a nonpolar or hydrophobic probe and monobromotrimethylammonium bimane being considered a polar probe. The reader is directed toward three recent studies on the use of these reagents for the study of sulfydryl group chemistry in proteins.[32,43,50] Martin et al.[43] have compared the reaction of ATP sulfurylase with various sulfydryl reagents, including bimane derivatives. Hydrophobic reagents were more effective than hydrophilic derivatives (i.e., N-phenylmaleimide > N-ethylmaleimide; dithionitropyridine > dithionitrobenzoate; monobromobimane > monobromotrimethylammonium bimane).

The conversion of cysteinyl residues to the S-cyanyl derivatives has also received considerable attention as the modification can be accomplished with a chromogenic reagent such as 2-nitro-5-thiocyanobenzoic acid. Although the formation of the S-cyano derivative (Figure 27) is the predominant reaction, Degani and Degani[64] have also demonstrated formation of the mixed disulfide with mercaptonitrobenzoate as well. These investigators studied the reaction of rabbit muscle creatine kinase with 2-nitro-5-thiocyanobenzoic acid in 0.02 M Tris, pH 7.8 containing 0.25 mM EDTA with a 2.5- to 10-fold molar excess of

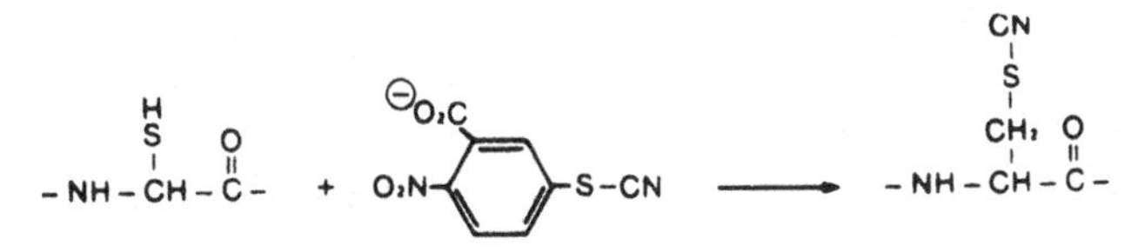

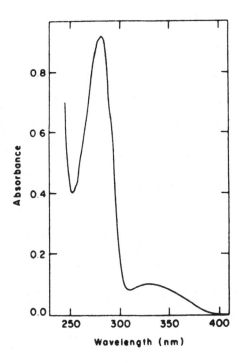

FIGURE 27. The reaction of 2-nitro-5-thiocyanobenzoic acid with sulfhydryl groups in proteins.

FIGURE 28. The UV absorption spectra of rabbit muscle creatine kinase after modification with 2-nitro-5-thiocyanobenzoic acid (NTCB). The spectra were obtained in 0.02 M Tris-acetate, pH 7.0. (From Degani, Y. and Degani, C., *Biochemistry*, 18, 5917, 1979. With permission.)

reagent. The expected reaction was that shown in Figure 27. While reaction of creatine kinase with 5,5′-dithiobis (2-nitrobenzoic acid) resulted in the modification of two sulfhydryl groups with greater than 99% loss of activity, reaction with 2-nitro-5-thiocyanobenzoic acid resulted in an equivalent loss of activity with apparent modification only at a single sulfhydryl residue as judged by the release of 2-mercapto-5-nitrobenzoic acid. There were not, however, any free sulfhydryl groups remaining after the reaction with 2-nitro-5-thiocyanobenzoic acid. Spectral analysis of the modified enzyme (Figure 28) was consistent with the incorporation of 1 mol of reagent per mol of protein (ϵ_{330} = 7500) as would result from the reaction shown in Figure 29. The denatured enzyme showed only the S-cyanylation reaction. Reaction of the modified protein with cyanate (0.11 M potassium cyanate, pH 9.5) resulted in the conversion to the cyanylated derivative with the return of 75% of the enzymatic activity of the native enzyme. Reaction of creatine kinase with 5,5′-dithiobis(2-nitrobenzoic acid) resulted in the modification of approximately 2 sulfhydryl groups (1.75 to 1.8 mol/mol of enzyme) with an almost complete loss of enzyme activity (greater than 99.5% loss of activity).

The formation of 2-mercapto-5-nitrobenzoic acid, which occurs with the reaction of 2-nitrothiocyanobenzoic acid with thiols to form S-cyano derivatives, can be used for the

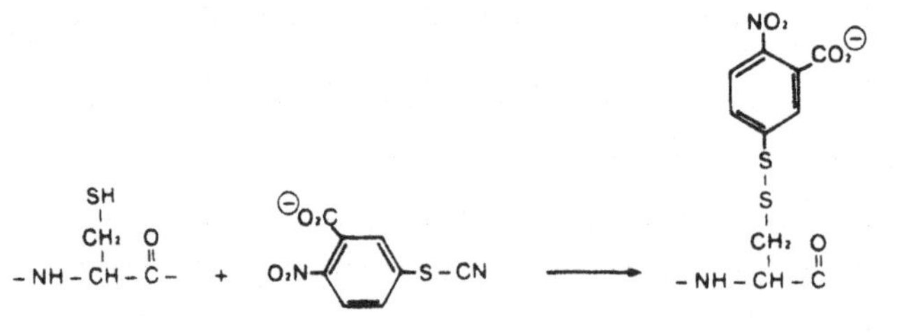

FIGURE 29.   The formation of a mixed disulfide between cysteine and 2-nitro-5-thiocyanobenzoic acid.

quantitative determination of sulfhydryl groups. 2-Mercapto-5-nitrobenzoic acid has an absorbance maximum at 412 nm with a molar extinction coefficient of 13,600 M^{-1} cm^{-1}.[65] Pecci and co-workers[66] have characterized the reaction of rhodanese with 2-nitrothiocyanobenzoic acid. These investigators used a 1.3 molar excess of reagent in 0.050 M phosphate buffer, pH 8.0 at 18°C. The reaction was followed spectrophotometrically by the release of 2-mercapto-5-nitrobenzoic acid and was complete after 6 h.

Cleavage at S-cyano-cysteinyl residues was first studied by Vanaman and Stark.[67] S-Cyanocysteine was first generated from the mixed disulfide of cysteine and 5-thio-2-nitrobenzoic acid by reaction with KCN (0.05 M) at pH 8.2 (0.2 M Tris-acetate with 20 mM EDTA).

Cleavage at S-cyano residues has also been reported by Marshall and Cohen.[68] In these studies the enzyme was first reacted with 5,5'-dithiobis (2-nitrobenzoic acid) in 0.020 M 4-morpholinepropanesulfonic acid-0.1 M KCl, pH 7.1 for 3 h at 25°C. Conversion to the 5-cyano derivative was accomplished by reaction in 0.2 M KCN, pH 8.1. Cleavage was accomplished by incubation at pH 8.0 at 50°C for 24 h. The reaction of 2-nitro-5-thiocyanobenzoic acid with phosphofructokinase has been studied by Ogilvie.[69] Approximately 1 mol of cysteine is available for modification in the native enzyme with an approximately stoichiometric excess of reagent (1.06 mol 2-nitro-5-thiocyanobenzoic acid per mole enzyme protomer) (Figure 30). The modification with 2-nitro-5-thiocyanobenzoic acid was performed in 0.025 M glycylglycine — 0.025 M sodium phosphate, pH 7.2 (containing 1 mM EDTA, 0.4 mM fructose-6-phosphate, and 0.1 mM ATP) at 24°C. Cleavage at the S-cyanocysteinyl residue is accomplished by incubation of the modified protein in 0.2 M Tris-acetate, pH 8.1 containing 2% sodium dodecyl sulfate at 37°C. Approximately 20% of the total phosphofructokinase was cleaved after 48 h of incubation at 37°C. This would correspond to approximately 40% cleavage of the S-cyanylated protein. Cleavage at S-cyano derivatives of cysteine is covered in detail in Chapter 5.

Kindman and Jencks[70] have reported interesting observations on the reaction of 2-nitrothiocyanobenzoic acid with succinyl-CoA:3 ketoacid coenzyme A transferase. These investigators conclude that the thiol group which reacts with this reagent to form the S-cyano derivative was not essential to activity. Reaction of the enzyme with 2-nitrothiocyanobenzoic acid was performed in 0.2 M potassium borate, pH 8.1 (Tris buffers as well as other buffers with nucleophilic characteristics should be avoided because of reaction with the reagent). While the reaction to yield the S-cyano derivative had no effect on catalytic activity, the formation of a mixed disulfide with 2-mercapto-5-nitrobenzoic acid via either 5,5'-dithiobis-(2-nitrobenzoic acid) or 2-nitrothiocyanobenzoic acid (2-nitro-5-(thiocyanato) benzoic acid) resulted in an inactive enzyme (Figure 31).

One of the most popular reagents for the modification and determination of the sulfhydryl group has evolved from the early studies of Ellman[65,71] on 5,5'-dithiobis-(2-nitrobenzoic) acid (Figure 32). Reaction with sulfhydryl groups in proteins results in the release of 2-nitro-5-mercaptobenzoic acid (Figure 33), which has a molar extinction coefficient of

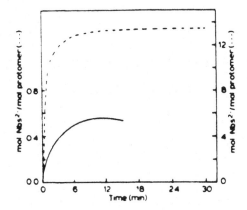

FIGURE 30. The release of 5-mercapto-2-nitrobenzoate dianion (Nbs^{2-}) during the sequential reaction of phosphofructokinase with 2-nitro-5-thiocyanobenzoic acid and 5,5'-dithiobis(2-nitrobenzoic acid) as determined by the increase in absorbance at 412 nm. The solid line (left ordinate) represents the results of the reaction of 2-nitro-5-thiobenzoic acid with phosphofructokinase (1.06 mol/mol protomer) at pH 7.2 resulting in the cyanylation of 0.57 mol/mol of cysteine per mol of protomer. The dashed line (right ordinate) represents the results of the reaction of 5,5'-dithiobis(2-nitrobenzoic acid) (60-fold molar excess with respect to protomer) in 2% sodium dodecyl sulfate (SDS), pH 7.2 with phosphofructokinase containing 0.57 mol of cyanylated cysteine per mole of protomer. (From Ogilvie, J. W., *Biochim. Biophys. Acta*, 622, 277, 1980. With permission.)

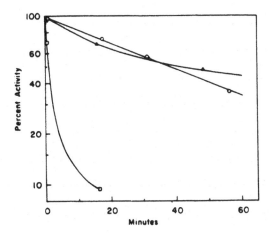

FIGURE 31. 5,5'-dithiobis(2-nitrobenzoic acid) (DTNB) inactivation of succinyl-CoA:3-ketoacid coenzyme A transferase previously modified with 2-nitro-5-(thiocyanato)benzoic acid (NTCB) (△), NTCB-modified enzyme separated from reagent by gel filtration (○), and NTCB-modified enzyme preincubated with 0.095 M dithiothreitol for 1 h in 0.2 M Tris-sulfate, pH 8.1 prior to gel filtration (□). (From Kindman, L. A. and Jencks, W. P., *Biochemistry*, 20, 5183, 1981. With permission.)

13,600 M^{-1} cm^{-1} at 410 nm. Recent examples of the use of this reagent have included studies on *E. coli* citrate synthase[72] and D-amino acid transaminase[73] (0.1 M Tris, 0.002 M EDTA, pH 7.5). The study on the reaction of 5,5'-dithiobis(2-nitrobenzoic acid) with the bacterial citrate synthase is worth considering in greater detail. Figure 34 shows the time for the reaction of this reagent with citrate synthase. Potassium chloride stimulates the rate

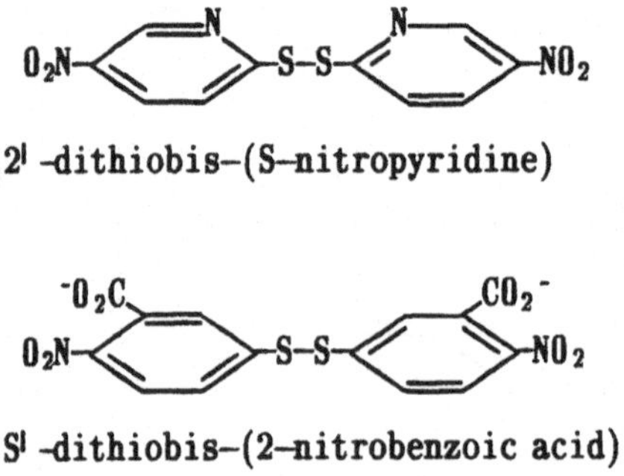

2,2'-dithiobis-(S-nitropyridine)

S,S'-dithiobis-(2-nitrobenzoic acid)

FIGURE 32.   The structure of 2,2'-dithiobis(5-nitropyridine) which is relatively hydrophobic compared to 5,5'-dithiobis(2-nitrobenzoic acid).

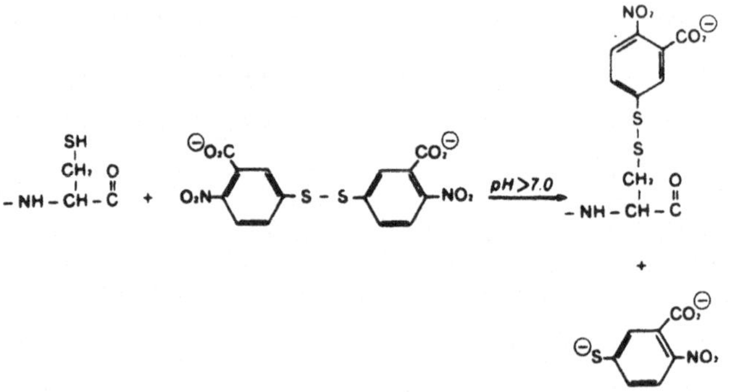

FIGURE 33.   The reaction of 5,5'-dithiobis(2-nitrobenzoic acid) with cysteinyl residues in proteins.

of reaction apparently by a direct effect on the velocity of the reaction as opposed to a change in the affinity of the protein for the reagent. A maximum increase of 85-fold with KCl is observed in 0.02 M Tris buffer, pH 7.8 (containing 1.0 M EDTA). The effect of salt is not a general effect on the reactivity of sulfhydryl groups since 0.1 M KCl decreases the rate of reaction of 5,5'-dithiobis-(2-nitrobenzoic acid) with coenzyme A. It is of interest that there is the release of 5-thio-2-nitrobenzoate from the modified enzyme after removal of reagents by gel filtration as shown in Figure 35. This release presumably reflects the formation of a cystine disulfide in the protein as there are two fewer sulfhydryl groups in the modified protein as compared to the control. These investigators also reported on the modification of citrate synthase with 4,4'-dithiodipyridine. This reagent is similar to 5,5'-dithiobis-(5-nitrobenzoic acid) in that a mixed disulfide is formed between a cysteinyl residue in the protein and the reagent with the concomitant release of pyridine-4-thione. The reaction of 4,4'-dithiodipyridine with protein sulfhydryl groups can be followed by spectroscopy ($\epsilon_{324\ nm} = 19,800\ M^{-1}\ cm^{-1}$). The reaction is readily reversed by the addition of a reducing agent such as dithiothreitol. The reaction of citrate synthase and 4,4'-dithiodipyridine in 0.02 M Tris, pH 7.8 at 21°C is shown in Figure 36. Figure 37 shows the effect of prior reaction of citrate synthase with one of the above reagents on subsequent reactivity with the other reagent. Modification of one sulfhydryl group with either reagent greatly reduced both the rate and extent of subsequent reaction with the other reagent. The reaction of 5,5'-dithiobis(2-nitrobenzoic acid) with D-amino acid transaminase also provides an illustration of the use of this reagent.[73] These studies were performed in 0.1 M Tris, pH 7.5; the results are shown in Figure 38. An extinction coefficient of 14,140 M^{-1} cm^{-1} for the 2-nitro-5-thiobenzoate anion was used in these studies. Approximately one half of the sulfhydryl

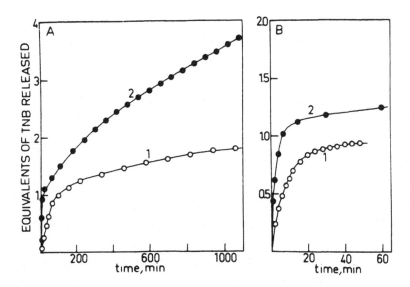

FIGURE 34. The reaction of *Escherichia coli* citrate synthase with 5,5'-dithiobis(2-nitrobenzoic acid) (DTNB). The reaction was performed at pH 7.8. In panel A, KCl was not present; experiment 1 contained 50 μM DTNB and 13.4 μM enzyme and experiment 2 contained 1500 μM DTNB and 132 μM enzyme. In panel B, 0.1 M KCl was present; experiment 1 contained 100 μM DTNB and 30.7 μM enzyme and experiment 2 contained 1100 μM DTNB and 293 μM enzyme. The extent of reaction was monitored by the release of the thiophenolate anion of 5-thio-2-nitrobenzoic acid (TNB). (From Talgoy, M. M., Bell, A. W., and Duckworth, H. W., *Can. J. Biochem.*, 57, 822, 1979. With permission.)

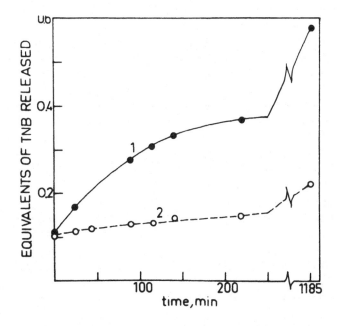

FIGURE 35. The spontaneous release of TNB from DTNB-modified citrate synthase after the removal of reagents by gel filtration. The solvent was 0.02 M Tris-HCl, pH 7.8-1 mM EDTA. In experiment 2 the solvent also contained 0.1 M KCl. The release of TNB was monitored by the increase in absorbance at 412 nm. (From Talgoy, M. M., Bell, A. W., and Duckworth, H. W., *Can. J. Biochem.*, 57, 822, 1979. With permission.)

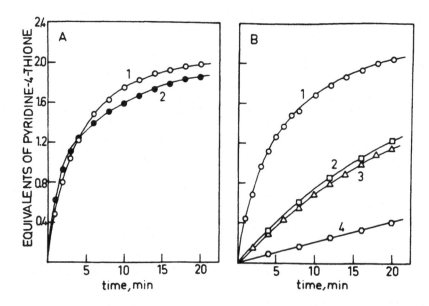

FIGURE 36.   The reaction of citrate synthase with 4,4′-dithiodipyridine (4,4′-PDS). The reactions were performed at pH 7.8 in 0.02 M Tris-HCl, 1 mM EDTA. In panel A, KCl was absent in curve 1 and present at a concentration of 0.1 M in curve 2. In panel B, curve 1 contains only the Tris-EDTA buffer, curve 2 contains 1.66 mM 5′-AMP, curve 3 contains 32 μM NADH, and curve 4 contains 2.94 mM ADP-ribose. The enzyme concentration was 21.8 μM in all experiments while the concentration of 4,4′-PDS was 50 μM. (From Talgoy, M. M., Bell, A. W., and Duckworth, W., *Can J. Biochem.*, 57, 822, 1979. With permission.)

groups are available for reaction with this reagent in the native enzyme. Reaction with 5,5′-dithiobis(2-nitrobenzoic acid) does result in the loss of activity and this loss of activity appears to be correlated with the modification of one of the more slowly reacting cysteinyl residues. Other proteins which have been studied with this reagent include rat brain nicotinic-like acetylcholine receptors[74] (calcium-containing Ringers solution, pH 7.4), lipophilin from human myelin[75] (0.001 M glycylglycine — 0.0001 M EDTA, pH 8.0), and human hemoglobin.[76] The latter study followed the changes in absorbance at 450 nm to monitor the release of the 2-nitro-5-mercaptobenzoic acid. The molar extinction coefficients obtained at 450 nm were 5550 M^{-1} cm^{-1} (pH 6.0); 6510 M^{-1} cm^{-1} (pH 7.0); 6810 M^{-1} cm^{-1} (pH 8.0); 6940 M^{-1} cm^{-1} (pH 9.0); and 7010 M^{-1} cm^{-1} (pH 9.5). The synthesis of a selenium analog of this class of reagents, 6,6-diselenobis(3-nitrobenzoic acid), has been reported.[77] The selenium-containing reagent has the same reaction characteristics as the sulfur-containing compound in terms of specificity of reaction with cysteinyl residues in proteins. The reaction is monitored by spectroscopy following the release of 6-seleno-3-nitrobenzoate which has a maximum at 432 nm (Figure 39). The extinction coefficient for the 6-seleno-3-nitrobenzoate anion varies slightly from 9532 M^{-1} cm^{-1} (with excess reagent) to 10,200 M^{-1} cm^{-1} (with either excess cysteine or excess β-mercaptoethanol).

More recent studies on the use of DTNB to modify sulfydryl groups in proteins have included the modification of ATP sulfurylase,[43] oncomodulin,[78] glutathione synthetase,[79] fibronectin,[80] and streptococcal NADH peroxidase.[81] In studies on the modification of ATP sulfurylase,[43] it was observed that DTNB was less potent than the more hydrophobic dithionitropyridine derivative (see Figure 32).

The above reagents (5,5′-dithiobis-(1-nitrobenzoic acid), 4,4′-dithiodipyridine, etc.) utilize mixed disulfide formation with reagent to obtain modification at cysteinyl residues. There are several other examples of this approach which are worth further consideration.

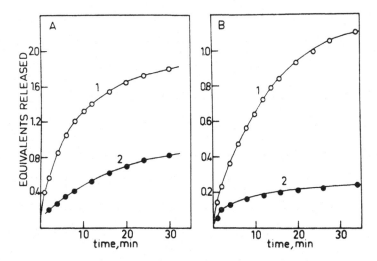

FIGURE 37. The effect of the prior modification of citrate synthase with one sulfhydryl reagent upon subsequent reaction with a different reagent. In panel A curve 1 represents the time course of the modification of citrate synthase with 4,4'-PDS; curve 2 represents a preparation of citrate synthase which was first modified with DTNB in the presence of 0.1 M KCl, subjected to gel filtration and allowed to react with 4,4'-PDS as in curve 1. At 32 min the difference between curve 1 and curve 2 is 0.99 groups per subunit. In panel B, curve 1 represents the time course for the reaction of citrate synthase with DTNB in the presence of 0.1 M KCl; curve 2 represents the time course of reaction of a preparation of citrate synthase previously modified with 4,4'-PDS, subjected to gel filtration and then allowed to react with DTNB under the same conditions as curve 1. At 34 min, the difference between curves 1 and 2 is 0.86 groups per subunit. (From Talgoy, M. M., Bell, A. W., and Duckworth, H. W., *Can. J. Biochem.*, 57, 822, 1979. With permission.)

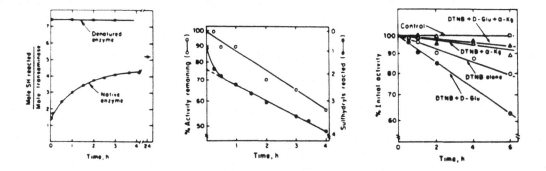

FIGURE 38. The left figure shows the time course for the modification of the sulfhydryl groups of D-amino acid transaminase with DTNB in 0.1 M Tris, pH 7.2-2.0 mM EDTA. The absorption at 412 nm was followed as a function of time and the number of sulfhydryl groups modified was determined using an extinction coefficient of 14,140. The experiment with the denatured enzyme was performed in the presence of 6.4 M guanidine hydrochloride. The center figure represents the temporal correlation between the extent of sulfhydryl group modification and loss of D-amino acid transaminase activity. The right-hand figure shows the effect of substrates on the inactivation of D-amino acid transaminase by DTNB. (From Soper, T. S., Jones, W. M., and Manning, J. M., *J. Biol. Chem.*, 245, 10901, 1979. With permission.)

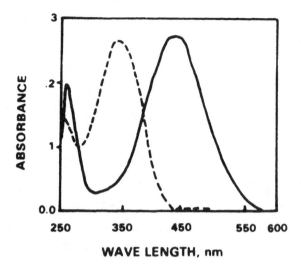

FIGURE 39. The UV absorption spectrum of 6-selenobis(3-nitrobenzoic acid) (SNB^{2-}) (25.9 μM) and 6,6-diselenobis(3-nitrobenzoic acid) (DSNB) (12.9 μM) in 0.2 M Tris-HCl, pH 8.2, 1 mM EDTA. (From Luthra, M. P., Dunlap, R. B., and Odom, J. D., *Anal. Biochem.,* 117, 94, 1981. With permission.)

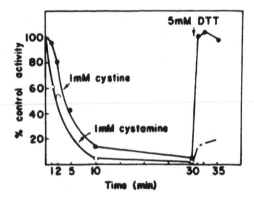

FIGURE 40. The effect of mixed disulfide formation on guanylate cyclase activity. Guanylate cylase was incubated with either 1 mM cystine or 1 mM cystamine in 0.02 M Tris-HCl, pH 7.6, 1 mM dithiothreitol, 10% sucrose. After 30 min of incubation, dithiothreitol was added to a final concentration of 5 mM. (From Brandwein, J., Lewicki, J., and Murad, F., *J. Biol. Chem.,* 256, 2958, 1981. With permission.)

Cystine or cystamine have proved effective in the modification of guanylate cyclase[83] as shown in Figure 40. Note the ready reversibility of the modification on the addition of dithiothreitol. Kaiser and co-workers[84] introduced methyl 3-nitro-2-pyridyl disulfide and methyl 2-pyridyl disulfide. Both of these reagents modify sulfhydryl groups forming the thiomethyl derivative. Figure 41 shows the spectra of methyl-3-nitro-2-pyridyl disulfide (NPySSMe) and 3-nitro-2-pyridone (NPySH) with determinations of the latter compared at several different conditions of pH. The spectrum of 3-nitro-2-pyridone is pH dependent. There is an isosbestic point at 310.4 nm which can be used to determine the extent of the

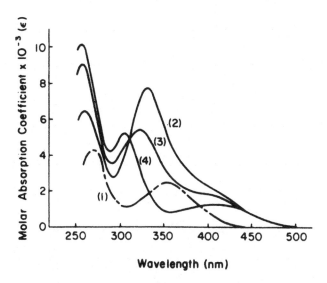

FIGURE 41. The UV absorption spectra of methyl-3-nitro-2-pyridyl disulfide (NPySSMe) and 3-nitro-2-pyridone (NPySH) in 0.050 M sodium phosphate: NPySSMe at pH 4.8 (curve 1), NPySH at pH 4.0, 4.6 (curve 2), pH 6.4 (curve 3), and pH 8.4, 8.8 (curve 4). (From Kimura, T., Matsueda, R., Nakagawa, Y., and Kaiser, E. T., *Anal. Biochem.*, 122, 274, 1982. With permission.)

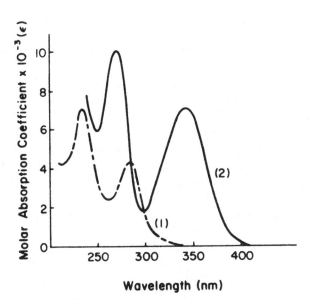

FIGURE 42. The UV absorption spectra of methyl-2-pyridyl disulfide (PySSMe) and 2-thiopyridone (PySH) in 0.050 M sodium phosphate, pH 7.5. Curve 1 is that for PySSMe and curve 2 for PySH. (From Kimura, T., Matsueda, R., Nakagawa, Y., and Kaiser, E. T., *Anal. Biochem.*, 122, 274, 1982. With permission.)

reaction of methyl 3-nitro-2-pyridyl disulfide with sulfhydryl groups. Similar spectral studies for methyl 2-pyridyl disulfide (PySSMe) and 2-thiopyridone (PySH) are shown in Figure 42. The difference in spectrum obtained does not show the pH dependence of the nitropyridyl derivative (see Figure 41). At 343 nm, the change in extinction coefficient is 7,060 M^{-1} cm^{-1}. Confirmation of S-methylcysteine and 2-thiopyridone as the reaction products from

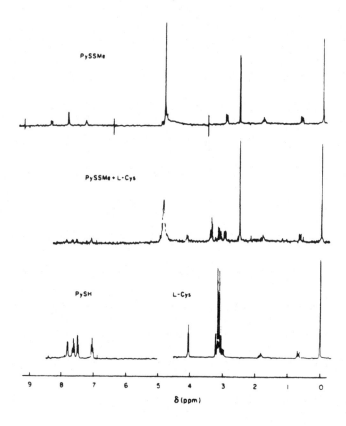

FIGURE 43.   The nuclear magnetic resonance spectra of methyl-2-pyridyl disulfide (PySSMe), a mixture of PySSMe and cysteine (L-Cys) and a mixture of 2-thiopyridone (PySH) and cysteine (L-Cys). (From Kimura, T., Matsueda, R., Nakagawa, Y., and Kaiser, E. T., *Anal. Biochem.*, 122, 274, 1982. With permission.)

L-cysteine and methyl-2-pyridyl disulfide was obtained from NMR spectroscopy (Figure 43). The time course for the reaction of methyl-2-pyridyl disulfide with glutathione or papain is shown in Figure 44. Note the differences in the rate of the reaction of methyl-2-pyridyl disulfide with the cystinyl residue in glutathione and papain.

The reaction of the single cysteinyl residue in albumin with 2,2'-dithiopyridine has been studied by Pederson and Jacobsen.[85] The suggested reaction mechanism and the spectra of 2,2'-dithiodipyridine and 2-thiopyridinone are shown in Figure 45. The extinction coefficient ($7600\ M^{-1}\ cm^{-1}$) of the 2-thiopyridinone at 343 nm is relatively stable from pH 3 to pH 8.0. Above pH 8.0 there is a marked decrease reflecting the loss of a proton. Reaction with the sulfhydryl group in the protein clearly proceeds more rapidly at alkaline pH.

In a related study, Drews and Faulstich[82] prepared 2,4-dinitrophenyl-^{14}C-cysteinyl disulfide (Figure 46) via a facile synthetic method as a means for introducing radiolabeled cysteine into proteins via disulfide exchange with free thiols. The reaction can be monitored by following the release of 2,4-dinitrophenol at 408 nm ($408\ =\ 12,700\ M^{-1}\ cm^{-1}$). The specificity of this reagent corresponded to that obtained with DTNB. Reaction with the sulfydryl groups of papain was more rapid than that observed with DTNB. The resulting derivative can be easily reversed with thiols but is stable to cyanogen bromide degradation and peptide purification.

p-Hydroxymercuribenzoate continues to be of use for the modification of sulfhydryl groups in proteins. The reagent is obtained as *p*-chloromercuribenzoate but is instantaneously converted to the hydroxy derivative in aqueous solution. This reagent was originally described

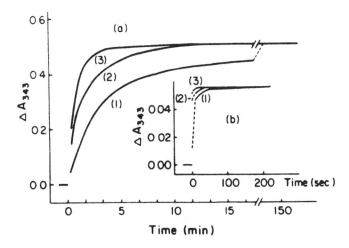

FIGURE 44. Time course studies of the formation of 2-thiopyridone resulting from the reaction of methyl-2-pyridyl disulfide (PySSMe) with glutathione (a) or papain (b). In the experiments with glutathione (a), the concentration of glutathione was 71.7 μM and the ratio of PySSMe to glutathione was 1.04 (1), 1.57 (2), and 3.13 (3). In the experiments with papain (b), the concentration of papain was 8.29 μM and the ratio of PySSMe to papain was 1.02 (1), 1.70 (2), and 3.41(3). (From Kimura, T., Matsueda, R., Nakagawa, Y., and Kaiser, E. T., *Anal. Biochem.*, 122, 274, 1982. With permission.)

by Boyer.[86] The absorbance change at 255 nm upon modification is 6200 M^{-1} cm^{-1} at pH 4.6 and 7600 M^{-1} cm^{-1} at pH 7.0. Bai and Hayashi[87] have examined the reaction of organic mercurials with yeast carboxypeptidase (carboxypeptidase Y). The titration of the catalytically essential cysteinyl residue in carboxypeptidase Y with p-hydroxymercuribenzoate is shown in Figure 47. Treatment of the modified enzyme with millimolar cysteine resulted in virtually complete recovery of catalytic activity. The inactivation of chalcone isomerase by p-chloromercuribenzoate and mercuric chloride has been studied by Bednar et al.[6] The modified protein could be readily reactivated by treatment with either thiols or KCN. The reactivation by KCN is based on the formation of a tight complex between cyanide and either organic or inorganic mercurials. The modification by mercuric chloride can be monitored by the increase in absorbance at 250 nm. Ojcius and Solomon[88] have examined the inhibition of erythrocyte urea and water transport by p-chloromercuribenzoate. Other studies with this reagent have included dissociation of erythrocyte membrane proteins,[89] NADH peroxidase,[25] and sulfobromophthalein transport protein.[45]

2-Chloromercuri-4-nitrophenol is a compound related to the organic mercurial described above. It has proved useful as a "reporter" group in the study of microenvironmental changes in the modified protein.[41,42] An excellent example of this is provided from the studies of Marshall and Cohen[90] on the properties of ornithine transcarbamylase modified with 2-chloromercuri-4-nitrophenol. The enzyme from *S. faecalis* was modified in 0.1 M MOPS, 0.1 M KCl, pH 7.5 using changes in absorbance at 403 nm to follow the extent of modification. The pH dependence of the spectrum of the modified *S. faecalis* enzyme is shown in Figure 48. The bovine enzyme is carboxamido methylated on a nonessential sulfhydryl group before reaction with the organic mercurial. Modification of the bovine enzyme with 2-chloromercuri-4-nitrophenol is performed in 0.020 M MOPS, 0.1 M KCl, pH 7.11 at 25°C. The modification was followed by the change in absorbance at 405 nm. The effect of pH on the spectrum of the modified bovine enzyme is shown in Figure 49. Baines and Brocklehurst[91] have reported the synthesis and characterization of 2-(2'-pyridylmercapto)-mercuri-4-nitrophenol, a reagent which does have certain advantages. In particular, the

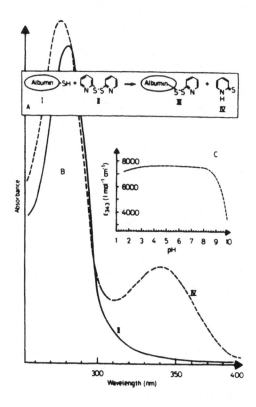

FIGURE 45.   (A) A scheme for the reaction of 2,2'-
dithiopyridine and mercaptalbumin; (B) The UV absorption spectra for 2,2'-dithiodipyridine (solid line, II)
and 2-thiopyridinone (dashed line, IV) in 0.1 *M* sodium
phosphate, pH 7.0; (C) the molar extinction coefficient
at 343 nm for 2-thiopyridinone as a function of pH.
(From Pedersen, A. O. and Jacobsen, J., *Eur. J.
Biochem.*, 106, 291, 1980. With permission.)

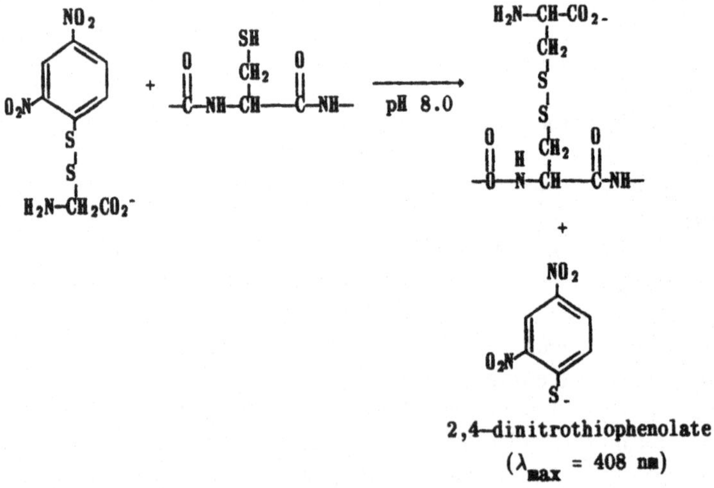

FIGURE 46.   The reaction of 2,4-dinitrophenyl cysteinyl disulfide with cysteine in
proteins.

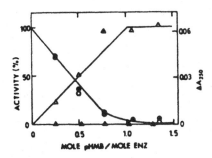

FIGURE 47. The spectrophotometric titration of native and DIP-carboxypeptidase Y with p-hydroxymercuribenzoate (p-HMB). The reaction with the protein was accomplished in 0.08 M sodium phosphate, pH 7.0. Increments of p-HMB were added to the protein preparations and allowed to stand for 20 min at which time absorbance at 250 nm was determined as catalytic activity (Z-Phe-Leu or Ac-Phe-OEt). The open circles indicate activity toward Ac-Phe-OEt, the closed circles indicate activity toward Z-Phe-Leu, the open triangles represent the absorbance at 250 nm of the native carboxypeptidase Y, and the closed triangles the absorbance at 250 nm of carboxypeptidase Y previously reacted with diisopropylphosphorofluoridate (DIP-carboxypeptidase Y). (From Bai, Y. and Hayashi, R., *J. Biol. Chem.*, 254, 8473, 1979. With permission.)

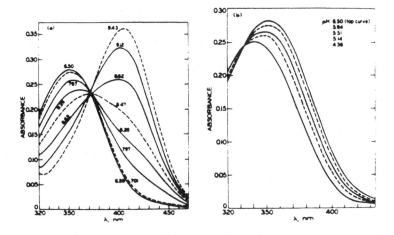

FIGURE 48. The effect of pH on the spectrum of the 2-chloro-mercuri-4-nitrophenol derivate of ornithine transcarbamylase. Panel a represents the results obtained in the pH range of 9.43 to 6.50. Panel b represents the results obtained in the pH range of 6.5 (top curve) to 4.36 (bottom curve). (From Marshall, M. and Cohen, P. P., *J. Biol. Chem.*, 225, 7296, 1980. With permission.)

spectral changes occurring on modification (Figure 50) permit the more facile *in situ* determination of the extent of reaction.

A number of other modifications of sulfhydryl groups have proved useful. *O*-Methylisourea reacts with cysteinyl residues to form the *S*-methyl derivative (Figure 51).[92] Cyanate also can modify sulfhydryl groups as shown in Table 2.[93] The carbamoyl derivative of cysteine is stable at acid pH but rapidly decomposes at alkaline pH.

4-Chloro-7-nitrobenzo-2-oxa-1,3-diazole (4-chloro-7-nitrobenzofurazan; Nbf-Cl) (Figure 52) is a reagent developed for the modification of amino groups.[94] It has also found application in the modification of sulfhydryl groups and is useful in that it introduces a fluorescent probe.[96-99] Nitta and co-workers[98] have noted that there are other possible reaction products of Nbf-Cl including the possibility of reaction products with sulfhydryl groups. The

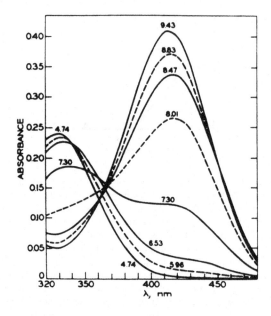

FIGURE 49. The effect of pH on the UV absorption spectrum of the 2-chloromercuri-4-nitrophenol derivative of the monocarboxamidomethyl bovine liver ornithine transcarbamylase. (From Marshall, M. and Cohen, P. P., *J. Biol. Chem.*, 255, 7296, 1980. With permission.)

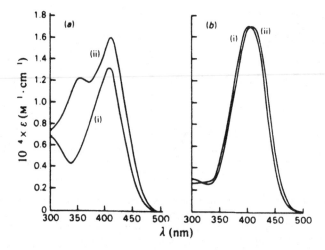

FIGURE 50. The UV absorption spectra of (a) 2-(2′-pyridylmercapto)mercuri-4-nitrophenol and (b) 2-chloromercuri-4-nitrophenol before (i) and after (ii) the addition of an excess of β-mercaptoethanol. The solvent was sodium/potassium phosphate (ionic strength = 0.1) containing 13% (v/v) ethanol. The reaction of the mercurial (concentration = 10 μM) with β-mercaptoethanol (concentration = 45 mM) was complete after 5 min of reaction. (From Baines, B. S. and Brocklehurst, K., *Biochem. J.*, 179, 701, 1979. With permission.)

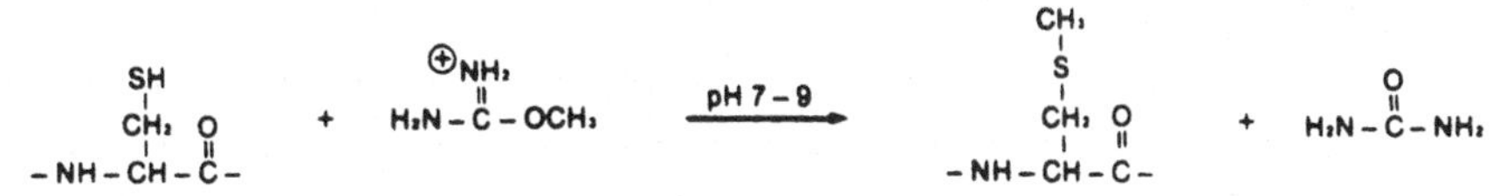

FIGURE 51. The reaction of *O*-methylisourea with cysteine.

Table 2
REACTION OF CYANATE WITH
FUNCTIONAL GROUPS IN PROTEINS

Functional group	pKa	$M^{-1} min^{-1}$
Alpha amino	7.8—8.2	1.4×10^{-1}
Epsilon amino	10.5—10.8	2×10^{-3}
Sulfhydryl	8.3—8.5	4.0
Imidazole	7.0—7.2	1.8×10^{-1}

From Stark, G. R., *Meth. Enzymol.*, 11, 590, 1967. With permission.

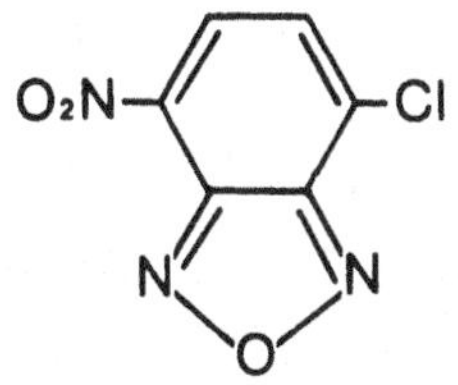

FIGURE 52. The structure of 4-chloro-7-nitrobenzo-2-oxa-1,3-diazole (4-chloro-7-nitrobenzofurazan, NBF-Cl).

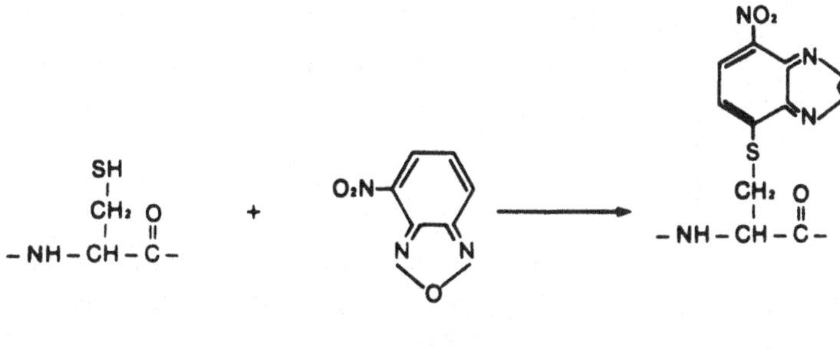

FIGURE 53. The reaction of 4-chloro-7-nitrobenzo-2-oxa-1,3-diazole with cysteine.

modification of the sulfhydryl group with concomitant reaction at the 4-position yields a derivative with molar absorption coefficient of 13,000 (Figure 53).[99] The reaction of Nbf-Cl with sulfhydryl groups in glutathione reductase and lipoamide dehydrogenase has also been reported.[100] Nitta and co-workers[98] have examined the chemistry of the reaction of Nbf-Cl with model sulfhydryl compounds in some detail. The spectra of the reagent (Nbf-Cl) and product of reaction with 2-mercaptoethanol (4-(2'-hydroxy-ethylthio)-7-nitro-benzofuran; Nbf-OHEtS) are presented in Figure 54. These data should be compared with that presented in Figure 55. Note the dependence of the different spectra on sulfhydryl concentration and pH/solvent species. The data in Figure 55 (I) were obtained in trietha-

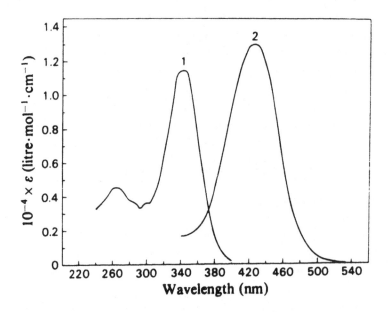

FIGURE 54.   The UV absorption spectra of 4-chloro-7-nitrobenzo-2-oxa-1,3-diazole (Nbf-Cl) (curve 1) and the reaction product between Nbf-Cl and β-mercaptoethanol (curve 2). The solvent was water adjusted to pH 7.1. (From Nitta, K., Bratcher, S. C., and Kronman, M. J., *Biochem. J.*, 177, 385, 1979. With permission.)

nolamine, pH 7.5 with an approximate 20-fold molar excess of β-mercaptoethanol while that in part II was obtained with an approximate 200-fold molar excess. Experimental series part III was performed with a 20-fold molar excess of β-mercaptoethanol in sodium citrate buffer, pH 5.0. Similar spectral changes are seen with dithiothreitol in Figure 56. The data in experimental series I were obtained at an Nbf-Cl concentration of 0.148 nM and a dithiothreitol concentration of 0.0097 mM while the data in experimental series III were obtained at an Nbf-Cl concentration of 0.0742 mM and a dithiothreitol concentration of 9.38 mM. The variety of potential products in this reaction requires that considerable caution be used in the interpretation of spectra data obtained with this reagent.

Toyo'oka and Imai[101] have reported the synthesis of a related compound, 4-(aminosulfonyl-7-fluoro-2,1,3-benzoxadiazole (Figure 57) which is a fluorogenic reagent for sulfhydryl groups. In a subsequent study, Kirby[102] has used this compound to label cysteinyl residues in proteins. Reaction readily occurred at pH 8.0 (100 mM borate-2 mM EDTA with 3% SDS).

The modification of cysteinyl residues in proteins with 2-bromoethane sulfonate has been reported.[103] This derivatization procedure was developed in response to a need for a strongly hydrophilic substituent in samples for the Edman degradation. The modification time is longer than for the corresponding carboxymethyl derivatives, taking 12 h for lysozyme, 24 h for insulin, and 48 h for glutathione. This derivative has considerable utility since the *S*-sulfoethylated lysozyme derivative is soluble between pH 5.0 and 10.0 while the *S*-carboxymethylated derivative is not. This procedure has potential for primary structure analysis.

A derivatization procedure that has proved useful in the primary structure analysis of protein has been the reaction of ethyleneimine (Figure 58) with sulfhydryl groups in proteins.[104] This reaction produces *S*-aminoethyl cysteine which provides an additional point of tryptic cleavage in proteins.[105] With bovine pancreatic ribonuclease A, with a 1/100 ratio of trypsin at pH 8.0, 83% cleavage of arginyl and lysyl bonds was obtained while 56%

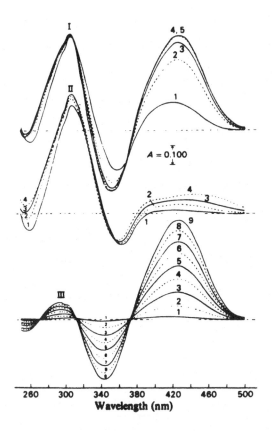

FIGURE 55. Different spectra of mixtures of 4-chloro-7-nitrobenzofurazan (Nbf-Cl) and β-mercaptoethanol at ambient temperature. The spectra were scanned at a rate of 30 nm/min from high to low wavelength. The times given below are for the initial wavelength in the scan. The solution containing the Nbf-Cl + β-mercaptoethanol was in the sample beam. The spectra in set I were obtained in 0.05 M triethanolamine HCl/NaOH, pH 7.5 at an Nbf-Cl concentration of 0.102 mM and a β-mercaptoethanol concentration of 2.28 mM. The times for the individual curves in set I were 2 min (curve 1), 12 min (curve 2), 22 min (curve 3), 42 min (curve 4), and 72 min (curve 5). The spectra in set II were obtained in 0.05 M triethanolamine HCl/NaOH buffer, pH 7.5, at an Nbf-Cl concentration of 0.104 mM and a β-mercaptoethanol concentration of 22.8 mM. The times for the individual curves in set II were 3 min (curve 1), 15 min (curve 2), 35 min (curve 3), and 60 min (curve 4). The spectra in set III were obtained in 0.05 M sodium citrate/citric acid, pH 5.0 at an Nbf-Cl concentration of 0.112 mM. The times for the individual curves of set III were 3 min (curve 1), 27 min (curve 2), 57 min (curve 3), 87 min (curve 4), 117 min (curve 5), 147 min (curve 6), 177 min (curve 7), 207 min (curve 8), and 237 min (curve 9). (From Nitta, K., Bratcher, S. C., and Kronman, M. J., *Biochem. J.*, 177, 385, 1979. With permission.)

cleavage was obtained at S-aminoethyl cysteine. This chemistry has been used to introduce a dansyl label into oncomodulin via modification of a cysteinyl residue with dansylaziridine (Figure 59).[78] Since the aziridines are photosensitive compounds (see Chapter 16), reaction proceeded in the dark. A 100-fold molar excess of reagent (dissolved in either dimethylformamide or dimethylsulfoxide) at pH 7.5 (Tris or HEPES) was used. The reaction was allowed to proceed for 16 to 20 h with rocking (most of the dansylaziridine is insoluble) and reagent removed by centrifugation.

Mutus et al.[106] have introduced 1-p-chorophenyl-4,4-dimethyl-5-diethylamino-1-pentene-3-one hydrobromide (Figure 60) as a reagent for the modification of thiol groups. This reagent readily and reversibly reacts with low molecular weight thiols such as cysteine or glutathione with a large decrease in absorbance at 310 nM (= 21,000 M^{-1} cm^{-1}). The reaction with larger thiol-containing molecules such as proteins appears to be irreversible.

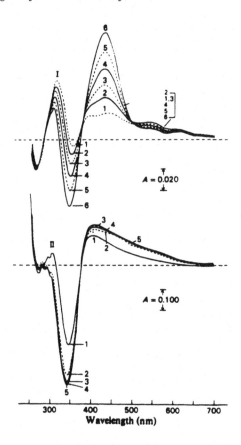

FIGURE 56.   Different spectra of mixtures of 4-chloro-7-nitrobenzofurazan(Nbf-Cl) and dithiothreitol at ambient temperature. Spectra were scanned at the rate of 30 nm/min from high to low wavelength. The times given below were for the initial wavelength in the scan. The solution of Nbf-Cl + thiol compound was in the sample beam. The buffer used was 0.05 N triethanolamine HCl/NaOH (pH 7.5). The spectra of set I were obtained at an Nbf-Cl concentration of 0.148 mM and a dithiothreitol concentration of 9.97 μM at 3 min (curve 1), 13 min (curve 2), 23 min (curve 3), 38 min (curve 4), 58 min (curve 5), and 88 min (curve 6). The spectra in set II were obtained at an Nbf-Cl concentration of 9.389 mM at 2 min (curve 1), 12 min (curve 2), 22 min (curve 3), 42 min (curve 4), and 72 min (curve 5). (From Nitta, K., Bratcher, S. C., and Kronman, M. J., *Biochem. J.*, 177, 385, 1979. With permission.)

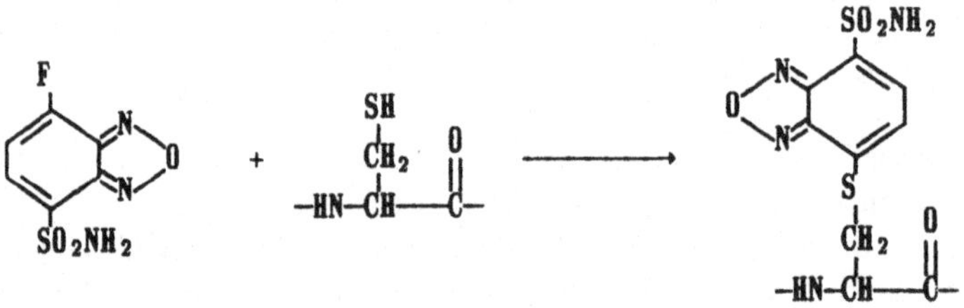

FIGURE 57.   The structure of 4-(aminosulfonyl)-7-fluoro-2,1,3-benzoxadiazole (ABD-F), a fluorogenic reagent for the modification of cysteine residues in proteins.

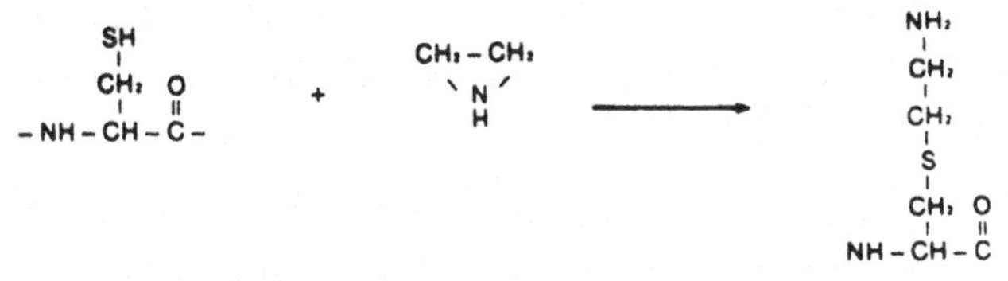

FIGURE 58. The reaction of ethyleneimine with cysteine.

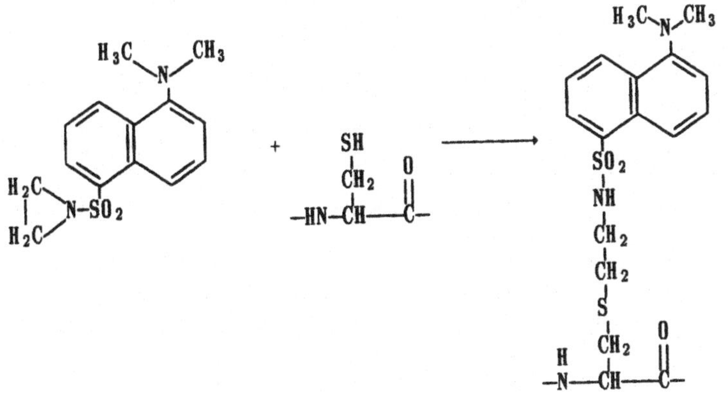

FIGURE 59. The reaction of cysteine with dansyl aziridine.

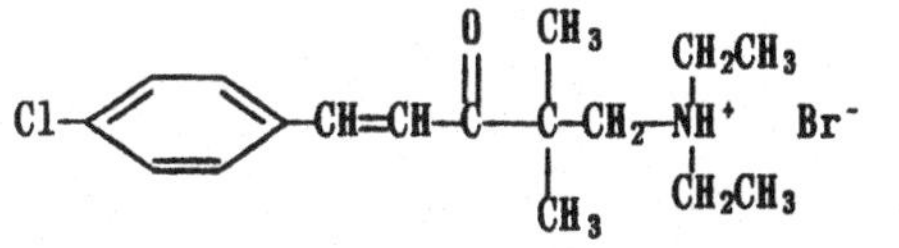

1–p–chlorophenyl–4,4–dimethyl–5–diethylamino–1–penten–3–one hydrobromide

FIGURE 60. The structure of a novel sulfydryl reagent.

REFERENCES

1. **Liu, T.-Y.,** The role of sulfur in proteins, *The Proteins,* Vol. 3, 3rd ed., Neurath, H. and Hill, R. L., Eds., Academic Press, New York, 1977, 240.
2. **Kenyon, G. L. and Bruice, T. W.,** Novel sulfydryl reagents, *Meth. Enzymol.,* 47, 407, 1977.
3. **Poole, L. B. and Claiborne, A.,** The non-flavin redox center of the streptococcal NADH peroxidase. II. Evidence for a stabilized cysteine-sulfenic acid, *J. Biol. Chem.,* 264, 12330, 1989.
4. **Pihl, A. and Lange, R.,** The interaction of oxidized glutathione, cystamine monosulfoxide, and tetrathionate with the -SH groups of rabbit muscle D-glyceraldehyde 3-phosphate dehydrogenase, *J. Biol. Chem.,* 237, 1356, 1962.
5. **Bednar, R. A., Fried, W. B., Lock, Y. W., and Pramanik, B.,** Chemical modification of chalcone isomerase by mercurials and tetrathionate. Evidence for a single cysteine residue in the active site, *J. Biol. Chem.,* 264, 14272, 1989.
6. **Smith, D. J., Maggio, E. T., and Kenyon, G. L.,** Simple alkane thiol groups for temporary blocking of sulfydryl groups of enzymes, *Biochemistry,* 14, 766, 1975.
7. **Bruice, T. W. and Kenyon, G. L.,** Novel alkyl alkanethiolsulfonate sulfydryl reagents. Modification of derivatives of L-cysteine, *J. Protein Chem.,* 1, 47, 1982.

8. **Bech, L. M. and Breddam, K.**, Chemical modification of a cysteinyl residue introduced in the binding site of carboxypeptidase Y by site-directed mutagenesis, *Carlsberg Res. Commun.*, 53, 381, 1988.

9. **Gerwin, B. I.**, Properties of the single sulfhydryl group of streptococcal proteinase. A comparison of the rates of alkylation by chloroacetic acid and chloroacetamide, *J. Biol. Chem.*, 242, 451, 1967.

10. **Liu, T. Y.**, Demonstration of the presence of a histidine residue at the active site of streptococcal proteinase, *J. Biol. Chem.*, 242, 4029, 1967.

11. **Chaiken, I. M. and Smith, E. L.**, Reaction of chloroacetamide with the sulfhydryl group of papain, *J. Biol. Chem.*, 244, 5087, 1969.

12. **Chaiken, I. M. and Smith, E. L.**, Reaction of the sulfhydryl group of papain with chloroacetic acid, *J. Biol. Chem.*, 244, 5095, 1969.

13. **Jörnvall, H., Fowler, A. V., and Zabin, I.**, Probe of β-galactosidase structure with iodoacetate. Differential reactivity of thiol groups in wild-type and mutant forms of β-galactosidase, *Biochemistry*, 17, 5160, 1978.

14. **Kalimi, M. and Love, K.**, Role of chemical reagents in the activation of rat hepatic glucocorticoid-receptor complex, *J. Biol. Chem.*, 255, 4687, 1980.

15. **Kallis, G.-B. and Holmgren, A.**, Differential reactivity of the functional sulfhydryl groups of cysteine-32 and cysteine-35 present in the reduced form of thioredoxin from *Escherichia coli*, *J. Biol. Chem.*, 255, 10261, 1980.

16. **Mikami, B., Aibara, S., and Morita, Y.**, Chemical modification of sulfhydryl groups in soybean β-amylase, *J. Biochem.*, 88, 103, 1980.

17. **Hempel, J. D. and Pietruszko, R.**, Selective chemical modification of human liver aldehyde and dehydrogenases E_1 and E_2 by iodoacetamide, *J. Biol. Chem.*, 256, 10889, 1981.

18. **Crestfield, A. M., Moore, S., and Stein, W. H.**, The preparation and enzymatic hydrolysis of reduced and S-carboxymethylated proteins, *J. Biol. Chem.*, 238, 622, 1963.

19. **Friedman, M., Krull, L. H., and Cavins, J. F.**, The chromatographic determination of cystine and cysteine residues in proteins as S-β-(4-pyridyl-ethyl) cysteine, *J. Biol. Chem.*, 245, 3868, 1970.

20. **Mak, A. S. and Jones, B. L.**, Application of S-pyridylethylation of cysteine to the sequence analysis of proteins, *Anal. Biochem.*, 84, 432, 1978.

21. **Dahl, K. S. and McKinley-McKee, J. S.**, The reactivity of affinity labels: a kinetic study of the reaction of alkyl halides with thiolate anions — a model reaction for protein alkylation, *Bioorganic Chem.*, 10, 329, 1981.

22. **Soper, T. S., Ueno, H., and Manning, J. M.**, Substrate-induced changes in sulfydryl reactivity of bacterial D-amino acid transaminase, *Arch. Biochem. Biophys.*, 240, 1, 1985.

23. **Kaslow, H. R., Schlotterbeck, J. D., Mar, V. L., and Burnette, W. N.**, Alkylation of cysteine 41, but not cysteine 200, decreases the ADP-ribosyltransferase activity of the S1 subunit of pertussis toxin, *J. Biol. Chem.*, 264, 6386, 1989.

24. **Makinen, A. L. and Nowak, T.**, A reactive cysteine in avian liver phosphoenolpyruvate carboxykinase, *J. Biol. Chem.*, 264, 12148, 1989.

25. **Poole, L. B. and Claiborne, A.**, The non-flavin redox center of the streptococcal NADH peroxidase. I. Thiol reactivity and redox behavior in the presence of urea, *J. Biol. Chem.*, 264, 12322, 1989.

26. **Wu, H., Yao, Q.-Z., and Tsou, C.-L.**, Creatine kinase is modified by 2-chloromercuri-4-nitrophenol at the active site thiols with complete inactivation, *Biochim. Biophys. Acta*, 997, 78, 1989.

27. **Wang, Z.-X., Preiss, B., and Tsou, C.-L.**, Kinetics of inactivation of creatine kinase during modification of its thiol groups, *Biochemistry*, 27, 5095, 1988.

28. **Seifried, S. E., Wang, Y., and Von Hippel, P. H.**, Fluorescent modification of the cysteine 202 residue of *Escherichia coli* transcription termination factor rho, *J. Biol. Chem.*, 263, 13511, 1988.

29. **Pardo, J. P. and Slayman, C. W.**, Cysteine 532 and cysteine 545 are the *N*-ethylmaleimide-reactive residues of the *Neurospora* plasma membrane H^+ [T-ATPase, *J. Biol. Chem.*, 264, 9373, 1989.

30. **Miyanishi, T. and Borejdo, J.**, Differential behavior of two cysteine residues on the myosin head in muscle fibers, *Biochemistry*, 28, 1287, 1989.

31. **Bishop, J. E., Squier, T. C., Bigelow, D. J., and Inesi, G.**, (Iodoacetamido) fluorescein labels a pair of proximal cysteines on the Ca^{2+} [T-ATPase of sarcoplasmic reticulum, *Biochemistry*, 27, 5233, 1988.

32. **First, E. A. and Taylor, S. S.**, Selective modification of the catalytic subunit of cAMP-dependent protein kinase with sulfhydryl-specific fluorescent probes, *Biochemistry*, 28, 3598, 1989.

33. **Gregory, J. D.**, The stability of *N*-ethylmaleimide and its reaction with sulfhydryl groups, *J. Am. Chem. Soc.*, 77, 3922, 1955.

34. **Leslie, J.**, Spectral shifts in the reaction of *N*-ethylmaleimide with proteins, *Anal. Biochem.*, 10, 162, 1965.

35. **Gorin, G., Martic, P. A., and Doughty, G.**, Kinetics of the reaction of *N*-ethylmaleimide with cysteine and some congeners, *Arch. Biochem. Biophys.*, 115, 593, 1966.

36. **Smyth, D. G., Blumenfeld, O. O., and Konigsberg, W.**, Reaction of *N*-ethylmaleimide with peptides and amino acids, *Biochem. J.*, 91, 589, 1964.

37. **Portanova, J. P. and Shrift, A.**, Usefulness of N-ethylmaleimide in the identification of ^{75}Se-labeled selenocysteine, *J. Chromatogr.*, 139, 391, 1977.

38. **Gehring, H. and Christen, P.**, A diagonal procedure for isolating sulfhydryl peptides alkylated with N-ethylmaleimide, *Anal. Biochem.*, 107, 358, 1980.

39. **Brown, R. D. and Matthews, K. S.**, Chemical modification of lactose repressor proteins using N-substituted maleimides, *J. Biol. Chem.*, 254, 5128, 1979.

40. **Brown, R. D. and Matthews, K. S.**, Spectral studies on *Lac* repressor modified with N-substituted maleimide probes, *J. Biol. Chem.*, 254, 5135, 1979.

41. **Quiocho, F. E. and Thomson, J. W.**, Substrate binding to an active creatine kinase with a thiol-bound mercurinitrophenol chromophoric probe, *Proc. Natl. Acad. Sci. U.S.A.*, 70, 2858, 1973.

42. **Quiocho, F. A. and Olson, J. S.**, The reaction of creatine kinase with 2-chloromercuri-4-nitrophenol, *J. Biol. Chem.*, 249, 5885, 1974.

43. **Martin, R. L., Daley, L. A., Lovric, Z., Wailes, L. M., Renosto, F., and Segel, I. H.**, The "regulatory" sulfhydryl group of *Penicillium chrysogenum* ATP sulfurylase. Cooperative ligand binding after SH modification; chemical and thermodynamic properties, *J. Biol. Chem.*, 264, 11768, 1989.

44. **Werner, P. K., Lieberman, D. M., and Reithmeier, R. A. F.**, Accessibility of the N-ethylmaleimide-unreactive sulfhydryl of human erythrocyte band 3, *Biochim. Biophys. Acta*, 982, 309, 1989.

45. **Passamonti, S. and Sottocasa, G. L.**, The role of sulfhydryl groups in sulfobromophthalein transport in rat liver plasma membrane vesicles, *Biochim. Biophys. Acta*, 979, 294, 1989.

46. **Pfister, K. K., Wagner, M. C., Bloom, G. S., and Brady, S. T.**, Modification of the microtubule-binding and ATPase activities of kinesin by N-ethylmaleimide (NEM) suggests a role for sulfhydryls in fast axonal transport, *Biochemistry*, 28, 9006, 1989.

47. **Perussi, J. R., Tinto, M. H., Nascimento, O. R., and Tabak, M.**, Characterization of protein spin labeling by maleimide: evidence for nitroxide reduction, *Anal. Biochem.*, 173, 289, 1988.

48. **Marquez, J., Iriarte, A., and Martinez-Carrion, M.**, Covalent modification of a critical sulfhydryl group in the acetylcholine receptor: cysteine-222 of the -subunit, *Biochemistry*, 28, 7433, 1989.

49. **Mills, J. S., Walsh, M. P., Nemcek, K., and Johnson, J. D.**, Biologically active fluorescent derivatives of spinach calmodulin that report calmodulin target protein binding, *Biochemistry*, 27, 991, 1988.

50. **Jezek, P. and Drahota, Z.**, Sulfhydryl groups of the uncoupling protein of brown adipose tissue mitochondria — distinction between sulfhydryl groups of the H^+ [T channel and the nucleotide binding site, *Eur. J. Biochem.*, 183, 89, 1989.

51. **Le-Quoc, K., Le-Quoc, D., and Gaudemer, Y.**, Evidence for the existence of two classes of sulfhydryl groups essential for membrane-bound succinate dehydrogenase activity, *Biochemistry*, 20, 1705, 1981.

52. **Rial, E., Aréchaga, I., Sainz-de-la-Maza, E., and Nicholls, D. G.**, Effect of hydrophobic sulphydryl reagents on the uncoupling protein and inner-membrane anion channel of brown-adipose-tissue mitochondria, *Eur. J. Biochem.*, 182, 187, 1989.

53. **Yee, A. S., Corley, D. E., and McNamee, M. G.**, Thiol-group modification of *Torpedo californica* acetylcholine receptor: subunit localization and effects on function, *Biochemistry*, 25, 2110, 1986.

54. **Pradier, L., Yee, A. S., and McNamee, M. G.**, Use of chemical modifications and site-directed mutagenesis to probe the functional role of thiol groups on the gamma subunit of *Torpedo californica* acetylcholine receptor, *Biochemistry*, 28, 6562, 1989.

55. **Abbott, R. E. and Schachter, D.**, Topography and functions of sulfhydryl groups of the human erythrocyte glucose transport mechanism, *Mol. Cell. Biochem.*, 82, 85, 1988.

56. **May, J. M.**, Reaction of an exofacial sulfhydryl group on the erythrocyte hexose carrier with an impermeant maleimide. Relevance to the mechanism of hexose transport, *J. Biol. Chem.*, 263, 13635, 1988.

57. **May, J. M.**, Interaction of a permeant maleimide derivative of cysteine with the erythrocyte glucose carrier. Differential labelling of an exofacial carrier thiol group and its role in the transport mechanism, *Biochem. J.*, 263, 875, 1989.

58. **Abbott, R. E. and Schachter, D.**, Impermeant maleimides. Oriented probes of erythrocyte membrane proteins, *J. Biol. Chem.*, 251, 7176, 1976.

59. **May, J. M.**, Selective labeling of the erythrocyte hexose carrier with a maleimide derivative of glucosamine: relationship of an exofacial sulfhydryl to carrier conformation and structure, *Biochemistry*, 28, 1718, 1989.

60. **Falke, J. J., Dernburg, A. F., Sternberg, D. A., Zalkin, N., Milligan, D. L., and Koshland, D. E., Jr.**, Structure of a bacterial sensory receptor. A site-directed sulfhydryl study, *J. Biol. Chem.*, 263, 14850, 1988.

61. **Lepke, S., Fasold, H., Pring, M., and Passow, H.**, A study of the relationship between inhibition of anion exchange and binding to the red blood cell membrane of 4,4'-dithiocyano stilbene-2,2'-disulfonic acid (DIDS) and its dihydro derivative (H_2DIDS), *J. Membrane Biol.*, 29, 147, 1976.

62. **Bettendorff, L., Wins, P., and Schoffeniels, E.**, Thiamine triphosphatase from *electrophorus* electric organ is anion-dependent and irreversibly inhibited by 4,4'-diisothiocyanostilbene-2,2'-disulfonic acid, *Biochem. Biophys. Res. Commun.*, 154, 942, 1988.

63. **Speth, M. and Schulze, H.-U.,** On the nature of the interaction between 4,4'-diisothiocyanostilbene 2,2'-disulfonic acid and microsomal glucose-6-phosphatase. Evidence for the involvement of sulfhydryl groups of the phosphohydrolase, *Eur. J. Biochem.,* 174, 111, 1988.

64. **Degani, Y. and Degani, C.,** Subunit-selective chemical modifications of creatine kinase. Evidence for asymmetrical association of the subunits, *Biochemistry,* 18, 5917, 1979.

65. **Ellman, G. L.,** Tissue sulfhydryl groups, *Arch. Biochem. Biophys.,* 82, 70, 1959.

66. **Pecci, L., Cannella, C., Pensa, B., Costa, M., and Cavallini, D.,** Cyanylation of rhodanese by 2-nitro-5-thiocyanobenzoic acid, *Biochim. Biophys. Acta,* 623, 348, 1980.

67. **Vanaman, T. C. and Stark, G. C.,** A study of the sulfydryl groups of the catalytic subunit of *Escherichia coli* aspartate transcarbamylase. The use of enzyme-5-thio-2-nitrobenzoate mixed disulfides as intermediates in modifying enzyme sulfydryl groups, *J. Biol. Chem.,* 245, 3565, 1970.

68. **Marshall, M. and Cohen, P. P.,** Ornithine transcarbamylases. Ordering of S-cyanopeptides and location of characteristically reactive cysteinyl residues within the sequence, *J. Biol. Chem.,* 255, 7287, 1980.

69. **Ogilvie, J. W.,** Cleavage of phosphofructokinase at S-cyanylated cysteine residues, *Biochim. Biophys. Acta,* 622, 277, 1980.

70. **Kindman, L. A. and Jencks, W. P.,** Modification and inactivation of CoA transferase by 2-nitro-5-(thiocyanato) benzoate, *Biochemistry,* 20, 5183, 1981.

71. **Habeeb, A. F. S. A.,** Reaction of protein sulfydryl groups with Ellman's reagent, *Meth. Enzymol.,* 25, 457, 1972.

72. **Talgoy, M. M., Bell, A. W., and Duckworth, H. W.,** The reactions of *Escherichia coli* citrate synthase with the sulfhydryl reagents 5,5'-dithiobis-(2-nitrobenzoic acid) and 4,4'-dithiodipyridine, *Can. J. Biochem.,* 57, 822, 1979.

73. **Soper, T. S., Jones, W. M., and Manning, J. M.,** Effects of substrates on the selective modification of the cysteinyl residues of D-amino acid transaminase, *J. Biol. Chem.,* 254, 10901, 1979.

74. **Lukas, R. J. and Bennett, E. L.,** Chemical modification and reactivity of sulfhydryls and disulfides of rat brain nicotinic-like acetylcholine receptors, *J. Biol. Chem.,* 255, 5573, 1980.

75. **Cockle, S. A., Epand, R. M., Stollery, J. G., and Moscarello, M. A.,** Nature of the cysteinyl residues in lipophilin from human myelin, *J. Biol. Chem.,* 255, 9182, 1980.

76. **Hallaway, B. E., Hedlund, B. E., and Benson, E. S.,** Studies of the effect of reagent and protein charges on reactivity of the β93 sulfhydryl group of human hemoglobin using selected mutations, *Arch. Biochem. Biophys.,* 203, 332, 1980.

77. **Luthra, M. P., Dunlap, R. B., and Odom, J. D.,** Characterization of a new sulfhydryl group reagent: 6,6'-diselenobis-(3-nitrobenzoic acid), a selenium analog of Ellman's reagent, *Anal. Biochem.,* 117, 94, 1981.

78. **Clayshulte, T. M., Taylor, D. F., and Henzl, M. T.,** Reactivity of cysteine 18 in oncomodulin, *J. Biol. Chem.,* 265, 1800, 1990.

79. **Kato, H., Tanaka, T., Nishioka, T., Kimura, A., and Oda, J.,** Role of cysteine residues in glutathione synthetase from *Escherichia coli* B. Chemical modification and oligonucleotide site-directed mutagenesis, *J. Biol. Chem.,* 263, 11646, 1988.

80. **Narasimhan, C., Lai, C.-S., Haas, A., and McCarthy, J.,** One free sulfhydryl group of plasma fibronectin becomes titratable upon binding of the protein to solid substrates, *Biochemistry,* 27, 4970, 1988.

81. **Poole, L. B. and Claiborne, A.,** Evidence for a single active-site cysteinyl residue in the streptococcal NADH peroxidase, *Biochem. Biophys. Res. Commun.,* 153, 261, 1988.

82. **Drewes, G. and Faulstich, H.,** 2,4-Dinitrophenyl[¹⁴C]cysteinyl disulfide allows selective radiolabeling of protein thiols under spectrophotometric control, *Anal. Biochem.,* 188, 109, 1990.

83. **Brandwein, H. J., Lewicki, J. A., and Murad, F.,** Reversible inactivation of guanylate cyclase by mixed disulfide formation, *J. Biol. Chem.,* 256, 2958, 1981.

84. **Kimura, T., Matsueda, R., Nakagawa, Y., and Kaiser, E. T.,** New reagents for the introduction of the thiomethyl group at sulfhydryl residues of proteins with concomitant spectrophotometric titration of the sulfhydryl: methyl 3-nitro-2-pyridyl disulfide and methyl 2-pyridyl disulfide, *Anal. Biochem.,* 122, 274, 1982.

85. **Pedersen, A. O. and Jacobsen, J.,** Reactivity of the thiol group in human and bovine albumin at pH 3-9, as measured by exchange with 2,2'-dithiodipyridine, *Eur. J. Biochem.,* 106, 291, 1980.

86. **Boyer, P. D.,** Spectrophotometric study of the reaction of protein sulfhydryl groups with organic mercurials, *J. Am. Chem. Soc.,* 76, 4331, 1954.

87. **Bai, Y. and Hayashi, R.,** Properties of the single sulfhydryl group of carboxypeptidase Y. Effects of alkyl and aromatic mercurials on activities toward various synthetic substrates, *J. Biol. Chem.,* 254, 8473, 1979.

88. **Ojcius, D. M. and Solomon, A. K.,** Sites of p-chloromercuribenzenesulfonate inhibition of red cell urea and water transport, *Biochim. Biophys. Acta,* 942, 73, 1988.

89. **Clark, S. J. and Ralston, G. B.,** The dissociation of peripheral proteins from erythrocyte membranes brought about by p-mercuribenzenesulfonate, *Biochim. Biophys. Acta,* 1021, 141, 1990.

90. **Marshall, M. and Cohen, P. P.**, The essential sulfhydryl group of ornithine transcarbamylases-pH dependence of the spectra of its 2-mercuri-4-nitrophenol derivative, *J. Biol. Chem.*, 255, 7296, 1980.

91. **Baines, B. S. and Brocklehurst, K.**, A thiol-labelling reagent and reactivity probe containing electrophilic mercury and a chromophoric leaving group, *Biochem. J.*, 179, 701, 1979.

92. **Banks, T. E. and Shafer, J. A.**, Inactivation of papain by S-methylation of its cysteinyl residue with O-methylisourea, *Biochemistry*, 11, 110, 1972.

93. **Stark, G.**, Modification of proteins with cyanate, *Meth. Enzymol.*, 11, 590, 1967.

94. **Ghosh, P. B. and Whitehouse, M. W.**, 7-Chloro-4-nitrobenzo-2-oxa-1,3-diazole: a new fluorigenic reagent for amino acids and other amines, *Biochem. J.*, 108, 155, 1968.

95. **Birkett, D. J., Price, N. D., Radda, G. K., and Salmon, A. G.**, The reactivity of SH groups with a fluorogenic reagent, *FEBS Lett.*, 6, 346, 1970.

96. **Birkett, D. J., Dwek, R. A., Radda, G. K., Richards, R. E., and Salmon, A. G.**, Probes for the conformational transitions of phosphorylase b. Effect of ligands studied by proton relaxation enhancement, fluorescence and chemical reactivities, *Eur. J. Biochem.*, 20, 494, 1971.

97. **Lad, P. M., Wolfman, N. M., and Hammes, G. G.**, Properties of rabbit muscle phosphofructokinase modified with 7-chloro-4-nitrobenzo-2-oxa-1,3-diazole, *Biochemistry*, 16, 4802, 1977.

98. **Nitta, K., Bratcher, S. C., and Kronman, M. J.**, Anomalous reaction of 4-chloro-7-nitrobenzofurazan with thiol compounds, *Biochem. J.*, 177, 385, 1979.

99. **Dwek, R. A., Radda, G. A., Richards, R. E., and Salmon, A. G.**, Probes for the conformational transitions of phosphorylase a. Effect of ligands studied by proton-relaxation enhancement, and chemical reactivities, *Eur. J. Biochem.*, 29, 509, 1972.

100. **Carlberg, I. and Mannervik, B.**, Interaction of 2,4,6-trinitrobenzenesulfonate and 4-chloro-7-nitrobenzo-2-oxa-1,3-diazole with the active sites of glutathione reductase and lipoamide dehydrogenase, *Acta Chem. Scand.*, B34, 144, 1980.

101. **Toyo'oka, T. and Imai, K.**, New fluorogenic reagent having halogenbenzofurazan structure for thiols: 4-(aminosulfonyl)-7-flouro-2,1,3-benzoxadiazole, *Anal. Chem.*, 56, 1984.

102. **Kirley, T. L.**, Reduction and fluorescent labeling of cyst(e)ine-containing proteins for subsequent structural analyses, *Anal. Biochem.*, 180, 231, 1989.

103. **Niketic, V., Thomsen, J., and Kristiansen, K.**, Modification of cysteine residues with 2-bromoethane-sulfonate. The application of S-sulfoethylated peptides in automatic Edman degradation, *Eur. J. Biochem.*, 46, 547, 1974.

104. **Raftery, M. A. and Cole, R. D.**, On the aminoethylation of proteins, *J. Biol. Chem.*, 241, 3457, 1966.

105. **Plapp, B. V., Raftery, M. A., and Cole, R. D.**, The tryptic digestion of S-aminoethylated ribonuclease, *J. Biol. Chem.*, 242, 265, 1967.

106. **Mutus, B., Wagner, J. D., Talpas, C. J., Dimmock, J. R., Phillips, O. A., and Reid, R. S.**, 1-*p*-Chlorophenyl-4,4-dimethyl-5-diethylamino-1-penten-3-one hydrobromide, a sulfhydryl-specific compound which reacts irreversibly with protein thiols but reversibly with small molecular weight thiols, *Anal Biochem.*, 177, 237, 1989.

Chapter 7

THE MODIFICATION OF CYSTINE — CLEAVAGE OF DISULFIDE BONDS

There are several approaches to the cleavage of disulfide bonds in proteins. The majority of studies involve the cleavage of the disulfide bond of cystine to the free thiol group of cysteine by reduction. Reduction has been generally accomplished with a mild reducing agent such as β-mercaptoethanol or cysteine. Gorin and co-workers[1] have examined the rate of reaction of lysozyme with various thiols. At pH 10.0 (0.025 M borate), the relative rates of reaction were β-mercaptoethanol (2-mercaptoethanol), 0.2; dithiothreitol, 1.0; 3-mercaptopropionate, 0.4; and 2-aminoethanol, 0.01. The results with aminoethanethiol were somewhat surprising since the reaction (disulfide exchange) involves the thiolate anion and 2-aminoethanethiol would be more extensively ionized than the other mercaptans. Dithiothreitol has been a useful reagent in the reduction of disulfide bonds in proteins[2] as introduced by Cleland. Dithiothreitol and the isomeric form, dithioerythritol, are each capable of the quantitative reduction of disulfide bonds in proteins. Furthermore, the oxidized form of dithiothreitol has an absorbance maximum at 283 nm ($\Delta\epsilon = 273$) which can be used to determine the extent of disulfide bond cleavage.[2] The UV spectra of dithiothreitol and oxidized dithiothreitol are shown in Figure 1. Insolubilized dihydrolipoic acid has also been proposed for use in the quantitative reduction of disulfide bonds.[4]

Reduction of disulfide bonds can be controlled by various factors. Homandberg and Wai[5] recently demonstrated that the reduction of urokinase by dithiothreitol in the presence of arginine allows the selective reduction of a disulfide bond joining the catalytically active chain to a nonessential 13 amino acid peptide. A synthetic peptide may then be coupled to the free sulfydryl group.

In most proteins, the free sulfhydryl groups (cysteine) derived from the reduction of cystine will, at alkaline pH, fairly rapidly undergo reoxidation to form the original disulfide bonds. This process can be accelerated by the sulfhydryl-disulfide interchange enzyme[6,7] or sulfhydryl oxidase.[8] Thus, it is necessary to "block" the new sulfhydryl groups by alkylation, arylation or reaction with dithionite (see Chapter 6).

A novel reaction has been developed by Neumann and co-workers[10] which allows for the reduction of disulfide bonds under mild conditions. Phosphorothioate reacts with disulfide bonds to yield the S-phosphorothioate derivatives. The reaction proceeds optimally at alkaline pH (pH optimum 9.7) and the reaction product, S-phosphorothioate cysteine, has an absorbance maximum at 250 nm ($\epsilon = 631$ M^{-1} cm^{-1}) as shown in Figure 2. Phosphorothioate does not absorb at this wavelength. This reagent has been used to study the reactivity of disulfide bonds in ribonuclease.[10] In the absence of a denaturing agent (reaction conditions: tenfold molar acess of reagent, pH 9.0, 16 h at 25°C), two specific disulfide bonds (Cys$_{65}$ – Cys$_{72}$; Cys$_{58}$– Cys$_{110}$) are converted to phosphorothioate derivatives. The resultant derivative of ribonuclease is fully active in hydrolysis of RNA and has increased activity in the hydrolysis of cyclic cytidylic acid. The synthesis of radiolabeled phosphorothioate from either [P^{32}] or [S^{35}] thiophosphoryl chloride was reported in this study.

Light and co-workers have examined the susceptibility of disulfide bonds in trypsinogen to reduction.[11] At pH 9.0 (0.1 M sodium borate), a single disulfide bond (Cys$_{179}$ – Cys$_{203}$) is cleaved in trypsinogen by 0.1 M NaBH$_4$. The resulting sulfhydryl groups are "blocked" by alkylation. The characterization of the modified protein has been performed by the same group.[12] The disulfide bond which is modified under these conditions is critical in establishing the structure of the primary specificity site in trypsin.

From the above studies, there is little doubt that the various disulfide bonds in a protein show different reactivity toward reducing agents. These differences in reactivity can be explored with various reagents and can be utilized with the aid of partial reduction followed

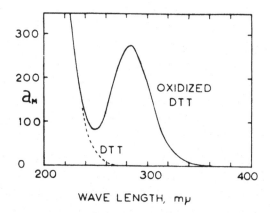

FIGURE 1. The absorption spectra of dithiothreitol (DTT) and oxidized dithiothreitol (oxidized DTT) in aqueous solution. (From Cleland, W. W., *Biochemistry*, 3, 480, 1964. With permission.)

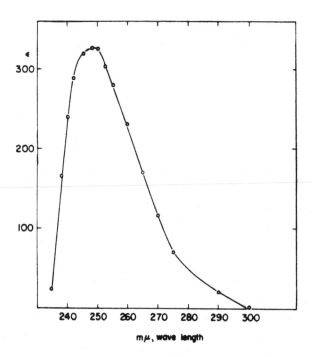

FIGURE 2. The absorption spectrum of the reaction product formed from cystine and phosphorothioate (PS). (From Neumann, H. and Smith, R. L., *Arch. Biochem. Biophys.*, 122, 354, 1967. With permission.)

by alkylation with radiolabeled iodoacetate to determine the position of disulfide bonds in proteins.[13]

Gorin and Godwin[14] have reported that cystine can be quantitatively converted to cysteic acid by reaction with iodate in 0.1 to 1.0 M HCl. This reaction has been applied to insulin. The reaction product was not completely characterized, but given the relationship between iodate consumption and the cystine residues in insulin, the primary reaction is the oxidation

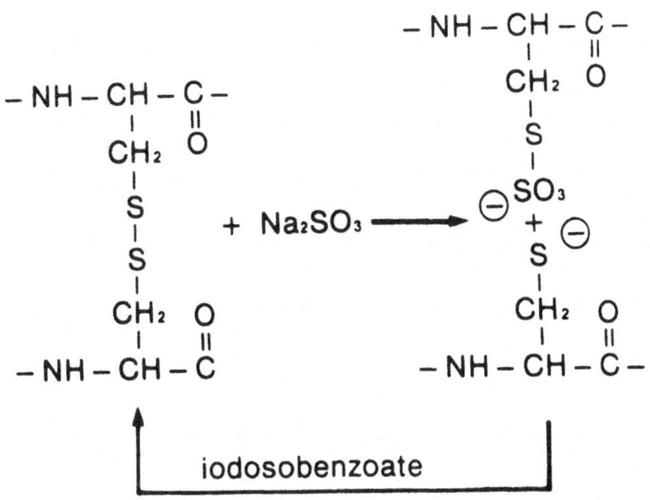

FIGURE 3.   The cleavage of disulfide bonds by sodium sulfite to form the S-sulfo derivative.

of disulfide bonds. This reaction was complete in 15 to 30 min. After longer periods of reaction, the iodination of tyrosine residues occurred.

Disulfide bonds are somewhat unstable at alkaline pH (pH ≥ 13.0). This has been examined by Donovan in some detail.[15] With protein-bound cystine, there is change in the spectrum with an increase in absorbance at 300 nm. This problem has been more recently studied by Florence.[16] This investigation presented evidence to suggest that cleavage of disulfide bonds in proteins by base proceeds via β-elimination to form dehydroalanine and a persulfide intermediate which can decompose to form several products.

The electrolytic reduction of proteins has been explored by Leach and co-workers.[17] These investigators recognized that although small peptides containing disulfide bonds could be reduced using cathodic reduction, there would likely be problems with proteins because of size and tertiary structure considerations. Therefore, a small thiol was used as a catalyst for the reduction.

Tri-n-butylphosphine will reduce disulfide bonds in proteins.[18] The reaction is generally performed under alkaline conditions (pH 8.0, 0.1 M Tris or 0.5 M bicarbonate). n-Propanol is added to dissolve the tri-n-butylphosphine. This procedure has recently been used to reduce disulfide bonds in various proteins prior to reaction with 4-(aminosulfonyl)-7-fluoro-2,1,3-benzodiazole.[19]

Finally, disulfide bonds can be cleaved by sulfite to form the S-sulfonate derivative as shown in Figure 3. The chemistry of this reaction has been reviewed by Cole.[20] The reaction proceeds optimally at alkaline pH (pH 9.0). It is necessary to include an oxidizing agent such as cupric ions, or as shown in Figure 3, o-iodosobenzoate to ensure effective conversion of all cystine residues to the corresponding S-sulfonate derivatives. The reaction is reversible to form cysteine upon treatment with a suitable mercaptan such as β-mercaptoethanol.

This reaction has been adapted to the controlled reduction of disulfide bonds in proteins in the absence of denaturing agents.[21] In the example presented, the disulfide bonds of bovine serum albumin were cleaved at pH 7.0 (0.1 M phosphate) at 40°C in the presence of 0.1 M sodium sulfite and simultaneously converted to the S-sulfo derivatives with oxygen and 0.4 mM cupric sulfate. The rate of reaction decreased markedly above pH 7.0.

REFERENCES

1. **Gorin, G., Fulford, R., and Deonier, R. C.,** Reaction of lysozyme with dithiothreitol and with other mercaptans, *Experientia,* 24, 26, 1968.
2. **Cleland, W. W.,** Dithiothreitol, a new protective reagent for SH groups, *Biochemistry,* 3, 480, 1964.
3. **Iyer, K. S. and Klee, W. A.,** Direct spectrophotometric measurement of the rate of reduction of disulfide bonds. The reactivity of the disulfide bonds of bovine α-lactalbumin, *J. Biol. Chem.,* 248, 707, 1973.
4. **Gorecki, M. and Patchornik, A.,** Polymer-bound dihydrolipoic acid: a new insoluble reducing agent for disulfides, *Biochim. Biophys. Acta,* 303, 36, 1973.
5. **Homandberg, G. A. and Wai, T.,** Reduction of disulfides in urokinase and insertion of a synthetic peptide, *Biochim. Biophys. Acta,* 1038, 209, 1990.
6. **Fuchs, S., DeLorenzo, F., and Anfinsen, C. B.,** Studies on the mechanism of the enzymic catalysis of disulfide interchange in proteins, *J. Biol. Chem.,* 242, 398, 1967.
7. **Creighton, T. E., Hillson, D. A., and Freedman, R. B.,** Catalysis by protein-disulphide isomerase of the unfolding and refolding of proteins with disulphide bonds, *J. Mol. Biol.,* 142, 43, 1980.
8. **Janolino, V. G., Sliwkowski, M. Y., Swaisgood, H. F., and Horton, H. R.,** Catalytic effect of sulfhydryl oxidase on the formation of three-dimensional structure in chymotrypsinogen A, *Arch. Biochem. Biophys.,* 191, 269, 1978.
9. **Neumann, H. and Smith, R. L.,** Cleavage of the disulfide bonds of cystine and oxidized glutathione by phosphorothioate, *Arch. Biochem. Biophys.,* 122, 354, 1967.
10. **Neumann, H., Steinberg, J. Z., Brown, J. R., Goldberger, R. F., and Sela, M.,** On the non-essentiality of two specific disulphide bonds in ribonuclease for its biological activity, *Eur. J. Biochem.,* 3, 171, 1967.
11. **Light, A., Hardwick, B. C., Hatfield, L. M., and Sondack, D. L.,** Modification of a single disulfide bond in trypsinogen and the activation of the carboxymethyl derivative, *J. Biol. Chem.,* 244, 6289, 1969.
12. **Knights, R. J. and Light, A.,** Disulfide bond-modified trypsinogen. Role of disulfide 179-203 on the specificity characteristics of bovine trypsin toward synthetic substrates, *J. Biol. Chem.,* 251, 222, 1976.
13. **Mise, T. and Bahl, O. P.,** Assignment of disulfide bonds in the α-subunit of human chorionic gonadotropin, *J. Biol. Chem.,* 255, 8516, 1980.
14. **Gorin, G. and Godwin, W. E.,** The reaction of iodate with cystine and with insulin, *Biochem. Biophys. Res. Commun.,* 25, 227, 1966.
15. **Donovan, J. W.,** Spectrophotometric observation of the alkaline hydrolysis of protein disulfide bonds, *Biochem. Biophys. Res. Commun.,* 29, 734, 1967.
16. **Florence, T. M.,** Degradation of protein disulphide bonds in dilute alkali, *Biochem. J.,* 189, 507, 1980.
17. **Leach, S. J., Meschers, A., and Swanepoel, O. A.,** The electrolytic reduction of proteins, *Biochemistry,* 4, 23, 1965.
18. **Ruegg, U. Th. and Rudingder, J.,** Reductive cleavage of cystine disulfides with tributylphosphine, *Meth. Enzymol.,* 47, 111, 1977.
19. **Kirley, T. L.,** Reduction and fluorescent labeling of cyst(e)ine-containing proteins for subsequent structural analysis, *Anal. Biochem.,* 180, 231, 1989.
20. **Cole, R. D.,** Sulfitolysis, *Meth. Enzymol.,* 11, 206, 1967.
21. **Kella, N. K. D. and Kinsella, J. E.,** A method for the controlled cleavage of disulfide bonds in proteins in the absence of denaturants, *J. Biochem. Biophys. Meth.,* 11, 251, 1985.

Chapter 8

THE MODIFICATION OF METHIONINE

The site-specific modification of methionine (Figure 1) in proteins and peptides is somewhat difficult to achieve under relatively mild conditions. Methionine contains a thioether functional group connected to the peptide chain backbone via a relatively hydrophobic two-carbon segment. The sulfur which is present in a thioether linkage is a relatively weak nucleophile and is unprotonated over a wide pH range. As a reflection of the hydrophobic character of methionine, it is generally a "buried" residue as opposed to a "surface" residue. Since the dissociation of a proton from the sulfur nucleophile is unnecessary, relatively specific derivatization by alkylating agents can be accomplished at acidic pH. Indeed, it has been suggested that the selective modification of methionine via alkylation in proteins is possible at low pH as other potential nucleophiles in a protein are unreactive.[1]

Oxidation of methionine to methionine sulfoxide (Figure 2) can occur under a variety of conditions. Reagents for the "selective" oxidation of methionine which have attracted recent attention include chloramine T[2,3] (0.1 M phosphate, pH 7.0 or 0.1 M Tris, pH 8.4), sodium periodate[3] (0.1 M sodium acetate, pH 5.0), and hydrogen peroxide.[4] The reaction of methionine with chloramine T can be followed spectrophotometrically.[2] The reaction of chloramine T with methionine (Figure 3) results in a significant change in the spectrum of chloramine T as shown in Figure 4. The use of this spectral change in the determination of methionine is shown in Figure 5. Cysteine interfered with this determination but other amino acids (i.e., tyrosine, tryptophan, histidine, serine) did not have any effect on the accuracy of analysis for methionine. It is noted that the oxidation of methionine is a possible side-reaction of the treatment of proteins with N-bromosuccinimide.[5] Oda and Tokushige[1] have studied the oxidation of tryptophanyl residues in tryptophanase by chloramine T. When the native enzyme is treated with chloroamine T (20 mM potassium phosphate, pH 8.5, 0°C), sulfhydryl groups and methionine residues are oxidized with loss of catalytic activity. With prior modification of the sulfhydryl groups with 5,5'-dithiobis(2-nitrobenzoic acid), 4-5/16 methionyl residues are modified with further loss of catalytic activity. In an earlier study, Sakurai and Nagahara[6] compared the relative sensitivity of amino acids in epsilon toxin to oxidation by N-bromosuccinimide (pH 5.0, 0.05 M acetate), N-chlorosuccinimide (pH 8.5, 0.05 M Tris) and chloramine T (pH 8.5, 0.05 M Tris). Methionine was totally lost with both chloramine T and N-chlorosuccinimide but 21% remained in the N-bromosuccinimide-treated sample. The opposite was found for tryptophan with total loss with either N-bromosuccinimide or N-chlorosuccinimide but no loss with chloramine T.

It is possible to convert methionine sulfoxide to methionine under relatively mild conditions[7] thus providing for the reversibility of the oxidative reactions described above (Figure 6). This can be accomplished through both nonenzymatic and enzymatic methods. The nonenzymatic approaches have, in general, proved to be of greater value. A systematic study has shown that of four reducing agents tested, mercaptoacetic acid, β-mercaptoethanol, dithiothreitol, and N-methylmercaptoacetamide, the latter reagent, N-methylmercaptoacetamide was the most effective. The reactions demonstrated little pH dependence but did not proceed well at concentrations of acetic acid above 50% (v/v). Complete regeneration of methionine could be accomplished with 0.7 to 2.8 M reagent at 37° for 21 h. An enzymatic system for the reduction of methionine sulfoxide has been reported.[8]

Methionine can be modified with various alkylation agents such as the α-halo acetic acids and their derivatives (Figure 7). The reaction of iodacetate with methionine has been examined in some detail by Moore, Stein, and Gundlach.[9] The reaction of iodacetate with methionine does not appear to be pH dependent and proceeds much slower than the reaction with cysteine under the mildly alkaline conditions used for reduction and carboxymethylation.

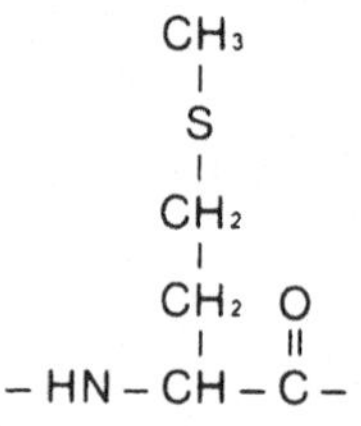
CH3
S
CH2
CH2 O
– HN – CH – C –

FIGURE 1. The structure of methionine.

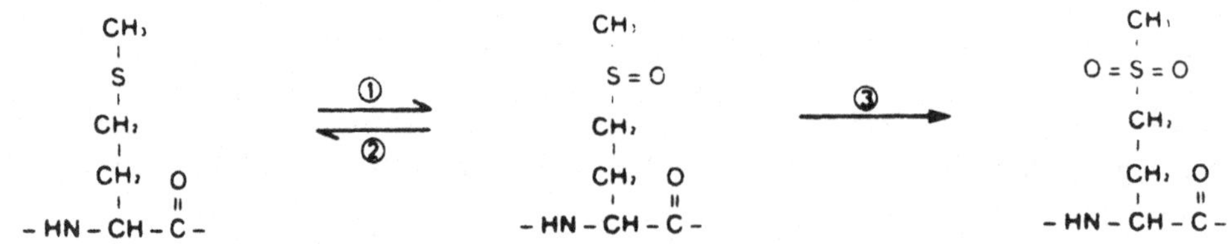
CH3
S
CH2
CH2 O
- HN - CH - C -
①
②
CH3
S = O
CH2
CH2 O
- HN - CH - C -
③
CH3
O = S = O
CH2
CH2 O
- HN - CH - C -

FIGURE 2. The oxidation of methionine to methionine sulfoxide (step 1) which is reversible (step 2, see Figure 6), and subsequently to methionine sulfone.

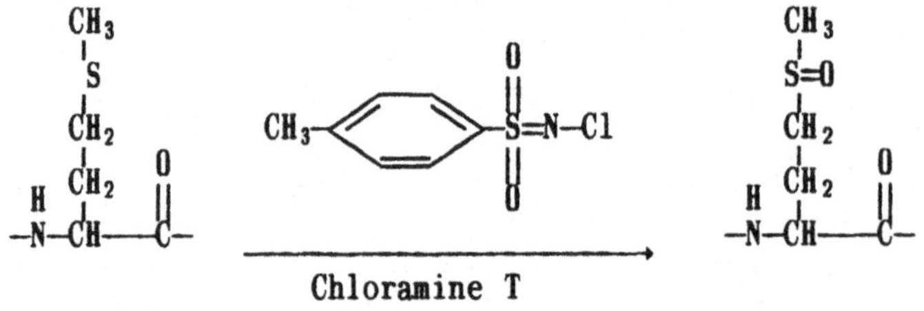
CH3
S
CH2
CH2
H
N
CH
C
O
CH3
S=N–Cl
O
O
Chloramine T
CH3
S=O
CH2
CH2
H
N
CH
C
O

FIGURE 3. A scheme for the oxidation of methionine by chloramine T.

The resulting sulfonium salt yields homoserine and homoserine lactone when heated at 100°C at pH 6.5. On acid hydrolysis (6 *N* HCl, 110°C, 22 h), a mixture of methionine and *S*-carboxymethyl homocysteine together with a small amount of homoserine lactone was obtained. In general, methionine residues only react with the α-haloacids after the disruption of the secondary and tertiary structure of a protein.[10] Selectivity in the modification of methionine in proteins by α-halo acids can be achieved by performing the reaction at acid pH (pH 3.0 or less). The modification of methionine by ethyleneimine has been reported in a reaction producing a sulfonium salt derivative.[11] The modification of methionine in azurin with bromoacetate has been reported.[12] In this protein, four of six methionine residues were modified at pH 4.0, while all methionine residues were reactive at pH 3.2. These modification reactions were performed in 0.1 *M* sodium formate at ambient temperature for 24 h with 0.16 *M* bromoacetate. The modification of methionine in porcine kidney acyl CoA-dehydrogenase occurs with iodoacetate (0.030 *M*) in 0.1 *M* phosphate, pH 6.6 at ambient temperature.[13] The identification of methionine as the residue modified by iodoacetate in this protein was supported by the comparison of the chromatogram of the acid hydrolyzate of the modified protein (reacted with ^{14}C-iodoacetate) with that of the acid hydrolyzate of synthetic *S*-([1-^{14}C]carboxymethyl)-methionine.[9] This is necessary since the *S*-carboxymethyl derivative yielded several different compounds on acid hydrolysis.[9,14]

Naider and Bohak[15] have reported that the sulfonium salt derivatives of methionine (e.g.,

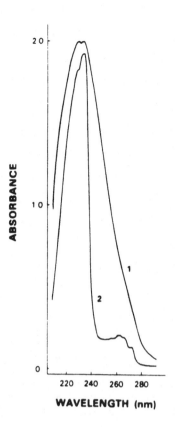

FIGURE 4.   The UV absorption spectrum of chloramine-T (93.1 μg) in 3.0 ml 0.1 *M* sodium phosphaate, pH 7.0 before (curve 1) and after (curve 2) the addition of 99.4 μg methionine. The major change in the spectrum of chloramine-T resulting from the interaction with methionine is a decrease in the width of the peak with λ_{max} 234 nm resulting in a decrease in absorbance which is maximal between 244 and 248 nm. (From Trout, G. E., *Anal. Biochem.*, 93, 419, 1979. With permission.)

S-carboxymethyl methionine, the reaction product of methionine and iodoacetic acid) can be converted to methionine by reaction with a suitable nucleophile. For example, reaction of *S*-carboxamidomethyl methionine (in the peptide Gly-Met-Gly) with a sixfold molar excess of mercaptoethanol at pH 8.9 at a temperature of 30°C resulted in the complete regeneration of methionine after 24 h of reaction. The *S*-phenacyl derivative of methionine (in the peptide Gly-Met-Gly) was converted to methionine in 1 h under the same reaction conditions. These investigators also showed that chymotrypsin previously treated with phenacyl bromide under conditions which inactivate the enzyme concomitant with the alkylation of methionine-192[16] could be reactivated by treatment with β-mercaptoethanol at pH 7.5 (sodium phosphate). It is of interest that the *S*-phenacyl methionine in chymotrypsin is converted to methionine at a substantially faster rate than the tripeptide derivative. The authors speculate that the increased reactivity of the chymotrypsin derivative is a reflection of interaction of the phenacyl moiety with the substrate-binding site.

Alkylation of methionyl residues in pituitary thyrotropin and lutropin with iodoacetic acid has been reported.[17] Differential reactivity of various methionyl residues was reported on reaction with iodoacetate in 0.2 *M* formate, pH 3.0 for 18 h at 37°C.

The reversible alkylation of methionine by iodoacetate in dehydroquinase has been reported by Kleanthous et al.[18] In this reaction, iodoacetate behaves kinetically as an affinity label with a K_i of 30 μ*M* and a k_{inact} of 0.014 min^{-1} at pH 7.0 (50 m*M* potassium phosphate).

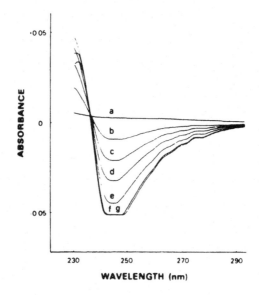

FIGURE 5. The effect of increasing concentration of chloramine-T on the difference spectrum resulting from the interaction of chloramine-T with methionine as shown in Figure 3. Curve a is the spectrum of 24.9 μg methionine in 3.0 ml of 0.1 M phosphate, pH 7.0. Spectra b through g were obtained from the successive additions of 10-μl portions of 10.0 mM chloramine-T. (From Trout, G. E., *Anal. Biochem.*, 93, 419, 1979. With permission.)

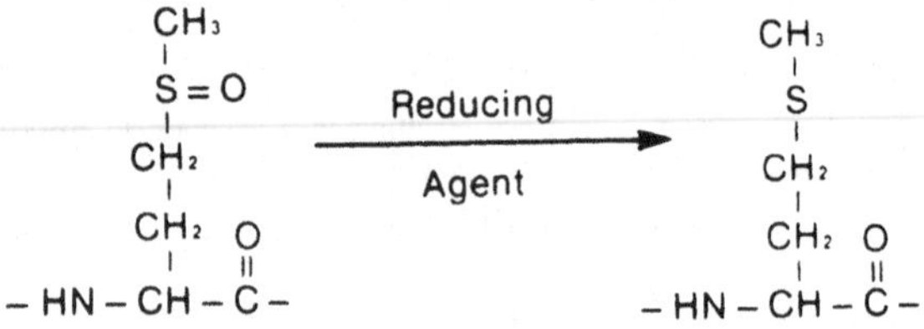

FIGURE 6. The conversion of methionine sulfoxide to methionine in the presence of a reducing agent.

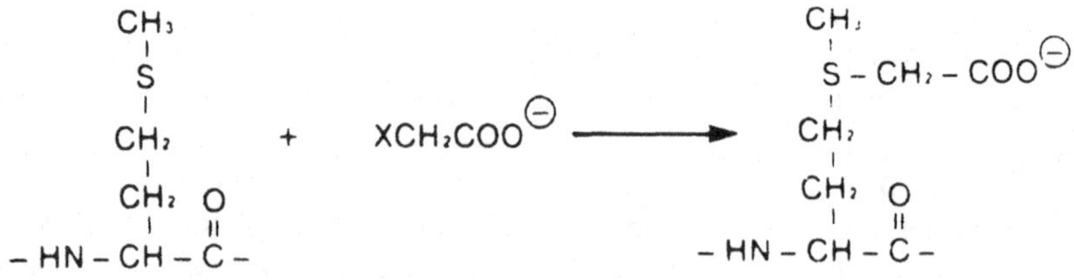

FIGURE 7. The alkylation of methionine with an α-haloacid, such as iodoacetic acid, to form the sulfonium salt derivative.

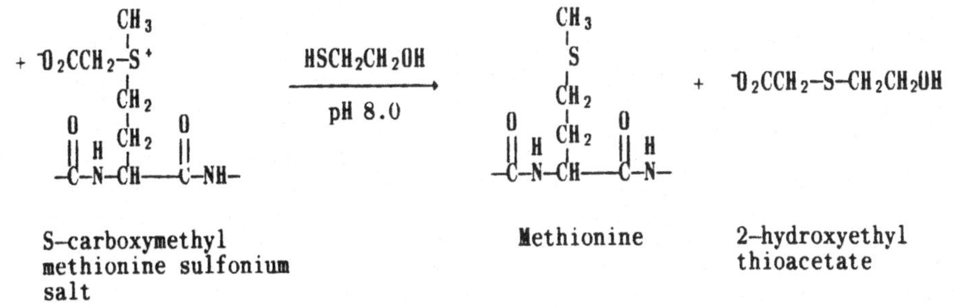

FIGURE 8. Facilitated regeneration of methionine from S-carboxymethyl methionine sulfonium salt in the presence of 2-mercaptoethanol.

There is no reaction with iodoacetamide. Two methionyl residues are modified during the reaction of dehydroquinase with iodoacetate. In a companion study, Kleanthous and Coggins[19] demonstrated that 2-mercaptoethanol treatment under alkaline conditions (0.5% ammonium bicarbonate, 37°C) could reverse modification at one of the two residues. If the modified protein is denatured, there is no reversal of modification at either residue. The results are interpreted in terms of the proximity of a positive charge (i.e., lysine) in close proximity to one of the two methionyl residues which (1) provides the basis for the affinity labeling; and (2) provides the basis for the 2-mercaptoethanol-mediated reversal of modification.

REFERENCES

1. **Oda, T. and Tokushige, M.,** Chemical modification of tryptophanase by chloramine T: a possible involvement of the methionine residue in enzyme activity, *J. Biochem.,* 104, 178, 1988.
2. **Trout, G. E.,** The estimation of microgram amounts of methionine by reaction with chloroamine-T, *Anal. Biochem.,* 93, 419, 1979.
3. **de la Llosa, P., El Abed., A., and Roy, M.,** Oxidation of methionine residues in lutropin, *Can. J. Biochem.,* 58, 745, 1980.
4. **Caldwell, P., Luk, D. C., Weissbach, H., and Brot, N.,** Oxidation of the methionine residues of *Escherichia coli* ribosomal protein L12 decreases the protein's biological activity, *Proc. Natl. Acad. Sci. U.S.A.,* 75, 5349, 1978.
5. **Spande, T. F. and Witkop, B.,** Determination of the tryptophan content of proteins with N-bromosuccinimide, *Meth. Enzymol.,* 11, 498, 1967.
6. **Sakurai, J. and Nagahama, M.,** Role of one tryptophan residue in the lethal activity of *Clostridium perfringens* epsilon toxin, *Biochem. Biophys. Res. Commun.,* 128, 760, 1985.
7. **Houghten, R. A. and Li, C. H.,** Reduction of sulfoxides in peptides and proteins, *Anal. Biochem.,* 98, 36, 1979.
8. **Brot, N., Weissbach, L., Werth, J., and Weissbach, H.,** Enzymatic reduction of protein-bound methionine sulfoxide, *Proc. Natl. Acad. Sci. U.S.A.,* 78, 2155, 1981.
9. **Gundlach, H. G., Moore, S., and Stein, W. H.,** The reaction of iodoacetate with methionine, *J. Biol. Chem.,* 234, 1761, 1959.
10. **Gurd, F. R. N.,** Carboxymethylation, *Meth. Enzymol.,* 11, 532, 1967.
11. **Schroeder, W. A., Shelton, J. R., and Robberson, B.,** Modification of methionyl residues during aminoethylation, *Biochim. Biophys. Acta,* 147, 590, 1967.
12. **Marks, R. H. L. and Miller, R. D.,** Chemical modification of methionine residues in azurin, *Biochem. Biophys. Res. Commun.,* 88, 661, 1979.
13. **Mizzer, J. P. and Thorpe, C.,** An essential methionine in pig kidney general acyl-CoA dehydrogenase, *Biochemistry,* 19, 5500, 1980.
14. **Goren, H. J., Glick, D. M., and Barnard, E. A.,** Analysis of carboxymethylated residues in proteins by an isotopic method and its application to the bromoacetate-ribonuclease reaction, *Arch. Biochem. Biophys.,* 126, 607, 1968.

15. **Naider, F. and Bohak, Z.,** Regeneration of methionyl residues from their sulfonium salts in peptides and proteins, *Biochemistry,* 11, 3208, 1972.
16. **Schramm, H. J. and Lawson, W. B.,** Über das activ Zentrum von Chymotrypsin. II. Modifizierung eines Methioninrestes in Chymotrypsin durch einfache Benzolderivate, *Hoppe-Seyler's Z. Physiol. Chem.,* 332, 97, 1963.
17. **Goverman, J. M. and Pierce, J. G.,** Differential effects of alkylation of methionine residues on the activities of pituitary thyrotropin and lutropin, *J. Biol. Chem.,* 256, 9431, 1981.
18. **Kleanthous, C., Campbell, D. G. and Coggins, J. R.,** Active site labeling of the shikimate pathway enzyme, dehydroquinase. Evidence for a common substrate binding site within dehydroquinase and dehydroquinate synthase, *J. Biol. Chem.,* 265, 10929, 1990.
19. **Kleanthous, C. and Coggins, J. R.,** Reversible alkylation of an active site methionine residue in dehydroquinase, *J. Biol. Chem.,* 265, 10935, 1990.

Chapter 9

THE MODIFICATION OF HISTIDINE RESIDUES

Photooxidation was used early for the modification of proteins,[1] but it was not until the work of Ray and Koshland[2,3] that it proved possible to relate the modification of a specific residue to changes in biological activity. The technique of photooxidation has not proved to be of extensive value because of problems with the specificity of modification. Histidine, methionine, and tryptophan are quite sensitive to photooxidation while tyrosine, serine, and threonine are somewhat less sensitive.[2-4] Despite these difficulties, photooxidation is still used by investigators to explore the role of various functional groups in proteins and protein-protein complexes. Photooxidation was used to identify the protein(s) at the peptidyltransferase site of a bacterial ribosomal subunit.[5,6] Rose bengal dye was used in these experiments. Histidine is the only amino acid modified under the reaction conditions. The time course for the loss of the various biological activities of reconstituted ribosomes on photooxidation is shown in Figure 1. Figure 2 shows the rate of histidine loss during photooxidation. The data are shown to be a summation of a minimum of three separate first-order reactions upon analysis as described by Ray and Koshland.[2] The rates of histidine loss were then compared to the rate of biological activity loss during photooxidation as shown in Figure 3. With the exception of EF-G·GTP binding activity, the loss of biological activity (see Figure 1 for symbols) is most closely related to the "fast" histidine loss. In subsequent experiments, methylene blue dye (Eastman, dye content 91%) was used.[7] Peptidyltransferase activity was lost at a more rapid rate in the presence of methylene blue than rose bengal but data are not presented regarding any differences in residues modified or whether amino acid residues other than histidine are modified in the presence of methylene blue. Other investigators have also explored the effects of photooxidation on peptidyltransferase activity in *Escherichia coli* ribosomes.[8] These experiments were performed in $0.030\ M$ Tris, $0.020\ M$ $MgCl_2$, 0.220 KCl, pH 7.5 (9 mg ribosomes in 0.300 ml) with either eosin or rose bengal as the photooxidation agent. Irradiation was performed at 0 to 4°C using a 500 W slide projector (26 cm from condensor lens to sample) for 20 min. Photooxidation has also been used to study the role of histidine residues in polypeptide chain elongation factor Tu from *E. coli*.[9] The reaction is performed in $0.05\ M$ Tris, $0.010\ M$ Hg $(OAc)_2$, $0.005\ M$ β-mercaptoethanol, 10% glycerol, pH 7.9. Irradiation is performed at 0 to 4°C with gentle stirring using a 375 W tungsten lamp at a distance of 15 cm. A glass plate was placed in the light beam to eliminate UV irradiation. The rose bengal dye is removed after 5 to 30 min from the reaction by chromatography on DEAE-Sephadex A-25 or A-50 equilibrated with $0.050\ M$ Tris, pH 7.9, $0.010\ M$ Mg $(OAc)_2$, $0.005\ M$ β-mercaptoethanol, 10% glycerol. Amino acid analysis after acid hydrolysis (6 N HCl, 22 h, 110°C, or 4 M methanesulfonic acid, 0.2% 2-aminoethylindol, 115°C, 24 h for the determination of tryptophan) demonstrated that only histidine is modified (approximately 5/10 residues are modified; only one residue is modified in the presence of guanosine diphosphate). In a more recent study, photooxidation with methylene blue (25 mM Tris, pH 7.9, 0.05% methylene blue; 8°C) abolished placental anticoagulant protein activity with loss only of histidine residues (based on amino acid analysis).[10] Diol dehydrase was inactivated with first-order kinetics by photooxidation in the presence of either rose bengal or methylene blue.[11] In these experiments, the substitution of an helium atmosphere markedly decreased the rate of enzyme inactivation. There was a difference in the pH dependence of the photooxidation reaction performed in the presence of rose bengal (optimum pH 6.2) as compared to the reaction in the presence of methylene blue (optimum > pH 8.0). The pH dependence for the rose bengal reaction was suggested to reflect the charge status of this compound.

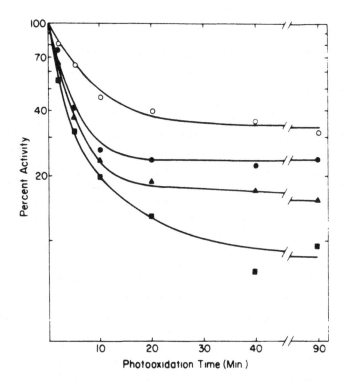

FIGURE 1.   The inactivation of biological activity of ribosome reconstituted with photooxidized ribosomal protein BL3. Ribosomal protein BL3
was photooxidized as the B-13-23 S RNA complex in the presence of rose
bengal. Samples of the purified reconstituted ribosomes were assayed for
EF-G·GTP binding (○), polyphenylalanine synthesis (●), peptidyltransferase activity (▲), and the ability to bind phenylalanyl-tRNA (■). (From
Auron, P. E., Erdelsky, K. J., and Fahnestock, S. R., *J. Biol. Chem.*,
253, 6893, 1978. With permission.)

Histidine residues can be modified by α-halo carboxylic acids and amides (Figure 4) (i.e.,
iodoacetate and iodacetamide). In general, the histidine residue must have either enhanced
nucleophilic character[12] or have been located in a unique microenvironment such as in
ribunoclease.[13-15] Another approach to the modification of histidyl residues at the active site
of certain enzymes (cf. serine proteases) has utilized peptide chloromethyl ketones[17-19] as
affinity labels.

A compound related to α-halo carboxylic acids is *p*-bromophenacyl bromide, which has
been demonstrated in several instances to modify histidyl residues in proteins. *p*-Bromophenacyl bromide modifies a single histidine residue in taipoxin with a 350-fold decrease
in neurotoxicity.[20] The modification was performed in 0.1 *M* sodium cacodylate, pH 6.0,
0.1 *M* NaCl with an eightfold molar excess of *p*-bromide* at 30°C for 22 h. The reaction
mixture was concentrated by lyophilization and subjected to gel filtration (G-25 Sephadex
in 0.1 *M* ammonium acetate) to remove excess reagent and buffer salts. The protein fraction
was taken to dryness as a salt-free preparation and subjected to a second reaction with
p-bromophenacyl bromide. The extent of modification was assessed by both amino acid
analysis (loss of histidine) and spectral analysis ($\Delta\epsilon$ 271 = 17,000 M^{-1} cm^{-1}).[21] Two of
seven histidine residues are modified (1 mol/mol in α-subunit; 1 mol/mol in β-subunit)
under these reaction conditions.

The basic phospholipase A$_2$ from *Naja nigrocollis* venom has been modified with

---

*   It has been the authors' experience that this reagent is somewhat unstable and preparations *must* be recrystallized.

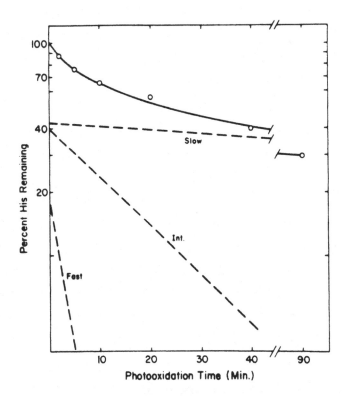

FIGURE 2. The loss of histidine residues occurring with photooxidation of BL3 in the presence of rose bengal dye. The loss of histidine was assessed by amino acid analysis after acid hydrolysis. Loss of amino acids other than histidine was not observed under these experimental conditions. The solid line (O) shows the rate of loss of histidine residues. These data can be fit to represent three different classes of histidine residues as indicated by the broken lines. (From Auron, P. E., Erdelsky, K. J., and Fahnestock. S. R., *J. Biol. Chem.*, 253, 6893, 1978. With permission.)

p-bromophenacyl bromide.[22] The modification was performed in 0.025 *M* Tris, pH 8.0 with a tenfold molar excess of reagent at 30°C. After 40 min of reaction, the mixture was taken to pH 4.0 with glacial acetic acid and taken through a G-25 Sephadex column. Amino acid analysis after acid hydrolysis showed the loss of 1 mol of histidine/mol enzyme with no other significant changes in composition. Subsequent analysis identified His[47] as the residue modified.

The reaction of *p*-bromophenacyl bromide with pancreatic phospholipase A_2 has also been studied.[23] The reaction was performed in 0.1 *M* sodium cacodylate, pH 6.0.[24] Only histidine residues are modified under these conditions and it has been established that His[48] is the residue modified. Under these reaction conditions the second-order rate constant for the reaction of *p*-bromophenacyl bromide with porcine pancreatic phospholipase A_2 is 125 M^{-1} min^{-1} as compared to 79 M^{-1} min^{-1} for phenacyl bromide and 75 M^{-1} min^{-1} for 1-bromooctan-2-one. No reaction was observed with iodoacetamide under these reaction conditions. This same study[23] also explored the methylation of His[48] at the N'-position on the imidazole ring with either methyl *p*-toluenesulfonate or methyl *p*-nitrobenzenesulfonate. Reaction with the latter reagent at pH 6.0 (0.050 *M* cacodylate) (40°C) is more rapid than with the former reagent.

Methyl *p*-nitrobenzenesulfonate has also been used to methylate histidine residue(s) in ribosomal peptidyl transferase.[25] In these experiments the ribosome preparation was modified by a 300-fold molar excess of methyl *p*-nitrobenzenesulfonate (from a stock solution dissolved

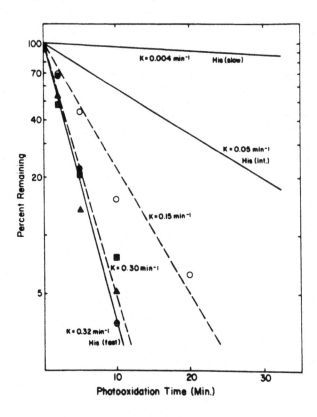

FIGURE 3.   A comparison of the rates of the loss of activity and histidine as a function of time of photooxidation. The solid lines represent the first-order rates for the loss of histidine replotted as a percentage of each class of reactive histidyl residues (see Figure 2). The broken line indicates the loss of activity (for symbols see Figure 1 caption). (From Auron, P. E., Erdelsky, K. J., and Fahnestock, S. R., *J. Biol. Chem.*, 253, 6893, 1978. With permission.)

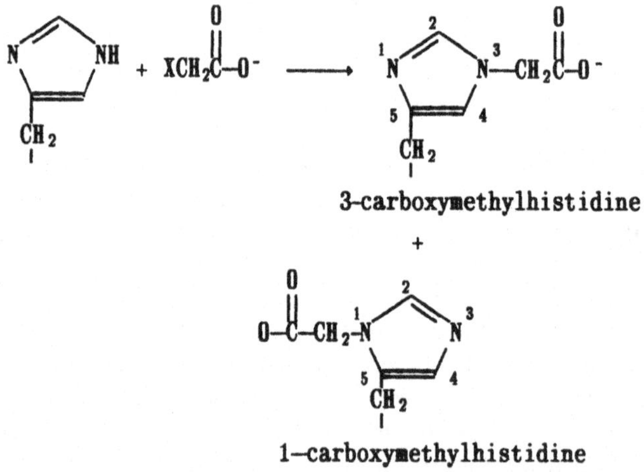

FIGURE 4.   A scheme for the carboxymethylation of histidine with iodoacetate resulting in the formation of 1-carboxymethylhistidine and 3-carboxymethylhistidine.

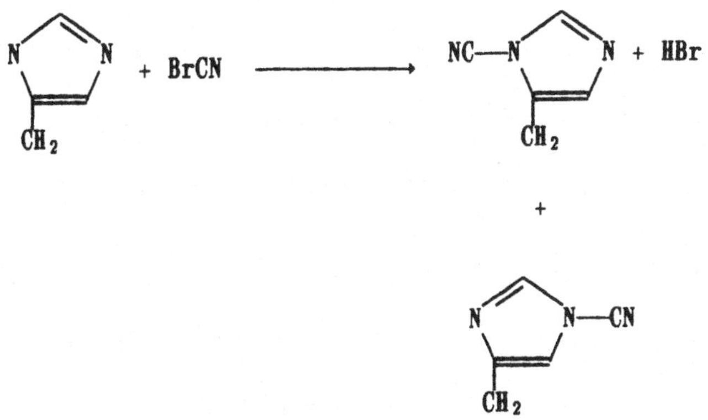

FIGURE 5. The reversible modification of histidine with cyanogen bromide.

in acetonitrile). The reaction took place in 0.01 M Tris, pH 7.4, 0.008 M MgCl$_2$, 0.05 M NH$_4$Cl, 1 μM puromycin at 24°C for 45 min. The author suggests only histidine residues are modified but definitive evidence on this point is absent.

Another example of the modification of histidine by reagents which, in general, react more avidly with other residues is the reaction of D-amino acid oxidase with dansyl chloride.[26] In this study, D-amino acid oxidase was allowed to react with a fivefold molar excess of dansyl chloride (from a stock solution in acetone; final concentration of acetone in the reaction mixture did not exceed 5% final volume) in 0.05 M phosphate, pH 6.6. The reaction was terminated by the addition of benzoate, insoluble material removed by centrifugation, and the mixture passed through a G-25 column equilibrated with 0.06 M phosphate, 0.010 M benzoate, pH 6.6. Reaction with dansyl chloride under these conditions resulted in virtually complete inactivation of the enzyme with the incorporation of 1.7 mol of reagent/ mol enzyme. Substantially complete reactivation occurred with 0.5 M hydroxylamine (NH$_2$OH) at pH 6.6. This reactivation excluded reaction with primary amino functional groups such as lysine, and amino acid analysis suggested the reaction had not occurred with an oxygen nucleophile such as tyrosine. Treatment of the enzyme with diethylpyrocarbonate also resulted in the loss of catalytic activity and reduced the amount of dansyl groups incorporated in a subsequent reaction suggesting that dansyl chloride reacts with the same functional group that reacted with diethylpyrocarbonate.

The cyanation of histidine residues (Figure 5) in myoglobin using an equimolar ratio of cyanogen bromide and protein at pH 7.0 has been reported.[27,28] This derivative is somewhat unstable but has proved useful in spectral studies (NMR, IR, UV-VIS) of this protein.

Competitive labeling (trace labeling; see Chapter 10 for full conceptual description of this technique) of the amino-terminal histidine residue in secretin with 1-fluoro-2,4-dinitrobenzene has been used to study the reactivity of this residue vs. other nucleophiles[29] in this protein. The amino-terminal functional group has a pKa of 8.83 and fivefold greater reactivity than the model compound (histidyl-glycine) while the imidazolium ring has a pKa value of 8.24 and a 26-fold greater reactivity than the model compound. These results were interpreted as reflecting a conformational state where the histidine is interacting with a carboxylate function.

Diethylpyrocarbonate (ethoxyformic anhydride) has become useful during the past 5 to 10 years for studies involving the specific modification of histidine. In the pH range from 5.5 to 7.5, diethylpyrocarbonate is reasonably specific for reaction with histidyl residues. There are several studies of the reaction under more acidic conditions.[30,31] In one of the studies, polymerization of ribonuclease was observed both in deionized water (presumably at acidic pH) and in 0.1 M Tris, pH 7.2. Maleylation of ribonuclease obviated polymerization,

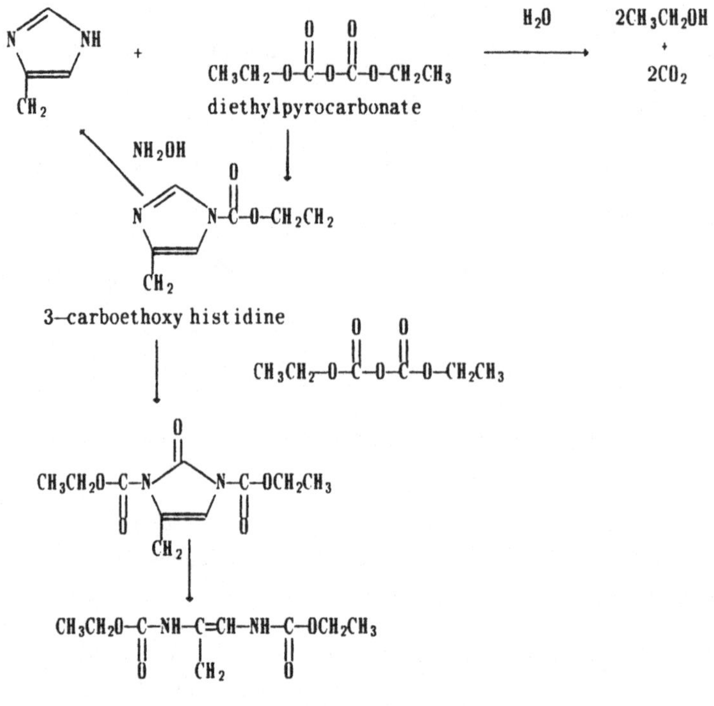

FIGURE 6.   A scheme for the reaction of diethylpyrocarbonate with histidine.

suggesting that the amino groups were involved in this cross-linking reaction. Work with diethylpyrocarbonate through 1975 has been reviewed by Miles.[32]

Reaction of diethylpyrocarbonate with histidine residues at a *moderate excess* of diethylpyrocarbonate results in substitution at one of the nitrogen positions on the imidazole ring (Figure 6). This reaction is associated with an increase in absorbance at 240 nm ($\Delta\epsilon$ = 3200 M^{-1} cm^{-1}). The modification is readily reversed at alkaline pH and, in particular, in the presence of nucleophiles such as Tris. Generally treatment with neutral hydroxylamine (0.1 to 1.0 M, pH 7.0) is used to regenerate histidine. As with the deacylation of O-acetyl tyrosine by neutral hydroxylamine (see Chapter 13), the higher the concentration of hydroxylamine, the more rapid the process of decarboxyethylation. Disubstitution on the imidazole ring, carboxyethylation at both the N_1 and N_3 positions, results in a derivative with altered spectral properties compared to the monosubstituted derivative. This derivative does not regenerate histidine and treatment with neutral hydroxylamine or base results in scission of the imidazole ring. With disubstitution, a loss of histidine is detected by amino acid analysis after acid hydrolysis. Sequence analysis using Edman degradation chemistry also shows the absence of histidine with the presence of a disubstituted derivative.[33] In these studies, a PTH derivative eluting near PTH-glycine was observed and the structure verified by mass spectroscopy. The monosubstituted derivative is unstable under conditions of acid hydrolysis and yields free histidine. Reaction can also occur with other nucleophiles such as cysteine, tyrosine, and primary amino groups. Modification at sulfhydryl residues, not well documented with protein-bound cysteine, can be determined by a decrease in free sulfhydryl groups. Reaction of tyrosine is easily assessed by a decrease in absorbance at 275 to 280 nm similar to that observed on O-acetylation with N-acetylimidazole (see Chapter 13). This modification is reversed by neutral hydroxylamine. Reaction at primary amino groups (α-amino groups; ϵ-amino groups of lysine) results in a derivative which is stable to hydroxylamine. An elegant study[34] has examined the reaction of diethylpyrocarbonate with histidyl residues in cytochrome b_5. Using NMR spectroscopy with this well-characterized protein it has been possible to identify factors influencing histidine modification with this reagent; three major factors include (1) the pKA of the individual histidine residue; (2) solvent exposure of the residue; and (3) hydrogen bonding of the imidazolium ring. Furthermore, these investigators point out that tautamerization of the imidazolium ring leads to heterogeneity of modification which, in turn, explains differences in the spectral properties of modified proteins.[32] Site-specific mutagenesis studies of subtilisin[35] have demonstrated the influence of neighboring charged groups on histidine ionization (and, hence, reactivity).

As described in some detail by Miles,[32] the reagent is very sensitive to base-catalyzed hydrolysis. At ambient temperature, the $T_{1/2}$ for the hydrolysis of diethylpyrocarbonate at pH 7.0 (phosphate) is less than 10 min and is markedly shorter with increasing pH. Increasing the pH not only decreases reagent stability (and thus the concentration of one component of a second-order reaction over the time period studied) but also increases the possibility of reaction at primary amine functional groups. In our laboratory we have found it convenient to use dilute (0.025 to 0.100 M) phosphate buffer, pH 6.0 for our studies. We prepare stock solutions of diethylpyrocarbonate in *anhydrous* ethanol. These solutions are used within a few hours and the actual concentration of reagent obtained by the stoichiometry of reaction with imidazole in the pH 6.0 buffer using the increase in absorbance at 230 nm to monitor the reaction ($\Delta\epsilon = 3 \times 10^3$ M^{-1} cm^{-1})[30,32] both before and after a given series of experiments. Morjana and Scarborough[36] have presented data on the rate of diethylpyrocarbonate hydrolysis and discussed the necessity of correcting for actual reagent concentration. It should be noted that there is not complete agreement regarding the magnitude of the spectral change as a result of carboxyethylation. The value $\Delta\epsilon = 3200$ M^{-1} cm^{-1} at 242 nm is given above. Other investigators have used the value of $\Delta\epsilon = 3600$ M^{-1} cm^{-1} at 240 nm.[37,38] A value of $\Delta\epsilon = 3500$ M^{-1} cm^{-1} at 242 nm has also been reported.[39] Most of these values have been obtained by the use of reaction with model compounds such as *N*-acetylhistidine. Neurath and co-workers[39] have noted that the use of spectral analysis of histidine modification with intact protein is greatly complicated if modification of tyrosine is occuring concomitantly. This situation results from the marked decrease in absorbance of tyrosine at 234 nm which will decrease the magnitude of the net absorbance increase in the 230 to 250 nm range resulting from histidine modification. Roosemont[40] has considered this problem in some detail. The greater the excess of diethylpyrocarbonate used the less reliable the value for $\Delta\epsilon$ obtained with *known* stoichiometric modification of model histidine (imidazole derivative) compounds. This is shown in Figure 7 where increasing the ratio of diethylpyrocarbonate to histidine results in species with increased absorbance. It is suggested that the commonly used $\Delta\epsilon = 3,200$ M^{-1} cm^{-1} can only be used at low concentrations of diethylpyrocarbonate.

A single histidine residue essential for catalysis by D-xylose isomerase has been identified by reaction with diethylpyrocarbonate.[41] Instability of *N*-carboethoxyhistidine has made unequivocal identification of the histidyl residues modified by diethylpyrocarbonate difficult. In this study, the protein was first denatured in 6.0 M guanidine hydrochloride (pH 7.0) and then digested with subtilisin in 2.0 M guanidine hydrochloride at pH 7.0/30°C for 2 h. A single peptide containing the modified histidine residue was purified by HPLC using dual wavelength detection. In this technique, effluent is monitored by absorbance at 238 nm (the maximum in the difference spectrum between the modified and native protein) and absorbance at 214 nm (peptide bond absorbance). The ratio of A_{238}/A_{214} was used to identify peptides containing the modified histidine residues.

Selected examples of the use of diethylpyrocarbonate to study the function of histidyl residues in proteins are presented in Table 1.

Neurath and co-workers[39] have examined the reaction of thermolysin with diethylpyrocarbonate (ethoxyformic anhydride) in some detail. The time course for the loss of catalytic

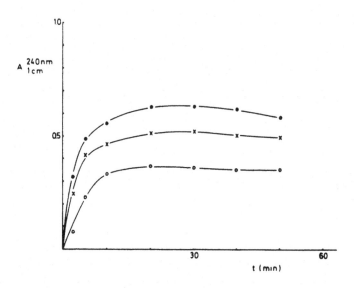

FIGURE 7.   The time course for the increase in absorbance at 240 nm occurring upon reaction between histidine and diethylpyrocarbonate (DEP) as a function of diethylpyrocarbonate concentration. The reaction mixtures were 0.1 mM with respect to histidine in 0.1 M acetate, pH 6.0 at 2.3 mM DEP (O), 11.5 mM DEP (x) and 23 mM DEP (●). (From Roosemont, J. L., *Anal. Biochem.*, 88, 314, 1978. With permission.)

activity by thermolysin upon reaction with diethylpyrocarbonate is shown in Figure 8. Also shown in Figure 8 is the recovery of activity upon reaction of the modified protein with hydroxylamine. Under these reaction conditions 13.4 carboethoxy groups were incorporated per mole of enzyme. The presence of carbobenzoxy-L-phenylalanine, a competitive inhibitor, protected the enzyme from inactivation and reduced the extent of modification to 12.5 mol/mol protein. It should be noted that the reaction demonstrated a pH dependence (Figure 9) consistent with the modification of histidine. Figure 10 shows the difference spectra of thermolysin (panel A) after reaction with diethylpyrocarbonate (solid line) and then after subsequent reaction with 0.020 M neutral hydroxylamine (broken line). This is compared with panel B where the difference spectrum obtained on the reaction of diethyl-pyrocarbonate with N-acetyl-L-tyrosine ethyl ester (solid line) or imidazole (broken line); the dotted line is the algebraic sum of the two reactions. The increase at 242 nm is consistent with the modification of histidine while the decrease at 278 to 280 nm is indicative of tyrosine modification. The tyrosyl residues modified during the reaction were *not* regenerated on reaction with 0.020 M hydroxylamine (Figure 11). These investigators also make the point that there is a significant decrease in the absorbance of N-acetyl-L-tyrosine ethyl ester at 234 nm (Figure 10, panel B) which would affect the accuracy of measurement at 240 to 242 nm for the determination of the extent of histidine modification. These investigators found it more accurate to determine the extent of histidine modification by spectral measurement during hydroxylamine reactivation.

McCormick and co-workers[42] have examined the reaction of diethylpyrocarbonate with pyridoxamine (pyridoxine)-5'-phosphate oxidase. The modification reaction was performed at pH 7.0 (0.1 M potassium phosphate containing 5% (v/v) EtOH) at 25°C generally in the presence of flavin mononucleotide (FMN). Figure 12 shows the time course for the modification of the oxidase under these experimental conditions. Also shown in Figure 12 is the dependence of the observed first-order rate constant on diethylpyrocarbonate concentration (panel B). The inset plot shows the reaction to be second-order with a rate constant of 12.5 $M^{-1} s^{-1}$.

Table 1
THE REACTION OF DIETHYLPYROCARBONATE WITH HISTIDYL RESIDUES IN PROTEINS

Protein	Solvent/temp.	Reagent excess[a]	Extent of modification[b]	Second-order rate constant[c] (1 M^{-1} min^{-1})	Other amino acid modified	Ref.
Thermolysin	0.05 M CaCl$_2$, 0.1 M NaCl, 0.025 M HEPES, pH 7.2/25°C	—	2/[d]	—	Tyr (2), Lys (8)	1
Thermolysin	0.05 M CaCl$_2$ 0.025 M HEPES, pH 5.7/25°C	—	1/[d]	—	Tyr (1), Lys (2)	1
Bacterial luciferase	0.1 M phosphate/pH 6.1/0°C	600	3/	146[e]	—	2
Crotoxin	Half-saturated NaOAc	1,000	—	7[e]	—	3
Prostatic acid phosphatase	0.025 M sodium barbital, 0.15 M NaCl, pH 6.9/25°C	5,000	12/27		f	
Pyridoxamine-5'-phosphate oxidase	0.1 M phosphate, pH 7.0/25°C	500	4/7	750[g]	Cys (1/6)[h]	5
Yeast enolase	0.050 M ADA, 0.001 M MgCl$_2$, 0.01 mM EDTA, pH 6.1/0°C	1,390	6/[i]	55.0[j] 10.7[i]	k	6
Fructose bisphosphatase	0.050 M acetate, pH 6.5	4,000 8,000 40,000	5.3/13 8.8/13 13/13[l]	—	l	7
Ribulose bisphosphate carboxylase	0.050 or Tris, 0.001 M EDTA, 0.020 M MgCl$_2$ pH 7.0/30°C	—	2/2	m	n	8
Escherichia coli elongation factor Tu	—[o]	—	—	—	—	10
L-α-Hydroxy acid oxidase	0.020 M MES, pH 7.0/25°C	—	2/[p]	690[q]	r	11
Thiamin binding protein from Saccharomyces cerevisiae	0.050 M sodium phosphate, pH 7.0/25°C	—	—	120.5[s]	—	12
Clostridium histolyticum collagenase	0.050 M HEPES 0.010 M CaCl$_2$, p 17.5/22°C	—	—	—	—	13
Lactate dehydrogenase	0.1 M sodium pyrophosphate, pH 7.2/10°C	—	—	10380 522[t]	—	14
Mitochondrial nicotinamide nucleotide transhydrogenase	0.025 M sucrose, 0.020 M MES, pH 5.9/23°C	—	—	—	—	15
Alcohol oxidase	0.050 M sodium, phosphate, pH 7.5/0°C	—	4/	25.2	w	16

Table 1 (continued)
THE REACTION OF DIETHYLPYROCARBONATE WITH HISTIDYL RESIDUES IN PROTEINS

Protein	Solvent/temp.	Reagent excess[a]	Extent of modification[b]	Second-order rate constant[c] ($1\ M^{-1}\ min^{-1}$)	Other amino acid modified	Ref.
D-β-hydroxybutyrate dehydrogenase	0.020 MES, 5 M rotenone, pH 6.0/	—	—	—	—	8
Benzodiazepine receptor	0.01 M sodium phosphate, 0.2 M NaCl, pH 6.0	—	—	—	—	19
Scrapie agent	0.020 M Tris, pH 7.4 containg 1 mM EDTA and 0.2% Sarkosyl/23°C	—	—	—	x	20
Succinate dehydrogenase	0.24 M sucrose, 0.100 M potassium phosphate, pH 6.0/0°C	—	—	—	y	21
Ribulose bis-phosphate carboxylase/oxygenase	0.050 M Tris, 0.001 M EDTA, 0.020 M MgCl₂, pH 7.0/21°C	—	3.4/[a]	2340	—	22
Transferrin	0.01 M potassium phosphate, 0.05 KCl, pH 6.1	—	54—72%[aa]	—	—	23
Dihydrofolate reductase	0.05 M Tris, pH 7.5/10°C	—	6/7	29	bb	24
RNA polymerase	100 mM phosphate, pH 6.0, ambient	50—500	—	—	—	25
A₁ Adenosine receptor	20 mM potassium phosphate, pH 7.0 ambient	—	—	—	—	26
Lysyl oxidase	200 mM potassium phosphate, pH 7.0, ambient	—	—	$2.5\ min^{-1}\ mM^{-1}$	—	27
Malic enzyme	50 mM acetate, pH 6.0 with 1.0 mM EDTA/25°C	—	2.8/5.0[cc] 1.8/5.0[cc]	—	—	28 28
Neurospora membrane ATPase	50 mM HEPES, pH 6.9 with 30% (V/V) glycerol	—	—	$385\text{—}420\ min^-\ M^{-1}$[dd]	—	29
Asparaginase	50 mM MES, pH 6.0, 25°C	—	—	—	—	30
Ampicillin acylase	10 mM sodium phosphate, pH 7.0	—	—	—	—	31
Pancreatic lipase	100 mM phosphate, pH 6.0/ambient	—	—	—	—	32
Lipase fragment	100 mM phosphate, pH 6.0/ambient	—	—	—	—	33
Phenol hydroxylase	50 mM potassium phosphate, pH 6.0, 4°C[ff]	—	—	[ee]	—	34
Lysolecithin-lysolecithin acyltransferase	100 mM phosphate, pH 6.5	—	—	$1.17\ min^{-1}\ mM^{-1}$[gg] $0.56\ min^{-1}\ mM^{-1}$	—	35

a Moles/mole of protein.

b Residues His modified/total His in protein.

c For reaction with histidine.

d Inactivation was demonstrated to result from the modification of a single histidine residue.

e Assuming loss of activity is a direct indication of a single histidine modification.

f There was only partial recovery of activity upon treatment with hydroxylamine (0.2 M, pH 7.0, 25°C). Two residues of histidine were lost as assessed by amino acid analysis after acid hydrolysis without loss of other amino acids suggesting that disubstitution has occurred on the imidazole ring of certain histidine residues.

g For inactivation of catalytic activity. A value of 51.6 M^{-1} sec^{-1} (3096 M^{-1} min^{-1}) was calculated for the pH-independent second order rate constant.

h No direct determination of primary amino modification is reported. Activity is recovered by neutral hydroxylamine (0.09 M). Direct determination of tryptophan and tyrosine revealed no loss of these residues.

i Obtained from reaction at either 0 or 25°C.

j Data obtained at pH 6.6 (0.050 M N-(2-acetamido) iminodiacetic acid, ADA), at 0°C. Two-phase reaction was observed.

k Spectral analysis did not indicate tyrosine modification. Possible primary amine modification was not determined. The loss in catalytic activity was reversed by 0.25 M hydroxylamine, pH 7.0.

l Addition of more diethylpyrocarbonate results in further increases in absorbance at 242 nm suggesting disubstitution on the imidazole ring of histidyl residues. Spectral analysis did not suggest modification of tyrosine under the reaction conditions. Possible modification of primary groups was not assessed.

m The reaction of diethylpyrocarbonate with ribulose bisphosphate carboxylase shows saturation kinetics (k = 7.3 mM) suggesting "specific" binding of diethylpyrocarbonate to the enzyme prior to the reaction resulting in inactivation. Data are not presented to show a similar phenomena with the actual reaction of histidyl residues in the enzyme.

n Activity was recovered by treatment with hydroxylamine (0.4 M NH$_2$OH, pH 7.0, 48 hr at 4°C increased activity from 55 to 89%; similar treatment at 25°C resulted in similar activity recovery in 1 hr). The authors note that reaction of diethylpyrocarbonate with cysteine (N-acetylcysteine) also results in an increase in absorbance at 240 nm that is reversed by hydroxylamine. This reaction apparently occurs only in carboxylate buffers (e.g. acetate or succinate) and has been noted by other investigators.[9] The reaction product of diethylpyrocarbonate with cysteine is considerably less stable than N-carbethoxyimidazole derivatives.

o The crystalline enzyme preparation (7 nmoles) [washed with 41% (NH$_4$)$_2$ SO$_4$] was dissolved in 0.600 mℓ, 0.010 M Tris, pH 7.0 containing 5 mM MgCl$_2$, 0.100 M KCl and 10 μM guanosine diphosphate. The pH of this solution was then adjusted to 6.0 with 1.0 M sodium cacodylate — 0.050 M MgCl$_2$.

p Per FMN (hence per dimer, therefore this would be 4 residues/tetramer).

q Determined from rate of loss of catalytic activity.

r No reaction at cysteine, tryptophan or tyrosine is observed under these reaction conditions.

s Determined from rate of loss of thiamine binding activity.

t Thiomethylated at cysteine-165 (reaction with methyl methanethiosulfonate). Enzyme remains catalytically active but with reduced affinity for pyruvate and lactate.

u The second order rate constant for the native enzyme is 10,920 M^{-1} min^{-1}. These values were obtained from the measurement of the rate of loss of enzyme activity. Virtually identical values were obtained from direct measurement of histidine modification by spectroscopy.

v Diethylpyrocarbonate introduced as acetonitrile solution.

w Incorporation of radiolabeled diethylpyrocarbonate was closely related to extent of histidine modification as assessed by spectroscopy ($\Delta\epsilon$ = 3900 M^{-1} cm^{-1} for monosubstituted derivative). Hydroxylamine treatment did not result in recovery of enzyme activity although radiolabel was lost. The enzyme was inactivated by 10 mM hydroxylamine at neutral pH, 0°C. This is not an infrequent observation from our consideration of the literature in this area. Although very few investigators (we have not found any report) have examined the possibility of peptide bond cleavage with hydroxylamine at neutral pH, the possibility cannot be disregarded considering the cleavage of Asn-Gly bonds under more alkaline conditions.[17]

Table 1 (continued)
THE REACTION OF DIETHYLPYROCARBONATE WITH HISTIDYL RESIDUES IN PROTEINS

x   Inactivation reversed by 0.100 to 0.5 M hydroxylamine. The pH of this reaction is not specified.

y   Submitochondrial particles were used in this study. The inactivation produced by diethylpyrocarbonate is partially reversed by neutral (pH 7.0) hydroxylamine. The extent of activity recovery was dependent on hydroxylamine with maximum activity recovery at 0.020 M hydroxylamine decreasing significantly at 0.115 M hydroxylamine.

z   Stoichiometry determined by spectral analysis ($\Delta\epsilon = 3200$ M^{-1} cm^{-1} at 240 nm) (3.4 residues modified) is in excellent agreement with amount of radiolabeled diethylpyrocarbonate incorporated (3.5).

aa Varied with species source of transferrin: human 14/7; rabbit, 14/18; human lactotransferrin, 7/9; bovine lactotransferrin, 7/10; chicken ovotransferrin, 9/14.

bb There is no reaction with tyrosine under these conditions. Reaction at primary amine functions was not excluded. Only partial reactivation is obtained upon treatment with hydroxylamine (approximately 50% recovery with 1.0 M hydroxylamine; no reaction at 0.1 M hydroxylamine).

cc Differences were noted between enzymes isolated from aged animals (old) and young animals (young). The difference in the extent of modification (5.0 residues are present in the native enzyme) is ascribed to oxidation occurring during the aging process.

dd Partial reactivation with hydroxylamine but no detectable modification at tyrosyl residues.

ee Fast (A) and slow (B) reaction and reaction at non-histidine residues as being involved in the loss of activity. K_A, 0.46 min^{-1}; K_B, 0.011 min^{-1}; and K_C, 0.031 min^{-1}.

ff Alternatively, 20 mM MES (pH 5.0 to 5.5) was used with 50 mM sodium phosphate.

gg Inactivation of hydrolytic reaction, 1.17 min^{-1} mM^{-1}; inactivation of transacylation, 0.56 min^{-1} mM.$^{-1}$ It was concluded that two different histidine residues are necessary for hydrolysis and only one histidine residue for transacylation.

References for Table 1

1. **Burstein, Y., Walsh, K. A., and Neurath, H.,** Evidence of an essential histidine residue in thermolysin, *Biochemistry,* 13, 205, 1974.
2. **Cousineau, J. and Meighen, E.,** Chemical modification of bacterial luciferase with ethoxyformic anhydride: evidence for an essential histidyl residue, *Biochemistry,* 15, 4992, 1976.
3. **Jeng, T.-W. and Fraenkel-Conrat, H.,** Chemical modification of histidine and lysine residues of crotoxin, *FEBS Lett.,* 87, 291, 1978.
4. **McTigue, J. J. and van Etten, R. L.,** An essential active-site histidine residue in human prostatic acid phosphatase. Ethoxyformylation by diethylpyrocarbonate and phosphorylation by a substrate, *Biochim. Biophys. Acta,* 523, 407, 1978.
5. **Horiike, K., Tsuge, H., and McCormick, D. B.,** Evidence for an essential histidyl residue at the active site of pyridoxamine (pyridoxine)-5'-phosphate oxidase from rabbit liver, *J. Biol. Chem.,* 254, 6638, 1979.
6. **George, A. L., Jr. and Borders, C. L., Jr.,** Chemical modification of histidyl and lysyl residues in yeast enolase, *Biochim. Biophys. Acta,* 569, 63, 1979.
7. **Demaine, M. M. and Benkovic, S. J.,** Selective modification of rabbit liver fructose bisphosphatase, *Arch. Biochem. Biophys.,* 205, 308, 1980.
8. **Saluja, A. K. and McFadden, B. A.,** Modification of histidine at the active site of spinach ribulose bisphosphate carboxylase, *Biochem. Biophys. Res. Commun.,* 94, 1091, 1980.
9. **Garrison, C. K. and Himes, R. H.,** The reaction between diethylpyrocarbonate and sulfhydryl groups in carboxylate buffers, *Biochem. Biophys. Res. Commun.,* 67, 1251, 1975.
10. **Jonák, J. and Rychlik, I.,** Chemical evidence for the involvement of histidyl residues in the functioning of *Escherichia coli* elongation factor Tu, *FEBS Lett.,* 117, 167, 1980.
11. **Meyer, S. E. and Cromartie, T. H.,** Role of essential histidine residues in L-α-hydroxy acid oxidase from rat kidney, *Biochemistry,* 19, 1874, 1980.
12. **Nishimura, H., Sempuku, K., and Iwashima, A.,** Possible functional roles of carboxyl and histidine residues in a soluble thiamine-binding protein of *Saccharomyces cerevisiae, Biochim. Biophys. Acta,* 668, 333, 1981.
13. **Bond, M. D., Steinbrink, D. R., and Van Wart, H. E.,** Identification of essential amino acid residues in *Clostridium histolyticum* collagenase using chemical modification reactions, *Biochem. Biophys. Res. Commun.,* 102, 243, 1981.
14. **Bloxham, D. P.,** The chemical reactivity of the histidine-195 residue in lactate dehydrogenase thiomethylated at the cysteine-165 residue, *Biochem. J.,* 193, 93, 1981.
15. **Phelps, D. C. and Hatefi, Y.,** Inhibition of the mitochondrial nicotinamide nucleotide transhydrogenase by dicyclohexylcarbodiimide and diethylpyrocarbonate, *J. Biol. Chem.,* 256, 8217, 1981.
16. **Cromartie, T. H.,** Sulfhydryl and histidinyl residues in the flavoenzyme alcohol oxidase from *Candida boidinii, Biochemistry,* 20, 5416, 1981.
17. **Bornstein, P. and Balian, G.,** Cleavage at Asn-Gly bonds with hydroxylamine, *Meth. Enzymol.,* 47, 132, 1977.
18. **Phelps, D. C. and Hatefi, Y.,** Inhibition of D-β-hydroxybutyrate dehydrogenase by butanedione, phenylglyoxal and diethyl pyrocarbonate, *Biochemistry,* 20, 459, 1981.
19. **Burch, T. P. and Ticku, M. K.,** Histidine modification with diethylpyrocarbonate shows heterogeneity of benzodiazepine receptors, *Proc. Natl. Acad. Sci. U.S.A.,* 78, 3945, 1981.
20. **McKinley, M. P., Masiarz, F. R., and Prusiner, S. B.,** Reversible chemical modification of the scrapie agent, *Science,* 214, 1259, 1981.
21. **Vik, S. B. and Hatefi, Y.,** Possible occurrence and role of an essential histidyl residue in succinate dehydrogenase, *Proc. Natl. Acad. Sci. U.S.A.,* 78, 6749, 1981.
22. **Saluja, A. K. and McFadden, B. A.,** Modification of the active site histidine in ribulosebisphosphate carboxylase/oxygenase, *Biochemistry,* 21, 89, 1982.
23. **Mazurier, J., Leger, D., Tordera, V., Montreuil, J., and Spik, G.,** Comparative study of the iron-binding properties of transferrins. Differences in the involvement of histidine residues as revealed by carbethoxylation, *Eur. J. Biochem.,* 119, 537, 1981.
24. **Daron, H. H. and Aull, J. L.,** Inactivation of dihydrofolate reductase from *Lactobacillus casei* by diethylpyrocarbonate, *Biochemistry,* 21, 737, 1982.
25. **Abdulwajid, A. W. and Wu, F. Y.-H.,** Chemical modification of *Escherichia coli* RNA polymerase by diethyl pyrocarbonate: evidence of histidine requirement for enzyme activity and intrinsic zinc binding, *Biochemistry,* 25, 8167, 1986.
26. **Klotz, K.-N., Lohse, M. J., and Schwabe, U.,** Chemical modification of A_1 adenosine receptors in rat brain membranes. Evidence for histidine in different domains of the ligand binding site, *J. Biol. Chem.,* 263, 17522, 1988.
27. **Gacheru, S. N., Trackman, P. C., and Kagan, H. M.,** Evidence for a functional role for histidine in lysyl oxidase catalysis, *J. Biol. Chem.,* 263, 16704, 1988.

References for Table 1 (continued)

28. **Gordillo, E., Ayala, A., F.-Lobato, M., Bautista, J., and Machado, A.,** Possible involvement of histidine residues in the loss of enzymatic activity of rat liver malic enzyme during aging, *J. Biol. Chem.*, 263, 8053, 1988.

29. **Morjana, N. A. and Scarborough, G. A.,** Evidence for an essential histidine residue in the *Neurospora crassa* plasma membrane H$^+$[T-ATPase, *Biochim. Biophys. Acta*, 985, 19, 1989.

30. **Bagert, U. and Röhm, K.-H.,** On the role of histidine and tyrosine residues in *E. coli* asparaginase. Chemical modification and ^{1}[TH-nuclear magnetic resonance studies, *Biochim. Biophys. Acta*, 999, 36, 1989.

31. **Kim, D. J. and Byun, S. M.,** Evidence for involvement of 2 histidine residues in the reaction of ampicillin acylase, *Biochem. Biophys. Res. Commun.*, 166, 904, 1990.

32. **De Caro, J. D., Guidoni, A. A., Bonicel, J. J., and Rovery, M.,** The histidines reacting with ethoxyformic anhydride in porcine pancreatic lipase: their relationships with enzyme activity, *Biochimie*, 71, 1211, 1989.

33. **De Caro, J. D., Rouimi, P., and Rovery, M.,** Hydrolysis of *p*-nitrophenyl acetate by the peptide chain fragment (335-449) of porcine pancreatic lipase, *Eur. J. Biochem.*, 158, 601, 1986.

34. **Sejlitz, T. and Neujahnr, H. Y.,** Chemical modification of phenol hydroxylase by ethoxyformic anhydride, *Eur. J. Biochem.*, 170, 351, 1987.

35. **Kinnunen, P. M., DeMichele, A., and Lange, L. G.,** Chemical modification of acyl-CoA:cholesterol *O*-acyltransferase. 1. Identification of acyl-CoA:cholesterol *O*-acyltransferase subtypes by differential diethyl pyrocarbonate sensitivity, *Biochemistry*, 27, 7344, 1988.

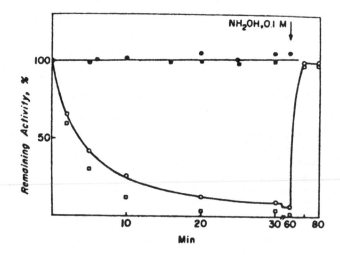

FIGURE 8. The inactivation of thermolysin (15 μ*M*) by diethylpyrocarbonate (3 m*M*) in 0.020 *M* HEPES, 0.005 *M* CaCl$_2$, pH 7.2 in the presence (●,■) or absence (○,□) of 5 m*M* Cbz-phenylalanine. Catalytic activity was determined with either furylacryloylglycyl-L-leucinamide (●,○) or casein (■,□). The arrow indicates the addition of neutral hydroxylamine (pH 7.2) to a final concentration of 0.1 *M*. (From Burstein, Y., Walsh, K. A., and Neurath, H., *Biochemistry*, 13, 205, 1974. With permission.)

Figure 13 shows the pH dependence for the inactivation process. The loss of catalytic activity appeared to be correlated with the modification of one of the four histidyl residues in this protein. This residue appears to be more accessible for modification as shown in Figure 14. Gordillo et al.[43] have used diethylpyrocarbonate reactivity to study the effects of aging on malic enzyme activity. Malic enzyme from "old" animals is 36% less active than that obtained from "young" animals. Reaction with diethylpyrocarbonate showed a decrease of approximately one residue in the "old" enzyme.

Kinnunen and co-workers[44] have been able to differentiate subtypes of acyl-CoA:cholesterol acyltransferase by reactivity with diethylpyrocarbonate (DEP). The liver enzyme (DEP-resistant) had an apparent Ki of 1500 μ*M* while the aortic enzyme (DEP-sensitive) had a Ki of 40 μ*M*.

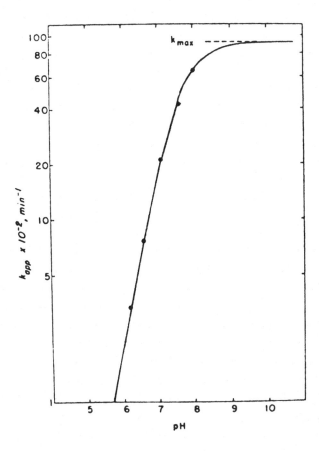

FIGURE 9. The pH dependence for the pseudo-first-order rate constant for the inactivation of thermolysin by diethylpyrocarbonate. The line is a theoretical curve calculated from

$$k_{app} = \frac{k_{max}}{1 + [H^+]K_a}$$

assuming a single ionizing group of pKa = 7.6 and k_{max} = 0.91 min^{-1}. (From Burstein, Y., Walsh, K. A., and Neurath, H., *Biochemistry*, 13, 205, 1974. With permission.)

Saluja and McFadden[45] have explored the reaction of diethylpyrocarbonate with spinach ribulose bisphosphate carboxylase. One interesting observation is that the plot of half-inactivation time vs. the reciprocal of diethylpyrocarbonate concentration suggested that saturation kinetics existed consistent with the "affinity" binding of reagent prior to protein modification. The solid line shows the change in absorbance at 242 nm (Figure 15) of the carboxylase upon reaction with diethylpyrocarbonate (the magnitude of the increase is consistent with the modification of 2.4 histidine residues per combination of small subunit and large subunit). This change is completely reversed on treatment with hydroxylamine. Also shown is the change in absorbance at 242 nm on the reaction of *N*-acetylcysteine with diethylpyrocarbonate in 0.1 *M* succinate pH 6.4. This spectral change occurs only in *carboxylate* buffers and is comparatively transient when compared to the protein reaction product. The study of Bloxham[46] on the reactivity of the active site histidine in lactate dehydrogenase is particularly fascinating. The rate of reaction of the histidine residue in the native enzyme was compared to the thiomethyl derivative (prepared by reaction with methyl methanethiosulfonate) as shown in Figure 16. There is a substantial decrease in the nucleophilic character of the active-site histidine (histidine-195). Cromartie[47] has examined the modification of alcohol oxidase with diethylpyrocarbonate in 0.050 *M* sodium phosphate, pH 7.5, at 0°C.

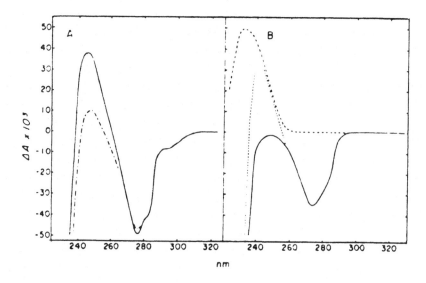

FIGURE 10.   (A) Difference UV absorption spectra of thermolysin after inactivation by diethylpyrocarbonate and reactivation by neutral hydroxylamine. Equal volumes (2.5 ml of enzyme (15 μM) in 0.02 M HEPES, 0.1 NaCl, 5 mM CaCl₂) were placed in two spectrophotometer cuvettes. Diethypyrocarbonate (25 μl of 0.3 M solution in ethanol) was added to one cuvette and an equal volume of ethanol added to the other cuvette. The difference spectra were determined after 40 min (solid line). Hydroxylamine (25 μl of a 2.0 M solution, pH 7.0) was then added to both cells and the difference spectra determined 40 min later (broken line). (B) Spectral changes of model compounds after treatment with diethylpyrocarbonate (15 μM) in 0.025 M HEPES, pH 7.0. The solid line is 50 μM N-acetyl-L-tyrosine ethyl ester while the broken line is 2 mM imidazole. The dotted line is the algebraic sum of the two difference spectra. (From Burstein, Y., Walsh, K. A., and Neurath, H., *Biochemistry*, 13, 205, 1974. With permission.)

The UV difference spectrum of the enzyme before (a) and after (b) the addition of diethyl-pyrocarbonate is shown in Figure 17. No evidence for tyrosine modification is seen under these reaction conditions. Further kinetic analysis supported the modification of histidine as the event responsible for inactivation of catalytic activity. It is, however, of interest to note that treatment with neutral hydroxylamine (0.010 to 0.100 M) did not result in the recovery of catalytic activity although most of the radiolabeled reagent was removed ([1-¹⁴C]-di-ethylpyrocarbonate). It was observed that 0.010 M hydroxylamine caused an 80% loss of alcohol oxidase activity at 0°C. As mentioned above, reaction of diethylpyrocarbonate at pH values above 7.0 does increase the possibility of amino group modification. This is demonstrated by the observation of Van Wart and co-workers[48] on the reaction of diethyl-pyrocarbonate with a bacterial collagenase. Reaction of the enzyme with diethylpyrocar-bonate results in the loss of catalytic activity. Reaction with hydroxylamine did not markedly restore enzymatic activity. Hydroxylamine by itself did not have a deleterious effect on catalytic activity as treatment with this reagent did restore activity lost on the modification of tyrosyl residues with N-acetylimidazole. These investigators consider modification of the ε-amino group(s) of lysine with diethylpyrocarbonate to be a more likely cause for the irreversible loss of enzymic activity. Daron and Aull[49] have studied the reaction of diethyl-pyrocarbonate with dihydrofolate reductase *(Lactobacillus casei)*. The UV spectra of the enzyme before and after reaction with diethylpyrocarbonate are shown in Figure 18. Catalytic activity is lost on reaction with diethylpyrocarbonate but is partially recovered on reaction with 1.0 M hydroxylamine (pH 7.5) but not with 0.1 M hydroxylamine (pH 7.5.) (Figure 19). Clearly the reaction of proteins with hydroxylamine after modification with diethyl-pyrocarbonate must be carefully studied in order to obtain meaningful results.

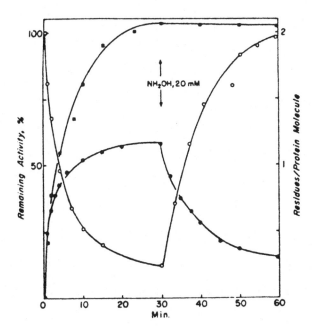

FIGURE 11. The results of the modification of thermolysin with diethylpyrocarbonate (ethoxyformic anhydride). Thermolysin (15 µ*M*) was allowed to react with DEP (3 m*M*) in 0.025 *M* HEPES, pH 7.2 followed by reaction with hydroxylamine (20 m*M*) indicated by the arrow. The open circles show the changes in catalytic activity. Modification of tyrosyl residues (■) was monitored by the decrease in absorbance at 278 nm using a $\Delta\epsilon = 1310$ M^{-1} cm^{-1}. Modification of histidyl residues was followed by the increase in absorbance at 242 nm using a $\Delta\epsilon = 3200$ M^{-1} cm^{-1}. (From Burstein, Y., Walsh, K. A., and Neurath, H., *Biochemistry*, 13, 205, 1974. With permission.)

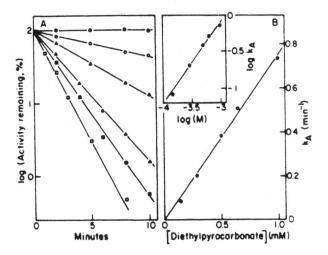

FIGURE 12. The inactivation of pyridoxamine-5'-phosphate oxidase by diethylpyrocarbonate. Panel A describes an experiment where the enzyme (2.32 µ*M*) was incubated in 0.1 *M* potassium phosphate, pH 7.0 containing 3.75 µ*M* riboflavin 5'-phosphate in the absence (●) or presence of diethylpyrocarbonate at the following concentrations 0.144 m*M* (○), 0.287 m*M* (▲), 0.501 m*M* (△), 0.644 m*M* (■), or 1.00 m*M* (□). Panel B shows the dependence of the pseudo-first-order rate constants for inactivation on the concentration of diethylpyrocarbonate. Values for k_A were determined from the slopes of the semilogarithmic plots of panel A. The inset in panel B shows a plot of k_A vs. log concentration of diethylpyrocarbonate. (From Horiike, K., Tsuge, H., and McCormick, D. B., *J. Biol. Chem.*, 254, 6638, 1979. With permission.)

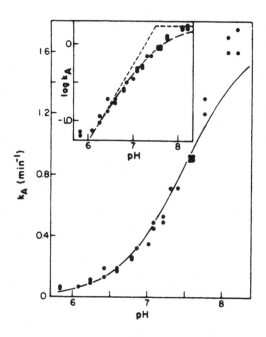

FIGURE 13.   The dependence of the rate constant (k_A; see Figure 9) for the inactivation of pyridoxamine-5'-phosphate oxidase by diethylpyrocarbonate. The pseudo-first-order rate constants (k_A) were calculated from the slopes of the semilogarithmic plots of activity vs. time (see Figure 9, panel A). The solid curve is drawn assuming there was no reaction between the protonated residue (pKa = 7.5). The second-order rate constant for the reaction of diethylpyrocarbonate with the unprotonated enzyme was 51.6 M^{-1} s^{-1}. The inset shows a plot of k_A vs. pH. (From Horiike, K., Tsuge, H., and McCormick, D. B., *J. Biol Chem.*, 254, 6638, 1979. With permission.)

In addition to the direct modifications of lysine, cysteine, and tyrosine by carboethoxylation which are occasionally observed as side reactions in the use of diethylpyrocarbonate for the modification of histidine residues in proteins, an additional side reaction involving lysyl residues has been observed. Sams and Matthews[50] reported isopeptide bond formation between the ε-amino group of lysine and an adjacent carboxylic acid. This reaction has been previously observed with ribonuclease.[31] A reaction mechanism has not been described but likely involves the transient diethylpyrocarbonate modification of the carboxyl group.[51]

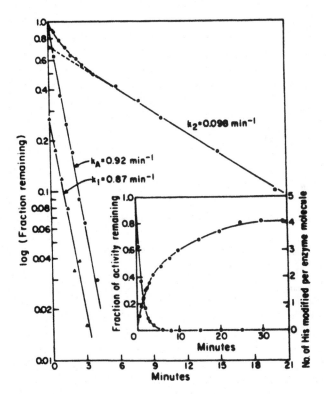

FIGURE 14. The relationship between the extent of histidine modification and the loss of catalytic activity of pyridoximine-5'-phosphate oxidase upon reaction with diethylpyrocarbonate. The holoenzyme (2.4 μM) was incubated with 1.2 mM diethylpyrocarbonate in 0.1 M potassium phosphate, pH 7.0. At the indicated times, the number of N-carboethoxyhistidyl residues was determined by spectrophotometric analysis and the fraction of remaining histidine residues (●) calculated by taking the total number of such modifiable residues (4.1) as unity and enzyme activity (○) determined. The fast phase of the modification (▲) was obtained by subtracting the contribution of the slow phase (dashed line) and replotting the differences. The solid curve is calculated on the basis of the following equation

$$x = (n - m)/n = 0.27\ e^{-0.87t} + 0.73\ e^{-0.098t}$$

where x is the total fraction of residues remaining after reaction, n is the total number of modifiable residues, m is the number of residues actually modified, and t is time. The inset shows a plot of activity remaining (○) and the number of histidyl residues modified per enzyme molecule (●) as a function of reaction time. (From Horiike, K., Tsuge, H., and McCormick, D. B., *J. Biol. Chem.*, 254, 6638, 1979. With permission.)

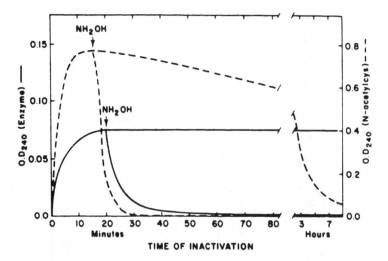

FIGURE 15. The reaction of spinach ribulose bisphosphate carboxylase with diethylpyrocarbonate in 0.1 M phosphate, pH 6.4 (solid line). The dashed line shows the reaction of diethylpyrocarbonate with N-acetylcysteine in 0.1 M succinate buffer, pH 6.4. The arrow indicates the point of addition of hydroxylamine, pH 7.0, to a final concentration of 0.4 M. A difference spectrum of the modified vs. unmodified enzyme (not shown) demonstrated an absorption maximum at 240 nm. (From Saluja, A. K. and McFadden, B. A., *Biochem. Biophys. Res. Commun.*, 94, 1091, 1980. With permission.)

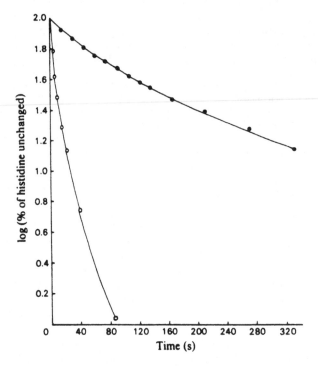

FIGURE 16. A comparison of the reaction rate of native (○) and thiomethylated (●) lactate dehydrogenase with diethylpyrocarbonate. The thiomethylated enzyme was prepared by reaction with methyl methanethiosulfonate. The proteins were in 0.1 M sodium phosphate, pH 7.2 at 10°C and allowed to react with 1 mM diethylpyrocarbonate. The extent of histidine modification was assessed by the increase in absorbance at 240 nm. ($\Delta\epsilon = 3600\ M^{-1}\ cm^{-1}$.) (From Bloxham, D. P., *Biochem. J.*, 193, 93, 1981. With permission.)

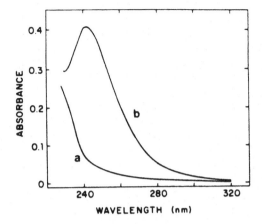

FIGURE 17. Ultraviolet difference spectrum for the reaction of *Candida boidinii* flavoenzyme alcohol oxidase with diethylpyrocarbonate in 0.05 *M* sodium phosphate, pH 7.5. Curve a was obtained before the addition of diethylpyrocarbonate while curve b was obtained after 30 min of reaction of protein in the sample cuvette with diethylpyrocarbonate. (From Cromartie, T. H., *Biochemistry*, 20, 5416, 1981. With permission.)

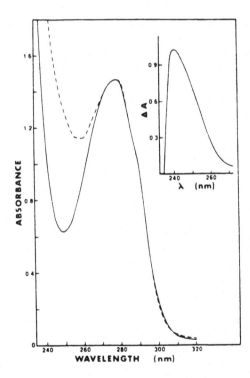

FIGURE 18. The UV absorption spectra of dihydrofolate reductase in the presence or absence of diethylpyrocarbonate. The reactions were performed in 0.05 *M* Tris-HCl, pH 7.5, in the presence (dashed line) or absence (solid line) of 3.24 m*M* diethylpyrocarbonate. (From Daron, H. H. and Aull, J. L., *Biochemistry*, 21, 737, 1982. With permission.)

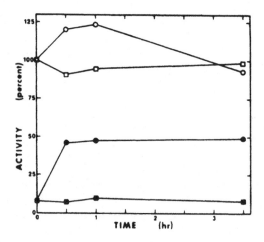

FIGURE 19.   Reaction of diethylpyrocarbonate-inactivated dihydrofolate reductase by hydroxylamine. The dihydrofolate reductase was incubated either in the presence ,olid symbols) or absence (closed symbols) of 6.9 m*M* diethylpyrocarbonate. The diethylpyrocarbonate-modified enzyme had 8% of the activity of the control enzyme preparation. The reaction mixtures were then treated with hydroxylamine (pH 7.5) at a final concentration of either 1.0 *M* (circles) or 0.1 *M* (squares). (From Daron, H. H., and Aull, J. L., *Biochemistry*, 21, 737, 1982. With permission.)

REFERENCES

1. **Weil, L., James, S., and Buchert, A. R.,** Photooxidation of crystalline chymotrypsin in the presence of methylene blue, *Arch. Biochem. Biophys.*, 46, 266, 1953.
2. **Ray, W. J., Jr. and Koshland, D. E., Jr.,** A method for characterizing the type and numbers of groups involved in enzyme action, *J. Biol. Chem.*, 236, 1973, 1961.
3. **Ray, W. J., Jr. and Koshland, D. E.,** Identification of amino acids involved in phosphoglucomutase action, *J. Biol. Chem.*, 237, 2493, 1962.
4. **Bond, J. S., Francis, S. H., and Park, J. H.,** An essential histidine in the catalytic activities of 3-phosphoglyceraldehyde dehydrogenase, *J. Biol. Chem.*, 245, 1041, 1970.
5. **Fahnestock, S. R.,** Evidence of the involvement of a 50S ribosomal protein in several active sites, *Biochemistry*, 14, 5321, 1975.
6. **Auron, P. E., Erdelsky, K. J., and Fahnestock, S. R.,** Chemical modification studies of a protein at the peptidyltransferase site of the *Bacillus stearothermophilus* ribosome. The 50S ribosomal subunit is a highly integrated functional unit, *J. Biol. Chem.*, 253, 6893, 1978.
7. **Dohme, F. and Fahnestock, S. R.,** Identification of proteins involved in the peptidyl transferase activity of ribosomes by chemical modification, *J. Mol. Biol.*, 129, 63, 1979.
8. **Cerna, J. and Rychlik, I.,** Photoinactivation of peptidyl transferase binding sites, *FEBS Lett.*, 102, 277, 1979.
9. **Nakamura, S. and Kaziro, Y.,** Selective photooxidation of histidine residues in polypeptide chain elongation factor Tu from *E. coli*, *J. Biochem. (Tokyo)*, 90, 1117, 1981.
10. **Funakoshi, T., Abe, M., Sakata, M., Shoji, S., and Kubota, Y.,** The functional site of placental anticoagulant protein: essential histidine residue of placental anticoagulant protein, *Biochem. Biophys. Res. Commun.*, 168, 125, 1990.
11. **Kuno, S., Fukui, S., and Toraya, T.,** Essential histidine residues in coenzyme B$_{12}$-dependent diol dehydrase: dye-sensitized photooxidation and ethoxycarbonylation, *Arch. Biochem. Biophys.*, 277, 211, 1990.
12. **Inagami, T. and Hatano, H.,** Effect of alkylguanidines on the inactivation of trypsin by alkylation and phosphorylation, *J. Biol. Chem.*, 244, 1176, 1969.

13. **Stark, G. R., Stein, W. H., and Moore, S.,** Relationships between the conformation of ribonuclease and its reactivity toward iodoacetate, *J. Biol. Chem.,* 236, 436, 1961.
14. **Heinrikson, R. L., Stein, W. H., Crestfield, A. M., and Moore, S.,** The reactivities of the histidine residues at the active site of ribonuclease toward halo acids of different structures, *J. Biol. Chem.,* 240, 2921, 1965.
15. **Fruchter, R. G. and Crestfield, A. M.,** The specific alkylation by iodoacetamide of histidine 12 in the active site of ribonuclease, *J. Biol. Chem.,* 242, 5807, 1967.
16. **Lin, M. C., Stein, W. H., and Moore, S.,** Further studies on the alkylation of the histidine residues of pancreatic ribonuclease, *J. Biol. Chem.,* 243, 6167, 1968.
17. **Schoellmann, G. and Shaw. E.,** Direct evidence for the presence of histidine in the active center of chymotrypsin, *Biochemistry,* 2, 252, 1963.
18. **Shaw, E., Mares-Guia, M., and Cohen, W.,** Evidence for an active center histidine in trypsin through use of a specific reagent, 1-chloro-3-tosylamido-7-amino-2-heptanone, the chloromethyl ketone derived from N^α-tosyl-L-lysine, *Biochemistry,* 4, 2219, 1965.
19. **Segal, D. M., Powers, J. C., Cohen, G. H., Davies, D. R., and Wilcox, P. E.,** Substrate binding site in bovine chymotrypsin Aγ. A crystallographic study using peptide chloromethyl ketones as site-specific inhibitors, *Biochemistry,* 10, 3728, 1971.
20. **Fohlman, J., Eaker, D., Dowdall, M. J., Lüllmann-Rauch, R., Sjödin, T., and Leander, S.,** Chemical modification of taipoxin and the consequences for phospholipase activity, pathophysiology, and inhibition of high-affinity choline uptake, *Eur. J. Biochem.,* 94, 531, 1979.
21. **Halpert, J., Eaker, D., and Karlsson, E.,** The role of phospholipase activity in the action of a presynaptic neurotoxin of *Notechis scutatus scutatus* (Australian Tiger Snake), *FEBS Lett.,* 61, 72, 1976.
22. **Yang, C. C. and King, K.,** Chemical modification of the histidine residue in basic phospholipase A$_2$ from the venom of *Naja nigricollis, Biochim. Biophys. Acta,* 614, 373, 1980.
23. **Verheij, H. M., Volwerk, J. J., Jansen, E. H. J. M., Puyk, W. C., Dijkstra, B. W., Drenth, J., and de Haas, G. H.,** Methylation of histidine-48 in pancreatic phospholipase A$_2$. Role of histidine and calcium ion in the catalytic mechanism, *Biochemistry,* 19, 743, 1980.
24. **Volwerk, J. J., Pieterson, W. A., and de Haas, G. H.,** Histidine at the active site of phospholipase A$_2$, *Biochemistry,* 13, 1446, 1974.
25. **Glick, B. R.,** The chemical modification of *Escherichia coli* ribosomes with methyl *p*-nitrobenzenesulfonate. Evidence for the involvement of a histidine residue in the functioning of the ribosomal peptidyl transferase, *Can. J. Biochem.,* 58, 1345, 1980.
26. **Nishino, T., Massey, V., and Williams, C. H., Jr.,** Chemical modifications of D-amino acid oxidase. Evidence for active site histidine, tyrosine, and arginine residues, *J. Biol. Chem.,* 255, 3610, 1980.
27. **Morishima, I., Shiro, Y., Adachi, S., Yano, Y., and Orii, Y.,** Effect of the distal histidine modification (cyanation) of myoglobin on the ligand binding kinetics and the heme environmental structures, *Biochemistry,* 28, 7582, 1989.
28. **Shiro, Y. and Morishima, I.,** Modification of the heme distal side chain in myoglobin by cyanogen bromide. Heme environmental structures and ligand binding properties of the modified myoglobin, *Biochemistry,* 23, 4879, 1984.
29. **Hefford, M. A. and Kaplan, H.,** Chemical properties of the histidine residue of secretin: evidence for a specific intramolecular interaction, *Biochim. Biophys. Acta,* 998, 267, 1989.
30. **Melchior, W. B. Jr. and Fahrney, D.,** Ethoxyformylation of proteins. Reaction of ethoxyformic anhydride with α-chymotrypsin, pepsin and pancreatic ribonuclease at pH 4, *Biochemistry,* 9, 251, 1970.
31. **Wolf, B., Lesnaw, J. A., and Reichmann, M. E.,** A mechanism of the irreversible inactivation of bovine pancreatic ribonuclease by diethylpyrocarbonate. A general reaction of diethylpyrocarbonate with proteins, *Eur. J. Biochem.,* 13, 519, 1970.
32. **Miles, E. W.,** Modification of histidyl residues in proteins by diethylpyrocarbonate, *Meth. Enzymol.,* 47, 431, 1977.
33. **Welsch, D. J. and Nelsestuen, G. L.,** Irreversible degradation of histidine-96 of prothrombin fragment 1 during protein acetylation: another unusually reactive site in the kringle, *Biochemistry,* 27, 7513, 1988.
34. **Altman, J., Lipka, J. J., Kuntz, I., and Waskell, L.,** Identification by proton nuclear magnetic resonance of the histidines in cytochrome b_5 modified by diethyl pyrocarbonate, *Biochemistry,* 28, 7516, 1989.
35. **Bycroft, M. and Fersht, A. R.,** Assignment of histidine resonances in the [TH NMR (500 MHz) spectrum of subtilisin BPN' using site-directed mutagenesis, *Biochemistry,* 27, 7390, 1988.
36. **Morjana, N. A. and Scarborough, G. A.,** Evidence for an essential histidine residue in the *Neurospora crassa* plasma membrane H$^+$[T-ATPase, *Biochim. Biophys. Acta,* 985, 19, 1989.
37. **Holbrook, J. J. and Ingram, V. A.,** Ionic properties of an essential histidine residue in pig heart lactate dehydrogenase, *Biochem. J.,* 131, 729, 1973.
38. **Cousineau, J. and Meighen, E.,** Chemical modification of bacterial luciferase with ethoxyformic anhydride: evidence for an essential histidyl residue, *Biochemistry,* 15, 4992, 1976.

39. **Burstein, Y., Walsh, K. A., and Neurath, H.,** Evidence of an essential histidine residue in thermolysin, *Biochemistry,* 13, 205, 1974.
40. **Roosemont, J. L.,** Reaction of histidine residues in proteins with diethylpyrocarbonate: differential molar absorptivities and reactivities, *Anal. Biochem.,* 88, 314, 1978.
41. **Vangrysperre, W., Ampe, C., Kersters-Hilderson, H., and Tempst, P.,** Single active-site histidine in D-xylose isomerase from *Streptomyces violaceoruber.* Identification by chemical derivatization and peptide mapping, *Biochem. J.,* 263, 195, 1989.
42. **Horiike, K., Tsuge, H., and McCormick, D. B.,** Evidence for an essential histidyl residue at the active site of pyridoxamine (pyridoxine)-5'-phosphate oxidase from rabbit liver, *J. Biol. Chem.,* 254, 6638, 1979.
43. **Gordillo, E., Ayala, A., F-Lobato, M., Bautista, J., and Machado, A.,** Possible involvement of histidine residues in the loss of enzymatic activity of rat liver malic enzyme during aging, *J. Biol. Chem.,* 263, 8053, 1988.
44. **Kinnunen, P. M., DeMichele, A., and Lange, L. G.,** Chemical modification of acyl-CoA:cholesterol *O*-acyltransferase. 1. Identification of acyl-CoA:cholesterol *O*-acyltransferase subtypes by differential diethyl pyrocarbonate sensitivity. *Biochemistry,* 27, 7344, 1988.
45. **Saluja, A. K. and McFadden, B. A.,** Modification of histidine at the active site of spinach ribulose bisphosphate carboxylase, *Biochem. Biophys. Res. Commun.,* 94, 1091, 1980.
46. **Bloxham, D. P.,** The chemical reactivity of the histidine-195 residue in lactate dehydrogenase thiomethylated at the cysteine-165 residue, *Biochem. J.,* 193, 93, 1981.
47. **Cromartie, T. H.,** Sulfhydryl and histidinyl residues in the flavoenzyme alcohol oxidase from *Candida boidinii, Biochemistry,* 20, 5416, 1981.
48. **Bond, M. D., Steinbrink, D. R., and Van Wart, H. E.,** Identification of essential amino acid residues in *Clostridium histolyticum* collagenase using chemical modification reactions, *Biochem. Biophys. Res. Commun.,* 102, 243, 1981.
49. **Daron, H. H. and Aull, J. L.,** Inactivation of dihydrofolate reductase from *Lactobacillus casei* by diethyl pyrocarbonate, *Biochemistry,* 21, 737, 1982.
50. **Sams, C. F. and Matthews, K. S.,** Diethyl pyrocarbonate reaction with the lactose repressor protein affects both inducer and DNA binding, *Biochemistry,* 27, 2277, 1988.
51. **Wold, F.,** Bifunctional reagents, *Meth. Enzymol.,* 25, 423, 1972.

Chapter 10

THE MODIFICATION OF LYSINE

The chemical modification of lysine residues in proteins is based upon the ability of the ε-amino group of this residue to react as a nucleophile. Under normal reaction conditions, lysyl residues are the second strongest nucleophiles in a protein molecule; cysteine is the most reactive nucleophile. However, for lysine to function optimally as a nucleophile, the proton usually bound to lysyl residues at physiological pH must be removed. This is shown in Figure 1. The protonated form is essentially unreactive. The pKa of an "average" lysyl residue in a protein is 10 (see Table 2 in Chapter 6). The majority of modification reactions are performed at pH 8.0 to 9.0.

It is somewhat difficult to selectively modify lysyl residues in proteins. A number of the reagents which are used to modify lysyl residues also have the potential to react with the N-terminal amino group(s), with tyrosyl residues and with cysteinyl residues.

Lysine residues can be modified by reaction with α-ketoalkyl halides such as iodoacetic acid.[8] Acylation can occur at pH greater than 7.0 but the rate of reaction is much slower than reaction with cysteinyl residues. Both the mono- and disubstituted derivatives have been reported. The monosubstituted derivative migrates close to methionine on amino acid analysis while the disubstituted derivative migrates near aspartic acid. It should be noted that reaction with α-ketoalkyl halides is not considered particularly useful for the modification of primary amino groups. This reaction can be a possible side reaction occurring during the reduction and carboxymethylation of proteins. The reactivity of a given lysyl residue is affected by the nature of surrounding amino residues.

Both fluoronitrobenzene and fluorodinitrobenzene have been of considerable value in protein chemistry since Sanger and Tuppy's work on the structure of insulin.[2] Carty and Hirs[3] developed the use of 4-sulfonyl-2-nitrofluorobenzene for the modification of amino groups in pancreatic ribonuclease (Figure 2). This is a particularly useful experiment since it is critical to understand that these investigators actually measured the amount of native protein remaining by chromatographic fractionation. As would be expected, the rate of modification increases with increasing pH. This reagent also is more stable than, for example, fluorodinitrobenzene under alkaline conditions, permitting more accurate measurement at pH greater than 9.0. The lysine residue at position 41 is the site of major substitution which is a reflection of the lower pKa for the ε-amino group of this residue. Use of this compound did not present the solubility and reactivity problems posed by the fluoronitrobenzene compounds. It was possible to qualitatively determine the classes of amino groups in ribonuclease; these were the α-amino group, nine "normal" amino groups and lysine 41. The reactivity of lysine 41 was influenced by neighboring functional groups. This effect was lost at pH greater than 11 or on thermal denaturation of the protein. The reaction of 1-dimethylaminonaphthalene-5-sulfonyl chloride (dansyl chloride) has been useful both in the structural analysis and amino group modification with proteins. In one study,[4] dansyl chloride (in acetone) is added to a solution of trypsin in 0.1 M phosphate, pH 8.0. The reaction is terminated after 24 h at 25°C by acidification to pH 3.0 with 1.0 M HCl. Insoluble material is removed by centrifugation and the supernatant fraction placed in dialysis. These investigators reported modification of the amino-terminal isoleucine and one lysine residue. The extent of modification was determined by absorbance at 336 nm ($\epsilon_m = 3.4 \times 10^4 \, M^{-1}$ cm^{-1}). Reaction of dansyl chloride with phosphoenolpyruvate carboxylase has been used to introduce a fluorescent probe into this protein.[5] A somewhat specific modification of one of the eight lysine residues was achieved. The extent of modification was determined by spectral analysis at 355 nm using an extinction coefficient of 3400 M^{-1} cm^{-1}.

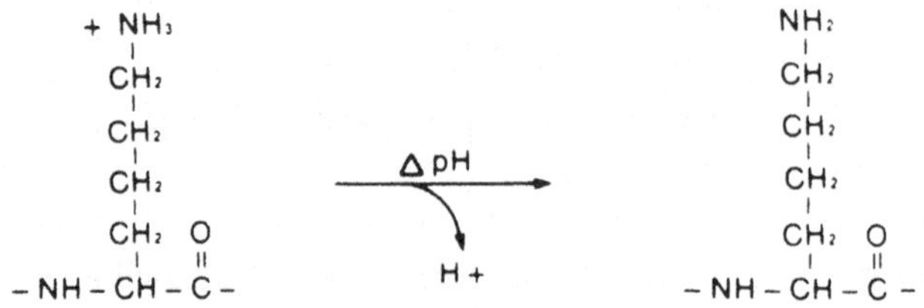

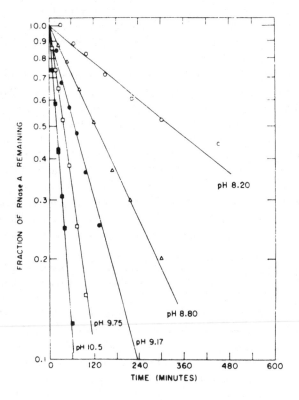

FIGURE 1.   The structure of lysine.

FIGURE 2.   The reaction of bovine pancreatic ribonuclease A with 4-sulfonyloxy-2-nitrofluorobenzene (potassium salt) as a function of pH. The pH was maintained by addition of 0.2 N NaOH during the course of the reaction at 28°C. The amount of ribonuclease remaining was determined by chromatographic analysis (Amerlite® IRC-50). (From Carty, R. P. and Hirs, C. H. W., *J. Biol. Chem.*, 243, 5254, 1968. With permission.)

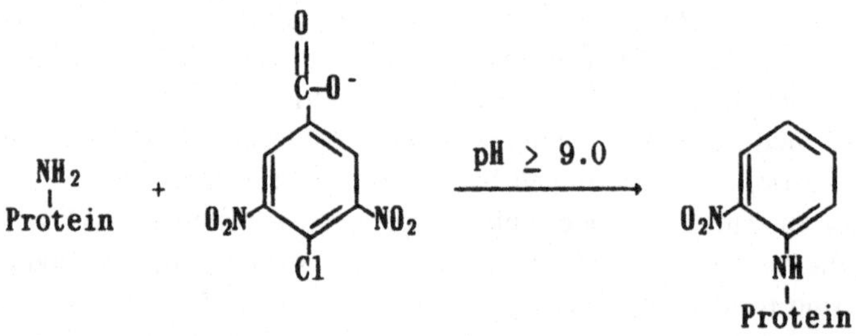

FIGURE 3.   The reaction of an amino group with 4-chloro-3,5-dinitrobenzoate.

The reaction of 2-carboxy-4,6-dinitrochlorobenzene with proteins (Figure 3) has been explored.[6,7] This reagent reacts with amino, sulfhydryl, and amino groups. This reagent has recently been used for the modification of specific lysine residues in cytochrome c.[8,9] The modification reaction (approximately 6-fold molar excess of reagent) was performed in 0.2 M sodium bicarbonate, pH 9.0 at ambient temperature for 24 h. The extent of modification was determined as described by Brautigan et al.[6] The absorbance maximum of derivatives formed with various alkylamines was 436 nm with an extinction coefficient of $6.9 \times 10^3 \, M^{-1} \, cm^{-1}$. Chromatographic fractionation of the modified protein (sulfoethylcellulose) yielded six fractions with major lysine group modification. Hiratsuka and Uchida[10] examined the reaction of N-methyl-2-anilino-6-naphthalenesulfonyl chloride with lysyl residues in cardiac myosin. There was a difference in the nature of the reaction in the presence and absence of divalent cation. N-methyl-2-anilino-6-naphthalenesulfonyl chloride has been suggested for use as a fluorescent probe for hydrophobic regions of protein molecules.[11-13] The extent of incorporation of the N-methyl-2-anilino-6-naphthalenesulfonyl moiety into protein can be determined by spectral analysis at 327 nm ($\Delta\epsilon = 2.0 \times 10^4 \, M^{-1} \, cm^{-1}$).[11,12] Modification of protein amino groups with isothiocyanate derivatives of various dyes has proved to be an effective means of introducing structural probes into proteins at specific sites.[13] Eosin isothiocyanate has been used to modify the lysyl residues in phosphoenolpyruvate carboxylase.[5] The reagent was dissolved in dimethylsulfoxide/50 mM HEPES, pH 8.0 (50/50) immediately prior to use and added to the protein (in 50 mM HEPES, pH 8.0). The modified derivatives were used to determine the spatial proximity of the modified lysine residues using resonance energy transfer. Fluorescein isothiocyanate has been used to modify cytochrome P-450 (reaction performed in 30 mM Tris, pH 8.0 containing 0.1% Tween 80; 2 h at 0°C in the dark),[14] actin (2 mM borate, pH 8.5; 3 h at ambient temperature then at 4°C for 16 h),[15] and ricin (pH 8.1, 6°C for 4 h).[16] The extent of modification with fluorescein isothiocyanate can be determining by spectroscopy using an extinction coefficient of 80,000 $M^{-1} \, cm^{-1}$ at 495 nm (1% SDS with 0.1 M NaOH)[14] or 74,500 $M^{-1} \, cm^{-1}$ (0.1 M Tris, pH 8.0).[15] Antibodies labeled with fluorescein have been used as targeted phototoxic agents.[17] In this approach, the fluorescein moiety is iodinated resulting in a photodynamic sensitizer.

Welches and Baldwin[18] have recently examined the reaction of bacterial luciferase with 2,4-dinitrofluorobenzene. The fluorescence of N-methyl-2-anilino-6-naphthalenesulfonyl derivatives is extremely sensitive to the polarity of the medium.[18] Modification was associated with inactivation at the rate of 157 $M^{-1} \, min^{-1}$ at pH 7.0 (0.05 M phosphate). Both lysyl and cysteinyl residues can be modified under the experimental conditions (0.05 M phosphate, pH 7.0 at 25°C) used in these studies. In order to assess the significance of reaction at primary amino groups, the cysteinyl residues were "blocked" with methyl methanethiosulfonate. Reaction of luciferase with methyl methanethiosulfonate resulted in greater than 95% loss of catalytic activity (twofold molar excess of methyl methanethiosulfonate in 0.02 M phosphate, pH 7.0 at 25°C). The loss of activity can be completely reversed with β-mercaptoethanol (97 mM). The small amount of residual activity present after treatment with methyl methanethiosulfonate is further reduced on treatment with 2,4-dinitrofluorobenzene and the recovery of activity subsequent to β-mercaptoethanol is greatly reduced (see Figure 4). Quantitative analysis was not performed but qualitative analysis suggested that the modification occurred at the α-amino group of methionine or the α- and/or β-subunits. The effects of pH on the reaction of fluorodinitrobenzene with luciferase is shown in Figure 5. It is of interest to compare the rate of reaction of fluorodinitrobenzene with model compounds and luciferase as has been done by these investigators as shown in Figure 6. Note that the rate of reaction with luciferase is much faster than with any of the model compounds. In a recent study, a combination of site-specific mutagenesis and site-specific chemical modification with 2,4-dinitroflurobenzene was used to study lysine residues in angiogenin.[20]

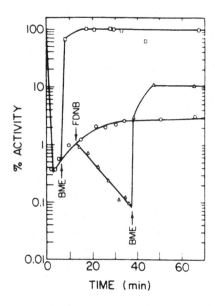

FIGURE 4.   Protection of the thiol functional group reactivity with 2,4-
dinitrofluorobenzene (FDNB) by prior reaction with methyl methanethiol-
sulfonate. Three portions of the methyl methanethiolsulfonate-luciferase
were studied: the control preparation (○), a second portion treated with
97 mM β-mercaptoethanol (BME) (□) (indicated by the BME arrow), and
a third portion (△) which was allowed to react with FDNB (indicated by
the FDNB arrow) which was allowed to proceed until 90% of the activity
had been lost at which point β-mercaptoethanol (97 mM) was added (indicated by the BME arrow at approximately 40 min). (From Welches, W.
R. and Baldwin, T. O., *Biochemistry*, 20, 512, 1981. With permission.)

Acylation of amino groups in proteins by reaction with carboxylic acid anhydrides has
been extensively used. Riordan and Vallee[21] have discussed the process of acetylation in
some detail. Acetylation is generally carried out with acetic anhydride at alkaline pH in
either a pH-stat or in saturated sodium acetate. Performing the modification reaction under
these latter conditions (saturated sodium acetate) results in increased specificity since
O-acetyl tyrosine is unstable in sodium acetate. Acetylation has been used to study calcitonin[22]
and a bacterial cytochrome.[23] Acetic and maleic anhydride have been used to study elastase.[24]
In these studies, the reaction was carried out in a pH-stat to maintain alkaline pH. Reaction
occurred at both lysyl and tyrosyl residues. It is relatively easy to differentiate between the
two sites of modification since O-acyl tyrosyl residues are unstable at pH ≥ 9.0. Studies
with maleic anhydride showed that the amino terminal valine was not available for modification at pH 8.0 to 9.0 but could be modified at pH 11.0. Modification of this residue
could be achieved in the presence of urea at a lower pH.

Competitive labeling (trace labeling) is a technique for determining the ionization state
or constant and intrinsic reactivity of individual amino groups in a protein.[25] The method
is based on the hypothesis that the individual amino groups will compete for a trace amount
of radiolabeled reagent (the reagent is selected on the basis of nonselective reactivity with
amino groups; with most studies, acetic anhydride has been the reagent of choice). The
extent of radiolabel incorporation into the protein at a given site will then be a function of
the pKa, microenvironment, and inherent nucleophilicity of that particular amino group.[25]
After the reaction with the radiolabeled reagent is complete, the protein is denatured and
complete modification at each amino group is achieved by the addition of an excess of
unlabeled reagent. A reproducible digestion method (i.e., tryptic or chymotryptic hydrolysis)
is used to obtain peptides from the completely modified protein. The peptides are separated
by a chromatographic technique and the extent of radiolabel at each site determined. The

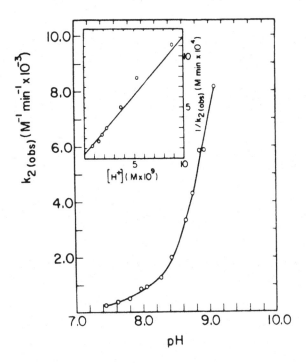

FIGURE 5. The pH dependence for the reaction of FDNB with luciferase. The observed second-order rate constant is plotted as a function of pH (0.05 M pyrophosphate). The inset shows a plot of the reciprocal of the observed second-order rate constant as a function of hydrogen ion concentration permitting the evaluation of the absolute second-order rate constant for the reaction (k_2) ($2.4 \times 10^5 \, M^{-1} \, min^{-1}$) and an apparent pKa of 9.4. (From Welches, W. R. and Baldwin, T. O., *Biochemistry*, 20, 512, 1981. With permission.)

reagent or protein	functional group	$\bar{k}_2$(obsd) ($M^{-1} \cdot min^{-1}$)
2-mercaptoethanol[a]	SH	5.5
N-acetylcysteine[a]	SH	6.3
N^{α}-acetyllysine[a]	NH_2	0.013
methionine[a]	NH_2	0.070
luciferase	NH_2	157

[a] Reactions were performed at pH 7.0, 20 °C, in 0.02 M phosphate buffer; the progress of the reaction was monitored spectrophotometrically.

FIGURE 6. The apparent second-order rate constants for the reaction of various functional groups with 2,4-dinitrofluorobenzene at pH 7.0 (0.02 M phosphate, 20°C). (From Welches, W. R. and Baldwin, T. O., *Biochemistry*, 20, 512, 1981. With permission.)

extent of radiolabel incorporation at a given site is a function of the reactivity of that individual amino group under the reaction conditions used at the radiolabel step. An alternative approach[26,27] involves a "trace" labeling step with tritiated acetic anhydride followed by complete modification with unlabeled acetic anhydride under denaturing conditions. This modified protein is then mixed with a preparation of the same protein which has been uniformly labeled with the ^{14}C-labeled acetic anhydride. Digestion and separation of peptide is performed by conventional techniques (see above) and the extent of radiolabeling is determined. The ratio of ^{3}H/^{14}C in peptides containing amino groups is an indication of functional group reactivity. This method is somewhat more sensitive than the original method. Reductive methylation (see below) has also been used.[28]

Although this is a laborious technique, the data obtained are excellent and provide considerable insight into the solution structure of proteins. There has been a consistent use of this technique for the study of troponin-T,[29] troponin-C,[30] troponin-I,[31] calmodulin,[32-34] and tropomyosin.[35] In particular, studies[32-35] which have used this technique to assess conformational change in solution have been particularly rewarding.

More recently, trifluoroacetylated derivatives have been of interest in the study of protein structure. In these studies, ethylthiotrifluoroacetate was used to modify cytochrome c in 0.14 M sodium phosphate, pH 8.0.[36,37] The pH was maintained at 8.0 using a pH-stat. Singly substituted derivatives of cytochrome c can be separated by chromatography on anion-exchange resin (Bio Rex 70) and carboxymethylcellulose. It is critical to avoid lyophilization during the preparation of the various derivatives. These derivatives have been subjected to further investigation[38,39] including the use of ^{19}F-containing derivatives for nuclear magnetic resonance probes.[40]

Succinic anhydride has also proved useful in the modification of lysine.[41] Modification of lysine residues with succinic anhydride results in charge reversal. Reaction with succinic anhydride frequently results in the dissociation of multimeric proteins and has also been used to "solubilize" insoluble proteins. Meighen and co-workers[42] have produced a "variant" form of bacterial luciferase through reaction with succinic anhydride. The succinylated protein retained the dimeric subunit structure of the native enzyme. By complementation experiments involving the mixing/hybridization of the modified and native enzyme, it was determined that succinylation of bacterial luciferase resulted in the inactivation of the α-subunit without markedly affecting the function of the β-subunit. Shetty and Rao[43] studied the reaction of succinic anhydride with arachin. In this study, reaction of the protein was performed in 0.1 M sodium phosphate, pH 7.8, with the pH maintained over the course of the reaction by the addition of 2.0 M NaOH. The extent of modification was determined by reaction of the unmodified primary amino groups on the protein with trinitrobenzene-sulfonic acid (see below). With a 200:1 molar excess of succinic anhydride, 82% of the available amino groups were succinylated with concomitant dissociation of the subunits of this protein. The reaction of chymotrypsinogen with succinic anhydride has been studied.[44] In these experiments, the reaction was performed under ambient conditions in 0.05 M sodium phosphate, pH 7.5. During the course of the reaction the pH was maintained at 7.5 by the addition of 1.0 M NaOH. Chymotrypsinogen (1 g) was dissolved in the sodium phosphate buffer and 50 mg of succinic anhydride was added over a 30-min period. Under these conditions, 8 of the 14 lysine residues were modified. A related reaction involves the trimesylation of amino groups in proteins (see Figure 7).[45] This reaction involves the modification of the protein with di(trimethysilyethyl)trimesic acid. Removal of the blocking groups results in an extremely polar derivative. The procedure is suggested to have value in the solubilization of membrane proteins.

Citraconic anhydride has proved useful since the modification of lysine residues with this reagent is a reversible reaction (Figure 8). Reaction conditions for the modification of lysine residues in proteins are similar to those described above for other carboxylic acid anhydrides. Atassi and Habeeb[46] have discussed the use of this reagent in some detail. As an example,

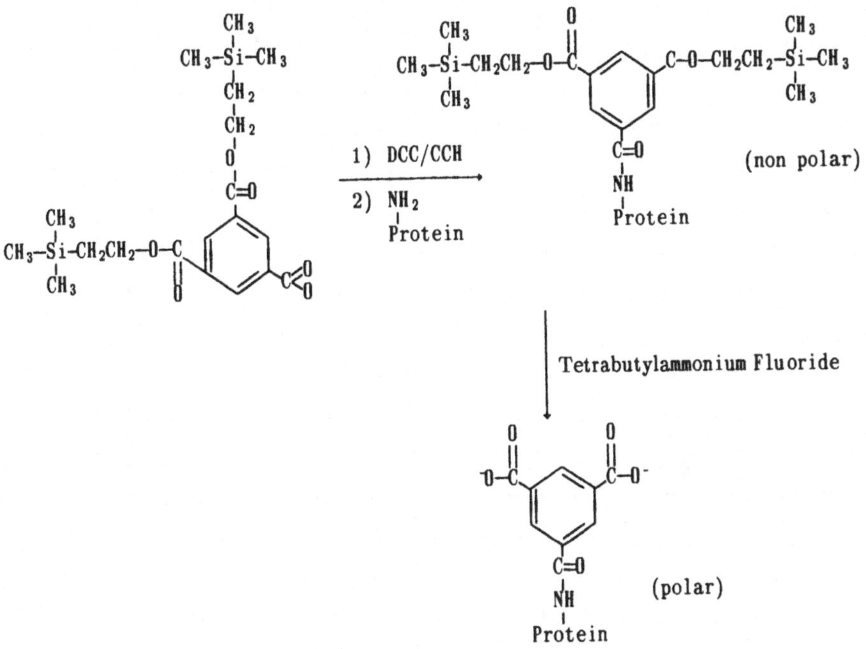

FIGURE 7. A scheme for the reaction of di(trimethylsilylethyl) trimesic acid with amino groups on protein and subsequent deprotection to produce a polar derivative.

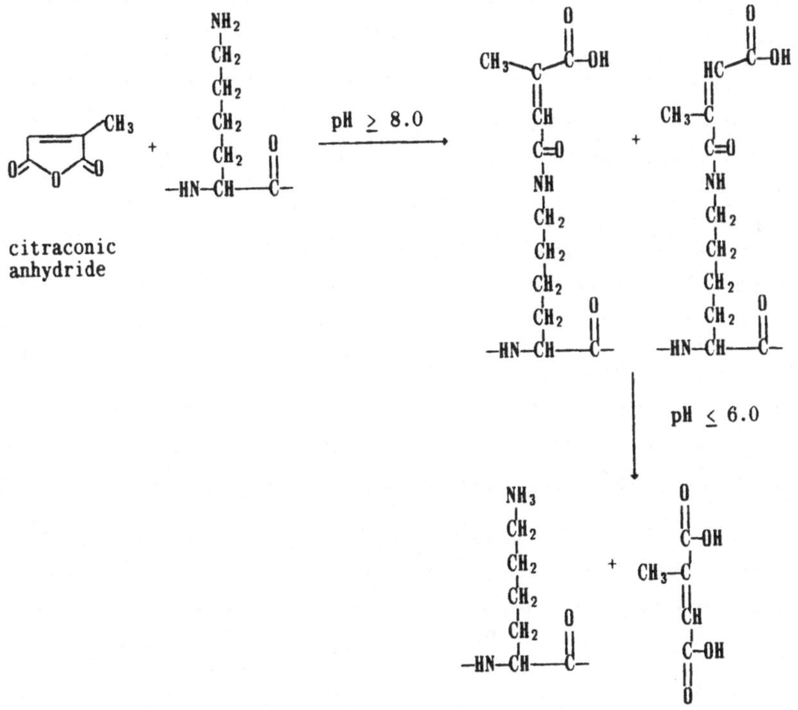

FIGURE 8. A scheme for the reversible reaction of lysine residues with citraconic anhydride.

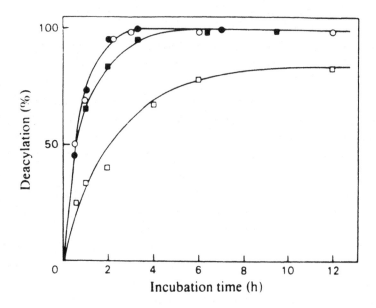

FIGURE 9.   The effect of pH on the rate of deacylation of the ε-amino groups of lysine in the citraconylated protein prepared from the nucleoprotein complex prepared from yeast. The reactions were performed at 30°C at pH 3.0 (●), pH 4.0 (○), pH 5.0 (■), and pH 6.0 (□). (From Shetty, J. K. and Kinsella, J. E., *Biochem. J.*, 191, 269, 1980. With permission.)

the reaction of egg white lysozyme with citraconic anhydride has been studied.[47] With multiple additions of reagent, all primary amino groups were modified at pH 8.2 (the pH of the reaction mixture was maintained with a pH-stat). The product of the reaction was heterogeneous as judged by polyacrylamide gel electrophoresis. All citraconyl groups could be removed by treatment with 1.0 *M* hydroxylamine at pH 10.0. This treatment also resulted in an electrophoretically homogeneous species. Complete removal of the citraconyl groups could also be achieved by incubation at pH 4.2 for 3 h at 40°C.

Reaction with citraconic anhydride has been used to dissociate nucleoprotein complexes.[48] Modification of the lysine residues with citraconic anhydride (pH 8.0 to 9.0 maintained with pH-stat) resulted in a marked change in the charge relationship between the ε-amino groups of lysine and the phosphate backbone of the nucleic acid, allowing subsequent separation of protein from nucleic acid. The citraconyl groups were subsequently removed from this protein by incubation at pH 3.0 to 4.0 at 30°C for 3 h (Figure 9).

Mahley and co-workers have prepared the acetoacetyl derivatives of lipoproteins by reaction with diketene in 0.3 borate, pH 8.5.[49,50] The modification of tyrosyl and seryl residues also can occur under these conditions, but the *O*-acetoacetyl groups can be removed by dialysis against a mild alkaline buffer such as bicarbonate. The modification at lysyl residues can be reversed by 0.5 *M* hydroxylamine, pH 7.0 at 37°C. A 0.06 *M* solution of diketene was prepared by taking 50 μl diketene into 10 ml 0.1 *M* sodium borate, pH 8.5. The modification was performed at pH 8.5. The extent of modification was determined by subsequent titration with fluorodinitrobenzene. The effect of the modification of lysine residues on the *in vivo* clearance of lipoproteins in rats has been investigated.[50]

Urabe and co-workers[51] prepared various mixed carboxylic acid anhydrides of tetradecanoic acid and oxa derivatives which varied in their "hydrophobicity". This represented an attempt to change the surface properties of the enzyme molecule, in this case, thermolysin. The carboxylic acid anhydrides were formed *in situ* from the corresponding acid and ethylchloroformate in dioxane with triethylamine. The modification reaction was performed in 0.013 *M* barbital, 0.013 *M* CaCl$_2$, pH 8.5 containing 39% (v/v) dioxane and was terminated

$$NCO^- \quad + \quad H_2N \sim\!\!\sim\!\!\sim \quad \longrightarrow \quad H_2N - \overset{\overset{\displaystyle O}{\|}}{C} - NH \sim\!\!\sim\!\!\sim$$

FIGURE 10. The reaction of primary amino groups with cyanate.

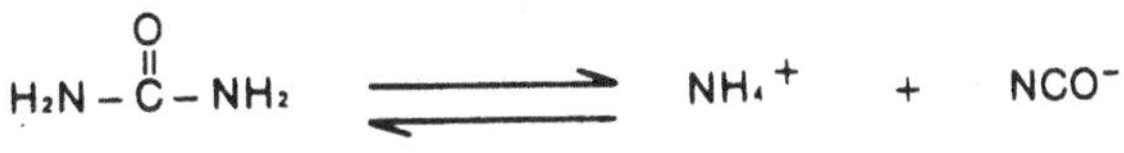

$$H_2N - \overset{\overset{\displaystyle O}{\|}}{C} - NH_2 \quad \underset{\longleftarrow}{\longrightarrow} \quad NH_4^+ \quad + \quad NCO^-$$

FIGURE 11. The formation of cyanate from urea.

with neutral hydroxylamine which also served to remove O-acyl derivatives. The extent of reaction was determined by titration with trinitrobenzenesulfonic acid. Derivatives obtained with tetradecanoic acid and 4-oxatetradecanoic acid were insoluble. Derivatives obtained with 4,7,10-trioxatetradecanoic acid and 4,7,10,13-tetraoxotetradecanoic acid both had approximately seven amino groups modified per mole of enzyme, showed little if any loss in either proteinase or esterase activity, and possessed enhanced thermal stability. Howlett and Wardrop[52] were able to dissociate the components of human erythrocyte membrane by the use of 3,4,5,6-tetrahydrophthalic anhydride. The reaction was performed in 0.02 M Tricine, pH 8.5. The 3,4,5,6-tetrahydrophthalic anhydride was introduced into the reaction mixture as a dioxane solution (a maximum of 0.10 ml/5 ml reaction mixture). The pH was maintained at pH 8.0 to 9.0 with 1.0 M NaOH. The reaction was considered complete when no further change in pH was observed. The extent of modification was determined by titration with trinitrobenzenesulfonic acid. The reaction could be reversed by incubation for 24 to 48 h at ambient temperature following the addition of an equal volume of 0.1 M potassium phosphate, pH 5.4 (the final pH of the reaction mixture was 6.0).

The reaction of primary amino groups in proteins with cyanate (Figure 10) has been a useful procedure for several decades. Stark and co-workers[53] pursued the observation that ribonuclease was inactivated by urea in a time-dependent reaction. It was established that this inactivation was a reflection of the content of cyanate in the urea preparation (Figure 11). This observation was subsequently developed into a method for the quantitative determination of amino-terminal residues in peptides and proteins.[54] The reaction of cyanate with amino acid residues has been reported by Stark.[55] The ϵ-amino group of lysine is the least reactive ($k = 2.0 \times 10^{-3} M^{-1} min^{-1}$) as compared to the α-amino group of glycylglycine ($k = 1.4 \times 10^{-1} M^{-1} min^{-1}$). The carbamyl derivative of histidine is quite unstable as is the corresponding derivative of cysteine. Concern should be given to reaction at residues other than amines. For example, the reaction of chymotrypsin with cyanate results in loss of catalytic activity associated with the carbamylation of the active-site serine residue.[56]

Manning and co-workers[57-60] established that the modification of sickle cell hemoglobin with cyanate increased the oxygen affinity of this protein. As with the studies of Stark and co-workers described above, interest in the use of cyanate derived from consideration of the effect of urea.[57] The modification of primary amino groups in hemoglobin has been considered in some detail. It has been established that the amino-terminal value of hemoglobin is more reactive to cyanate in deoxygenated blood than in partially deoxygenated blood. At pH 7.4, the amino-terminal valyl residues of oxyhemoglobin S are carbamylated 50 to 100 times faster than lysyl residues.[50] The rate of incorporation of radiolabeled cyanate into oxyhemoglobin S is shown in Figure 12. Analysis of this reaction after 5 min showed 1 mol valine modified per tetramer and 0.27 mol homocitrulline (the reaction product of cyanate with the ϵ-amino group of lysine) per mol tetramer. After 30 min of reaction, 3 of the 4 amino-terminal valine residues are carbamylated and 2 of 44 (total) lysine residues are modified. The rates of reaction of various hemoglobins and separated chains with cyanate are shown in Figure 13. Figure 14 shows the separation of the α- and β-chain of carbamylated

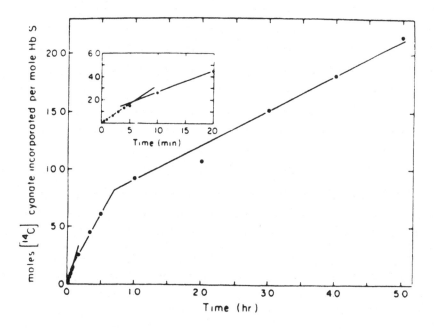

FIGURE 12.   The carbamylation of the α- and ε-amino groups of oxyhemoglobin S (sickle cell hemoglobin) as measured by the incorporation of [¹⁴C] sodium cyanate at pH 7.4 in a pH-stat. Portions were removed at the indicated periods of time, precipitated with cold 5% trichloroacetic acid. The inset describes the early phase of the reaction demonstrating that there are three distinct rates for the reaction. (From Lee, C. K. and Manning, J. M., *J. Biol. Chem.*, 248, 5861, 1973. With permission.)

hemoglobin S by countercurrent distribution. The same laboratory has examined the carbamylation of α-chain and β-chain in some detail.[59] With the deoxy protein, the ratio of radiolabel from ¹⁴C-cyanate on α-chain as compared to the β-chain is 1.7:1.0 while it is 1:1 with the oxy protein. The carbamylation of the amino-terminal valine residues of hemoglobin is approximately 2.5-fold greater in partially deoxygenated media as compared to fully oxygenated media. Thus, it would appear the reactivity of the amino-terminal valine is a sensitive index of conformational change.[60] It is also of interest that removal of Arg¹⁴¹ (α) with carboxypeptidase B abolishes the enhancement of carbamylation observed with the removal of oxygen from hemoglobin.

Mahley and co-workers[49] used carbamylation to explore the role of lysyl residues in the binding of plasma lipoprotein to fibroblasts. The reaction was performed in 0.3 *M* sodium borate, pH 8.0. The extent of modification was determined in two ways. In the first, the modified protein was subjected to acid hydrolysis. The amount of homocitrulline, the product of the reaction of the ε-amino group of lysine with cyanate, was considered equivalent to the number of lysine residues modified. However homocitrulline is partially degraded on acid hydrolysis to produce lysine (17 to 30%). In order to obviate this difficulty, these investigators removed a portion of the modified protein and reacted it under denaturing conditions with 2,4-dinitrifluorobenzene, yielding an acid-stable derivative. The number of lysine residues modified was therefore the sum of free lysine and homocitrulline obtained on amino acid analysis following acid hydrolysis.

In an elegant study by Plapp and co-workers,[61] the modification of lysyl residues in bovine pancreatic deoxyribonuclease A by several different reagents, including cyanate, was examined as shown in Figure 15. The modification with cyanate is performed at 37°C in

Protein	$k \times 10^3 \ min^{-1}$
CO-HbA	2.3
CO-HbS	2.4
Deoxy HbA	4.2
Deoxy HbS	4.0
CO-HMB-α_A	1.9
CO-HMB-α_B	1.6
CO-HMB-β_A	1.9
CO-HMB-β_B	1.6

FIGURE 13. pH dependence of first-order rate constants for the carbamylation of hemoglobin preparations with cyanate at pH 7.4. Carbonmonoxyhemoglobin solutions (9.6 μM as tetramer) were carbamylated with radiolabeled sodium cyanate. Deoxyhemoglobin solutions were prepared as 7.5 μM as tetramer with approximately 1 mg $Na_2S_2O_4$. After 5 min, $NaN^{14}CO$ (final concentration 20 mM) was added for initiation of the reaction. The rate constants are an average of four determinations for HbA and six determinations for HbS. The carbonmonoxy HMB-α and HMB-β chains of Hb, 30 μM, were incubated with 20 mM $NaN^{14}CO$. The precision of the kinetic constants is ± 0.50 for the deoxyhemoglobins. (From Lee, C. K. and Manning, J. M., *J. Biol. Chem.*, 248, 5861, 1973. With permission.)

1.0 M triethanolamine hydrochloride, pH 8.0. The extent of modification was determined by analysis for homocitrulline following acid hydrolysis. A time course of hydrolysis was utilized to provide for the accurate determination of homocitrulline since this amino acid slowly decomposes to form lysine during acid hydrolysis (see above). This modification was sensitive to the conformation of the protein since both the extent of modification and loss of catalytic activity depended on the presence or absence of calcium ions as shown in Figures 16 and 17.

Chollet and Anderson[62] have examined the modification of lysyl residues with potassium cyanate in the catalytic subunit of tobacco ribulose bisphosphate carboxylase. The modification was performed in 0.050 M HEPES, 0.025 M NaCl, pH 7.4. Stoichiometry was not established in this study but it was noted that modification occurred at both the amino terminal and the ϵ-amino groups of lysine.

The reaction of imidoesters with the primary amino groups of proteins has been the subject of considerable investigation in the past 10 to 20 years. The most extensive use of this class of reagents has been the covalent cross-linking of proteins (see Chapter 15). These reagents have the particular advantage that the charge of the lysine residue is maintained during the modification as shown for the reaction of lysine with methyl acetimidate in Figure 18. Ethyl acetimidate has been used to study the role of lysyl residues in thrombin.[63] The reaction was performed with a 1000-fold molar excess of reagent in 0.02 M sodium borate-0.15 M NaCl, pH 8.5. Amino acid analysis indicated that approximately 80% of the lysyl residues were modified under these conditions. The modification of a glutamine synthetase from *Bacillus stearothermophilus* with ethyl acetimidate has been studied by Sekiguchi and co-workers.[64] The modification was performed at pH 9.5 with 0.2 M phosphate for 1 h at 35°C and terminated by dialysis at pH 7.2. The extent of modification was determined by titration of the modified protein with trinitrobenzenesulfonic acid. As these investigators suggest, consideration must be given to the possibility of cross-linking occurring with this reagent under the conditions used.[65] Monneron and d'Alayer[66] examined the reaction of either methyl acetamidate or dimethyl suberimidate with particulate adenylate cyclase. The

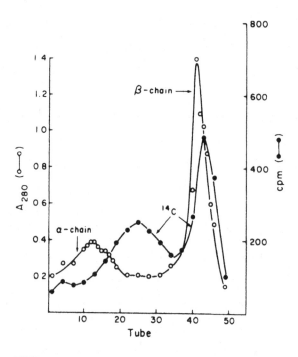

FIGURE 14.   Countercurrent distribution patterns for carbamylated HbS (sickle cell hemoglobin). Oxygenated erythrocytes
were incubated with 10 mM radiolabeled sodium cyanate for 1 h
at 37°C. Globin was prepared from the labeled erythrocytes and
subjected to 50 transfers in 1% dichloroacetic acid-2-butanol.
(From Lee, C. K. and Manning, J. M., *J. Biol. Chem.*, 248,
5861, 1973. With permission.)

reaction was performed in 0.05 M triethanolamine, 10% (w/v) sucrose, 0.005 M MgCl$_2$,
pH 8.1. Plapp and co-workers[61] examined the reaction of methyl picolinimidate with pancreatic deoxyribonuclease. Methyl picolinimidate is an imidoester which reacts with the
primary amino groups in proteins (Figure 19). The reaction was performed in 0.5 M triethanolamine hydrochloride, pH 8.0 containing 1 mM CaCl$_2$ with 0.1 M methyl picolinimidate
for 22 h at 25°C, then with 0.2 M methyl picolinimidate for an additional 8 h. The extent
of modification of a protein by methyl picolinimidate can be determined by spectral analysis
(see Figure 20). Under these conditions, essentially all of the primary amino groups in
deoxyribonuclease (nine lysine and one amino-terminal amino group) were modified but
there was no change in biological activity. The work on DNase modification forms a
particularly useful paper[61] because of its wealth of experimental detail as well as the comparison of the reaction of dexyribonuclease with four different reagents which modify primary
amino groups: O-methylisourea, methyl picolinimidate, cyanate, and trinitrobenzenesulfonic acid. As mentioned above, the reaction of methyl picolinimidate with deoxyribonuclease either in the presence or absence of calcium ions resulted in the modification of
essentially all of the primary amino groups without change in biological activity. Reaction
of deoxyribonuclease with cyanate in either the presence or absence of calcium ions eventually
resulted in the modification of all of the primary amino groups with the complete loss of
biological activity (see Figures 16 and 17). Modification of seven to eight amino groups
with trinitrobenzenesulfonic acid resulted in the loss of all biological activity (Figure 21),
while reaction of a similar number of residues with O-methylisourea only resulted in approximately 50% inactivation (see Figure 15). Plapp has also studied the reaction of methyl
picolinimidate with horse liver alcohol dehydrogenase.[67] This study was somewhat unique

Derivative	Substituent	CaCl₂ used in preparation	No. of amino groups modified	Activity
		mM		$\%$
Guanidino	⊕NH₂ ‖ H₂N—C—	0	8.8 ε, 0.1 α	40
		5	8.9 ε, 0.2 α	75
Picolinimidyl	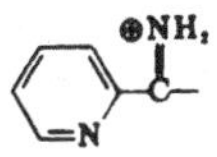 ⊕NH₂ C— =N	0	9.5 (ε + α)	100
		1	9 ε, 0.7 α	100
α-Picolinimidyl, ε-guanidino		5	9.0 ε, 0.9 α	65
Carbamyl	O ‖ H₂N—C—	0	7 ε, 1 α	55*
		0 or 10	7 ε, 1 α	90
		0 or 10	9 ε, 1 α	0
Trinitrophenyl	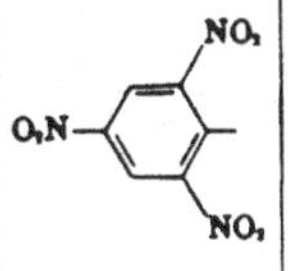 NO₂ O₂N— —NO₂	0	1	95*
		0	7–8	0*
		5	4–5	100
		5	7	0

* Assayed in the absence of Ca⁺⁺.

FIGURE 15. The modification of bovine pancreatic DNase I by various reagents specific for the modification of lysine residues. The extent of lysine modification was determined by homocitrulline formation for reaction with *O*-methylisourea (guanidation), radiolabeled sodium cyanate for carbamylation and spectroscopy for picolinimydilation or trinitrophenylation. Enzymatic activity is expressed as a percent of that of a control preparation of DNase. (From Plapp, B. V., Moore, S., and Stein, W. H., *J. Biol. Chem.*, 246, 939, 1971. With permission.)

in that modification of the enzyme resulted in enhanced catalytic activity reflecting more rapid dissociation of the enzyme-coenzyme complex. It should be noted that the derivatized lysine reverts to lysine (60% yield) under the normal conditions of acid hydrolysis.

A number of investigators have used pyridoxal-5′-phosphate to modify lysyl residues in proteins. Pyridoxal-5′-phosphate is the cofactor form of vitamin B₆ and plays an important role in biological catalysis.[68] Pyridoxal phosphate is useful for the modification of lysine because of selectivity of reaction, spectral properties of the modified residue, reversibility of reaction, and the establishment of stereochemistry by use of radiolabeled sodium borohydride (sodium borotritiide) to reduce the Schiff base initially formed on the reaction of pyridoxal phosphate with a primary amine. Pyridoxal phosphate will react with all primary amines (both ε-amino groups of lysine and the amino-terminal α-amino function) in a protein (Figure 22). In general, pyridoxal 5′-phosphate is far more reactive than pyridoxal because of intramolecular hemiacetal formation and the neighboring group effect of the phosphate moiety (Figure 23). Horecker and co-workers investigated the reaction of pyridoxal phosphate with rabbit muscle aldolase.[69] The initial reaction produced a species with an absorbance maximum at 430 to 435 nm reflecting the protonated Schiff base form of the pyridoxal phosphate-protein complex. After reduction with sodium borohydride, the absorbance maximum is at 325 nm which is characteristic of the reduced Schiff base. This is a quite useful

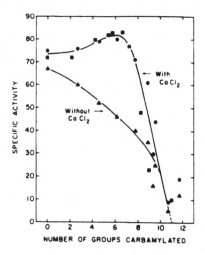

FIGURE 16.   The modification of bovine pancreatic DNase I with potassium cyanate in the presence (■) or absence (●) of 10 m*M* CaCl$_2$. The calcium-free DNase was assayed in the presence (●) or absence (▲) of 10 m*M* CaCl$_2$. (From Plapp, B. V., Moore, S., and Stein, W. H., *J. Biol. Chem.*, 246, 939, 1971. With permission.)

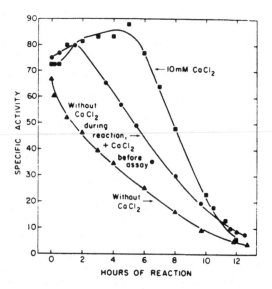

FIGURE 17.   The inactivation of bovine pancreatic DNase with cyanate. The reactions were performed at pH 8.0 (1.0 *M* triethanolamine) in the presence of 1.0 *M* potassium cyanate at 37°C. In the experiment described with the solid squares, 10 m*M* CaCl$_2$ was present during the reaction with potassium cyanate. In the experiment with the solid circles, the enzyme carbamylated in the absence of calcium ions was diluted into 10 m*M* CaCl$_2$ 15 min prior to assay as compared to the experiment described with the solid triangles where the DNase was carbamylated and assayed in the absence of CaCl$_2$. (From Plapp, B. V., Moore, S., and Stein, W. H., *J. Biol. Chem.*, 246, 939, 1971. With permission.)

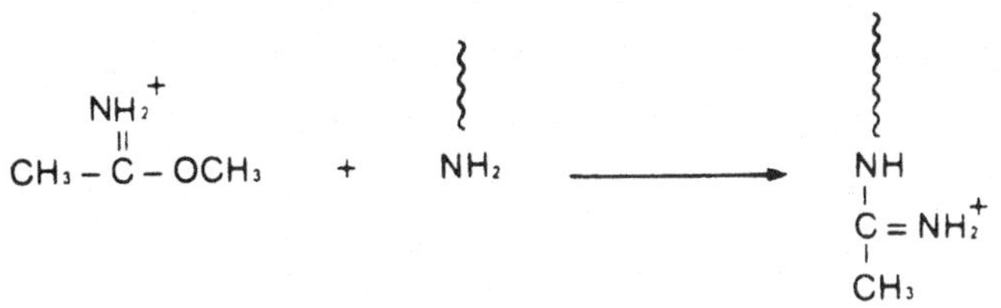

FIGURE 18. The reaction of lysine with methyl acetimidate.

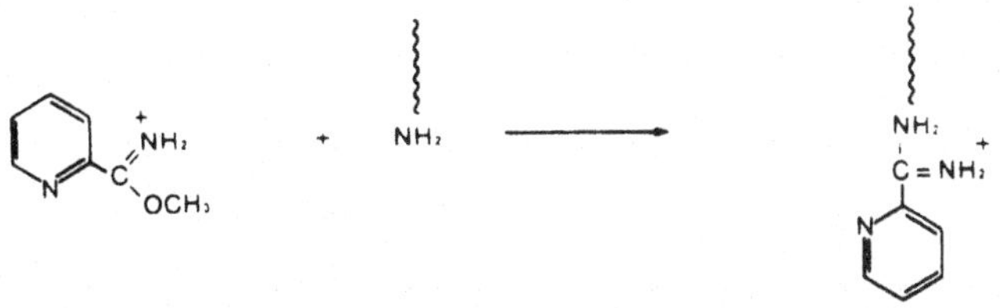

FIGURE 19. The reaction of amino groups with methyl picolinimidate.

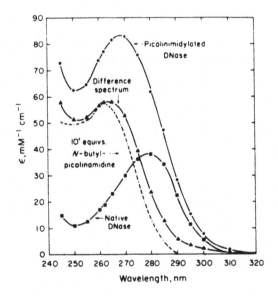

FIGURE 20. The UV spectra of native DNase and the picolinimidylated derivative. The spectra of picolinimidylated DNase (●) and native DNase (■) are presented together with the difference spectrum (▲). From the absorbance at 262 nm and the extinction coefficient for N-butylpicolinamidine (5700 M^{-1} cm^{-1}), it was calculated that the modified enzyme contained 10 picolinimidyl groups (the theoretical difference spectrum for this extent of modification is shown by the dashed line.) The proteins were dissolved in 0.05 M sodium acetate, 1 mM CaCl$_2$ and clarified by centrifugation prior to analysis. A molecular weight of 31,000 was assumed in the calculations. (From Plapp, B. V., Moore, S., and Stein, W. H., *J. Biol. Chem.*, 246, 939, 1971. With permission.)

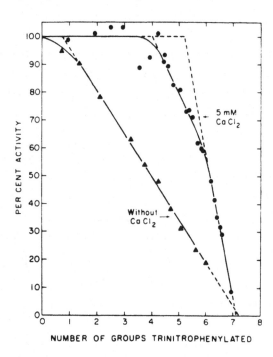

FIGURE 21.   The reaction of bovine pancreatic DNase by 2,4,6-trinitrobenzenesulfonic acid. Reaction was accomplished in 0.3 *M* sodium borate buffer, pH 9.5 in the dark for 5 h in absence of added metal ion (▲) or for 23 h in the presence of 5m*M* CaCl₂(●). The extent of modification with 2,4,6-trinitrobenzenesulfonic acid was assessed by absorbance at 367 nm. (From Plapp, B. V., Moore, S., and Stein, W. H., *J. Biol. Chem.*, 246, 939, 1971. With permission.)

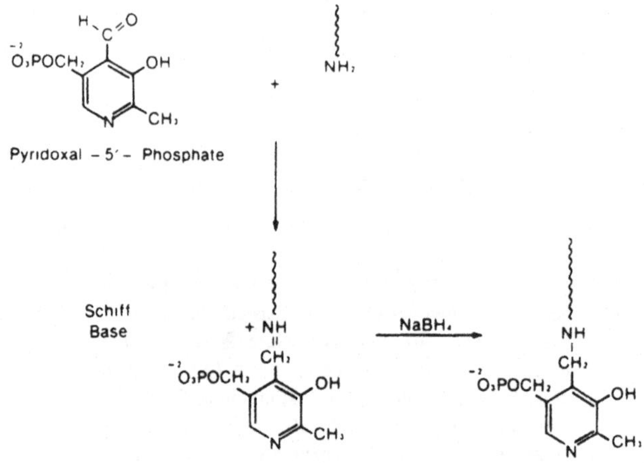

FIGURE 22.   The reaction of pyridoxal-5'-phosphate with amino groups in proteins.

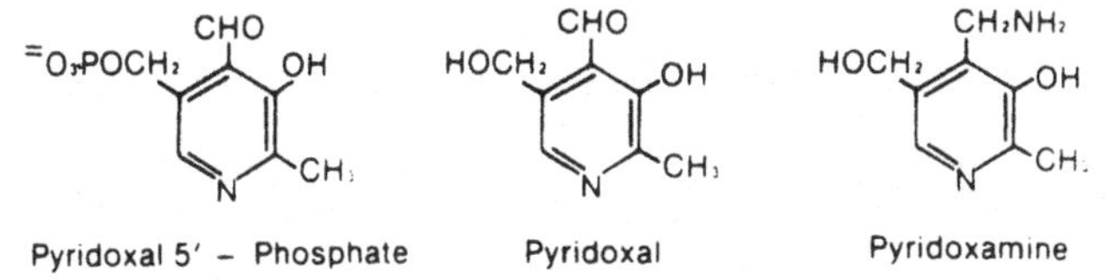

FIGURE 23. The structure of pyridoxal-5'-phosphate, pyridoxal, and pyridoxamine.

study in that the difference in reactivity between pyridoxal and pyridoxal-5'-phosphate is demonstrated as is the reversible nature of the initial complex. Schnackerz and Noltmann[70] compared the reaction of pyridoxal-5'-phosphate and other aldehydes in reaction with rabbit muscle phosphoglucose at pH 8.0. Pyridoxal-5'-phosphate (0.19 mM) resulted in 82% inactivation while the following results were obtained with other aldehydes: pyridoxal (8.4 mM), 16% inactivation; acetaldehyde (75 mM), 75% inactivation; and acetone (75 mM), 31% inactivation. This last reaction is of interest as many investigators are unaware that acetone can react with amino groups in proteins. The reaction of acetone with primary amino groups has been known for some time[71] and is discussed in further detail below within the topic of reductive alkylation. The reaction of ribulose 1,5-bisphosphate carboxylase/oxygenase with pyridoxal-5'-phosphate has been studied by Paech and Tolbert.[72] Pyridoxal-5'-phosphate inactivated the enzyme with or without reduction with NaBH$_4$. This reaction was performed in 0.1 M Bicine (N,N-(2-hydroxyethyl) glycine), 0.010 M MgCl$_2$, 0.2 mM EDTA, 0.001 M dithiothreitol. The reaction demonstrated an optimum at pH 8.4. Spectral studies showed the formation of a species absorbing at 432 nM. As is characteristic for the Schiff base derivative, this peak disappears on reduction to yield a species with an optimum at 325 nm ($\Delta\epsilon = 4800$ M^{-1} cm^{-1}). This supports the suggestion that the loss of activity observed on reaction with pyridoxal-5'-phosphate is due to the formation of a Schiff base which can be reduced with NaBH$_4$ to form a stable derivative, as opposed to the formation of a 2-azolidine ring with a second nucleophile as has been observed by other investigators.[73-75] Jones and Priest[76] have investigated the modification of apo-serine hydroxymethyltransferase with pyridoxal phosphate and the subsequent use of the enzyme-bound pyridoxal phosphate as a structural probe. Cortijo and co-workers[77] have suggested the use of the ratio of absorbance at 415 nm and 335 nm of enzyme-bound pyridoxal phosphate as an indication of the polarity of the medium. Cake and co-workers[78] have demonstrated that modification of activated hepatic glucorticoid receptor with pyridoxal-5'-phosphate obviated the binding of the receptor to DNA. Greatly reduced inhibition was seen with pyridoxamine-5'-phosphate, pyridoxamine, or pyridoxine (see Figure 24). Inhibition could be reversed by gel filtration or treatment with dithiothreitol while treatment with NaBH$_4$ resulted in irreversible inhibition of DNA binding. These investigators used 0.2 M borate, 0.25 M sucrose, 0.003 M MgCl$_2$ (pH 8.0) as the solvent for reaction with pyridoxal-5'-phosphate. Slebe and Martinez-Carrion[79] have introduced the use of phosphopyridoxal trifluoroethyl amine as a probe for pyridoxal phosphate binding sites in enzymes (Figure 25). Nishigori and Toft[80] explored the reaction of pyridoxal-5'-phosphate with the avian progesterone receptor. Reaction with pyridoxal-5'-phosphate was performed in 0.02 M barbital, 10% (v/v) glycerol, 0.005 mM dithiothreitol, 0.010 M KCl, pH 8.0. The modification was stabilized by NaBH$_4$. It is of interest that these investigators noted that the modification was readily reversed in Tris buffer unless stabilized by NaBH$_4$. Sugiyama and Mukohata[81] observed that modification with pyridoxal-5'-phosphate of the lysine residue in chloroplast coupling factor using 0.020 M Tricine, 0.001 M EDTA, 0.010 M MgCl$_2$, pH 8.0 resulted in complete inactivation of the ATPase activity. Peters and co-workers[82] reported on the inactivation of the ATPase activity in a bacterial coupling factor by reaction with pyridoxal-5'-phosphate. The modification was performed in 0.050 M morpholinosulfonic acid, pH 7.5. The inhibition was

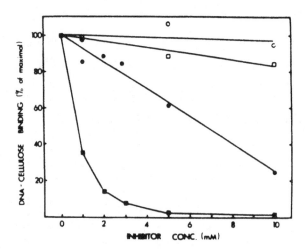

FIGURE 24.   The specificity of the effect of pyridoxal-5′-phos-
phate on the DNA binding site of activated hepatic glucocorticoid receptor. The reactions were performed in 0.2 *M* boric acid,
0.25 *M* sucrose, 3 m*M* NaCl$_2$, pH 18.0 at 0°C. The reactions
included either pyridoxal-5′-phosphate, 0.75 m*M* (■), 6.5 m*M*
pyridoxal (●), pyridoxamine-5′-phosphate (□), or pyridoxamine
(○). In data not shown, pyridoxine or phosphate ions were without effect in the inhibition of DNA binding by the activated
receptor. (From Cake, M. A., DiSorbo, D. M., and Litwack,
G., *J. Biol. Chem.*, 253, 4886, 1978. With permission.)

readily reversed by dilution or by 0.01 *M* lysine and was, as expected, stabilized by NaBH$_4$.
Gould and Engel[83] reported on the reaction of mouse testicular lactate dehydrogenase with
pyridoxal-5′-phosphate in 0.050 *M* sodium pyrophosphate, pH 8.7 at 25°C. This reaction
resulted in the inactivation of the dehydrogenase activity. The inactivation was reversed by
cysteine (Figure 26) and stabilized by NaBH$_4$. These investigators reported that the observed
absorption coefficient at 325 nm may be decreased as much as 50% with protein-bound
pyridoxal phosphate. Thus, estimation of the number of lysine residues modified using the
absorption coefficient obtained with model compounds might provide only a minimum value.
Ogawa and Fujioka[84] studied the reaction of pyridoxal-5′-phosphate with saccharopine
dehydrogenase in 0.1 *M* potassium phosphate, pH 6.8, at ambient temperature in the dark.
Both spectral analysis (Figure 27) and tritium incorporation from sodium borohydride reduction (Figure 28) were consistent with the modification of one lysine residue per mol of
enzyme being responsible for the loss of enzyme activity. A value of $1 \times 10^4 \ M^{-1} \ cm^{-1}$
for the extinction coefficient at 325 nm[85] was used in this study. It is of interest that this
study demonstrated that it is possible to establish an equilibrium between the native and
modified forms of the enzyme. The reversibility of the modification is shown in Figure 28.
Also shown in Figure 28 is a series of experiments designed to determine the equilibrium
constant for the reaction using a graphical method where the reciprocal of the concentration
of pyridoxal-5-phosphate is plotted vs. the activity at equilibrium (A_{eq}) divided by the value
obtained (A_o-A_{eq}) by subtracting the activity at equilibrium (A_{eq}) from the initial activity
(A_o). The slope of this graph provides the equilibrium constant (K_{eq}) for the reaction under
the experimental conditions (0.1 *M* potassium phosphate, pH 6.8 at 0°C). A value of 3.3
$\times 10^3 \ M^{-1}$ was obtained for the equilibrium constant as shown in Figure 29. Protection is
not provided by α-ketoglutarate in the absence of the reduced coenzyme. Pyridoxal was
much less effective than pyridoxal-5′-phosphate in the inactivation of saccharopine
dehydrogenase. The concentrations of pyridoxal and pyridoxal-5′-phosphate were determined

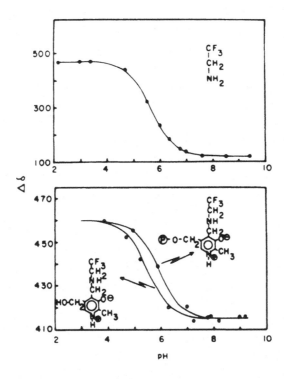

FIGURE 25. The pH dependence of the chemical shift response of ^{19}F nuclear magnetic resonance with fluorinated compounds in the absence of enzymes. The top panel shows 2,2,2-trifluoroethylamine (100 mM). The solid curve indicates a theoretical titration curve of a simple ionization group for a pKa of 5.65. The bottom panel shows phosphopyridoxal trifluoroethyl amine (10 mM) before (●) and after (○) treatment with alkaline phosphatase. The solid lines show theoretical titration curves for a single ionization with a pKa of 5.90 and 5.50 respectively. (From Slebe, J. C. and Martinez-Carrion, M., *J. Biol. Chem.*, 253, 2093, 1978. With permission.)

spectrophotometrically in 0.1 M NaOH using an extinction coefficient of $5.8 \times 10^3\ M^{-1}$ cm^{-1} at 300 nm and $6.6 \times 10^3\ M^{-1}$ cm^{-1} at 388 nm respectively.[86] Amine compounds have the potential to interfere in the reaction of pyridoxal-5′-phosphate with proteins. Moldoon and Cidlowski[87] demonstrate that 0.1 M Tris, pH 7.4 markedly interfered with the modification of rat uterine estrogen receptor with pyridoxal-5′-phosphate. These investigators also noted that, as in the other studies, 0.05 M lysine would block the modification reaction and could also reverse the modification if the Schiff base had not been reduced. Stock solutions of pyridoxal phosphate were prepared in 0.01 M NaOH to avoid acid decomposition. The importance of local environmental factors in the specificity of modification by pyridoxal phosphate is emphasized by Ohsawa and Gualerzi.[88] These investigators examined the modification of *Escherichia coli* initiation factor by pyridoxal phosphate in 0.020 M triethanolamine, 0.03 M KCl, pH 7.8. In the course of the studies, it was observed that pyridoxal phosphate will not react with poly (AUG). These investigators also reported the preparation of N^6-pyridoxal lysine by reaction of pyridoxal phosphate with polylysine in 0.01 M sodium phosphate, pH 7.2 at 37°C followed by reduction with NaBH$_4$. The reduction was terminated by the addition of acetic acid. Acid hydrolysis (6 N HCl, 110°C, 22 h) yielded N^6-pyridoxal-L-lysine. Bürger and Görisch[89] reported the inactivation of histidinol dehydrogenase upon reaction with pyridoxal phosphate in 0.02 M Tris, pH 7.6. This modification could be

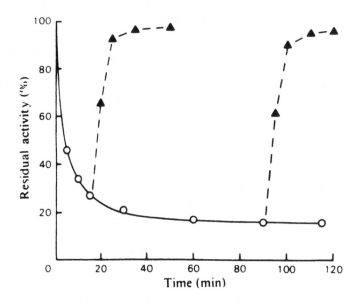

FIGURE 26.   The L-cysteine reversal of the inactivation of mouse C_4 lactate dehydrogenase inactivated by pyridoxal-5′-phosphate. Mouse C_4 lactate dehydrogenase was incubated with 1 mM pyridoxal-5′-phosphate in the dark at 25°C in 0.05 M sodium pyrophosphate, pH 8.7 (○). At 15 min and 90 min, 0.2 ml portions of the reaction mixture were removed and mixed with 10 μl of 1.0 M cysteine and assayed for enzyme activity at the time points indicated (▲). (From Gould, K. G. and Engel, P. C., *Biochem. J.*, 191, 365, 1980. With permission.)

reversed by dialysis unless the putative Schiff base was stabilized by reduction with NaH_4 (*n*-octyl alcohol added to prevent foaming). These investigators used a $\Delta\epsilon$ for ϵ-amino pyridoxal lysine of 1×10^4 M^{-1} cm^{-1} at 325 nm. Recent applications of pyridoxal-5′-phosphate modification has been used to study hydroxymethylbilane synthetase,[90] DNA polymerase I,[91] and rabbit glycogen synthase isozymes.[92] A novel affinity label (pyridoxal-5′-diphospho-5′-adenosine; see Figure 30) utilizing pyridoxal-5′-phosphate chemistry has been used to study the adenine nucleotide binding sites in yeast hexokinase.[93]

A substantial portion of the specificity of pyridoxal-5′-phosphate in protein modification arises from electrostatic interaction(s) via the phosphate group with positively charged groups (i.e., arginine) on the protein surface. A conceptually related compound is methyl acetyl phosphate (Figure 31). The reagent was originally developed as an affinity label for D-3-hydroxybutyrate dehydrogenase.[94] Manning and co-workers have examined the chemistry of the reaction of methyl acetyl phosphate with hemoglobin in some detail.[95,96] It appears to be an affinity label for the 2,3-diphosphoglycerate binding site.[95] More recent work suggests that this reagent may be a useful probe for other anion binding sites in proteins.[96]

The modification of primary amines in proteins by reductive alkylation has proved to be a useful reaction (Figure 32). This reaction has the advantage that the basic charge properties of the modified residue are preserved. The early work on this modification has been reviewed by Means and co-workers.[97] Both monosubstituted and disubstituted derivatives can be prepared depending upon reaction conditions and the nature of the carbonyl compound.

Rice and co-workers[98] reported the stabilization of trypsin by reductive methylation. This reaction utilized formaldehyde/sodium borohydride in 0.2 M sodium borate, pH 9.2 in the cold. Unsubstituted amino groups were present after the reaction as demonstrated by titration with trinitrobenzenesulfonic acid. The amino-terminal isoleucine residue was not modified

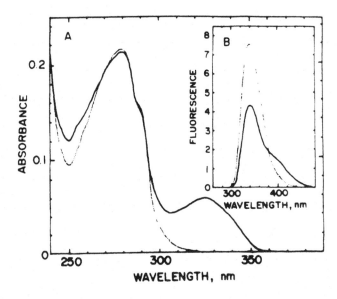

FIGURE 27.   The UV spectra and fluorescence spectra of native and pyridoxal-5′-treated saccharopine dehydrogenase (L-lysine forming). The enzyme preparation (17.9 nmol) was incubated with 0.5 mM pyridoxal-5′-phosphate in 0.1 M potassium phosphate, pH 6.8 followed by reduction with sodium borohydride and dialysis again with 0.1 M potassium phosphate, pH 6.8 in the dark. Panel A shows the UV absorption spectra for the native (dotted line) and modified enzyme (solid line). Panel B shows the fluorescence emission spectra for the native (dotted line) and the reduced enzyme (solid line). The excitation wavelength in the fluorescence spectra was 280 nm. The protein concentrations for the native and modified enzyme were identical in these experiments. (From Ogawa, H. and Fujioka, M., J. Biol. Chem., 255, 7420, 1980. With permission.)

under these conditions. Morris and co-workers[99] investigated the reductive methylation of monellin. The modification was performed in 0.2 M sodium borate, pH 8.0 with 1 mM monellin (11 mM) with respect to primary amino groups in the cold. Sodium borohydride was added to give a final concentration of 0.5 mg/ml, and 1 to 5 μl of 6 to 8 M formaldehyde was added per ml of solution. Tritiated formaldehyde was used to establish the extent of modification. One of the problems with the use of formaldehyde in this reaction is the presence of paraformaldehyde. Chen and Benoiton[100] obviated this difficulty by the in situ generation of formaldehyde from methanol.

The introduction of sodium cyanoborohydride as a reducing agent for this reaction represented a real advance. Sodium cyanoborohydride is stable in aqueous solution at pH 7.0. Unlike sodium borohydride which can reduce aldehydes and disulfide bonds, sodium cyanoborohydride only reduces the Schiff base formed in the initial process of reductive alkylation. The radiolabeling of proteins using ^{14}C-formaldehyde and sodium cyanoborohydride has been reported.[101] The modification was performed in 0.04 M phosphate, pH 7.0 at 25°C. The modification can be performed equally well at 0°C but, as would be expected, takes a longer period of time; there is no effect on the extent of the modification. In this regard, these authors estimated that the same extent of modification obtained in 1 h at 37°C could be achieved in 4 to 6 h at 25°C or 24 h at 0°C. Although the majority of experiments in this study were performed in phosphate buffer at pH 7.0, equivalent results can be obtained in Tris or HEPES (N-2-hydroxyethylpiperazine-N′-2-ethanesulfonic acid) buffer at pH 7.0. A greater extent of modification was observed with sodium cyanoborohydride at pH 7.0 than with sodium borohydride at pH 9.0.

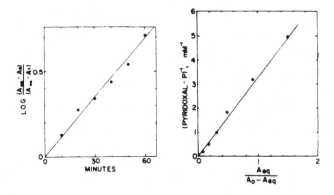

FIGURE 28.   Left panel shows recovery of activity of saccharopine dehydrogenase inactivated by pyridoxal-5′-phosphate. The enzyme (23 nmol) was inactivated by reaction in 0.2 ml of 0.1 M potassium phosphate buffer, pH 6.8 at 0°C. After 30 min, 10-μl portions were transferred to 1.7 ml 0.1 potassium phosphate, pH 6.8 at 0°C. At the indicated times, portions were reduced with sodium borohydride and assayed for enzyme activity. A_o indicates enzyme activity at zero time, A_t indicates enzyme activity at time t while A_{eq} indicates enzyme activity at equilibrium. The right panel shows a plot of the reciprocal of pyridoxal-5′-phosphate concentration vs. $A_{eq}/A_o - A_{eq}$. Saccaropine dehydrogenase (2 nmol) was incubated in 0.1 M potassium phosphate, pH 6.8 and residual enzyme activity determined at 24°C. (From Ogawa, H. and Fujioka, M., *J. Biol. Chem.*, 255, 7420, 1980. With permission.)

Reductive methylation with ³C-enriched formaldehyde has been used to introduce an NMR probe for the study of protein conformation.[102] A similar approach has been developed using deuterated acetone.[103]

The effect of carbonyl compounds of different size on the extent of reductive alkylation has been examined by Feeney and co-workers.[104] The extent of modification is more a reflection of the type of alkylating agent and reaction conditions than an intrinsic property of the protein under study. For example, nearly 100% disubstitution can be obtained with formaldehyde and approximately 35% disubstitution with *n*-butanol, while only monosubstitution can be obtained with acetone, cyclopentanone, cyclohexanone, and benzaldehyde. While most of the products of reductive alkylation retained solubility, the reaction products obtained with cyclohexanone and benzaldehyde tended to precipitate. Examination of the reductive alkylation of ovomucoid, lysozyme, and ovotransferrin with different aldehydes suggests that such modification occurs without major conformational change as judged by circular dichroism measurements.[105] The same study also examined the stability of the modified proteins by scanning differential calorimetry. The extensive modification of amino groups decreases thermal stability. The destabilization effect increases with increasing size (and hydrophobicity) of the modifying aldehyde.

In another study, the reversible reductive alkylation of proteins has been examined.[106] Both glycolaldehyde and acetol will react with the primary amino groups in proteins to yield derivatives which can be cleaved with periodate under mild basic condition to yield the free amine. Figure 33 shows the distribution of reaction products of lysine and glycolaldehyde as a function of pH with either sodium borohydride (A) or sodium cyanoborohydride (B) as the reducing agent. It is apparent that sodium cyanoborohydride is much more effective in the range of pH 6.0 to pH 8.0 while sodium borohydride is more effective under more alkaline conditions. Treatment of 30.0 mg lysozyme in 6.0 ml 0.2 M sodium borate, pH 9.0, with 60 mg glycoladehyde and 10 mg sodium borohydride at ambient temperature

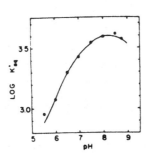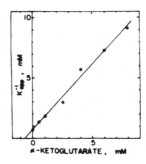

FIGURE 29. The left panel shows the effect of pH on the equilibrium constant for the inactivation of saccharopine dehydrogenase by pyridoxal-5′-phosphate. The enzyme (2.5 nmol) was incubated at 24°C with 0.1 M potassium phosphate at the indicated pH. Values for the equilibrium constant were calculated from the equation

$$K_{eq} = (A_o - A_{eq})/A_{eq}[P]$$

The points were determined experimentally and the line was calculated from the following equation:

$$\log K'_{eq} = \log K + \log \left(1 + \frac{[H^+]}{K_{3S}} \right.$$
$$+ \frac{[H^+]^2}{K_{2S}K_{3S}} + \frac{[H^+]^3}{K_{1S}K_{2S}K_{3S}}\left)\right.$$
$$- \log \left(1 + \frac{[H^+]}{K_{3P}} + \frac{[H^+]^2}{K_{2P}K_{3P}} + \frac{[H^+]^3}{K_{1P}K_{2P}K_{3P}}\right)$$
$$- \log \left(1 + \frac{[H^+]}{K_E}\right)$$

The right panel shows a plot of reciprocal apparent equilibrium constant vs. α-ketoglutarate concentration. The enzyme (2 nmol) was incubated with 1.0 mM pyridoxal-5′-phosphate containing 0.2 mM reduced nicotinamide-adenine dinucleotide (NADH) and α-ketoglutarate at the concentrations indicated. The values for the equilibrium constants were calculated using the equation described above. (From Ogawa, H. and Fujioka, M., *J. Biol. Chem.*, 255, 7420, 1980. With permission.)

FIGURE 30. The structure of pyridoxal-5′-diphospho-adenosine, an affinity label based on pyridoxal chemistry.

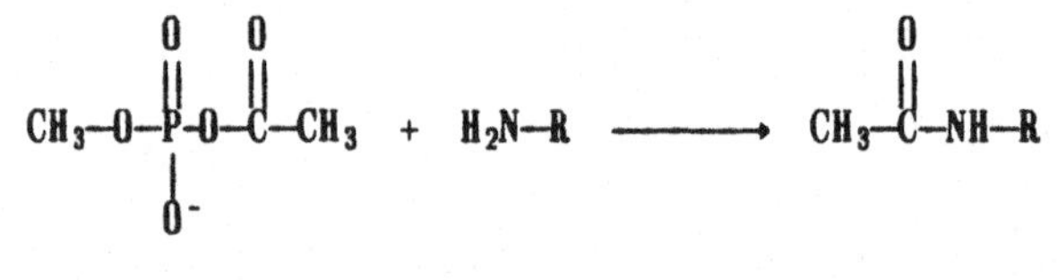

$$CH_3-O-\overset{\overset{\displaystyle O}{\|}}{\underset{\underset{\displaystyle O^-}{|}}{P}}-O-\overset{\overset{\displaystyle O}{\|}}{C}-CH_3 \; + \; H_2N-R \; \longrightarrow \; CH_3-\overset{\overset{\displaystyle O}{\|}}{C}-NH-R$$

FIGURE 31.   The structure of methyl acetyl phosphate, a site-specific reagent for the modification of lysine residues in proteins.

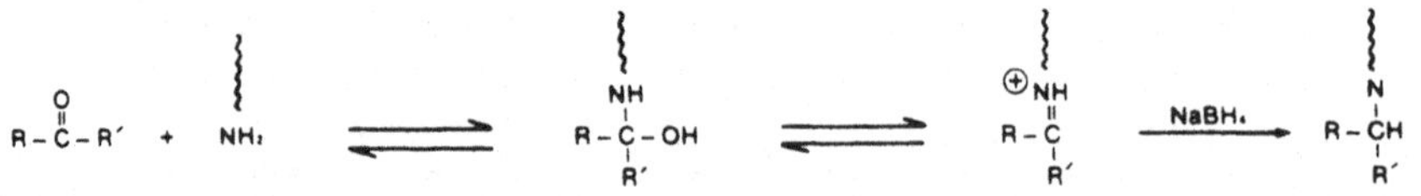

$$R-\overset{\overset{\displaystyle O}{\|}}{C}-R' \; + \; NH_2 \; \rightleftharpoons \; R-\overset{\overset{\displaystyle NH}{|}}{\underset{\underset{\displaystyle R'}{|}}{C}}-OH \; \rightleftharpoons \; R-\overset{\overset{\displaystyle \oplus NH}{\|}}{\underset{\underset{\displaystyle R'}{|}}{C}} \; \xrightarrow{NaBH_4} \; R-\overset{\overset{\displaystyle N}{|}}{\underset{\underset{\displaystyle R'}{|}}{CH}}$$

FIGURE 32.   The reductive alkylation of amino groups in proteins.

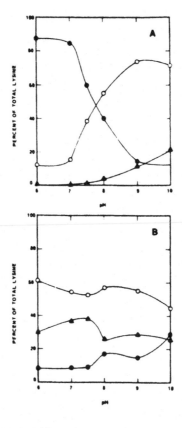

FIGURE 33.   The pH dependence of the reductive alkylation of α-L-lysine using two different reducing agents. In panel A sodium borohydride was used as the reducing agent while in panel B sodium cyanoborohydride was used as the reducing agent. The composition of the reaction products was determined after removal of the α-*N*-acetyl group by acid hydrolysis. The products shown are lysine (●), ε-*N*-(2-hydroxyethyl)lysine (○), and ε-*N*,*N*-bis-(2-hydroxyethyl)lysine (▲). (From Geoghegan, K. F., Cabacungan, J. C., Dixon, H. B. F., and Feeney, R. E., *Int. J. Peptide Protein Res.*, 17, 345, 1981. With permission.)

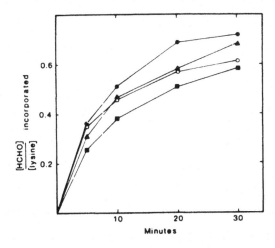

FIGURE 34.   The effect of sodium cyanoborohydride concentration on the rate of reductive methylation of albumin.
The reaction mixtures contained 1 mg/ml of albumin, 2 nm
[¹⁴C] formaldehyde in 0.1 *M* HEPES buffer, pH 7.5. The
reaction mixtures were maintained at 22°C and terminated
at the indicated points by the addition of trichloroacetic acid
and incorporated radiolabel determined. The concentration
of sodium cyanoborohydride used in the experiments were
10 m*M* (■), 25 m*M* (▲), 100 m*M* (●), and 250 m*M* (○).
(From Jentoft, N. and Dearborn, D. G., *J. Biol. Chem.*,
254, 4359, 1979. With permission.)

resulted in 60% 2-hydroxyethylation. Treatment of 20 mg ovomucoid in 2.0 ml 0.2 *M*
sodium borate, pH 9.0 with 10% acetol and 30 mg sodium borohydride (added in portions)
resulted in 55% hydroxyisopropylation. In both situations, the reaction was terminated by
adjustment of the pH to 5 with glacial acetic acid. The extent of modification was determined
either by titration with trinitrobenzenesulfonic acid and/or by amino acid analysis after acid
hydrolysis. Periodate oxidation could be accomplished with 0.015 *M* sodium periodate at
pH 7.9 for 30 min at ambient temperature.

The replacement of sodium borohydride with sodium cyanoborohydride appears to represent a significant advance in the stabilization of Schiff bases in proteins after reaction with
carbonyl compounds. There are several difficulties associated with the use of sodium borohydride in this reaction including the reduction of aldehydes to alcohols, the dependence
of reduction on pH, the reduction of disulfide bonds, and the possible cleavage of peptide
bonds. Jentoft and Dearborn have studied the use of sodium cyanoborohydride in some
detail.[107] In particular, the preparation of sodium cyanoborohydride is critical and most, if
not all, commercial preparations require recrystallization prior to use. This reflects the
presence of impurities which limit the extent of the reductive alkylation (see below). Recrystallization is accomplished by dissolving 11 g of sodium cyanoborohydride in 25 ml
acetonitrile. Insoluble material is removed by centrifugation. Crystallization is accomplished
by the addition of 150 ml methylene chloride and allowing to stand overnight at 4°C. The
recrystallized sodium cyanoborohydride is collected by filtration and stored in a vacuum
desiccator. A fresh solution of reagent is prepared daily. Using [¹⁴C]-formaldehyde and
sodium cyanoborohydride, the major product is ε-methylated lysine, with minor incorporation
of radiolabel into arginine and histidine. Figure 34 shows the effect of sodium cyanoborohydride incorporation on the extent of reductive methylation (¹⁴C-formaldehyde) in 0.1 *M*
HEPES buffer, pH 7.5. The rate of reductive methylation in this experiment with albumin
was not sensitive to cyanoborohydride concentration. The effect of pH on the reaction is

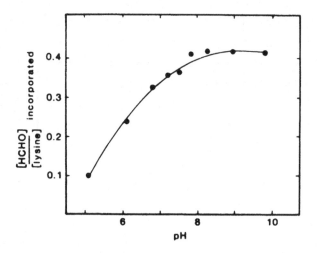

FIGURE 35.   The pH dependence for the reductive methylation of lysine residues in albumin. The reaction mixtures contained 0.86 mg/ml of protein, 20 m*M* sodium cyanoborohydride, and 2 m*M* [^{14}C] formaldehyde and were incubated for 10 min at 22°C. The extent of modification was determined by incorporation of radio-label. The buffers used were sodium acetate (pH 5.1), sodium phosphate (pH 6.1 and pH 6.8), HEPES (pH 7.2 and 8.25), and sodium borate (pH 9.0 and 9.8). (From Jentoft, N. and Dearborn, D. G., *J. Biol. Chem.*, 254, 4359, 1979. With permission.)

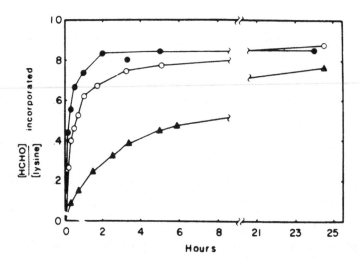

FIGURE 36.   The effect of time and temperature on the reductive methylation of albumin. The reaction mixture contained 1.0 mg/ml albumin in 0.2 *M* HEPES, pH 7.5 in the presence of 20 m*M* sodium cyanoborohydride, and 2 m*M* [^{14}C] formaldehyde. The reactions were incubated at 4°C (▲), 22°C (○), or 37°C (●) for the indicated periods of time. (From Jentoft, N. and Dearborn, D. G., *J. Biol. Chem.*, 254, 4359, 1979. With permission.)

shown in Figure 35. Optimal reductive methylation was obtained at pH values greater than 8.0 during a short-term (10 min) incubation. The effect of pH is much less pronounced at longer periods of incubation (1 to 2 h) with optimal reductive methylation occurring between pH 7.0 and pH 8.0. The effect of temperature on the rate of reaction at pH 7.5 (0.1 *M* HEPES) is shown in Figure 36. Note that although the reaction is much slower at 4°C, the

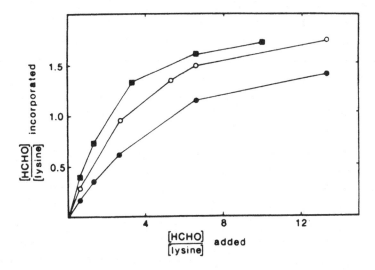

FIGURE 37.   The effect of formaldehyde concentration and protein concentration on the reductive methylation of albumin. The reaction mixtures contained 20 mM sodium cyanoborohydride, with varying amounts of formaldehyde and albumin in 0.1 M HEPES buffer, pH 7.5. In (●), the reaction mixture contained 0.43 mg/ml albumin, in (○), 1.07 mg/ml albumin and in (■), 3.41 mg/ml albumin. The reactions were maintained at 22°C for 2 h. The extent of modification was determined by measuring the extent of radiolabel incorporated [^{14}C] formaldehyde. (From Jentoft, N. and Dearborn, D. G., *J. Biol. Chem.*, 254, 4359, 1979. With permission.)

extent of modification is almost equivalent to that achieved at higher temperature. The effect of formaldehyde concentration and protein concentration on the extent of reductive methylation is shown in Figure 37. An examination of this data suggests that approximately 80% modification can be achieved at a protein (bovine serum albumin) concentration of greater than 1 mg/ml at a formaldehyde/lysine ratio of 8 while virtually quantitative modification was obtained at a ratio of 12. These investigators also noted that Tris, β-mercaptoethanol, dithiothreitol, ammonium ions (as ammonium sulfate), and guanidine (5 M) inhibited the reductive alkylation of albumin by formaldehyde and sodium cyanoborohydride in 0.1 M HEPES, pH 7.5. The use of [^{13}C] formaldehyde in the reductive alkylation of ribonuclease has been reported.[108] In a subsequent study,[109] Jentoft and Dearborn characterized the inhibition by cyanide of reductive alkylation with sodium cyanoborohydride (Figure 38). This is of some importance since cyanide is a product of reductive alkylation with sodium cyanoborohydride. Inhibition by cyanide can be blocked by nickel (II) or cobalt (III). The observation that nickel (II) can preclude the inhibition of reductive alkylation by cyanide was shown to obviate the previously observed necessity for recrystallization of the sodium cyanoborohydride. The effect of NiCl$_2$ or KCN on the time course of the reductive methylation of bovine serum albumin at pH 7.5 (0.050 M HEPES) is shown in Figure 39. Additional studies on the development of reagents alternative to sodium borohydride have been reported from other laboratories. Feeney and co-workers[110] compared sodium cyanoborohydride, dimethylamine borane, and trimethylamine borane (Figure 40) with respect to effectiveness in reductive alkylation. Reduction at disulfide bonds was not observed with any of the three reagents. Dimethylamine borane was only slightly less effective than sodium cyanoborohydride while trimethylamine borane was much less effective (Figure 41). This decrease in effectiveness in reductive alkylation is balanced by the absence of toxic byproducts such as cyanide evolving during the reaction. Figure 42 compares dimethylamine borane and trimethylamine borane in the reductive methylation of turkey ovomucoid in

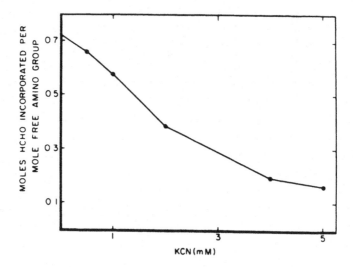

FIGURE 38. The effect of the addition of potassium cyanide (KCN) on the reductive methylation of albumin. Reaction mixtures contained 1.04 mg/ml bovine serum albumin, 2 mM [^{14}C] formaldehyde, 10 mM sodium cyanoborohydride in 0.05 M HEPES, pH 7.5 with varying amounts of KCN as indicated. The extent of modification was determined by measuring the amount of radiolabel incorporation. (From Jentoft, N. and Dearborn, D. G., *Anal. Biochem.*, 106, 186, 1980. With permission.)

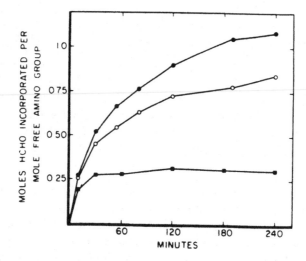

FIGURE 39. The effect of Ni (II) and KCN on the time course of the reductive methylation of albumin. The reactions were performed in 0.05 M HEPES, pH 7.5 with 10 mM sodium cyanoborohydride, and 2 mM [^{14}C] formaldehyde and incubated in the presence of either 2 mM NiCl$_2$ (●), 2 mM KCN (■), or no addition (○). (From Jentoft, N. and Dearborn, D. G., *Anal. Biochem.*, 106, 186, 1980. With permission.)

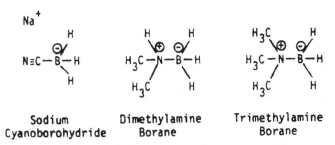

FIGURE 40.   The structure of sodium cyanoborohydride, dimethylamine borane, and trimethylamine borane. (From Geoghegan, K. F., Cabacungan, J. C., Dixon, H. B. F., and Feeney, R. E., *Int. J. Peptide Protein Res.*, 17, 345, 1981. With permission.)

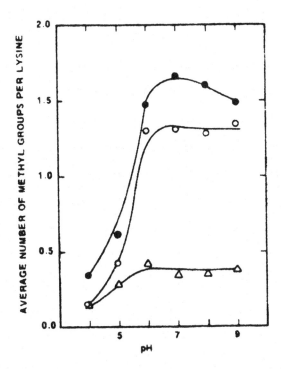

FIGURE 41.   The effect of pH on the reductive methylation of turkey ovomucoid in the presence of various reducing agents. The concentration of turkey ovomucoid was 5 mg/ml, the concentration of formaldehyde was 20 mM in the presence of either sodium cyanoborohydride (●), 15 mM, dimethylamine borane (○), 15 mM, or trimethylaminoborane (△), 15 mM. (From Geoghegan, K. F., Cabacungan, J. C., Dixon, H. B. F., and Feeney, R. E., *Int. J. Peptide Protein Res.*, 17, 345, 1981. With permission.)

0.2 M sodium phosphate, pH 7.0. Quantitative reductive methylation (equal to or greater than one methyl group per lysyl residue) is achieved at 10 mM formaldehyde with dimethylamine borane and at 50 mM formaldehyde with trimethylamine borane. It should be noted that a similar extent of modification is obtained with 5 mM formaldehyde using sodium cyanoborohydride. In a subsequent study[111] this laboratory reported the successful use of pyridine borane in the reductive alkylation of proteins. Wu and Means[112] have used reductive

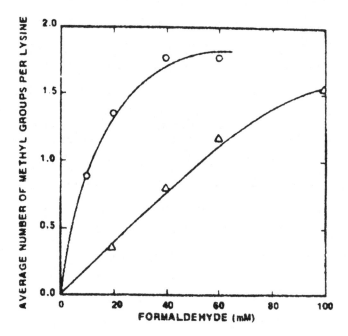

FIGURE 42.   The effect of formaldehyde concentration on the reductive methylation of turkey ovomucoid. The reaction was performed in 0.2 *M* sodium phosphate, pH 7.0 with a turkey ovomucoid concentration of 5 mg/ml. The reducing agents were used at a concentration of 15 m*M* and included dimethylamine borane (○) and trimethylamine borane (△) at 22°C. The reducing agents were dissolved in methanol at a concentration of 150 m*M* and diluted 1:10 in the reaction mixture such that the final concentration of methanol was 10% (v/v). (From Geoghegan, K. F., Cabacungan, J. C., Dixon, H. B. F., and Feeney, R. E., *Int. J. Peptide Protein Res.*, 17, 345, 1981. With permission.)

alkylation with a nonpolar aldehyde (dodecylaldehyde) to subsequently prepare insoluble proteins by binding of the modified protein to octyl-Sepharose.

The reaction of glyceraldehyde with carbonmonoxyhemoglobin S has been explored by Acharya and Manning.[113] This reaction was performed with 0.010 *M* glyceraldehyde in phosphate-buffered saline, pH 7.4, and the resultant Schiff bases were stabilized by reduction with sodium borohydride. Using radiolabeled glyceraldehyde, these investigators were able to obtain support for the concept that there is selectivity in the reaction of sugar aldehydes with hemoglobin. The reaction product between glyceraldehyde and hemoglobin S did have stability properties without reduction that were not consistent with only Schiff base products. These investigators suggested that the glyceraldehyde-hemoglobin Schiff base could undergo an Amadori rearrangement (Figure 43) to form a stable ketoamine adduct which could be reduced with sodium borohydride to form a product identical to that obtained by direct reduction of the Schiff base. In a subsequent study, these investigators did show that the glyceraldehyde-hemoglobin S Schiff base could rearrange to form a ketamine via an Amadori rearrangement.[114] These investigators were able to use reaction with phenylhydrazine to detect the protein-bound ketamine adduct as shown in Figure 44.

Another class of aldehydes that reacts with protein to give interesting products are simple monosaccharides which exist in solution in enol and keto forms (Figure 45). Wilson[115] showed that bovine pancreatic ribonuclease dimer would react with lactose in the presence of sodium cyanoborohydride to yield an active derivative that shows selectivity in uptake by the liver during *in vivo* experiments. The modification of ribonuclease dimer was performed in 0.2 *M* potassium phosphate, pH 7.4 (phosphate buffer was used to protect lysine-41

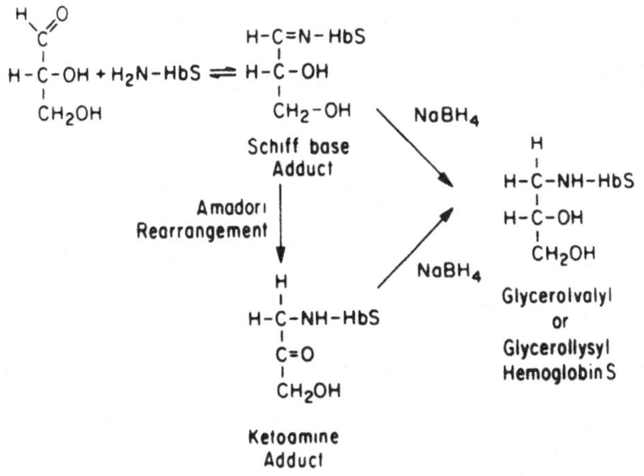

FIGURE 43. Schematic representation of the formation of glycerovaline or glycerollysine on the reaction of hemoglobin S with glyceraldehyde. (From Acharya, A. S. and Manning, J. M., *J. Biol. Chem.*, 255, 1406, 1980. With permission.)

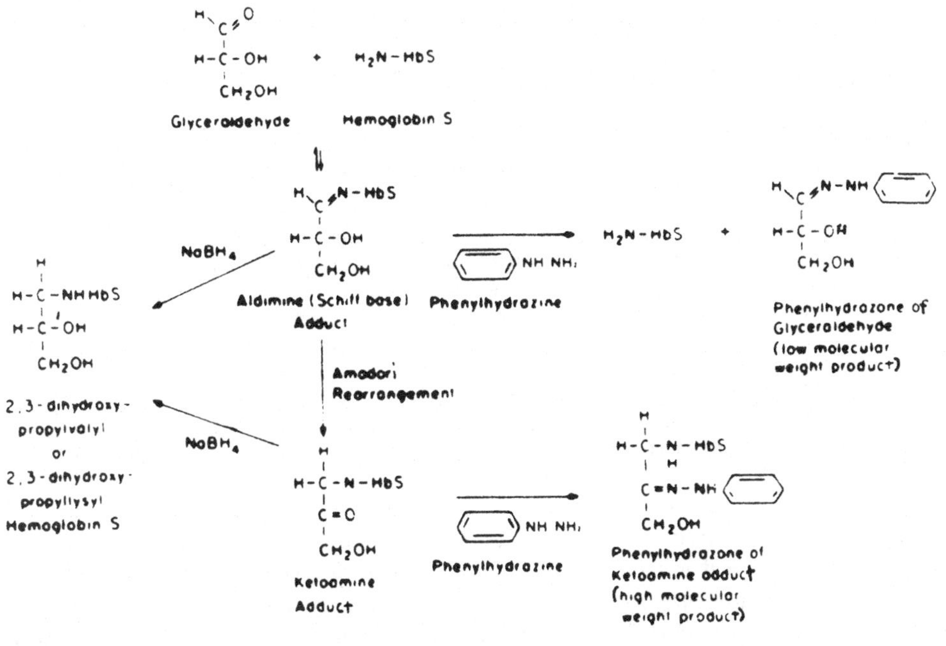

FIGURE 44. The reaction of the glyceraldehyde-hemoglobin adduct with either phenylhydrazine or sodium borohydride. (From Acharya, A. S. and Manning, J. M., *J. Biol. Chem.*, 255, 1406, 1980. With permission.)

from modification) at 37°C for 5 days with lactose and sodium cyanoborohydride. Under these conditions, 80% of the amino groups were modified. Bunn and Higgins[116] have explored the reaction of monosaccharides with protein amino groups in the presence of sodium cyanoborohydride in some detail. These investigators studied the reaction of hemoglobin with various monosaccharides in Krebs-Ringer phosphate buffer, pH 7.3 (Figure 46). The extent of modification was determined using tritiated sodium cyanoborohydride. The rate of modification was demonstrated to be a direct function of the amount of each sugar in the carbonyl (or keto) form (Figure 47). Thus the k_1 ($\times$ 10^{-3} mM^{-1} h^{-1}) for D-glucose is 0.6 with 0.002% in the carbonyl form while the k_1 ($\times$ 10^{-3} mM^{-1} h^{-1}) for D-ribose is 10.0 with 0.05% in the carbonyl form.

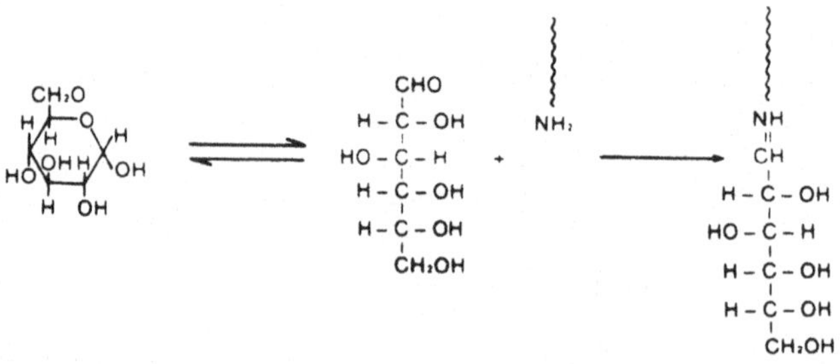

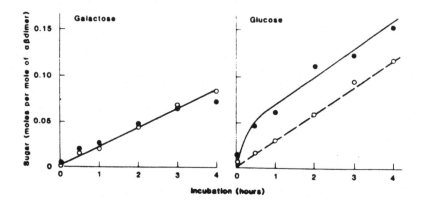

FIGURE 45.   A scheme for the reaction of a monosaccharide with a primary amino group.

FIGURE 46.   The measurement of the rate of condensation of monosaccharides with hemoglobin. The extent of reaction was measured either by incubation with unlabeled sugar followed by reduction of the aldimine linkage with tritiated sodium cyanoborohydride (open circles) or by incubation of the [^{14}C]-labeled sugar with hemoglobin followed by reduction with unlabeled sodium cyanoborohydride (closed circles). The left panel shows the rate of reaction with 42 mM D-galactose ($k_1 = 1.9 \times 10^{-3}$ mM^{-1} h^{-1}). The right panel shows the reaction with 42 mM D-glucose ($k_1 = 0.6 \times 10^{-3}$ mM^{-1} h^{-1}). The initial rapid rate of incorporation of D-[^{14}C] glucose can be explained by the small amount of rapidly reacting impurity remaining in the preparation. (From Bunn, H. F. and Higgins, R. J., *Science*, 213, 222, 1981. With permission.)

The reaction of trinitrobenzenesulfonic acid with amino groups has been of value in studying the function and reactivity of the ε-amino groups of lysyl residues in proteins.[117-119] The reaction of trinitrobenzenesulfonic acid with the primary amino groups in proteins is shown in Figure 48. The modification of amino groups with trinitrobenzenesulfonic acid is easy to monitor by spectral analysis. In the presence of an excess of sulfite, absorbance at 420 nm is the most sensitive index, having $\epsilon = 2.0 \times 10^4$ M^{-1} cm^{-1}. Absorbance at 420 nm is dependent upon the ability of the reaction product to form a complex with sulfite. It has proved convenient in our laboratories to use the fact that the spectrum of a trinitrobenzyl amino compound has an isosbestic point at 367 nm with $\epsilon = 1.05 \times 10^4$ M^{-1} cm^{-1}. As suggested by Fields,[120] we recrystallize trinitrobenzenesulfonic acid from 2.0 M HCl prior to use. We generally perform the modifications in phosphate buffer (pH 6.0 to 9.0). The derivatives of α-amino groups and ε-amino groups have similar spectra with the exception that α-amino derivatives have a slightly higher extinction coefficient at 420 nm ($\epsilon = 2.20 \times 10^4$ M^{-1} cm^{-1}) than ε-amino groups ($\epsilon = 1.92 \times 10^4$ M^{-1} cm^{-1}). Both of these derivatives have much higher extinction coefficients than the derivative obtained by reaction of trinitrobenzenesulfonic acid with cysteinyl residues ($\epsilon = 2.25 \times 10^3$ M^{-1} cm^{-1}). The α-amino and ε-amino derivatives can be differentiated by their stability to acid or base

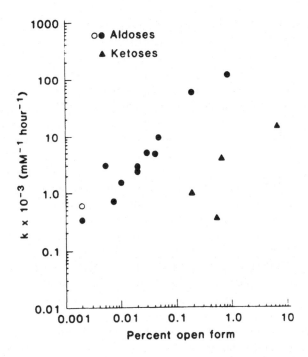

FIGURE 47. The relation between the rate of condensation of monosaccharide with hemoglobin and the equilibrium between the open and ring structures of the monosaccharide (l_1). The open circle is for glucose ($k_1 = 0.6 \times 10^{-3} \ mM^{-1} \ h^{-1}$). The closed circles represent data for other aldoses and the closed triangles for ketoses. (From Bunn, H. F. and Higgins, P. J., *Science*, 213, 222, 1981. With permission.)

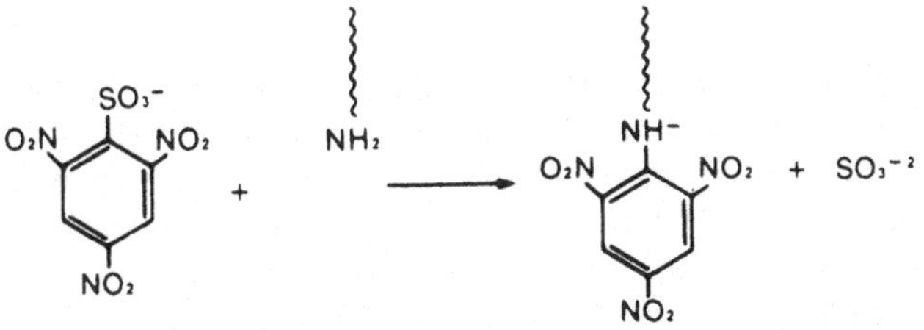

FIGURE 48. The reaction of 2,4,6-trinitrobenzenesulfonic acid with primary amines in proteins.

hydrolysis. The α-amino derivatives are unstable to acid hydrolysis (8 h at 110°C) or base hydrolysis.[121]

Frieden and co-workers have explored the reaction of trinitrobenzenesulfonic acid with bovine liver glutamate dehydrogenase.[122,123] In these studies, the modification was performed in 0.04 M potassium phosphate, pH 8.0. Under these reaction conditions, the cysteinyl residues were not modified. The preparative reactions were terminated by reaction with β-mercaptoethanol. It is of interest that under certain conditions (with reduced coenzyme), glutamate dehydrogenase catalyzed the conversion of trinitrobenzenesulfonic acid to trinitrobenzene.[124]

The reaction of trinitrobenzenesulfonic acid with simple amines and hydroxide ions has been studied in some detail by Means and co-workers.[125] The reaction of trinitrobenzenesulfonic acid with hydroxide is first-order with respect to both trinitrobenzenesulfonate and hydroxide ions. Reaction with amines was considered in some detail. In general, reactivity of trinitrobenzenesulfonate with amines increases with increasing basicity except that secondary amines and *t*-alkylamines are comparatively unreactive. The specific binding of trinitrobenzenesulfonate to proteins must be considered in the study of the reaction of this compound with proteins. Only amines with a pKa greater than 8.7 follow a simple rate law. These investigators presented the following considerations regarding the reaction of trinitrobenzenesulfonic acid with proteins. Reactivity is a sensitive measure of the basicity of an amino group. Adjacent charged groups have an influence on the rate of reaction with an increase observed with a positively charged group and a decrease with a negatively charged group. Proximity to surface hydrophobic regions which can bind trinitrobenzenesulfonic acid can increase the observed reactivity of a particular amino group.

Flügge and Heldt have explored the labeling of a specific membrane component with trinitrobenzenesulfonic acid[126] and pyridoxal-5'-phosphate.[127] The modification of the phosphate translocation protein in spinach chloroplasts with trinitrobenzenesulfonic acid was performed in 0.050 M HEPES, 0.33 M sorbitol, 0.001 M MgCl$_2$, 0.001 M MnCl$_2$, 0.002 M EDTA, pH 7.6 at 4°C for periods of time up to 15 min at which point tritiated sodium borohydride was added to both terminate the reaction and radiolabel the trinitrophenyl derivatives.[128] It is possible to label components on the surface of membranes with trinitrobenzenesulfonic acid as the sulfonate moiety does not permit membrane penetration. The same is true for pyridoxal-5'-phosphate.

On occasion, the modification of an amino acid residue in a protein is associated with an apparent increase in catalytic activity. This was the situation with the modification of 14S and 30S dynein adenosine triphosphatase activities with trinitrobenzenesulfonic acid.[129] In this study, the reaction was performed in 0.030 M barbital, pH 8.5 at 25°C. The extent of modification was determined spectrophotometrically at 345 nm ($\epsilon = 1.45 \times 10^4\ M^{-1}$ cm^{-1}). In studies similar to those obtained with glutamate dehydrogenase as discussed above,[124] glutathione reductase was demonstrated to reduce trinitrobenzenesulfonate.[130] Inhibition of glutathione reductase was noted at low concentration (0.05 μM) of trinitrobenzenesulfonate.

The reaction of trinitrobenzenesulfonic acid with ammonium has also been investigated by Whitaker and co-workers.[131] This reaction was performed in tetraborate buffer and 1 μM sulfite. The rate of the reaction was determined by following the increase in absorbance at 420 nm ($\epsilon = 2.02 \times 10^4\ M^{-1}$ cm^{-1}). The rate of reaction with ammonium (k = 0.128 min^{-1}) was slower than that with the average amine in a protein (k = 0.907 min^{-1} for enterotoxin) (Figure 49). The reaction with ammonium does, however, provide a sensitive assay for ammonia (as low as 6 nmol) with a precision of 1 to 2%.

The use of trinitrobenzenesulfonate in the selective modification of membrane surface components has been explored by Salem and co-workers.[132] This study involved the modification of intact cells with the trinitrobenzenesulfonic acid (dissolved in methyl alcohol) diluted to a 1% methanolic solution. As mentioned above, trinitrobenzenesulfonate does not pass across (or into) membranes, being more hydrophilic than, for example, fluorodinitrobenzene.

Haniu et al.[133] have examined the reaction of lysine residues in NAD(P)H:quinone reductase with trinitrobenzenesulfonic acid as compared to the reaction of tyrosine residues with *p*-nitrobenzenesulfonyl fluoride. Isolation and characterization of the peptides containing the modified residues showed that the modified tyrosyl residues are in hydrophobic regions of the protein while the modified lysine residues are in hydrophilic regions. Other recent examples of the use of trinitrobenzenesulfonic acid for the site-specific chemical modification of proteins include placental 17-β-dehydrogenase,[134] a snake venom phospholipase A$_2$[135], rat liver 6-phosphogluconate dehydrogenase,[136] luffin-a,[137] and myosin.[138] In this latter study,

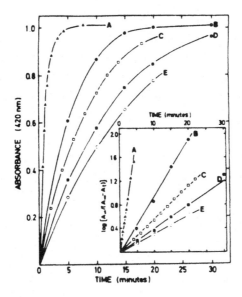

FIGURE 49.   The reaction of 2,4,6-trinitrobenzenesulfonic acid (TNBS) with ammonia and the available amino groups of enterotoxin. The basic experimental approach was that described by Fields.[90] The rate assay approach involves the addition of TNBS to a reference cuvette containing only reagent and cuvette containing the sample. The difference in the rate of increase in absorbance at 420 nm is recorded (the buffer contains sodium sulfite). In the endpoint method, the reaction is allowed to proceed for a period of time at which point it is terminated by the addition of 0.1 M NaH$_2$PO$_4$ containing 1.5 mM sodium sulfite. The absorbance at 420 nm is then determined. Experiment A used the rate assay method with 6.7 μM enterotoxin at 25°C. Curve B used the endpoint method with 50 μM ammonium sulfate at 35°C. Curve C used the rate assay method with 50 μM ammonium sulfate at 25°C. Curve D used the endpoint method with 50 μM ammonium sulfate at 25°C with twice the TNBS concentration used in the other experiments. Curve E used the endpoint method with 50 μM ammonium sulfate. The insert is a plot of the rate data according to the first-order rate equation. (From Whitaker, J. R., Granum, P. E., and Ausen, G., *Anal. Biochem.*, 108, 72, 1980. With permission.)

the peptides containing the modified lysine residues were isolated by immunoaffinity chromatography using an anti-trinitrophenyl antibody obtained from rabbits immunized with trinitrophenyl hemocyanin.

Guanidation of proteins is a reaction which is fairly specific for ε-amino groups.[139] This modification involves the reaction of O-methylisourea with lysyl residues at basic pH (pH >9) to yield homoarginine (Figure 50). This reaction is fairly slow and generally takes several days to go to completion. Bregman and co-workers[140] examined the modification of the single lysyl residue in glucagon. In this study 3.4 g O-methylisourea (O-methylisourea hydrogen sulfate) was dissolved in 20 ml H$_2$O and 6.0 g Ba(OH)$_2$ added followed by filtration or centrifugation to remove the resulting BaSO$_4$. The pH of the solution was adjusted to 11.0 and 200 mg glucagon added. The reaction was allowed to proceed for 8 h at 4°C and was terminated by the addition of glacial acetic acid. The products of the reaction were purified on Sulfopropyl-Sephadex. Guanidation of human recombinant erythropoietin has been accomplished with either O-methylisourea (Figure 50) or 1-guanyl-3,5-dimethylpyrazole (Figure 51).[141] Seven of the eight lysine residues were modified with O-methylisourea while all eight lysine residues were modified with 1-guanyl-3,5-dimethylpyrazole. Both derivatives demonstrated increased biological activity.

With the exception of the Boulton-Hunter reagent[142] (Figure 52), the use of N-hydroxysuccinimide ester derivatives to modify lysine residues has been somewhat restricted to crosslinking reagents as described in Chapter 15. However, the specificity demonstrated by this chemistry provides considerable potential for the introduction of structural probes and other unique functional groups into proteins. Yem et al.[143] have used N-hydroxysuccinimide chem-

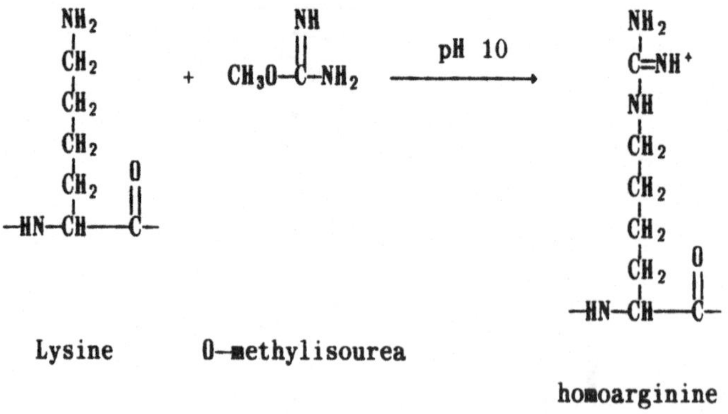

FIGURE 50.   A scheme for the guanidation of lysine residues in proteins to produce homoarginine.

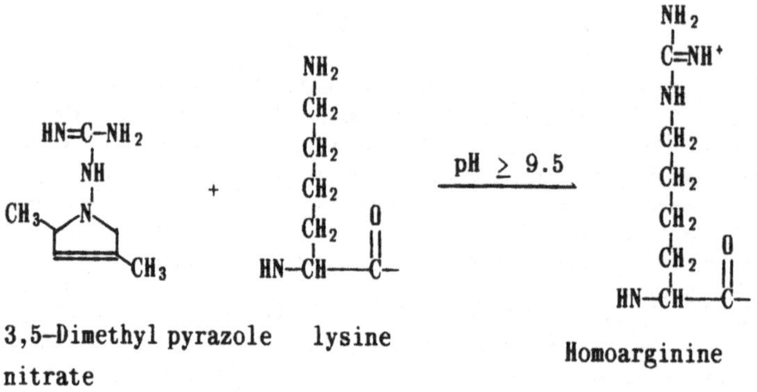

FIGURE 51.   A scheme for the reaction of lysine with guanyl-3,5-dimethyl pyrazole to produce homoarginine.

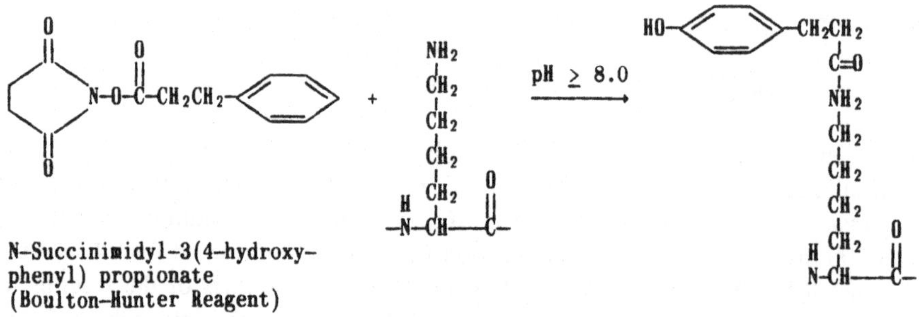

FIGURE 52.   The structure of *N*-succinimidyl-3-(4-hydroxyphenyl) propionate (Boulton-Hunter reagent) and its reaction with lysine residues in proteins.

istry to introduce biotin into recombinant interleukin-1-β (Figure 53). This is a fascinating technology with substantial promise.[144,145]

It is possible to selectively modify the α-amino groups of proteins by chemical transamination with glyoxylate (Figure 54) at slightly acid pH.[146,147] This modification has been applied to *Euglena* cytochrome C-552. This reaction was performed in 2.0 *M* sodium acetate, 0.10 *M* acetic acid, 0.005 *M* nickel sulfate, 0.2 *M* sodium glyoxylate and resulted in the

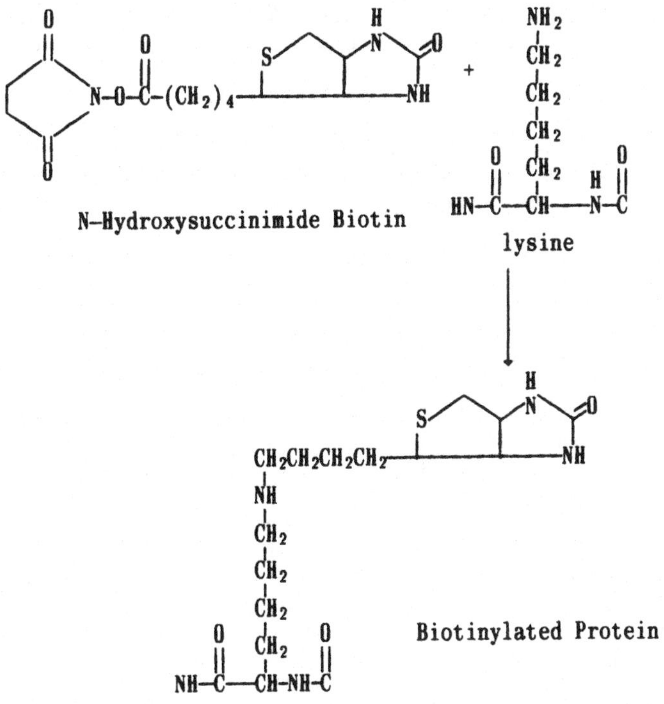

FIGURE 53. Incorporation of biotin into protein via reaction with an *N*-hydroxysuccinimide derivative.

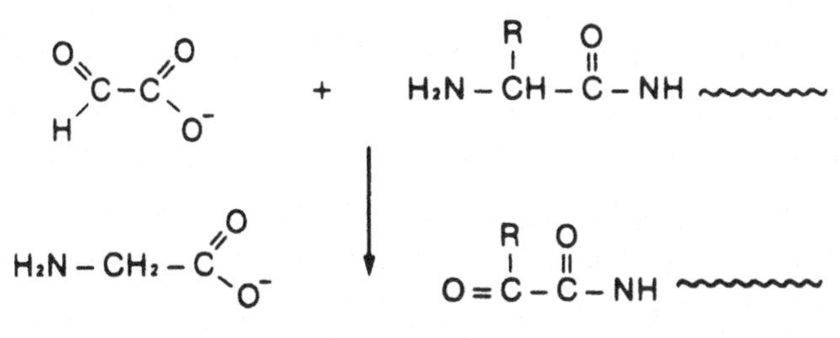

FIGURE 54. The modification of α-amino groups in proteins with glyoxylate.

complete loss of the amino-terminal residue. Snake venom phospholipase A_2 has been subjected to chemical transamination.[147] This reaction was performed in 2.0 *M* sodium acetate, 0.4 *M* acetic acid, 0.010 *M* cupric ions, 0.1 *M* glyoxylic acid, pH 5.5.

REFERENCES

1. **Gurd, F. R. N.,** Carboxymethylation, *Meth. Enzymol.,* 11, 532, 1967.
2. **Sanger, F. and Tuppy, H.,** The amino acid sequence in the phenylalanyl chain of insulin. I. The identification of lower peptides from partial hydrolysates, *Biochem. J.,* 49, 463, 1951.
3. **Carty, R. P. and Hirs, C. H. W.,** Modification of bovine pancreatic ribonuclease A with 4-sulfonyloxy-2-nitrofluorobenzene, *J. Biol. Chem.,* 243, 5254, 1968.
4. **Franklin, J. G. and Leslie, J.,** Some enzymatic properties of trypsin after reaction with 1-dimethylaminonaphthalene-5-sulfonyl chloride, *Can. J. Biochem.,* 49, 516, 1971.

5. **Wagner, R., Podestá, F. E., González, D. H., and Andreo, C. S.,** Proximity between fluorescent probes attached to four essential lysyl residues in phospho*enol*pyruvate carboxylase — a resonance energy transfer study, *Eur. J. Biochem.,* 173, 561, 1988.

6. **Brautigan, D. L., Ferguson-Miller, S., and Margoliuash, E.,** Definition of cytochrome c binding domains by chemical modification. I. Reaction with 4-chloro-3,5-dinitrobenzoate and chromatographic separation of singly substituted derivatives, *J. Biol. Chem.,* 253, 130, 1978.

7. **Bello, J., Iijima, H., and Kartha, G.,** A new arylating agent, 2-carboxy-4,6-dinitrochlorobenzene. Reaction with model compounds and bovine pancreatic ribonuclease, *Int. J. Peptide Protein Res.,* 14, 199, 1979.

8. **Hall, J., Zha, X., Yu, L., Yu, C.-A., and Millett, F.,** Role of specific lysine residues in the reaction of *Rhodobacter sphaeroides* cytochrome c_2 with the cytochrome bc_1 complex, *Biochemistry,* 28, 2568, 1989.

9. **Long, J. E., Durham, B., Okamura, M., and Millett, F.,** Role of specific lysine residues in binding cytochrome c_2 to the *Rhodobacter sphaeroides* reaction center in optimal orientation for rapid electron transfer, *Biochemistry,* 28, 6970, 1989.

10. **Hiratsuka, T. and Uchida, K.,** Lysyl residues of cardiac myosin accessible to labeling with a fluorescent reagent, N-methyl-2-anilino-6-naphthalenesulfonyl chloride, *J. Biochem.,* 88, 1437, 1980.

11. **Onondera, M., Shiokawa, H., and Takagi, T.,** Flourescent probes for antibody active sites. I. Production of antibodies specific to the N-methyl-2-anilinonapthalene-6-sulfonate group in rabbits and some fluorescent properties of the hapten bound to the antibodies. *J. Biochem.,* 79, 195, 1976.

12. **Cory, R. P., Becker, R. R., Rosenbluth, R., and Isenberg, I.,** Synthesis and fluorescent properties of some N-methyl-2-anilino-6-naphthalensulfonyl derivatives, *J. Am. Chem. Soc.,* 90, 1643, 1968.

13. **Haugland, R. P.,** *Molecular Probes. Handbook of Fluorescent Probes and Research Chemicals,* Molecular Probes, Inc., Eugene, OR, 1989, 37.

14. **Tuls, J., Geren, L., and Millett, F.,** Fluorescein isothiocyanate specifically modifies lysine 338 of cytochrome P-450$_{scc}$ and inhibits adrenodoxin binding, *J. Biol. Chem.,* 264, 16421, 1989.

15. **Miki, M.,** Interaction of Lys-61 labeled actin with myosin subfragment-1 and the regulatory proteins, *J. Biochem. (Tokyo),* 106, 651, 1989.

16. **Bellelli, A., Ippoliti, R., Brunori, M., Kam, Z., Benveniste, M., Emmanuel, F., Turpin, E., Alfsen, A., and Fency, J. P.,** Binding and internalization of ricin labelled with fluorescein isothiocyanate, *Biochem. Biophys. Res. Commun.,* 169, 602, 1990.

17. **Devanathan, S., Dahl, T. A., Midden, W. R., and Neckers, D. C.,** Readily available fluorescein isothiocyanate-conjugated antibodies can be easily converted into targeted phototoxic agents for antibacterial, antiviral, and anticancer therapy, *Proc. Natl. Acad. Sci. U.S.A.,* 87, 2980, 1990.

18. **Turner, D. C. and Brand, L.,** Quantitative estimation of protein binding site polarity. Fluorescence of N-arylaminonaphthalenesulfonates, *Biochemistry,* 7, 3381, 1968.

19. **Welches, W. R. and Baldwin, T. O.,** Active center studies on bacterial luciferase: modification of the enzyme with 2,4-dinitrofluorobenzene, *Biochemistry,* 20, 512, 1981.

20. **Shapiro, R., Fox, E. A., and Riordan, J. F.,** Role of lysines in human angiogenin: chemical modification and site-directed mutagenesis, *Biochemistry,* 28, 1726, 1989.

21. **Riordan, J. F. and Vallee, B. L.,** Acetylation, *Meth. Enzymol.,* 11, 565, 1967.

22. **Merle, M., Lefevre, G., Staub, J. F., Raulais, D., and Milhaud, G.,** Acylation of porcine and bovine calcitonin: effects on hypocalcemic activity in the rat, *Biochem. Biophys. Res. Commun.,* 79, 1071, 1977.

23. **Aviram, I.,** The role of lysines in *Euglena* cytochrome C-552. Chemical modification studies, *Arch. Biochem. Biophys.,* 181, 199, 1977.

24. **Karibian, D., Jones, C., Gertler, A., Dorrington, K. J., and Hofmann, T.,** On the reaction of acetic and maleic anhydrides with elastase. Evidence for a role of the NH$_2$-terminal valine, *Biochemistry,* 13, 2891, 1974.

25. **Kaplan, H., Stevenson, K. J., and Hartley, B. S.,** Competitive labeling, a method for determining the reactivity of individual groups in proteins. The amino groups of porcine elastin, *Biochem. J.,* 124, 289, 1971.

26. **Bosshard, H. R., Koch, G. L. E., and Hartley, B. S.,** The aminoacyl tRNA synthetase-tRNA complex: detection by differential labeling of lysine residues involved in complex formation, *J. Mol. Biol.,* 119, 125, 1978.

27. **Richardson, R. H. and Brew, K.,** Lactose synthase. An investigation of the interaction site of alpha-lactalbumin for galactosyltransferase by differential kinetic labeling, *J. Biol. Chem.,* 255, 3377, 1980.

28. **Rieder, R. and Bosshard, H. R.,** The cytochrome c oxidase binding site on cytochrome c. Differential chemical modification of lysine residues in free and oxidase-bound cytochrome c, *J. Biol. Chem.,* 253, 6045, 1978.

29. **Hitchcock, S. E., Zimmerman, C. J., and Smalley, C.,** Study of the structure of troponin-T by measuring the relative reactivities of lysines with acetic anhydride, *J. Mol. Biol.,* 147, 125, 1981.

30. **Hitchcock, S. E.,** Study of the structure of troponin-C by measuring the relative reactivities of lysines with acetic anhydride, *J. Mol. Biol.,* 147, 153, 1981.

31. **Hitchcock-De Gregori, S. E.,** Study of the structure of troponin-I by measuring the relative reactivities of lysine with acetic anhydride, *J. Biol. Chem.,* 257, 7372, 1982.

32. **Giedroc, D. P., Sinha, S. K., Brew, K., and Puett, D.,** Differential trace labeling of calmodulin: investigation of binding sites and conformational states by individual lysine reactivities. Effects of beta-endorphin, trifluoperazine, and ethylene glycol bis(beta-aminoethyl ether)-$N,N,N'N$-tetraacetic acid, *J. Biol. Chem.,* 260, 13406, 1985.

33. **Wei, Q., Jackson, A. E., Pervaiz, S., Carrawy, K. L., III, Lee, E. Y. C., Puett, D., and Brew, K.,** Effects of interactions of with calcineurin of the reactivities of calmodulin lysines, *J. Biol. Chem.,* 263, 19541, 1988.

34. **Winkler, M. A., Fried, V. A., Merat, D. L., and Cheung, W. Y.,** Differential reactivities of lysines in calmodulin complexed to phosphatase, *J. Biol. Chem.,* 262, 15466, 1987.

35. **Hitchcock-De Gregori, S. E., Lewis, S. F., and Mistrik, M.,** Lysine reactivities of tropomyosin complexed with troponin, *Arch. Biochem. Biophys.,* 264, 410, 1988.

36. **Staudenmayer, N., Smith, M. B., Smith, H. T., Spies, F. K., Jr., and Millett, F.,** An enzyme kinetics and ^{19}F nuclear magnetic resonance study of selectively trifluoroacetylated cytochrome c derivatives, *Biochemistry,* 15, 3198, 1976.

37. **Smith, M. B., Stonehuerner, J., Ahmed, A. J., Staudenmayer, N., and Millett, F.,** Use of specific trifluoroacetylation of lysine residues in cytochrome C to study the reaction with cytochrome b$_5$, cytochrome c$_1$ and cytochrome oxidase, *Biochim. Biophys. Acta,* 592, 303, 1980.

38. **Webb, M., Stonehuerner, J., and Millett, F.,** The use of specific lysine modifications to locate the reaction site of cytochrome C with sulfite oxidase, *Biochim. Biophys. Acta,* 593, 290, 1980.

39. **Ahmed, A. J. and Millett, F.,** Use of specific lysine modifications to identify the site of reaction between cytochrome C and ferricyanide, *J. Biol. Chem.,* 256, 1611, 1981.

40. **Smith, M. B. and Millett, F.,** A ^{19}F nuclear magnetic resonance study of the interaction between cytochrome C and cytochrome C peroxidase, *Biochim. Biophys. Acta,* 626, 64, 1980.

41. **Klotz, I. M.,** Succinylation, *Meth. Enzymol.,* 11, 576, 1967.

42. **Meighen, E. A., Nicolim, M. Z., and Hustings, J. W.,** Hybridization of bacterial luciferase with a variant produced by chemical modification, *Biochemistry,* 10, 4062, 1971.

43. **Shetty, K. J. and Rao, M. S. N.,** Effect of succinylation on the oligomeric structure of arachin, *Int. J. Peptide Protein Res.,* 11, 305, 1978.

44. **Shiao, D. D. F., Lumry, R., and Rajender, S.,** Modification of protein properties by change in charge. Succinylated chymotrypsinogen, *Eur. J. Biochem.,* 29, 377, 1972.

45. **Morton, R. C. and Gerber, G. E.,** Water solubilization of membrane proteins. Extensive derivatization with a novel polar derivatizing reagent, *J. Biol. Chem.,* 263, 7989, 1988.

46. **Atassi, M. Z. and Habeeb, A. F. S. A.,** Reaction of protein with citraconic anhydride, *Meth. Enzymol.,* 25, 546, 1972.

47. **Habeeb, A. F. S. A. and Atassi, M. Z.,** Enzymic and immunochemical properties of lysozyme. Evaluation of several amino group reversible blocking reagents, *Biochemistry,* 9, 4939, 1970.

48. **Shetty, J. K. and Kinsella, J. E.,** Ready separation of proteins from nucleoprotein complexes by reversible modification of lysine residues, *Biochem. J.,* 191, 269, 1980.

49. **Weisgraber, K. H., Innerarity, T. L., and Mahley, R. W.,** Role of the lysine residues of plasma lipoproteins in high affinity binding to cell surface receptors on human fibroblasts, *J. Biol. Chem.,* 253, 9053, 1978.

50. **Mahley, R. W., Weisgraber, K. H., Innerarity, T. L., and Windmueller, H. G.,** Accelerated clearance of low-density and high-density lipoproteins and retarded clearance of E apoprotein-containing lipoproteins from the plasma of rats after modification of lysine residues, *Proc. Natl. Acad. Sci. U.S.A.,* 76, 1746, 1979.

51. **Urabe, I., Yamamoto, M., Yamada, Y., and Okada, H.,** Effect of hydrophobicity of acyl groups on the activity and stability of acylated thermolysin, *Biochim. Biophys. Acta,* 524, 435, 1978.

52. **Howlett, G. J. and Wardrop, A. J.,** Dissociation and reconstitution of human erythrocyte membrane proteins using 3,4,5,6-tetrahydrophthalic anhydride, *Arch. Biochem. Biophys.,* 188, 429, 1978.

53. **Stark, G. R., Stein, W. H., and Moore, S.,** Reaction of the cyanate present in aqueous urea with amino acids and proteins, *J. Biol. Chem.,* 235, 3177, 1960.

54. **Stark, G. R. and Smyth, D. G.,** The use of cyanate for the determination of NH$_2$-terminal residues in proteins, *J. Biol. Chem.,* 238, 214, 1963.

55. **Stark, G. R.,** Modification of proteins with cyanate, *Meth. Enzymol.,* 25, 579, 1972.

56. **Shaw, D. C., Stein, W. H., and Moore, S.,** Inactivation of chymotrypsin by cyanate, *J. Biol. Chem.,* 239, PC 671, 1964.

57. **Cerami, A. and Manning, J. M.,** Potassium cyanate as an inhibitor of the sickling of erythrocytes *in vitro, Proc. Natl. Acad. Sci. U.S.A.,* 68, 1180, 1971.

58. **Lee, C. K. and Manning, J. M.,** Kinetics of the carbamylation of the amino groups of sickle cell hemoglobin by cyanate, *J. Biol. Chem.,* 248, 5861, 1973.

59. **Njikam, N., Jones, W. M., Nigen, A. M., Gillette, P. N., Williams. R. C., Jr., and Manning, J. M.,** Carbamylation of the chains of hemoglobin S by cyanate *in vitro* and *in vivo, J. Biol. Chem.,* 248, 8052, 1973.

60. **Nigen, A. M., Bass, B. D., and Manning, J. M.,** Reactivity of cyanate with valine-1 (α) of hemoglobin. A probe of conformational change and anion binding, *J. Biol. Chem.,* 251, 7638, 1976.

61. **Plapp, B. V., Moore, S., and Stein, W. H.,** Activity of bovine pancreatic deoxyribonuclease A with modified amino groups, *J. Biol. Chem.,* 246, 939, 1971.

62. **Chollet, R. and Anderson, L. L.,** Cyanate modification of essential lysyl residues in the catalytic subunit of tobacco ribulosebisphosphate carboxylase, *Biochim. Biophys. Acta,* 525, 455, 1978.

63. **Kang, E. P.,** Amidinated thrombin: preparation and peptidase activity, *Thromb. Res.,* 12, 177, 1977.

64. **Sekiguchi, T., Oshiro, S., Goingo, E. M., and Nosoh, Y.,** Chemical modification of ϵ-amino groups in glutamine synthetase from *Bacillus stearothermophilus* with ethyl acetimidate, *J. Biochem.,* 85, 75, 1979.

65. **Browne, D. J. and Kent, S. B. H.,** Formation of non-amidine products in the reaction of primary amines with imido esters, *Biochem. Biophys. Res. Commun.,* 67, 126, 1975.

66. **Monneron, A. and d'Alayer, J.,** Effects of imido-esters on membrane-bound adenylate cyclase, *FEBS Lett.,* 122, 241, 1980.

67. **Plapp, B. V.,** Enhancement of the activity of horse liver alcohol dehydrogenase by modification of amino groups at the active sites, *J. Biol. Chem.,* 245, 1727, 1970.

68. **Dunathan, H. C.,** Stereochemical aspects of pyridoxal phosphate catalysis, in *Adv. Enzymol.,* 35, 79, 1971.

69. **Shapiro, S., Enser, M., Pugh, E., and Horecker, B. L.,** The effect of pyridoxal phosphate on rabbit muscle aldolase, *Arch. Biochem. Biophys.,* 128, 554, 1968.

70. **Schnackerz, K. D. and Noltmann, E. A.,** Pyridoxal-5'-phosphate as a site-specific protein reagent for a catalytically critical lysine residue in rabbit muscle phosphoglucose isomerase, *Biochemistry,* 10, 4837, 1971.

71. **Havran, R. T. and du Vigneaud, V.,** The structure of acetone-lysine vasopressin as established through its synthesis from the acetone derivative of S-benzyl-L-cysteinyl-L-tyrosine, *J. Am. Chem. Soc.,* 91, 2696, 1969.

72. **Paech, C. and Tolbert, N. E.,** Active site studies of ribulose-1,5-bisphosphate carboxylase/oxygenase with pyridoxal-5'-phosphate, *J. Biol. Chem.,* 253, 7864, 1978.

73. **Kent, A. B., Krebs, E. G., and Fischer, E. H.,** Properties of crystalline phosphorylase b, *J. Biol Chem.,* 232, 549, 1958.

74. **Wimmer, M. J., Mo, T., Sawyers, D. L., and Harrison, J. H.,** Biphasic inactivation of porcine heart mitochondrial malate dehydrogenase by pyridoxal-5'-phosphate, *J. Biol. Chem.,* 250, 710, 1975.

75. **Bleile, D. M., Jameson, J. L., and Harrison, J. H.,** Inactivation of porcine heart cytoplasmic malate dehydrogenase by pyridoxal-5'-phosphate, *J. Biol. Chem.,* 251, 6304, 1976.

76. **Jones, C. W., III and Priest, D. G.,** Interaction of pyridoxal-5'-phosphate with apo-serine hydroxymethyltransferase, *Biochim. Biophys. Acta,* 526, 369, 1978.

77. **Cortijo, M., Jimenez, J. S., and Lior, J.,** Criteria to recognize the structure and micropolarity of pyridoxal-5'-phosphate binding sites in proteins, *Biochem. J.,* 171, 497, 1978.

78. **Cake, M. A., DiSorbo, D. M., and Litwack, G.,** Effect of pyridoxal phosphate on the DNA binding site of activated hepatic glucocorticoid receptor, *J. Biol. Chem.,* 253, 4886, 1978.

79. **Slebe, J. C. and Martinez-Carrion, M.,** Selective chemical modification and ¹⁹F NMR in the assignment of a pK value to the active site lysyl residue in aspartate transaminase, *J. Biol. Chem.,* 253, 2093, 1978.

80. **Nishigori, H. and Toft, D.,** Chemical modification of the avian progesterone receptor by pyridoxal-5'-phosphate, *J. Biol. Chem.,* 254, 9155, 1979.

81. **Sugiyama, Y. and Mukohata, Y.,** Modification of one lysine by pyridoxal phosphate completely inactivates chloroplast coupling factor 1 ATPase, *FEBS Lett.,* 98, 276, 1979.

82. **Peters, H., Risi, S., and Dose, K.,** Evidence for essential primary amino groups in a bacterial coupling factor F_1 ATPase, *Biochem. Biophys. Res. Commun.,* 97, 1215, 1980.

83. **Gould, K. G. and Engel, P. C.,** Modification of mouse testicular lactate dehydrogenase by pyridoxal 5'-phosphate, *Biochem. J.,* 191, 365, 1980.

84. **Ogawa, H. and Fujioka, M.,** The reaction of pyridoxal-5'-phosphate with an essential lysine residue of saccharopine dehydrogenase (L-lysine-forming), *J. Biol. Chem.,* 255, 7420, 1980.

85. **Forrey, A. W., Olsgaard, R. B., Nolan, C., and Fischer, E. H.,** Synthesis and properties of α- and ϵ-pyridoxyl lysines and their phosphorylated derivatives, *Biochimie,* 53, 269, 1971.

86. **Sober, H. A.,** in *Handbook of Biochemistry,* 2nd ed., The Chemical Rubber Company, Cleveland, Ohio, 1970.

87. **Moldoon, T. G. and Cidlowski, J. A.,** Specific modifications of rat uterine estrogen receptor by pyridoxal-5'-phosphate, *J. Biol. Chem.,* 2, 55, 3100, 1980.

88. **Ohsawa, H., and Gualerzi, C.,** Structure-function relationship in *Escherichia coli* inhibition factors. Identification of a lysine residue in the ribosomal binding site of initiation factor by site-specific chemical modification with pyrodixal phosphate, *J. Biol. Chem.,* 256, 4905, 1981.

89. **Bürger, E. and Görisch, H.,** Evidence for an essential lysine at the active site of L-histidinol:NAD$^+$ oxidoreductase, a bifunctional dehydrogenase, *Eur. J. Biochem.,* 118, 125, 1981.

90. **Miller, A. D., Packman, L. C., Hart, G. J., Alefounder, P. R., Abell, C., and Battersby, A. R.,** Evidence that pyridoxal phosphate modification of lysine residues (Lys-55 and Lys-59) causes inactivation of hydroxymethylbilane synthase (porphobilinogen deaminase), *Biochem. J.,* 262, 119, 1989.

91. **Basu, S., Basu, A., and Modak, M. J.,** Pyridoxal 5'-phosphate mediated inactivation of *Escherichia coli* DNA polymerase I: Identification of lysine-635 as an essential residue for the processive mode of DNA synthesis, *Biochemistry,* 27, 6710, 1988.

92. **Mahrenholz, A. M., Wang, Y., and Roach, P. J.,** Catalytic site of rabbit glycogen synthase isozymes. Identification of an active site lysine close to the amino terminus of the subunit, *J. Biol. Chem.,* 263, 10561, 1988.

93. **Tamura, J. K., LaDine, J. R., and Cross, R. L.,** The adenine nucleotide binding site on yeast hexokinase PII. Affinity labeling of Lys-111 by pyridoxal 5'-diphospho-5'-adenosine, *J. Biol. Chem.,* 263, 7907, 1988.

94. **Kluger, R.,** Methyl acetyl phosphate. A small anionic acetylating agent, *J. Org. Chem.,* 45, 2733, 1980.

95. **Ueno, H., Pospishchil, M. A., Manning, J. M., and Kluger, R.,** Site-specific modification of hemoglobin by methyl acetyl phosphate, *Arch. Biochem. Biophys.,* 244, 795, 1986.

96. **Ueno, H., Pospischil, M. A., and Manning, J. M.,** Methyl acetyl phosphate as a covalent probe for anion-binding sites in human and bovine hemoglobins, *J. Biol. Chem.,* 264, 12344, 1989.

97. **Means, G. E.,** Reductive alkylation of amino groups, *Meth. Enzymol.,* 47, 469, 1977.

98. **Rice, R. H., Means, G. E., and Brown, W. D.,** Stabilization of bovine trypsin by reductive methylation, *Biochim. Biophys. Acta,* 492, 316, 1977.

99. **Morris, R. W., Cagan, R. H., Martenson, R. E., and Deibler, G.,** Methylation of the lysine residues of monellin, *Proc. Soc. Exp. Biol. Med.,* 157, 194, 1978.

100. **Chen, F. M. F. and Benoiton, N. L.,** Reductive *N,N*-dimethylation of amino acid and peptide derivatives using methanol as the carbonyl source, *Can. J. Biochem.,* 56, 150, 1978.

101. **Dottavio-Martin, D. and Ravel, J. M.,** Radiolabeling of proteins by reductive alkylation with [^{14}C] formaldehyde and sodium cyanoborohydride, *Anal. Biochem.,* 87, 562, 1978.

102. **Dick, L. R., Geraldes, C. F. G. C., Sherry, A., D., Gray, C. W., and Gray, D. M.,** ^{13}[TC NMR of methylated lysines of fd gene 5 protein: evidence for a conformational change involving lysine 24 upon binding of a negatively charged lanthanide chelate, *Biochemistry,* 28, 7896, 1989.

103. **Brown, E. M., Pfeffer, P. E., Kumosinski, T. F., and Greenberg, R.,** Accessibility and mobility of lysine residues in β-lactoglobulin, *Biochemistry,* 27, 5601, 1988.

104. **Fretheim, K., Iwai, S., and Feeney, R. F.,** Extensive modification of protein amino groups by reductive addition of different sized substituents, *Int. J. Peptide Protein Res.,* 14, 451, 1979.

105. **Fretheim, K., Edelandsdal, B., and Harbitz, O.,** Effect of alkylation with different size substituents on the conformation of ovomucoid, lysozyme and ovotransferrin, *Int. J. Peptide Protein Res.,* 25, 601, 1985.

106. **Geoghegan, K. F., Ybarra, D. M., and Feeney, R. E.,** Reversible reductive alkylation of amino groups in proteins, *Biochemistry,* 18, 5392, 1979.

107. **Jentoft, N. and Dearborn, D. G.,** Labeling of proteins by reductive methylation using sodium cyanoborohydride, *J. Biol. Chem.,* 254, 4359, 1979.

108. **Jentoft, J. E., Jentoft, N., Gerken, T. A., and Dearborn, D. G.,** ^{13}C NMR studies of ribonuclease A methylated with [^{13}C] formaldehyde, *J. Biol. Chem.,* 254, 4366, 1979.

109. **Jentoft, N. and Dearborn, D. G.,** Protein labeling by reductive methylation with sodium cyanoborohydride: effect of cyanide and metal ions on the reaction, *Anal. Biochem.,* 106, 186, 1980.

110. **Geoghegan, K. F., Cabacungan, J. C., Dixon, H. B. F., and Feeney, R. E.,** Alternative reducing agents for reductive methylation of amino groups in proteins, *Int. J. Peptide Protein Res.,* 17, 345, 1981.

111. **Cabacungan, J. C., Ahmed, A. J., and Feeney, R. E.,** Amine boranes as alternative reducing agents for reductive alkylation of proteins, *Anal. Biochem.,* 124, 272, 1982.

112. **Wu, H.-L. and Means, G. E.,** Immobilization of proteins by reductive alkylation with hydrophobic aldehydes, *Biotechnol. Bioeng.,* 23, 855, 1981.

113. **Acharya, A. S. and Manning, J. M.,** Reactivity of the amino groups of carbonmonoxyhemoglobin S with glyceraldehyde, *J. Biol. Chem.,* 255, 1406, 1980.

114. **Acharya, A. S. and Manning, J. M.,** Amadori rearrangement of glyceraldehyde-hemoglobin Schiff base adducts. A new procedure for the determination of ketoamine adducts in proteins, *J. Biol. Chem.,* 255, 7218, 1980.

115. **Wilson, G.,** Effect of reductive lactosamination on the hepatic uptake of bovine pancreatic ribunoclease A dimer, *J. Biol. Chem.,* 253, 2070, 1978.

116. **Bunn, H. F. and Higgins, P. J.,** Reaction of monosaccharides with proteins: possible evolutionary significance, *Science,* 213, 222, 1981.

117. **Goldfarb, A. R.**, A kinetic study of the reactions of amino acids and peptides with trinitrobenzenesulfonic acid, *Biochemistry*, 5, 2570, 1966.

118. **Goldfarb, A. R.**, Heterogeneity of amino groups in proteins. I. Human serum albumin, *Biochemistry*, 5, 2574, 1966.

119. **Habeeb, A. F. S. A.**, Determination of free amino groups in proteins by trinitrobenzenesulfonic acid, *Anal. Biochem.*, 14, 328, 1966.

120. **Fields, R.**, The rapid determination of amino groups with TNBS, *Meth. Enzymol.*, 25, 464, 1972.

121. **Kotaki, A. and Satake, K.**, Acid and alkaline degradation of the TNP-amino acids and peptides, *J. Biochem.*, 56, 299, 1964.

122. **Coffee, C. J., Bradshaw, R. A., Goldin, B. R., and Frieden, C.**, Identification of the sites of modification of bovine liver glutamate dehydrogenase reacted with trinitrobenzenesulfonate, *Biochemistry*, 10, 3516, 1971.

123. **Goldin, B. R. and Frieden, C.**, Effects of trinitrophenylation of specific lysyl residues on the catalytic, regulatory and molecular properties of bovine liver glutamate dehydrogenase, *Biochemistry*, 10, 3527, 1971.

124. **Bates, D. J., Goldin, B. R., and Frieden, C.**, A new reaction of glutamate dehydrogenase: the enzyme-catalyzed formation of trinitrobenzene from TNBS in the presence of reduced coenzyme, *Biochem. Biophys. Res. Commun.*, 39, 502, 1970.

125. **Means, G. E., Congdon, W. I., and Bender, M. L.**, Reactions of 2,4,6-trinitrobenzenesulfonate ion with amines and hydroxide ion, *Biochemistry*, 11, 3564, 1972.

126. **Flügge, U. I. and Heldt, H. W.**, Specific labelling of the active site of the phosphate translocator in spinach chloroplasts by 2,4,6-trinitrobenzene sulfonate, *Biochem. Biophys. Res. Commun.*, 84, 37, 1978.

127. **Flügge, U. I. and Heldt, H. W.**, Specific labelling of a protein involved in phosphate transport of chloroplasts by pyridoxal-5'-phosphate, *FEBS Lett.*, 82, 29, 1977.

128. **Parrott, C. L. and Shifrin, S.**, A spectrophotometric study of the reaction of borohydride with trinitrophenyl derivatives of amino acids and proteins, *Biochim. Biophys. Acta*, 491, 114, 1977.

129. **Shimizu, T.**, Enhancement of 14S and 30S dynein adenosine triphosphatase activities by modification of amino groups with trinitrobenzenesulfonate. A comparison with modification of SH groups, *J. Biochem.*, 85, 1421, 1979.

130. **Carlberg, I. and Mannervik, B.**, Interaction of 2,4,6-trinitrobenzene sulfonate and 4-chloro-7-nitrobenzo-2-oxa-1,3-diazole with the active sites of glutathione reductase and lipoamide dehydrogenase, *Acta Chem. Scand.*, B34, 144, 1980.

131. **Whitaker, J. R., Granum, P. E., and Aasen, G.**, Reaction of ammonia with trinitrobenzene sulfonic acid, *Anal. Biochem.*, 108, 72, 1980.

132. **Salem, N., Jr., Lauter, C. J., and Trams, E. G.**, Selective chemical modification of plasma membrane ectoenzymes, *Biochim. Biophys. Acta*, 641, 366, 1981.

133. **Haniu, M., Yuan, H., Chen, S., Iyanagi, T., Lee, T. D., and Shively, J. E.**, Structure-function relationship of NAD(P)H:quinone reductase: characterization of NH_2-terminal blocking group and essential tyrosine and lysine residues, *Biochemistry*, 27, 6877, 1988.

134. **Inano, H.**, Chemical modification of lysine residues at active-site of human placental estradiol 17β-dehydrogenase, *Biochem. Biophys. Res. Commun.*, 152, 789, 1988.

135. **Yang, C.-C. and Chang, L.-S.**, Studies on the status of lysine residues in phospholipase A_2 from *Naja naja atra* (Taiwan cobra) snake venom, *Biochem. J.*, 262, 855, 1989.

136. **Gordillo, E., Ayala, A., Bautista, J., and Machado, A.**, Implication of lysine residues in the loss of enzymatic activity in rat liver 6-phosphogluconate dehydrogenase found in aging, *J. Biol. Chem.*, 264, 17024, 1989.

137. **Watanabe, K., Suemasu, Y., and Funatsu, G.**, Identification of lysine residue at or near active site of luffin-a, a ribosome-inactivating protein from seeds of *Luffa cylindrica*, *J. Biochem. (Tokyo)*, 106, 977, 1989.

138. **Dan-Goor, M., Kessel, M., and Muhlrad, A.**, Anti-TNP antibody localization of the reactive lysine residues in myosin, *Biochim. Biophys. Acta*, 1038, 269, 1990.

139. **Kimmel, J. R.**, Guanidination of proteins, *Meth. Enzymol.*, 11, 584, 1967.

140. **Bregman, M. D., Trivedi, D., and Hruby, V. J.**, Glucagon amino groups. Evaluation of modification leading to antagonism and agonism, *J. Biol. Chem.*, 255, 11725, 1980.

141. **Satake, R., Kozutsumi, H., Takeuchi, M., and Asano, K.**, Chemical modification of erythropoietin: an increase in *in vitro* activity by guanidination, *Biochim. Biophys. Acta: Protein Structure and Molecular Enzymology*, 1038 125, 1990.

142. **Boulton, A. E. and Hunter, W. M.**, The labelling of proteins to high specific radioactivities by conjugation to a ^{125}I-containing acylating agent, *Biochem. J.*, 133, 529, 1973.

143. **Yem, A. W., Zurcher-Neely, H. A., Richard, K. A., Staite, N. D., Heinrikson, R. L., and Deibel, M. R., Jr.**, Biotinylation of reactive amino groups in native recombinant human interleukin-1β, *J. Biol. Chem.*, 264, 17691, 1989.

144. **Wilchek, M. and Bayer, E.**, Biotin-containing reagents, *Meth. Enzymol.*, 184, 123, 1990.

145. **Bayer, E. and Wilchek, M.**, Protein Biotinylation, *Meth. Enzymol.*, 184, 148, 1990.

146. **Dixon, H. B. F. and Fields, R.**, Specific modification of NH$_2$-terminal residues by transamination, *Meth. Enzymol.*, 25, 409, 1972.

147. **Verheij, H. M., Egmond, M. R., and de Haas, G. H.**, Chemical modification of the α-amino group in snake venom phospholipases A$_2$. A comparison of the interaction of pancreatic and venom phospholipases with lipid-water interfaces, *Biochemistry*, 20, 94, 1981.

Chapter 11

THE MODIFICATION OF ARGININE

Until approximately 20 years ago the specific chemical modification of arginine was relatively difficult to achieve. The high pKa of the guanidine functional group (pKa ≃ 12 to 13) necessitated fairly drastic reaction conditions (pH ≥12) to generate an effective nucleophile. Most proteins are not stable to extreme alkaline pH. The modification of arginyl residues was however possible and the early efforts in this area have been previously reviewed.[1]

It is reasonable to suggest that the recent advances in the study of the function of arginine residues in proteins stem from the work of Takahashi[2] on the use of phenylglyoxal as a reagent for the specific modification of arginine although observations on the use of 2,3-butanedione[3] and glyoxal[4] appeared at approximately the same time. The greatly increased interest in the elucidation of functional arginyl residues probably arises from the suggestion of Riordan and co-workers[5] that arginyl residues function as "general" anion recognition sites in proteins. Patthy and Thész[6] extended this concept by suggesting that the pKa of arginyl residues at anion binding sites (Figure 1) is lower than that of other arginine residues which would explain the specificity of the dicarbonyl residues which will be discussed below.

This chapter will primarily consider the reaction of arginyl residues in proteins with three different reagents; phenylglyoxal, 2,3-butanedione, and 1,2-cyclohexanedione since the vast majority of reports during the past decade have used these reagents. It is noted that several other reagents have been used for the modification of arginine. The modification of arginyl residues with ninhydrin occurs under relatively mild conditions (pH 8.0, 25°C, 0.1 M N-ethylmorpholine acetate, pH 8.0) as described by Takahashi.[7] The modification of pancreatic ribonuclease A or ribonuclease T by ninhydrin is shown in Figure 2. The reaction proceeds quite rapidly at pH 8.0 with the modification of both arginyl and lysyl residues. Reducing the pH to 5.5 (0.1 M sodium acetate, pH 5.5) reduced the rate of inactivation but did not increase the specificity of the modification. The UV spectra of ribonuclease T, before and after modification with ninhydrin are presented in Figure 3. Takahashi[7] achieved specificity of modification by first modifying available lysyl residues with a reagent such as methyl-maleic anhydride (citraconic anhydride) which can subsequently be removed under conditions where the arginine derivative is stable (pH 3.6). The arginine derivative is unstable under basic conditions (1% piperidine, ambient temperature, 34 h) and arginine was regenerated. Under the conditions commonly used for the preparation of protein samples for amino acid analysis (6 N HCl 110°C, 24 h), the ninhydrin-arginine derivative was destroyed with the partial regeneration of free arginine. The structure of the ninhydrin-arginine derivative (Figure 4) is similar to that proposed for the α,α'-dicarbonyl compounds such as phenylglyoxal[2] or 1,2-cyclohexanedione.[8] At the same time a report by Chaplin[9] appeared proposing the use of ninhydrin for the reversible modification of arginine residues in proteins. The study suggested that at pH 9.1 (0.1 M sodium phosphate), 37°C, the rate of reaction at arginine residues is approximately 100-fold more rapid than at lysine residues but reaction at cysteinyl residues is approximately 100-fold more rapid than at arginine. The extent of reaction was determined by measuring the decrease in the absorbance of ninhydrin at 232 nm (ϵ = 3.4 × 10^4 M^{-1} cm^{-1}). As noted by Takahashi,[7] the ninhydrin-arginine derivative is unstable under alkaline conditions and can be used for the reversible modification of arginine residues. The fluorescence properties of the reaction product between ninhydrin and guanidino compounds such as arginine have provided the basis for the use of ninhydrin for the detection of guanidine compounds in biological fluids (plasma) following separation by high-performance liquid chromatography.[10]

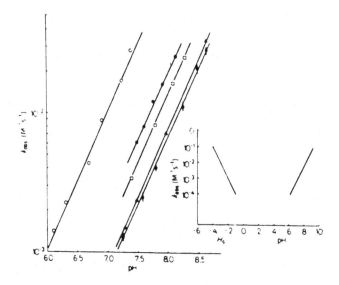

FIGURE 1.   Dependence of the reaction of arginine with dicarbonyl compounds on pH. Shown are second-order rate constants for the reaction of phenylglyoxal (○———○), hydroxypyruvaldehyde (□———□), glyoxal (▲———▲), and 1,2-cyclohexanedione (●———●) with free arginine at 25°C at the indicated pH (the buffers were 0.1 M sodium phosphate for pH 6 to 8; 0.1 M triethanolamine-HCl for pH 7 to 9 and in HCl solutions (H_o-4-0). Also included are the rate constants for the reaction of 1,2-cyclohexanedione with aldolase determined in 0.1 M triethanolamine-HCl buffers at 25°C (●———●). The inset shows the second-order rate constants for the arginine-glyoxal reaction over a wider pH range. (From Patthy, L. and Thész, J., *Eur. J. Biochem.*, 105, 387, 1980. With permission.)

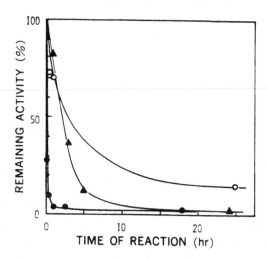

FIGURE 2.   Rates of inactivation of ribonucleases A and T_1 by ninhydrin. The reaction was performed at 25°C in the dark either at pH 8.0 in 0.1 M N-ethylmorpholine acetate, or at pH 5.5 in 0.1 M sodium acetate, at a protein concentration of 0.5% and a ninhydrin concentration of 1.5%. pH 8.0: ●, ribonuclease A; ▲, ribonuclease T_1. pH 5.5: ○, ribonuclease A. (From Takahashi, K., *J. Biochem.*, 80, 1173, 1976. With permission.)

The modification of arginyl residues with glyoxal has also been proposed.[11] Specificity of reaction is a problem with reaction also at primary amine groups and sulfhydryl groups. For example, reaction of glyoxal with bovine serum albumin at pH 9.0 resulted in modification of greater than 80% of the arginine residues with approximately 30% modification of lysine residues.[11] Glass and Pelzig[12] have examined the reversible modification of arginyl residues with glyoxal in some detail. Several products are formed from the reaction of glyoxal and arginine at alkaline pH. One of these derivatives is markedly stable in strong

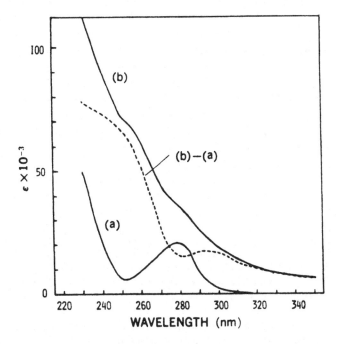

FIGURE 3. Changes in the UV absorption spectrum of ribonuclease T$_1$ on reaction with ninhydrin. The spectra were measured in 0.01 *M* ammonium acetate. ———: (a) native ezyme; (b) ninhydrin-modified enzyme. - - - -: difference, (b) − (a). (From Takahashi, K., *J. Biochem.*, 80, 1173, 1976. With permission.)

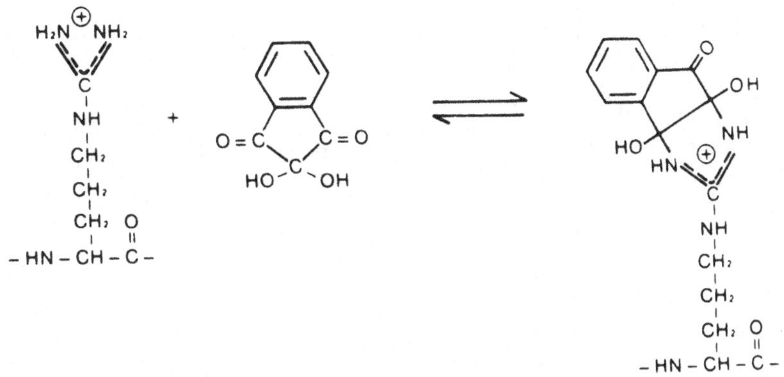

FIGURE 4. A scheme for the reaction of ninhydrin with arginine.

acid (12 *M* HCl) at ambient temperature but is rapidly degraded to form free arginine in the presence of *O*-phenylenediamine (0.16 *M*) at pH 8.1 to 8.3. More alkaline conditions resulted in more rapid decomposition of the glyoxal-arginine derivative and ninhydrin-positive compounds other than arginine were formed. Reaction of arginine with glyoxal in borate buffer also yields the product described above. The same research group has reported on the reversible modification of arginine residues with camphorquinone-10-sulfonic acid and derivatives such as camphorquinone-10-sulfonylnorleucine.[13] The synthesis of the parent compounds and various derivatives is reported. The sulfonic acid function provides a basis for the attachment of a "tag" such as norleucine which can be used for determining the extent of modification.[14] Reaction with arginine occurs in 0.2 *M* sodium borate, pH 9.0. Under

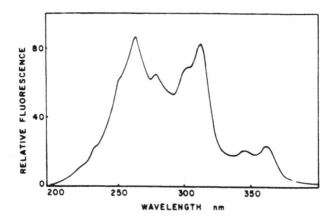

FIGURE 5. The fluorescence excitation spectrum of the condensation product of arginine and 9,10-phenanthrenequinone. Arginine (90 μg/ml) was reacted with 9,10-phenanthrenequinone (68 μ*M*) in 70% aqueous ethanol containing 0.2 *M* NaOH at 30°C for 60 min. The reaction mixture was then diluted with an equal volume of 1.2 *M* HCl and the spectrum recorded. The spectrum was recorded using an emission wavelength of 400 nm and a 2.5-nm slit width. (From Smith, R. E. and McQuarrie, R., *Anal. Biochem.*, 90, 246, 1978. With permission.)

these conditions, reaction of camphorquinone-sulfonic acid with an amino acid analysis standard showed a greater than 90% loss of arginine and a 25% loss of cystine. Loss of cystine was not observed in the proteins studied (soybean trypsin inhibitor, ribonuclease S-peptide). The arginine derivative is stable for 24 h in trifluoroacetic acid and under other mild acid conditions. The derivative is stable to 0.5 *M* hydroxylamine, pH 7.0, conditions under which the cyclohexanedione derivative of arginine decomposes[8] but arginine is regenerated in 0.2 *M* o-phenylenediamine, pH 8.5 (approximately 75% after 4 h; complete after 16 h).

The modification of arginyl residues with hydrazine (aqueous conditions) results in the formation of ornithine but also results in peptide bond cleavage (predominantly at gly-X, X-gly, asn-X, and X-ser peptide bonds).[15]

The determination of the extent of arginine modification is generally determined by amino acid analysis after acid hydrolysis but conditions generally need to be modified to prevent loss of the arginine derivative.[8] This will be discussed for each of the reagents discussed below. The Sakaguchi reaction[16] continues to be useful with recent modifications[17,18] and has recently been used, after acid hydrolysis, to determine the extent of arginine modification by 2,3-butanedione.[19] The use of ninhydrin as a fluorometric reagent for arginine has been described above.[10] Another fluorometric method for the determination of arginine using 9,10-phenanthrenequinone[20] has been described. Figure 5 shows the excitation spectrum for the reaction product of arginine and phenanthrenequinone, while the emission spectrum is shown in Figure 6. The time course for the reaction with free arginine is shown in Figure 7 while the time course for the reaction with arginyl residues in proteins is shown in Figure 8. This method is some 1000-fold more sensitive than the Sakaguchi reaction but some concern remains concerning the absolute accuracy of the reagent for determination of arginine in peptide linkage. This is also true of the other reagents.

The use of phenylglyoxal (Figure 9) was developed by Takahashi[2] and has since been applied to the study of the role of arginyl residues in proteins as shown in Table 1 and Figure 10. The use of this reagent has been somewhat limited in the last six years but there has been interest in modifying residues involved in ion transport. Unfortunately, many of these studies fail to recognize that phenylglyoxal, like glyoxal, will react with α-amino groups at a significant rate[2] (Figure 11). The rate of inactivation of ribonuclease A by phenylglyoxal at different values of pH is shown in Figure 12. Polymerization was noted in a sample

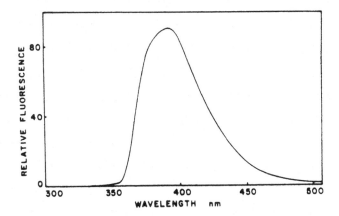

FIGURE 6. The fluorescence emission spectrum of the condensation product of arginine and 9,10-phenanthrenequinone. The reaction conditions are described in Figure 4. The spectrum was recorded using an excitation wavelength of 260 nm and a 2.5-nm slit width. (From Smith, R. E. and McQuarrie, R., *Anal. Biochem.*, 90, 246, 1978. With permission.)

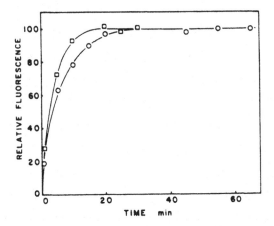

FIGURE 7. The development of fluorescence as a function of the time of reaction of arginine and 9,10-phenanthrenequinone. The reaction was initiated by mixing 1 ml of arginine (8 μg) in water with 3 ml of 50 μM 9,10-phenanthrenequinone in ethanol and 0.5 ml of 2 M NaOH at either 30°C (●) or 44°C (■). At the indicated times, portions were withdrawn and mixed with an equal volume of 1.2 N HCl. The fluorescence was recorded using an excitation wavelength of 312 nm and an emission wavelength of 392 nm. A 5-nm slit width was used. (From Smith, R. E. and McQuarrie, R., *Anal. Biochem.*, 90, 246, 1978. With permission.)

incubated for 21 h. The amino-terminal lysine residue was rapidly modified under these conditions. The possible effect of light on the reaction of phenylglyoxal with arginine as has been reported for 2,3-butanedione[21-23] has not been studied. As noted by Takahashi, the stoichiometry of the reaction involves the reaction of 2 mol of phenylglyoxal with 1 mol of arginine (Figure 9). The [14C]-labeled reagent can be easily prepared.[2,24] A facile modification of the original Riley and Gray[24] method which omits the vacuum distillation step has been reported by Hartman and co-workers.[25] Radiolabeled acetophenone was added to an equal amount (on the basis of weight) of selenium dioxide in dioxane-water (30:1). The mixture was refluxed for 3 h after which solvent was removed under a stream of nitrogen. The residue was taken up in boiling water and activated charcoal added. The hot slurry was filtered through Celite. The phenylglyoxal crystallized spontaneously from the filtrate on cooling.

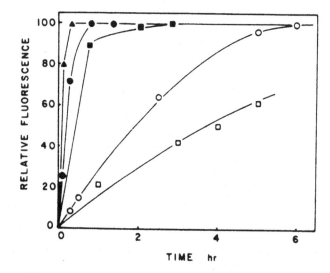

FIGURE 8.   The development of fluorescence as a function of time of reaction of proteins with 9,10-phenanth-renequinone. The reaction was initiated by mixing 1 ml of protein (100 μg) in 50 mM borate, pH 8.5, with 3 ml of 50 μM 9,10-phenanthrenequinone in ethanol and 0.5 ml of 2 M NaOH. At the indicated times, portions were removed and mixed with an equal volume of 1.2 N HCl. The fluorescence was recorded using an excitation wavelength of 312 nm and an emission wavelength of 392 nm with a 5-nm slit width. The reactions were performed either at 30°C (open symbols) or 60°C (closed symbols). The proteins used were bovine serum albumin (□), lysozyme (○), and the β-chain of insulin (△). (From Smith, R. E. and McQuarrie, R., *Anal. Biochem.*, 90, 246, 1978. With permission.)

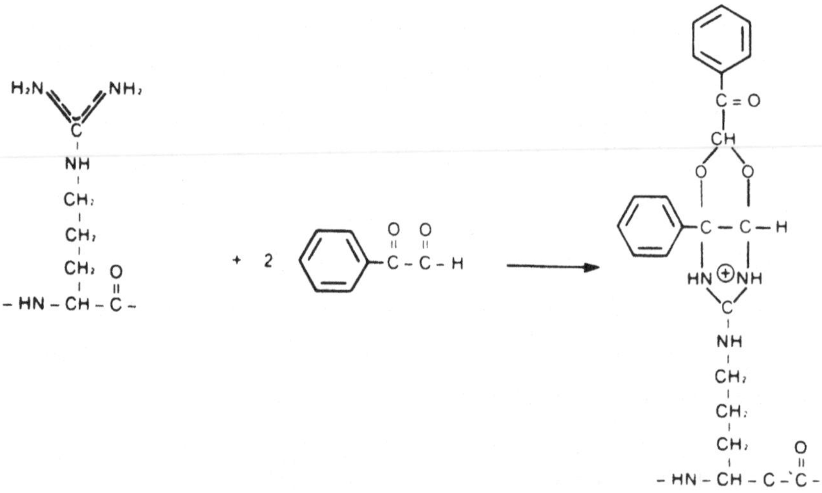

FIGURE 9.   A scheme for the reaction of phenylglyoxal with arginine.

The synthesis of phenyl [2-³H] glyoxal[26] has been reported. Borders and co-workers[27] have reported the synthesis of a chromophoric derivative, 4-hydroxy-3-nitrophenylglyoxal, which should prove quite useful in the study of arginyl residues. *p*-Hydroxylphenylglyoxal[28] has also been used as a spectrophotometric reagent for the study of this reaction.

Of particular interest has been the observations of Fonda and Cheung[29] that the reaction of arginine with phenylglyoxal is greatly accelerated in bicarbonate-carbonate buffer systems. Figure 13 shows the reaction of phenylglyoxal with *N*-acetylarginine, *N*-acetyllysine and *N*-acetylcysteine in 0.083 M sodium bicarbonate, pH 7.5. Reaction is only seen, for all practical purposes, with the arginine derivative. L-Arginine reacted in the same manner suggesting that modification of the α-amino group did not occur under these conditions. Figure 14

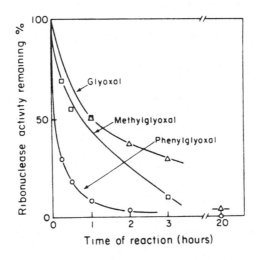

FIGURE 10. The rate of inactivation of ribonuclease A by reaction with phenylglyoxal and related compounds. The reactions were performed in 0.2 M N-ethylmorpholine acetate, pH 8.0, at 25°C. The protein concentration was 0.5% with either 1.5% phenylglyoxal hydrate, 1.5% methylglyoxal, or 1.5% glyoxal hydrate as indicated in the figure. (From Takahashi, K., *J. Biol. Chem.*, 243, 6171, 1968. With permission.)

Table 1
REACTION OF PHENYLGLYOXAL WITH ARGINYL RESIDUES IN PEPTIDES AND PROTEINS

Protein	Solvent	Reagent excess[a]	Extent of modification	Ref.
Pancreatic RNase	0.1 M N-ethylmorpholine acetate, pH 8.0	—	2—3/4[b,c]	1
Porcine carboxypeptidase B	0.3 M borate, pH 7.9	200[d]	1/[e]	2
Aspartate transcarbamylase	0.125 M potassium bicarbonate, pH 8.3 or 0.1 M N-ethylmorpholine, pH 8.3	—	2.2/[f,g]	3
Pyruvate kinase	0.1 M triethanolamine, pH 7.0	—	3/28.33[h]	4
Horse liver alcohol dehydrogenase	—	—	—	5, 6
Mitochondrial ATPase	0.097 M sodium borate, 0.097 M EDTA, pH 8.0	—	4/[i]	7
Adenylate kinase	0.1 M triethanolamine ·HCl, pH 7.0	—	/[j]	8, 9
Rhodospirillum rubrum chromatophores	0.05 M borate, pH 8.0	—	/[k]	10
Glutamic acid decarboxylase	0.05 M sodium borate[l]	—	—	11
Ribulose bisphosphate carboxylase	0.066 M sodium[m] bicarbonate, 0.050 M bicine, 0.1 M EDTA, pH 8.0	—	2—3/35[n]	12
Yeast hexokinase	0.035 M Veronal, pH 7.5	—	1/18[o]	13
Propionyl CoA carboxylase	0.050 M borate, pH 8.0	—	—	14
β-Methylcrotonyl CoA carboxylase	0.050 M borate pH 8.0	—	—	14
Superoxide dismutase	0.125 M sodium bicarbonate, pH 8.0	—	1/4[p]	15

Table 1 (continued)
REACTION OF PHENYLGLYOXAL WITH ARGINYL RESIDUES IN PEPTIDES AND PROTEINS

Protein	Solvent	Reagent excess[a]	Extent of modification	Ref.
Myosin (subfragment 1)	0.1 M potassium bicarbonate, pH 8.0	—	1.7/35[q]	16
Thymidylate synthetase	0.125 M bicarbonate, pH 8.0[r]	—	3.6/12	17
Glutamate apodecarboxylase	0.125 M sodium[s] bicarbonate, pH 7.5	—	1/23[t]	18
Adenylate[u] kinase (yeast)	0.025 M HEPES, pH 7.5	—	—	19
Cardiac myosin S-1	0.1 M N-ethylmorpholine acetate, pH 7.6	—	2.8/42[v]	20
Cystathionase	0.125 M bicarbonate, pH 7.9	—	18/45	21
Fatty acid synthetase	0.1 M sodium phosphate, 0.0005 M dithioerythritol, 0.001 M EDTA, pH 7.6	—	4/106	22
Yeast inorganic pyrophosphatase	0.08 M N-ethylmorpholine acetate, pH 7.0	—	1/6	23
Porcine phospholipase A	0.125 M potassium bicarbonate, pH 8.5	—	1.4/4[w]	24
Superoxide dismutase[x]	0.100 M sodium bicarbonate, pH 8.3	50—100	0.88/4.0[y]	25, 26[z]
p-Hydroxybenzoate hydroxylase	0.050 M potassium phosphate, pH 8.0	250	2—3/24[aa]	27
Thymidylate synthetase	0.200 M N-ethylmorpholine, pH 7.4[bb]	65	2/12[cc]	28
Acetylcholine esterase	0.025 M borate, 0.005 phosphate, 0.050 M NaCl, pH 7.0	—	3/31[dd]	29
γ-Aminobutyrate aminotransferase	0.05 M Tris, pH 8.5	—	—	30
D-β-Hydroxybutyrate dehydrogenase	0.05 M HEPES, pH 7.5	—	—[ee]	31
Ornithine transcarboxylase	0.05 M Bicine, 0.1 M KCl, 0.0001 M EDTA, pH 8.05	—	—[ff]	32
Coenzyme B$_{12}$-dependent diol dehydrase	0.05 M borate, pH 8.0	—	—	33
Transketolase	0.125 M sodium bicarbonate, pH 7.6	—	4/34[gg]	34
ATP citrate lyase	0.050 M HEPES,[hh] pH 8.0	—	8.5/40	36
Malic enzyme	0.037 M borate,[ii] pH 7.5	—	—	37
Pyridoxamine-5'-phosphate oxidase	0.1 M potassium phosphate, pH 8.0, containing 5% ETOH	—[jj]	6/40	38
Ornithine transcarboxylase	0.125 M potassium bicarbonate, pH 8.3	—[kk]	1.5/[ll]	39
Acetate kinase	0.050 M triethanolamine, pH 7.6	—[mm]	—[nn]	40
Pancreatic phospholipase A$_2$	0.2 M N-ethylmorpholine, pH 8.0	30	1.0—1.2/[oo]	41
Phosphatidylcholine transfer protein	0.1 M sodium bicarbonate, pH 8.0	—	4/10[pp]	42
Aldehyde reductase	0.020 M phosphate[qq] pH 7.0	—	0.6/16[rr]	43
Choline acetyltransferase	0.050 M HEPES, pH 7.8	—	—[ss]	44
ADP-glucose synthetase	0.05 M potassium phosphate, 0.00025 M EDTA, pH 7.5	110	1/[tt]	45

Table 1 (continued)
REACTION OF PHENYLGLYOXAL WITH ARGINYL RESIDUES IN PEPTIDES AND PROTEINS

Protein	Solvent	Reagent excess[a]	Extent of modification	Ref.
Pyruvate oxidase	0.1 M sodium phosphate, 0.010 M magnesium chloride, pH 7.8	—	2.5/5[uu]	46
Calcineurin	50 mM Tris, pH 7.5, with 0.1 M EDTA, 0.1 mM NiCl$_2$ and 0.3 mM CaCl$_2$	10,000[vv]	—	47
Carbon monoxide	20 mM sodium phosphate, pH 8.2 with 4 mM dithiothreitol	—	—	48
Epithelial sodium channel	pH 8.1[ww]	—	—	49
Calcium "pump"	100 mM N-ethylmorpholine-40 mM KCl-6 mM HEPES-0.7 mM MgCl$_2$-0.2 mM EGTA, pH 7.7	—	—	50
Calmodulin-dependent	40 mM HEPES, pH 7.5 with 7% glycerol, 0.1 M EDTA and 0.3 mM CaCl$_2$	333[xx]	—	51

[a] Reagent/protein.
[b] After 3 h at 25°C.
[c] Had modification of α-amino group and lysine residues.
[d] Reagent/arginine.
[e] After 1 h at 37°C.
[f] After 3 h at 25°C.
[g] 1.3/8 In regulatory chain.
[h] 20 Min at 37°C with 23.8 mM phenylglyoxal, protein 1 mg/ml.
[i] 30 Min of reaction at 30°C; the presence of efrapeptin, a low-molecular weight antibiotic which is a potent inhibitor of oxidative phosphorylation, prevented the modification of one "fast-reacting" arginyl residue.
[j] A single arginine residue is modified (Arg-97).
[k] A single site appeared to be modified with a second-order rate constant of 1.6 M^{-1} min^{-1}.
[l] pH Not given; reaction at 23°C, kinetic evidence for stoichiometric inactivation.
[m] Solvent made metal-free using BioRad Chelex; reaction performed with and without MgCl$_2$.
[n] Analysis of sulfhydryl groups after phenylglyoxal modification showed no loss of cysteine. These investigations noted the modification with phenylglyoxal is apparently more specific than 2,3-butanedione.
[o] The authors claim 1:1 stoichiometry of phenylglyoxal with the arginyl residue from analysis of dependence of pseudo first-order rate constant vs. reciprocal of reagent (phenylglyoxal concentration). Partial reactivation of modified enzyme was observed reflecting lability of modified arginine residues. Reaction also shows saturation kinetics reflecting "specific" affinity of reagent for enzyme possibly from hydrophobic interaction. These authors suggest that this phenomenon is observed with the reaction of other hydrophobic reagents with this enzyme. A similar phenomenon has been observed with trinitrobenzenesulfonic acid (see Chapter 10).
[p] 25°C, 1 h.
[q] 25°C, 3 mM phenylglyoxal, 3 min.
[r] Rates of enzyme inactivation were dependent upon buffer; at 5.9 mM phenylglyoxal, the following data were obtained, bicarbonate ($T_{1/2}$ = 6.0 min), MOPS ($T_{1/2}$ = 11.5 min), borate ($T_{1/2}$ = 34.0), and phosphate ($T_{1/2}$ = 48.0 min) at 25°C.
[s] These investigators noted a significant buffer effect on the reaction which is more thoroughly explored in Reference 29 of Chapter 11. In this study the following second-order rate constants were obtained with the following reagent/solvent conditions (reactions performed at 23°C): 0.69 M^{-1} min^{-1} with 2,3-butanedione/0.050 M borate, pH 8.0; 33.78 M^{-1} min^{-1} with glyoxal/0.125 M sodium bicarbonate, pH 8.0; 31.00 M^{-1} min^{-1} with methylglyoxal/0.125 M sodium bicarbonate, pH 8.0); and 107.68 M^{-1} min^{-1} with phenylglyoxal/0.125 M sodium bicarbonate, pH 8.0.
[t] 300-Fold excess of reagent, 0.083 M sodium bicarbonate, pH 8.1, 7 min, 23°C.
[u] See more complete discussion of this work in Table 2. 2,3-Butanedione or 1,2-cyclohexanedione appeared to be more effective than phenylglyoxal in this system.

Table 1 (continued)

ᵛ 6 Min, 22°C, 50% loss of activity.

ʷ Determined at 99% inactivation (25°C) of phospholipase activity (release of fatty acid from egg yolk in water with 3 mM CaCl$_2$ and 1.4 mM sodium deoxycholate. These investigators (see Reference 24, Table 1) did examine the possibility of amino-terminal alanine modification: no loss of alanine was observed with 75% inactivation (0.9 mol Arg modified/mol protein) while enzyme samples with a greater extent of inactivation did have some loss of amino-terminal alanine (quantity not given). These investigators did examine the pH dependence of enzyme inactivation by phenylglyoxal (presumably a direct measure of the rate of arginine modification) and reported the following second-order rate constants (M^{-1} min^{-1}): pH 6.5, 0.3; pH 7.5, 1.5; pH 8.5, 3.3; and pH 9.5, 3.9. These investigators also showed that phenylglyoxal (T$_{1/2}$ = 1 min) was more effective than 2,3-butanedione (T$_{1/2}$ = 20 min) and 1,2-cyclohexanedione (T$_{1/2}$ = 120 min).

ˣ Cu, Zn superoxide dismutase from *Saccharomyces cerevisiae*.

ʸ Determined at 80% loss of enzymatic acitivity using reaction of the modified enzyme with 9,10-phenanthrenequinone. This value corresponded to that determined by the incorporation of radiolabeled phenylglyoxal assuming 2:1 adduct. Amino acid analysis with samples prepared using normal hydrolytic conditions (6 N HCl, 110°C, 20 h) suggested only approximately 50% of this extent of arginine modification. When thioglycolic acid was included during the hydrolysis, values for the extent of arginine modification approached those determined by the fluorescence technique and radiolabel incorporation.

ᶻ The study is an extension of the observation reported in Reference 25 and uses reaction with 4-hydroxy-3-nitrophenylglyoxal, a chromophoric derivative of phenylglyoxal, to identify the specific arginine residue modified. It is of some interest that the rate of reaction with this derivative is approximately sixfold less than that with the parent phenylglyoxal.

ᵃᵃ Reaction at 25°C for 60 to 120 min. Loss of lysine residues was not observed under these reaction conditions. Amino acid analysis (hydrolysis in 6 N HCl, 110°C, 24 h) correlated well with radiolabeled phenylglyoxal incorporation assuming 2:1 stoichiometry (i.e., amino acid analysis gave 3.6 mol Arg lost/mol enzyme while 7.54 mol radiolabel was incorporated).

ᵇᵇ These investigators (see Reference 28, Table 1) examined the reaction at pH 7.4 (rate of inactivation of 32 M^{-1} min^{-1}). An approximate 100-fold increase in the rate of inactivation.

ᶜᶜ The presence of substrate, 2′-deoxyuridylate, prevents the modification of 1 mol of arginine per mole of enzyme. It is noted that these results differ from those reported in Reference 17. There were differences in solvent conditions. It is not clear why this would account for the differences observed in these two studies. It is noted that the investigators in Reference 17 obtained similar stoichiometry with 2,3-butanedione.

ᶠᶠ See more complete discussion of this study under Table 2. For inactivation by phenylglyoxal, a second-order rate constant of 56 M^{-1} min^{-1} was obtained at pH 8.04. The reactions were performed in the dark.

ᵍᵍ Analysis of Tsou plots[35] indicates at least two classes of residues react at different rates.

ʰʰ Most studies were performed in this solvent at 30°C with a second-order rate constant of 0.33 M^{-1} s^{-1}. The rate was reduced in potassium phosphate (k = 0.25 M^{-1} s^{-1}) and borate (k = 0.078 M^{-1} s^{-1}).

ⁱⁱ Under these conditions at 24°C, a second-order rate constant of k = 7.08 M^{-1} min^{-1} assuming that the rate of inactivation is directly related to the modification of arginine. With 2,3-butanedione in 0.048 M borate a second-order rate constant of k = 5.4 M^{-1} min^{-1} is compared to 1.69 M^{-1} min^{-1} with methylglyoxal and 0.032 M^{-1} min^{-1} with 2,4-pentanedione.

ʲʲ The rate of inactivation at 25°C for the apoenzyme was determined to be 3.7 M^{-1} min^{-1} and 11.1 M^{-1} min^{-1} for the holoenzyme.

ᵏᵏ A second-order rate constant of k = 4.6 M^{-1} min^{-1} at 25°C was obtained under these conditions.

ˡˡ Based on incorporation of radiolabeled phenylglyoxal, 1.5 arginine residues are modified per 35,000 chain after 3 h of reaction. There are likely different classes of reactive arginyl residues where the more reactive group(s) directly associated with catalytic activity.

ᵐᵐ Saturation kinetics are observed with phenylglyoxal suggesting the formation of an enzyme-inhibitor complex prior to reaction with an arginine residue(s).

ⁿⁿ With 95% loss of catalytic activity there is 94% modification of arginine.

ᵒᵒ See Reference 24 for somewhat differing results. This study shows that this level of arginine modification is associated with 80% loss of amino-terminal alanine. It was necessary to protect the α-amino group of the amino-terminal alanine with a *t*-butyloxycarbonyl group to avoid modification under these reaction conditions. The use of radiolabeled cyclohexandedione established Arg-6 as the primary site of modification.

ᵖᵖ 30 Min at 25°C. Extent of modification based on radiolabel incorporation and amino acid analysis.

ᑫᑫ For reaction at 30°C, a second-order rate constant of k = 2.6 M^{-1} min^{-1} assuming that the loss of activity seen with phenylglyoxal directly reflected the loss of an arginine residue(s).

ʳʳ Determined from both amino acid analysis and radiolabel incorporation.

ˢˢ Phenylglyoxal was much more effective than 2,3-butanedione or camphorquinone-10-sulfonic acid.

ᵗᵗ Assuming 2:1 stoichiometry of phenylglyoxal to arginine; reaction at 25°C. Phenylglyoxal is much more effective than 1,2-cyclohexanedione (twofold molar excess of 1,2-cyclohexanedione had T$_{1/2}$ = 24 min).

Table 1 (continued)

uu From radiolabel incorporation assuming 2:1 stoichiometry. There are clearly at least two classes of reactive arginine residue. When the reaction is performed at pH 6.0, inactivation with phenylglyoxal can be partially reversed on dilution in pH 6.0 buffer.

vv Inactivation rate constant of $1.5\ M^{-1}$ min^{-1} at pH $7.5/30°C$.

ww Reaction performed with an undefined quantity of Tris buffer. The inactivation reaction was markedly increased by the presence of sodium ions.

xx Inactivation rate constant of $132\ M^{-1}$ min^{-1} at pH 7.5

References for Table 1

1. **Takahashi, K.**, The reaction of phenylglyoxal with arginine residues in proteins, *J. Biol. Chem.*, 243, 6171, 1968.
2. **Werber, M. M. and Sokolovsky, M.**, Chemical evidence for a functional arginine residue in carboxypeptidase B, *Biochem. Biophys. Res. Commun.*, 48, 384, 1972.
3. **Kantrowitz, E. R. and Lipscomb, W. N.**, Functionally important arginine residues of aspartate transcarbamylase, *J. Biol. Chem.*, 252, 2873, 1977.
4. **Berghäuser, J.**, Modifizierung von argininresten in pyruvat-kinase, *Hoppe-Seyler's Physiol. Chem.*, 358, 1565, 1977.
5. **Lange, L. G., III, Riordan, J. F., and Vallee, B. L.**, Functional argininyl residues as NADH binding sites of alcohol dehydrogenases, *Biochemistry*, 13, 4361, 1974.
6. **Jörnvall, H., Lange, L. G., III, Riordan, J. F., and Vallee, B. L.**, Identification of a reactive arginyl residue in horse liver alcohol dehydrogenase, *Biochem. Biophys. Res. Commun.*, 77, 73, 1977.
7. **Kohlbrenner, W. E. and Cross, R. L.**, Efrapeptin prevents modification by phenylglyoxal of an essential arginyl residue in mitochondrial adenosine triphosphatase, *J. Biol. Chem.*, 253, 7609, 1978.
8. **Berghäuser, J.**, A reactive arginine in adenylate kinase, *Biochim. Biophys. Acta*, 397, 370, 1975.
9. **Berghäuser, J. and Schirmer, R. H.**, Properties of adenylate kinase after modification of Arg-97 by phenylglyoxal, *Biochim. Biophys. Acta*, 537, 428, 1978.
10. **Vallejos, R. H., Lescano, W. I. M., and Lucero, H. A.**, Involvement of an essential arginyl residue in the coupling activity of *Rhodospirillum rubrum* chromatophores, *Arch. Biochem. Biophys.*, 190, 578, 1978.
11. **Tunnicliff, G. and Ngo, T. T.**, Functional role of arginine residues in glutamic acid decarboxylase from brain and bacteria, *Experientia*, 34, 989, 1978.
12. **Schloss, J. V., Norton, I. L., Stringer, C. D., and Hartman, F. C.**, Inactivation of ribulosebisphosphate carboxylase by modification of arginyl residues with phenylglyoxal, *Biochemistry*, 17, 5626, 1978.
13. **Philips, M., Pho, D. B., and Pradel, L.-A.**, An essential arginyl residue in yeast hexokinase, *Biochim. Biophys. Acta*, 566, 296, 1979.
14. **Wolf, B., Kalousek, F., and Rosenberg, L. E.**, Essential arginine residues in the active sites of propionyl CoA carboxylase and beta-methylcrotonyl CoA carboxylase, *Enzyme*, 24, 302, 1979.
15. **Malinowski, D. P. and Fridovich, I.**, Chemical modification of arginine at the active site of the bovine erythrocyte superoxide dismutase, *Biochemistry*, 18, 5909, 1979.
16. **Mornet, D., Pantel, P., Audemard, E., and Kassab, R.**, Involvement of an arginyl residue in the catalytic activity of myosin heads, *Eur. J. Biochem.*, 100, 421, 1979.
17. **Cipollo, K. L. and Dunlap, R. B.**, Essential arginyl residues in thymidylate synthetase from amethopterin-resistant *Lactobacillus casei*, *Biochemistry*, 18, 5537, 1979.
18. **Cheung, S.-T. and Fonda, M. L.**, Kinetics of the inactivation of *Escherichia coli* glutamate apodecarboxylase by phenylglyoxal, *Arch. Biochem. Biophys.*, 198, 541, 1979.
19. **Varimo, K. and Londesborough, J.**, Evidence for essential arginine in yeast adenylate cyclase, *FEBS Lett.*, 106, 153, 1979.
20. **Morkin, E., Flink, I. L., and Banerjee, S. K.**, Phenylglyoxal modification of cardiac myosin S-1. Evidence for essential arginine residues at the active site, *J. Biol. Chem.*, 254, 12647, 1979.
21. **Portemer, C., Pierre, Y., Loriette, C., and Chatagner, F.**, Number of arginine residues in the substrate binding sites of rat liver cystathionase, *FEBS Lett.*, 108, 419, 1979.
22. **Poulose, A. J. and Kolattukudy, P. E.**, Presence of one essential arginine that specifically binds the 2'-phosphate of NADPH on each of the ketoacyl reductase and enoyl reductase active sites of fatty acid synthetase, *Arch. Biochem. Biophys.*, 199, 457, 1980.
23. **Bond, M. W., Chiu, N. Y., and Cooperman, B. S.**, Identification of an arginine residue important for enzymatic activity within the covalent structure of yeast inorganic pyrophosphatase, *Biochemistry*, 19, 94, 1980.
24. **Vensel, L. A. and Kantrowitz, E. R.**, An essential arginine residue in porcine phospholipase A_2, *J. Biol. Chem.*, 255, 7306, 1980.

References for Table 1 (continued)

25. **Borders, C. L., Jr. and Johansen, J. T.**, Essential arginyl residues in Cu, Zn superoxide dismutase from *Saccharomyces cerevisiae*, *Carlsberg Res. Commun.*, 45, 185, 1980.
26. **Borders, C. L., Jr. and Johansen, J. T.**, Identification of Arg-143 as the essential arginyl residue in yeast Cu, Zn superoxide dismutase by the use of a chromophoric arginine reagent, *Biochem. Biophys. Res. Commun.*, 96, 1071, 1980.
27. **Shoun, H., Beppu, T., and Arima, K.**, An essential arginine residue at the substrate-binding site of *p*-hydroxybenzoate hydroxylase, *J. Biol. Chem.*, 255, 9319, 1980.
28. **Belfort, M., Maley, G. F., and Maley, F.**, A single functional arginyl residue involved in the catalysis promoted by *Lactobacillus casei* thymidylate synthetase, *Arch. Biochem. Biophys.*, 204, 340, 1980.
29. **Lu, H. S., Talent, J. M., and Gracy, R. W.**, Chemical modification of critical catalytic residues of lysine, arginine and tryptophan in human glucose phosphate isomerase, *J. Biol. Chem.*, 256, 785, 1981.
30. **Fujioka, M. and Takata, Y.**, Role of arginine residue in saccharopine dehydrogenase (L-Lysine Forming) from baker's yeast, *Biochemistry*, 20, 468, 1981.
31. **El Kebbaj, M. S., Latruffe, N., and Gaudemer, Y.**, Presence of an essential arginine residue in D-β-hydroxybutyrate dehydrogenase from mitochondrial inner membrane, *Biochem. Biophys. Res. Commun.*, 96, 1569, 1980.
32. **Marshall, M. and Cohen, P. P.**, Evidence for an exceptionally reactive arginyl residue at the binding site for carbamyl phosphate in bovine ornithine transcarbamylase, *J. Biol. Chem.*, 255, 7301, 1980.
33. **Kuno, S., Toraya, T., and Fukui, S.**, Coenzyme B_{12}-dependent diol dehydrase: chemical modification with 2,3-butanedione and phenylglyoxal, *Arch. Biochem. Biophys.*, 205, 240, 1980.
34. **Kremer, A. B., Egan, R. M., and Sable, H. Z.**, The active site of transketolase. Two arginine residues are essential for activity, *J. Biol. Chem.*, 255, 2405, 1980.
35. **Tsou, C.-L.**, Relation between modification of functional groups of proteins and their biological activity. I. A graphical method for the determination of the number and type of essential groups, *Sci. Sin.*, 11, 1535, 1962.
36. **Ramakrishna, S. and Benjamin, W. B.**, Evidence for an essential arginine residue at the active site of ATP citrate lyase from rat liver, *Biochem. J.*, 195, 735, 1981.
37. **Chang, G.-G. and Huang, T.-M.**, Modification of essential arginine residues of pigeon liver malic enzyme, *Biochim. Biophys. Acta*, 660, 341, 1981.
38. **Choi, J.-D. and McCormick, D. B.**, Roles of arginyl residues in pyridoxamine-5′-phosphate oxidase from rabbit liver, *Biochemistry*, 20, 5722, 1981.
39. **Fortin, A. F., Hauber, J. M., and Kantrowitz, E. R.**, Comparison of the essential arginine residue in *Escherichia coli* ornithine and aspartate transcarbamylases, *Biochim. Biophys. Acta*, 662, 8, 1981.
40. **Wong, S. S. and Wong, L.-J.**, Evidence for an essential arginine residue at the active site of *Escherichia coli* acetate kinase, *Biochim. Biophys. Acta*, 660, 142, 1981.
41. **Fleer, E. A. M., Puijk, W. C., Slotboom, A. J., and DeHaas, G. H.**, Modification of arginine residues in porcine pancreatic phospholipase A_2, *Eur. J. Biochem.*, 116, 277, 1981.
42. **Akeroyd, R., Lange, L. G., Westerman, J., and Wirtz, K. W. A.**, Modification of the phosphatidyl-choline-transfer protein from bovine liver with butanedione and phenylglyoxal. Evidence for one essential arginine residue, *Eur. J. Biochem.*, 121, 77, 1981.
43. **Branlant, G., Tritsch, D., and Biellmann, J.-F.**, Evidence for the presence of anion-recognition sites in pig-liver aldehyde reductase. Modification by phenylglyoxal and *p*-carboxyphenyl glyoxal of an arginyl residue located close to the substrate-binding site, *Eur. J. Biochem.*, 116, 505, 1981.
44. **Mautner, H. G., Pakyla, A. A., and Merrill, R. E.**, Evidence for presence of an arginine residue in the coenzyme A binding site of choline acetyltransferase, *Proc. Natl. Acad. Sci. U.S.A.*, 78, 7449, 1981.
45. **Carlson, C. A. and Preiss, J.**, Involvement of arginine residues in the allosteric activation of *Escherichia coli* ADP–glucose synthetase, *Biochemistry*, 21, 1929, 1982.
46. **Koland, J. G., O'Brien, T. A., and Gennis, R. B.**, Role of arginine in the binding of thiamin pyrophosphate to *Escherichia coli* pyruvate oxidase, *Biochemistry*, 21, 2656, 1982.
47. **King, M. M. and Heiny, L. P.**, Chemical modification of the calmodulin-stimulated phosphatase, calcineurin, by phenylglyoxal, *J. Biol. Chem.*, 262, 10658, 1987.
48. **Shanmugasundaram, T., Kumar, G. K., Shenoy, B. C., and Wood, H. G.**, Chemical modification of the functional arginine residues of carbon monoxide dehydrogenase from *Clostridium thermoaceticum*, *Biochemistry*, 28, 7112, 1989.
49. **Garty, H., Yeger, O., and Asher, C.**, Sodium-dependent inhibition of the epithelial sodium channel by an arginyl-specific reagent, *J. Biol. Chem.*, 263, 5550, 1988.
50. **Missiaen, L., Raeymaekers, L., Droogmans, G., Wuytack, F., and Casteels, R.**, Role of arginine residues in the stimulation of the smooth-muscle plasma-membrane Ca^{2+} [T pump by negatively charged phospholipids, *Biochem. J.*, 264, 609, 1989.
51. **King, M. M.**, Conformation-sensitive modification of the type II calmodulin-dependent protein kinase by phenylglyoxal, *J. Biol. Chem.*, 263, 4754, 1988.

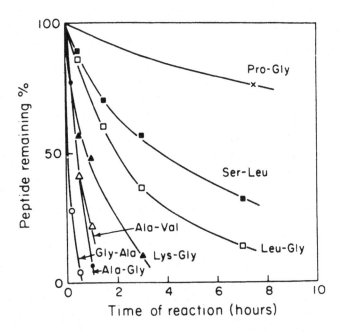

FIGURE 11. The rate of reaction of phenylglyoxal with various dipeptides. The reactions were performed in 0.2 *M N*–ethylmorpholine acetate, pH 8.0, at 25°C. The concentration of peptide was 0.017% and the concentration of phenylglyoxal hydrate was 1.25%. At the indicated times a 50-μl portion was withdrawn from the reaction mixture, diluted into 1.2 ml sodium citrate, pH 2.2, and stored at −10°C until analysis for residual peptide on the amino acid analyzer and for amino acids after acid hydrolysis. (From Takahashi, K., *J. Biol. Chem.*, 243, 6171, 1968. With permission.)

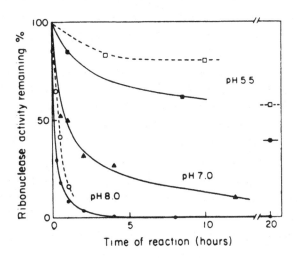

FIGURE 12. The rate of inactivation of bovine pancreatic ribonuclease A by phenylglyoxal as a function of pH. The concentration of protein was 0.5% and the concentration of phenylglyoxal hydrate was 1.5% at 25°C under the following conditions: ○- - - -○, pH 8.0 (0.1 *M N*-ethylmorpholine acetate; ●——●, pH 8.0 (0.1 *M N*-ethylmorpholine acetate with 0.6% 2′(3′)-cytidylic acid); ▲——▲, pH 7.0 (0.1 *M* sodium phosphate); □- - - -□, pH 5.5 (0.1 *M* sodium acetate); ■——■, pH 5.5 (0.1 *M* sodium acetate with 0.6% 2′(3′)-cytidylic acid. (From Takahashi, K., *J. Biol. Chem.*, 243, 6171, 1968. With permission.)

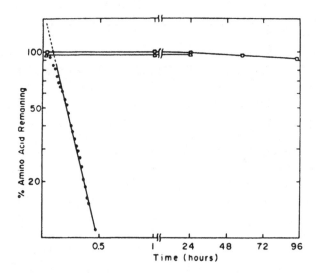

FIGURE 13.   The modification of amino acid derivatives with phenylglyoxal in bicarbonate buffer. Shown is the time course for the reaction of *N*-acetylarginine (●), *N*-acetyllysine (□), and *N*-acetylcysteine (△) with phenylglyoxal in 83 m*M* bicarbonate buffer, pH 7.5, at 23°C. The reaction with *N*-acetylarginine was monitored by the increase in absorbance at 340 nm. The amounts of unreacted *N*-acetyllysine and *N*-acetylcysteine were determined by reaction with 2,4,6-trinitrobenzenesulfonic acid. (From Cheung, S.-T. and Fonda, M. L., *Biochem. Biophys. Res. Commun.*, 90, 940, 1979. With permission.)

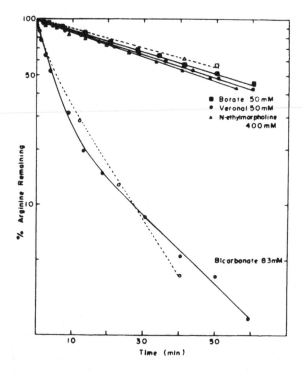

FIGURE 14.   The reaction of arginine with phenylglyoxal in various buffers. The reactions mixtures contained 5 m*M* L-arginine and 25 m*M* phenylglyoxal in the designated buffer at pH 7.5 and 25°C. Portions were removed at the indicated times, and the arginine concentrations were determined by the Sakaguchi test (solid lines and closed symbols) or by amino acid analysis (dashed lines and open symbols). (From Cheung, S.-T. and Fonda, M. L., *Biochem. Biophys. Res. Commun.*, 90, 940, 1979. With permission.)

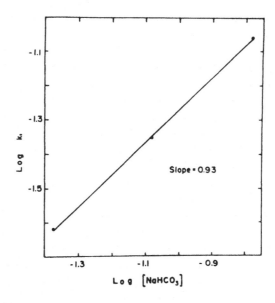

FIGURE 15. The effect of bicarbonate concentration on the rate of reaction of arginine with phenylglyoxal. Shown is a plot of logarithm apparent first-order rate constants vs. logarithm bicarbonate concentrations. The reaction mixtures contained 5 mM N-acetylarginine and 25 mM phenylglyoxal in sodium bicarbonate, pH 7.5, at 25°C. The absorbance at 340 nm was recorded, and the rate constants were obtained from the slopes of the plots of ln (A$_x$-A$_t$) vs. time. The slope of the line obtained in this figure is 0.93 suggesting that the reaction is first order with respect to bicarbonate. (From Cheung, S.-T. and Fonda, M. L., *Biochem. Biophys. Res. Commun.*, 90, 940, 1979. With permission.)

compares the rate of reaction of phenylglyoxal with arginine in bicarbonate buffer with that in other buffer systems (borate, Veronal, N-ethylmorpholine). The reaction appears to be first order with respect to bicarbonate (Figure 15). The reaction of methylglyoxal with arginine is also enhanced by bicarbonate (Figure 16) while a similar effect is not seen with either glyoxal or 2,3-butanedione. The molecular basis for this specific buffer effect is not clear at this time nor is it known whether reaction with α-amino functional groups occurs at a different rate than with other solvent systems used for this modification of arginine with phenylglyoxal. Feeney and co-workers[30] reported that p-nitrophenylglyoxal (prepared from p-nitroacetophenone — see Reference 31) reacts with arginine in 0.17 sodium pyrophosphate — 0.15 M sodium ascorbate, pH 9.0 to yield a derivative which absorbs at 475 nm. There is also reaction with histidine (the imidazole ring is critical for this reaction in that the 1-methyl derivative yielded a derivative which absorbed at 475 nm while the 3-methyl derivative did not). Free sulfhydryl groups also yielded a product with absorbance at 475 nm, but its absorbance was only 3% of that of the arginine. Branlant and co-workers[32] have used p-carboxyphenyl glyoxal in bicarbonate buffer at pH 8.0 to modify aldehyde reductase. Saturation kinetics were noted with the use of this reagent.

Eun[33] has examined the effect of borate on the reaction of arginine with phenylglyoxal and p-hydroxyphenylglyoxal. The base buffer of these studies was 0.1 M sodium pyrophosphate, pH 9.0. Spectroscopy was used to follow the rate of arginine modification. The rate of modification of either free arginine or N-acetyl-L-arginine with phenylglyoxal was 10 to 15 times faster than that of p-hydroxyphenylglyoxal in the base buffer system. The inclusion of sodium borate (10 to 50 mM) markedly increased the rate of the reaction (approximately 20-fold) of p-hydroxyphenylglyoxal with either arginine or N-acetyl-L-arginine while there was only a slight enhancement of the phenylglyoxal reaction. In a related study,[34] the effect of phenylglyoxal on sodium-channel gating in frog myelinated nerve was compared with that of p-hydroxyphenylglyoxal or p-nitrophenylglyoxal. Both p-hydroxy-

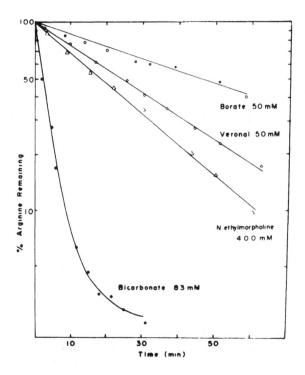

FIGURE 16.   The effect of various buffers on the rate of reaction of arginine with methylglyoxal. The reaction mixtures contained 5 mM arginine and 25 mM methylglyoxal in the buffers indicated. Portions were removed at the indicated times for the determination of the amount of arginine remaining by the Sakaguchi test. (From Cheung, S.-T. and Fonda, M. L., *Biochem. Biophys. Res. Commun.*, 90, 940, 1979. With permission.)

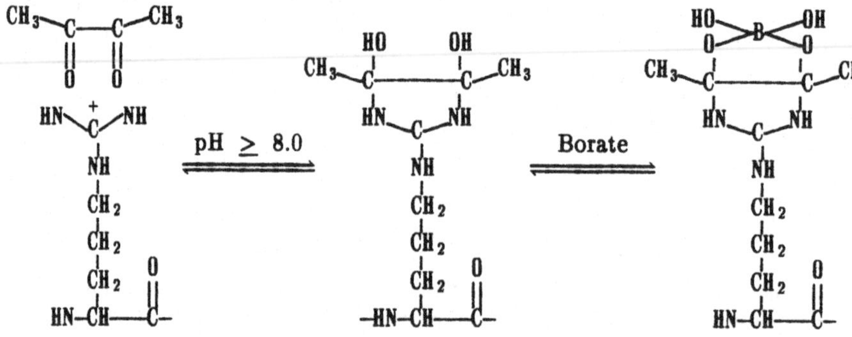

FIGURE 17.   A scheme for the reaction of arginine with 2,3-butanedione.

phenylglyoxal and p-nitrophenylglyoxal had less effect than phenylglyoxal in reduced sodium current. The results are discussed in terms of the differences in hydrophobicity of the reagents but it is clear that the intrinsic difference in reagent effectiveness described by Eun may be responsible, in part, for the observed differences.

2,3-Butanedione is a second well-characterized reagent for the selective modification of arginyl residues in proteins. Yankeelov and co-workers introduced the use of this reagent.[3,35] There were problems with the specificity of the reaction (c.f. Reference 35) and the time required for modification until the observation of Riordan[36] that borate had a significant effect on the nature of the reaction of 2,3-butanedione with arginyl residues in proteins (Figure 17). Figure 18 shows the effect of borate (0.05 M borate, 1.0 M NaCl, pH 7.5) on

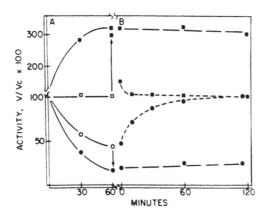

FIGURE 18.   The modification of carboxypeptidase A with 2,3-butanedione in borate buffer. (A) Changes in esterase (□, ■) and peptidase (○, ●) activities on modification of carboxypeptidase A (0.15 mM) with 2,3-butanedione in 0.05 M borate — 1 M NaCl, pH 7.5 (9 mM reagent, closed symbols), or in 0.02 M Veronal — 1.0 M NaCl, pH 7.5 (75 mM reagent, open symbols) at 20°C. The changes in the activity immediately on addition of borate after 1 h to the sample reacted in Veronal buffer are indicated by the arrows. (B) Changes in activities of the samples reacted in borate buffer subsequent to gel filtration through Bio-Gel P-4 equilibrated either with 0.05 M borate — 1.0 M NaCl, pH 7.5 (— — —), or with 0.02 M Veronal — 1.0 M NaCl, pH 7.5 (- - - -). (From Riordan, J. F., *Biochemistry*, 12, 3915, 1973. With permission.)

the changes in biological activity occurring on the reaction of carboxypeptidase A (0.15 mM) with 2,3-butanedione (freshly distilled). Note that in particular, the enhancement of esterase activity in the presence of butanedione is dependent on the presence of borate buffer as no significant change is seen with butanedione in 0.02 M Veronal, 1.0 M NaCl, pH 7.5. The removal of borate by gel filtration results in the recovery of activity.

The ability of 2,3-butanedione to act as a photosensitizing agent for the destruction of amino acids and proteins in the presence of oxygen was emphasized in work by Fliss and Viswanatha.[21] Figure 19 shows the destruction of certain amino acids in the presence of 2,3-butanedione and oxygen at pH 6.0 (phosphate) 36°C upon irradiation at 350 to 375 nm ("Blak-Lite" UV-Lamp, 100 W bulb, 20 cm from sample contained in a quartz cuvette). As would be expected from consideration of early photooxidation work, tryptophan and histidine are lost most rapidly with methionine; cystine and tyrosine are lost at a much slower rate. Loss is not seen on irradiation in the absence of 2,3-butanedione (open symbols). Azide (10 mM), a singlet oxygen scavenger, greatly reduced the rate of loss of amino acids. The absence of oxygen also greatly reduces the rate of loss of sensitive amino acids.

These observations have been confirmed and extended by other laboratories.[22,23] An examination of recent studies using 2,3-butanedione to modify arginyl residues in proteins is presented in Table 2.

The use of 1,2-cyclohexanedione under very basic conditions to modify arginyl residues was demonstrated in 1967.[37] However, it was not until Patthy and Smith[8] reported on the reaction of 1,2-cyclohexanedione in borate with arginyl residues in proteins that the use of this reagent became practical. These investigators reported that 1,2-cyclohexanedione reacted with arginyl residues in 0.2 M borate, pH 9.0. At alkaline pH, reaction of 1,2-cyclohexanedione with arginine (Figure 20) forms N^5-(4-oxo-1,3-diazaspiro[4,4]non-2-yliodene)-L-ornithine (CHD-arginine), a reaction which cannot be reversed. Between pH 7.0 and pH 9.0 a compound is formed from arginine and 1,2-cyclohexanedione, N^7-N^8-(1,2-dihydroxycyclohex-1,2-ylene)-L-arginine (DHCH-arginine). This compound is stabilized by the presence of borate and is unstable in the presence of buffers such as Tris. This compound is readily converted back to free arginine in 0.5 M hydroxylamine, pH 7.0 (Figure 21).

These authors have subsequently used this reagent to identify functional residues in bovine pancreatic ribonuclease A and egg white lysozyme.[39] Extent of modification of arginine

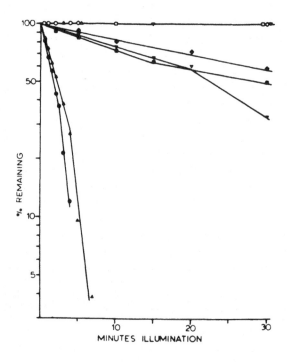

FIGURE 19. 2,3-Butanedione-sensitized destruction of α-amino acids. ●, tryptophan (99.5 μ*M*); ■, tyrosine (333 μ*M*); ▲, histidine (92 μ*M*); ▼, methionine (1000 μ*M*); and ◆, cystine (33.3 μ*M*) in the presence of 2,3-butanedione (9580 μ*M*) and continuous oxygenation were irradiated at pH 6.0 (irradiation was performed in quartz cuvettes 20 cm from a ''Blak-Lite'' UV light source, Canlab catalog No. L6093-1, equipped with a 100 W lamp emitting light almost exclusively in the range of 350 to 375 nm) at 36°C. Open symbols represent preparations of amino acids (at the same concentrations as the experiments described above) irradiated in the absence of 2,3-butanedione. The above experiments used freshly distilled monomer preparation of 2,3-butanedione. (From Fliss, H. and Viswanatha, T., *Can. J. Biochem.*, 57, 1267, 1979. With permission.)

Table 2
USE OF 2,3-BUTANEDIONE TO MODIFY ARGINYL RESIDUES IN PROTEINS

Protein	Solvent	Reagent excess[a]	Stoichiometry	Ref.
Carboxypeptidase A	0.05 *M* borate, 1.0 *M* NaCl, pH 7.5	—[b]	2/10	1
Chymotrypsin	0.1 *M* phosphate, pH 6.0	100[c]	1/3[d]	2
Thymidylate synthetase	0.050 *M* borate, pH 8.0	—	—[e]	3
Prostatic acid phosphatase	0.050 *M* borate, pH 8.0	—	—[f]	4
Purine nucleoside phosphorylase	0.0165 *M* borate, pH 8.0	—	—[g]	5
Yeast hexokinase PII	0.050 *M* borate, pH 8.3	—	4.2/18[h]	6
Isocitrate dehydrogenase	0.05 *M* MES, pH 6.2, 20% glycerol, 0.0021 *M* MnSO₄	—	1.6/13.4[i]	7
Stearylcoenzyme A desaturase	0.050 *M* sodium borate, pH 8.1	2500	2[j]	8
Superoxide dismutase	0.050 *M* borate, pH 9.0	—[k]	1.3/4[l]	9
Energy-independent transhydrogenase	0.050 *M* sodium[m] borate, pH 7.8	—	—	10
Enolase	0.050 *M* borate, pH 8.3, 0.001 *M* Mg (OAc)₂, 0.01 m*M* EDTA	260	3/16[n]	11
NADPH-dependent aldehyde reductase	0.050 *M* borate, pH 7.0	—[o]	1/18[p]	12

Table 2 (continued)
USE OF 2,3-BUTANEDIONE TO MODIFY ARGINYL RESIDUES IN PROTEINS

Protein	Solvent	Reagent excess[a]	Stoichiometry	Ref.
Aryl sulfatase A	0.050 M^q NaHCO$_3$, pH 8.0	—	—	13
Na$^+$, K$^+$-ATPase	0.04 M TES, 0.02 M borate, pH 7.4	—	—	14
Carbamate kinase	0.005 M triethanolamine, 0.050 M borate, pH 7.5	2000	1.2/3.0[r]	15
Thymidylate synthetase	0.050 M borate, 0.001 M EDTA, pH 8.0	1201	2.1/12[s]	16
(K$^+$ + H$^+$)-ATPase	0.125 M sodium borate, pH 7.0	—	—[t]	17
Cu, Zn superoxide dismutase	0.050 M borate, pH 8.3	—[u]	—	18
Fatty acid synthetase	0.020 M borate, 0.200 M KCl, 0.001 M dithiothreitol, 0.001 mM EDTA, pH 7.6	—	—[v]	19
Acetylcholinesterase	0.005 M phosphate, 0.025 M borate, 0.050 M NaCl, pH 7.0	—	4/31[w]	20
Coenzyme B$_{12}$-dependent diol dehydrase	0.050 M borate, pH 8.5	—	—[x]	21
Ornithine transcarbamylase	0.05 M bicine,[y] 0.1 mM EDTA, 0.1 M KCl, pH 7.67	—	0.88/11[z]	22
Glycogen phosphorylase	0.020 M sodium tetraborate, 1 mM EDTA, pH 7.5	—	—	23
Cytochrome c	0.05 M sodium bicarbonate, pH 7.5	9900[aa]	2/2[bb]	24
Bacteriorhodopsin	0.100 M borate, pH 8.2	66,700	4/79[cc]	25
α-Ketoglutarate dehydrogenase	0.050 M sodium borate, pH 8.0	—[dd]	—[ee]	26
Acetate kinase	0.050 M borate, pH 8.6	—	—	27
Malic enzyme	0.045 M borate,[ff] pH 7.5	—	—	28
Glucose phosphate isomerase	0.05 M sodium borate, pH 8.7	—	7.8/30[gg]	29
Saccharopine dehydrogenase	0.08 M HEPES, 0.2 M KCl, 0.01 M borate, pH 8.0	—[hh]	8/38[ii]	30
Testicular hyaluronidase	0.050 M borate, pH 8.3	—[jj]	3.6/28	31
Glutathione reductase	0.050 M sodium borate, pH 8.3, 1 mM EDTA	20,000	5.3/[kk]	32
E. coli fibrillar adhesins	100 mM sodium borate with 0.9% NaCl, pH 7.5	—	—	34
Inter-alpha trypsin inhibitor	10 mM HEPES-175 mM NaCl-100 mM sodium borate, pH 7.4	—	—	35
D-Glyceraldehyde-3-phosphate dehydrogenase	100 mM medinal[ll] buffer, pH 8.3 with 5 mM EDTA and 2 mM dithiothreitol	—	—	36

[a] Mole reagent per mole protein unless otherwise indicated.

[b] This study demonstrated that, in the presence of borate, there is essentially no difference in the reaction of 2,3-butanedione monomer and butadione trimer. It is noted that the commercially available 2,3-butanedione should be distilled immediately prior to use.

[c] This study used 2,3-butanedione trimer prepared by allowing 2,3-butanedione (40 ml) to stand with 80 g untreated Permutit under dry air (after shaking to obtain an even dispension of 2,3-butanedione in Permutit) for 4 to 6 weeks at ambient temperature. The mixture was extracted with anhydrous ether. The ether extract was taken to an oil with dry air. The oil was allowed to stand for 5 to 7 days to permit crystallization of the trimer.

Table 2 (continued)
USE OF 2,3-BUTANEDIONE TO MODIFY ARGINYL RESIDUES IN PROTEINS

d   In the absence of light, also some loss of lysine; no loss of catalytic activity. In the presence of sunlight there was rapid inactivation of the enzyme with loss of lysine, arginine (less than in the dark), and tyrosine. With the exception of tyrosine modification, the changes in amino acid composition in the reaction exposed to light were less than those for the dark reaction despite the more significant loss of activity. Study of the wavelength dependence demonstrates that light of 300 nm is most effective. 2,3-Butanedione monomer was not effective in this photoinactivation process.

e   Stoichiometry of reaction not established. Inactivation was reversed by gel filtration in 0.05 M Tris, 0.010 M β-mercaptoethanol, pH 8.0.

f   30°C.

g   Ambient temperature. Calf spleen enzyme had 26 Arg modified at 98% loss of activity. Reaction with arginyl residues (as judged by loss of catalytic activity) was 50% as rapid with 2,3-butanedione in borate ($T_{1/2}$ = 40.3 min) as with phenylglyoxal in Tris buffer ($T_{1/2}$ = 19.2 min).

h   Reaction at 25°C. Determined by amino acid analysis after acid hydrolysis (6 N HCl, 110°C, 18 h). MgATP (5 mM) did not protect against either modification or loss of enzymatic activity but MgATP and glucose reduced extent of modification from 3.3 arginine residues per subunit (65% inactivation) to 2.1 residues per subunit (20% inactivation). Inactivation was also observed with phenylglyoxal in 0.050 M BICINE, pH 8.3. Stoichiometry with this modification was not established.

i   Determined by amino acid analysis. As indicated, the maximum value obtained is 1.6 residues modified out of an average of 13.4 arginyl residues per subunit.

j   The modification was performed at 25°C. The presence of stearyl-CoA greatly decreased the rate and extent of inactivation by 2,3-butanedione. When the modified enzyme is taken into 0.020 Tris (acetate), 0.100 M NaCl, pH 8.1 by gel filtration there is the rapid recovery of activity and the concomitant decrease in the extent of arginine modification. A similar extent of modification and loss of catalytic activity was seen with 1,2-cyclohexanedione in 0.1 M sodium borate, pH 8.1.

k   Inactivation occurred at a rate of 10.9 M^{-1} min^{-1} under these conditions (compared to 4.0 M^{-1} min^{-1} with phenylglyoxal in bicarbonate/carbonate and 6.6 M^{-1} min^{-1} with 1,2-cyclohexanedione in 0.050 M borate, pH 9.0). Inactivation with 2,3-butanedione is not observed in 0.05 M bicarbonate/carbonate, pH 9.0 at 25°C; however there is reduced modification of arginine (0.4 residue per subunit as compared to 1.3 residues per subunit with 77% inactivation).

l   The majority of arginine modification could be reversed by the removal of reagent and borate solvent by dialysis vs. 0.05 M potassium phosphate, pH 7.8. Enzymic activity was also recovered as a result of the dialysis procedure. These investigators were able to obtain evidence supporting the selective modification of Arg[141] by either 2,3-butanedione, 1,2-cyclohexandione or phenylglyoxal.

m   The modification was performed at 22°C. These studies were performed with bacterial membrane preparations. Stoichiometry was not established. Analysis of the rates of inactivation suggested that inactivation was due to the modification of a single arginine residue. NADH, which stimulates the transhydrogenation of 3-acetylpyridine-NAD by NADPH, protects the enzyme from inactivation.

n   The modification was performed at 25°C. The extent of modification was determined by amino acid analysis after acid hydrolysis. The extent of modification reported was obtained after 75 min of reaction concomitant with 85% loss of activity. The presence of substrate, α-phosphoglycerate, reduced the extent of modification to 2 mol arginine per subunit with only 5% loss of catalytic activity.

o   A second-order rate constant of 0.0635 M^{-1} min^{-1} was obtained for the loss of enzymic activity upon reaction with 2,3-butanedione in 0.050 M borate, pH 7.0 at 25°C. This presumably reflects the modification of a single arginine residue (see Footnote p). The inactivation of the enzyme by 1,2-cyclohexanedione, methylglyoxal, and phenylglyoxal is compared with that by 2,3-butanedione (all at 10 mM in 0.05 M borate, pH 7.0). Butanedione is clearly most effective followed by phenylglyoxal, methylglyoxal, and 1,2-cyclohexanedione. The authors note that the enzyme under study, aldehyde reductase, can utilize methylglyoxal and phenylglyoxal as substrates, precluding their rigorous evaluation in this study.

p   Obtained by amino acid analysis after acid hydrolysis (6 N HCl, 110°C, 24 h). The control preparation yielded a value of 17.8 ± 1 Arg while the modified enzyme yielded a value of 16.7 ± 1 Arg. The presence of cofactor yielded a preparation with 17.5 ± 1 Arg.

q   The reactions are reported at 25°C. Borate buffers could not be used since borate is a competitive inhibitor of the enzyme and prevents inactivation in bicarbonate buffer. Reaction with phenylglyoxal in the same solvent.

r   Reaction performed at 25°C. Stoichiometry established by amino acid analysis after acid hydrolysis (6 N HCl, 100°C, 20 h). Arginine is the only amino acid modified under these reaction conditions. These values were obtained at 80% inactivation. The presence of ADP reduced activity loss to 55% with extent of arginine modification reduced to 0.4 to 0.5 residues.

s   Reaction performed at 25°C for 90 min. Stoichiometry determined by amino acid analysis after acid hydrolysis (6 N HCl, 110°C, 24 h).

Table 2 (continued)

USE OF 2,3-BUTANEDIONE TO MODIFY ARGINYL RESIDUES IN PROTEINS

t   The use of isolated "membrane fraction" prevented the establishment of stoichiometry in these studies. Analysis of the dependence of reaction rate on concentration of 2,3-butanedione is consistent with the modification of a single arginine residue. As expected, the stability of modification is dependent upon the presence of borate. Gel filtration into HEPES (0.125 M, pH 7.0) and subsequent inactivation at 37°C resulted in the recovery of a substantial amount of catalytic activity. Similar results were obtained with imidazole and Tris buffers under similar reaction conditions. This reactivation does not occur when the incubation following gel filtration is performed at 0°C instead of 37°C.

u   A reaction rate with a second-order rate constant of k = 5.2 M^{-1} min^{-1} is obtained at 25°C. Inactivation is dependent on the presence of borate as inactivation is not observed with use of BICINE buffer. Dialysis vs. 0.025 M phosphate, pH 7.0 for 21 h at 4°C results in an increase in activity of 14 to 85% while complete recovery of activity is achieved after 21 h of dialysis.

v   Stoichiometry was not established for the reaction with 2,3-butanedione. As shown in Table 1, reaction with phenylglyoxal modifies approximately 4 of the 106 arginyl residues in each subunit of fatty acid synthetase. The loss of the biological activity as determined either by fatty acid synthetase activity, ketoreductase activity, or enoylreductase activity was considerably more rapid with phenylglyoxal than with 2,3-butanedione. It is noted that these reactions are performed in borate buffer for the studies with 2,3-butanedione and phosphate buffer for the studies with phenylglyoxal, both buffers at pH 7.6 with the reactions performed at 30°C.

w   Reactions were performed at 25°C. The modification of arginyl residues is associated with an approximate 70% loss of enzymatic activity. The presence of N-phenylpyridinium-2-aldoxine iodide reduces the extent of arginine modification by approximately 1 mol/mol of enzyme with concomitant protection of enzymatic activity. It should be noted that modification of this enzyme with phenylglyoxal results in the modification of 3 mol of arginine/mol enzyme with 17% loss of enzymatic activity (see Table 1). It is not clear when modification of a particular arginyl residue with the two reagents is a mutually exclusive event.

x   Reactions were performed at 25°C. Rigorous evaluation of the stoichiometry of the reaction is not available. Analysis of the dependence of first-order rate constants on reagent concentration (double-logarithmic relationships) is consistent with the modification of a single arginyl residue. The inactivation was reversed by 100-fold dilution into 0.05 M potassium phosphate, pH 8.5, at 25°C.

y   The inactivation of ornithine transcarbamylase is readily reversible in this solvent; the presence of borate precludes reactivation observed on dilution of modified enzyme in solvent. A value of 179 M^{-1} min^{-1} for the second-order rate constant for reaction of 2,3-butanedione with ornithine transcarbamylase under these conditions was recorded.

z   Obtained at 88% inactivation.

aa   Reaction at 22°C.

bb   Determined by amino acid analysis. The reaction is readily reversible, even in the presence of borate.

cc   Determined by amino acid analysis. Constructed Scatchard plot shows that two residues were not available for modification with 2,3-butanedione.

dd   Second-order rate constant, k = 2.95 M^{-1} min^{-1} in this solvent, assuming that loss in catalytic activity is a measure of reaction with arginine.

ee   Stoichiometry was not established. Kinetic analysis suggests that inactivation of catalytic activity results from the modification of a single arginine residue.

ff   Modification reaction was performed at 24°C. Very little inactivation is observed if the reaction is performed in Tris buffer at the same pH. Reactivation of enzyme modified in borate buffer is observed when the inactivated enzyme is diluted in borate buffer.

gg   The reaction was performed at 25°C for 4 h. The presence of the competitive inhibitor, 6-phosphogluconate, protected 1 mol of arginine/mol of enzyme from modification suggesting that there is a single arginine residue critical for catalytic activity. A 20-fold increase in inhibitor concentration resulted in the modification of greater than 95% of the total arginine residues.

hh   Second-order rate constant of k = 7.5 M^{-1} min^{-1} at 25°C was obtained from the analysis of reaction rate data. pH Dependence study showed optimal rate of inactivation at pH 8.2.

ii   Determined by amino acid analysis on 95 + % inactivated enzyme. Plotting loss of activity vs. arginine residues modified suggests that inactivation is due to the modification of a single arginine residue. Inactivation occurs with loss of sulfhydryl content.

jj   Second-order rate constant of k = 13.57 M^{-1} min^{-1} obtained at 20°C. Inactivation much less rapid in 0.050 M HEPES, pH 8.3 ($T_{1/2}$ = 30 min in borate; 11.5 min in HEPES).

kk   Reactions performed at 30°C. Modification associated with 80 to 90% inactivation. Reaction with phenylglyoxal (0.050 M sodium phosphate, 1 mM EDTA, pH 7.6) at 2000-fold molar excess led to the modification of 2 arginyl residues at a level of 90% inactivation. The extent of arginine was determined by spectrophotometric analysis (increase in absorbance at 250 nm, $\Delta\epsilon$ = 11,000 M^{-1} cm^{-1}; see Reference 33).

ll   Reaction readily reversible, reflecting the absence of borate in the buffer.

References for Table 2

1. **Riordan, J. F.,** Functional arginyl residues in carboxypeptidase A. Modification with butanedione, *Biochemistry,* 12, 3915, 1973.
2. **Fliss, H., Tozer, N. M., and Viswanatha, T.,** The reaction of chymotrypsin with 2,3-butanedione trimer, *Can. J. Biochem.,* 53, 275, 1975.
3. **Cipollo, K. L. and Dunlap, R. B.,** Essential arginyl residues in thymidylate synthetase, *Biochem. Biophys. Res. Commun.,* 81, 1139, 1978.
4. **McTigue, J. J. and Van Etten, R. L.,** An essential arginine residue in human prostatic acid phosphatase, *Biochim. Biophys. Acta,* 523, 422, 1978.
5. **Jordan, F. and Wu, A.,** Inactivation of purine nucleoside phosphorylase by modification of arginine residues, *Arch. Biochem. Biophys.,* 190, 699, 1978.
6. **Borders, C. L., Jr., Cipollo, K. L., and Jordasky, J. F.,** Role of arginyl residues in yeast hexokinase PII, *Biochemistry,* 17, 2654, 1978.
7. **Hayman, S. and Colman, R. F.,** Effect of arginine modification on the catalytic activity and allosteric activation by adenosine diphosphate of the diphosphopyridine nucleotide specific isocitrate dehydrogenase of pig heart, *Biochemistry,* 17, 4161, 1978.
8. **Enoch, H. G. and Strittmatter, P.,** Role of tyrosyl and arginyl residues in rat liver microsomal stearyl-coenzyme A desaturase, *Biochemistry,* 17, 4927, 1978.
9. **Malinowski, D. P. and Fridovich, I.,** Chemical modification of arginine at the active site of the bovine erythrocyte superoxide dismutase, *Biochemistry,* 18, 5909, 1979.
10. **Homyk, M. and Bragg, P. D.,** Steady-state kinetics and the inactivation by 2,3-butanedione of the energy-independent transhydrogenase of *Escherichia coli* cell membranes, *Biochim. Biophys. Acta,* 571, 201, 1979.
11. **Borders, C. L., Jr. and Zurcher, J. A.,** Rabbit muscle enolase also has essential argininyl residues, *FEBS Lett.,* 108, 415, 1979.
12. **Davidson, W. S. and Flynn, T. G.,** A functional arginine residue in NADPH-dependent aldehyde reductase from pig kidney, *J. Biol. Chem.,* 254, 3724, 1979.
13. **James, G. T.,** Essential arginine residues in human liver arylsulfatase A, *Arch. Biochem. Biophys.,* 197, 57, 1979.
14. **Grisham, C. M.,** Characterization of essential arginyl residues in sheep kidney ($Na^+ + K^+$)-ATPase, *Biochem. Biophys. Res. Commun.,* 88, 229, 1979.
15. **Pillai, R. P., Marshall, M., and Villafranca, J. J.,** Modification of an essential arginine of carbamate kinase, *Arch. Biochem. Biophys.,* 199, 16, 1980.
16. **Cipollo, K. L. and Dunlap, R. B.,** Essential arginyl residues in thymidylate synthetase from amethopterin-resistant *Lactobacillus casei, Biochemistry,* 18, 5537, 1979.
17. **Schrijen, J. J., Luyben, W. A. H. M., DePont, J. J. H. M., and Bonting, S. L.,** Studies on ($K^+ + H^+$)-ATPase. I. Essential arginine residue in its substrate binding center, *Biochim. Biophys. Acta,* 597, 331, 1980.
18. **Belfort, M., Maley, G. F., and Maley, F.,** A single functional arginyl residue involved in the catalysis promoted by *Lactobacillus casei* thymidylate synthetase, *Arch. Biochem. Biophys.,* 204, 340, 1980.
19. **Poulose, A. J. and Kolattukudy, P. E.,** Presence of one essential arginine that specifically binds the 2'-phosphate of NADPH on each of the ketoacyl reductase and enoyl reductase active sites of fatty acid synthetase, *Arch. Biochem. Biophys.,* 199, 457, 1980.
20. **Müllner, H. and Sund, H.,** Essential arginine residue in acetylcholinesterase from *Torpedo californica, FEBS Lett.,* 119, 283, 1980.
21. **Kuno, S., Toraya, T., and Fukui, S.,** Coenzyme B_{12}-dependent diol dehydrase: chemical modification with 2,3-butanedione and phenylglyoxal, *Arch. Biochem. Biophys.,* 205, 240, 1980.
22. **Marshall, M. and Cohen, P. P.,** Evidence for an exceptionally reactive arginyl residue at the binding site for carbamyl phosphate in bovine ornithine transcarbamylase, *J. Biol. Chem.,* 255, 7301, 1980.
23. **Dreyfus, M., Vandenbunder, B., and Buc, H.,** Mechanism of allosteric activation of glycogen phosphorylase probed by the reactivity of essential arginyl residues. Physicochemical and kinetic studies, *Biochemistry,* 19, 3634, 1980.
24. **Pande, J. and Myer, Y. P.,** The arginines of cytochrome c. The reduction-binding site for 2,3-butanedione and ascorbate, *J. Biol. Chem.,* 255, 11094, 1980.
25. **Tristram-Nagle, S. and Packer, L.,** Effects of arginine modification on the photocycle and proton pumping of bacteriorhodopsin, *Biochem. Int.,* 3, 621, 1981.
26. **Gomazkova, V. S., Stafeeva, and Severin, S. E.,** The role of arginine residues in the functioning of α-ketoglutarate dehydrogenase from pigeon breast muscle, *Biochem. Int.,* 2, 51, 1981.
27. **Wong, S. S. and Wong, L.-J.,** Evidence for an essential arginine residue at the active site of *Escherichia coli* acetate kinase, *Biochim. Biophys. Acta,* 660, 142, 1981.
28. **Chang, G.-G. and Huang, T.-M.,** Modification of essential arginine residues of pigeon liver malic enzyme, *Biochim. Biophys. Acta,* 660, 341, 1981.

References for Table 2 (continued)

29. **Lu, H. S., Talent, J. M., and Gracy, R. W.,** Chemical modification of critical catalytic residues of lysine, arginine and tryptophan in human glucose phosphate isomerase, *J. Biol. Chem.,* 256, 785, 1981.
30. **Fujioka, M. and Takata, Y.,** Role of arginine residue in saccharopine dehydrogenase (L-Lysine Forming) from baker's yeast, *Biochemistry,* 20, 468, 1981.
31. **Gacesa, P., Savitsky, M. J., Dodgson, K. S., and Olavesen, A. H.,** Modification of functional arginine residues in purified bovine testicular hyaluronidase with butane-2,3-dione, *Biochim. Biophys. Acta,* 661, 205, 1981.
32. **Boggaram, V. and Mannervik, B.,** Essential arginine residues in the pyridine nucleotide binding sites of glutathione reductase, *Biochim. Biophys. Acta,* 701, 119, 1982.
33. **Takahashi, K.,** Further studies on the reactions of phenylgloxal and related reagents with proteins, *J. Biochem.,* 81, 403, 1977.
34. **Jacobs, A. A. C., van Mechelen, J. R., and De Graaf, F. K.,** Effect of chemical modification on the K99 and K88ab fibrillar adhesins of Escherichia coli, *Biochim. Biophys. Acta,* 832, 148, 1985.
35. **Swaim, M. W. and Pizzo, S. V.,** Modification of the tandem reactive centres of human inter-trypsin inhibitor with butanedione and *cis*-dichlorodiammineplatinum (II), *Biochem. J.,* 254, 171, 1988.
36. **Asryants, R. A., Kuzminskaya, E. V., Tishkov, V. I., Douzhenkova, I. V., and Nagradova, N. K.,** An examination of the role of arginine residues in the functioning of D-glyceraldehyde-3-phosphate dehydrogenase, *Biochim. Biophys. Acta,* 997, 159, 1989.

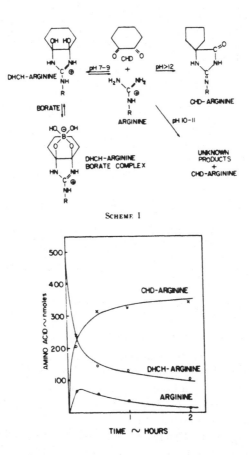

FIGURE 20. The reaction of arginine with 1,2-cyclohexanedione. Scheme I shows a representation of the reaction of 1,2-cyclohexanedione with arginine. The figure shows the conversion of DHCH-arginine to CHD-arginine in 0.5 *M* NaOH. Amino acids were determined on the amino acid analyzer. (From Patthy, L. and Smith, E. L., *J. Biol. Chem.,* 250, 557, 1975. With permission.)

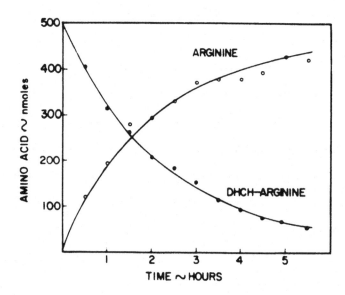

FIGURE 21.   Disappearance of DHCH-arginine and formation of arginine on treatment with neutral hydroxylamine. DHCH-arginine (0.1 *M*) was incubated in 0.5 *M* hydroxylamine, pH 7.0, at 37°C. The amino acids were determined on the amino acid analyzer. Both sets of data are first order with a half time of 100 min. (From Patthy, L. and Smith, E. L., *J. Biol. Chem.*, 250, 557, 1975. With permission.)

residues in protein by 1,2-cyclohexanedione is generally assessed by amino acid analysis after acid hydrolysis. Under the conditions normally used for acid hydrolysis (6 *N* HCl, 110°C, 24 h), the borate-stabilized reaction product between arginine and 1,2-cyclohexanedione is unstable and there is partial regeneration of arginine and the formation of unknown degradation products.[8] Acid hydrolysis in the presence of an excess of mercaptoacetic acid (20 μl/ml of hydrolysate) prevents the destruction of DHCD-arginine.[8] Table 3 lists some of the enzymes in which structure-function relationships have been studied by reaction with 1,2-cyclohexanedione and others are discussed below in comparison with phenylglyoxal and/or 2,3-butanedione. It is the purpose of the following section to discuss some selected studies on the use of the reagents discussed above for the modification of arginyl residues in proteins. We have chosen these particular studies *strictly on the basis* of the illustration of a *specific aspect* of the *chemistry* of a *given reagent(s)*. As will be apparent, a number of investigators use several reagents (e.g., phenylglyoxal and/or 2,3-butanedione) with a given protein.

Vallejos and co-workers[39] have examined the modification of a photophosphorylation factor in *Rhodospirillum rubrum* chromatophore with either 2,3-butanedione or phenylglyoxal as shown in Figure 22. The reactions were performed in 0.050 *M* borate, pH 7.8 (25°C). Stoichiometry is not reported but it is not unreasonable to suggest that the two reagents react at the same site, in which case phenylglyoxal is more effective. These reactions were performed in the dark. When the reaction with 2,3-butanedione is performed in the light there is an approximately 25-fold increase in the rate of inactivation. These investigators discuss this in terms of a conformational change in the chromatophore but do not consider possible photosensitization as described above. Homyk and Bragg[40] compared the effect of 2,3-butanedione and phenylglyoxal on the energy-independent transhydrogenase of *Escherichia coli*. The results of these experiments are shown in Figure 23. The reactions were performed in 0.050 *M* sodium borate, pH 7.8 at 22°C. Phenylglyoxal and 2,3-butanedione were of approximately equal effectiveness in reducing enzymatic activity. The insets show plots of the logarithm of the observed pseudo-first-order rate constants vs. the logarithm of

Table 3
REACTION OF ARGINYL RESIDUES IN PROTEINS WITH 1,2-CYCLOHEXANEDIONE

Protein	Solvent	Reagent excess	Extent of modification	Ref.
Ribonuclease A	0.2 M sodium borate, pH 9.0	50,000	3/4	1
Lysozyme	0.2 M sodium borate, pH 9.0	50,000	11/11	1
Kunitz bovine trypsin inhibitor	0.2 M sodium borate, pH 9.0	—	5.5/6	2
Threonine dehydrogenase	25 μM Triethanolamine-25 μM sodium borate with 2.5 μM 2-mercaptoethanol, pH 7.4	—	—[a]	3
Phosphoenolpyruvate carboxykinase	65 mM Tris-Cl, pH 7.4	—	—[b]	4

[a] Rate of inactivation with 1,2-cyclohexanedione less than that observed with corresponding molar excesses of either phenylglyoxal or 2,3-butanedione.
[b] Rate constant for inactivation of 0.313 M^{-1} min^{-1} at pH 7.4/22°C.

References for Table 3

1. **Patthy, L. and Smith, E. L.**, Identification of functional arginine residues in ribonuclease A and lysozyme, *J. Biol. Chem.*, 250, 565, 1975.
2. **Menegatti, E., Ferroni, R., Benassi, C. A., and Rocchi, R.**, Arginine modification in Kunitz bovine trypsin inhibitor through 1,2-cyclohexanedione, *Int. J. Pept. Protein Res.*, 10, 146, 1977.
3. **Epperly, B. R. and Dekker, E. E.**, Inactivation of *Escherichia coli* L-threonine dehydrogenase by 2,3-butanedione. Evidence for a catalytically essential arginine residue, *J. Biol. Chem.*, 264, 18296, 1989.
4. **Cheng, K.-C. and Nowak, T.**, Arginine residues at the active site of avian liver phosphoenolpyruvate carboxykinase, *J. Biol. Chem.*, 264, 3317, 1989.

the inhibitor concentration. In this type of analysis a straight line should be obtained with a slope equal to the number of inhibitor molecules reacting with each active site to yield an inactive enzyme.[41,42] The analysis for phenylglyoxal yielded a slope of 1.1 while that for 2,3-butanedione gave a slope of 0.8. Therefore these experiments are consistent with the loss in catalytic activity resulting from the modification of one arginyl residue per active site of the enzyme. Also shown in Figure 23 is the protection by substrates and substrate analogs on the rate of inactivation by 2,3-butanedione.

The modification of hexokinase[43] by phenylglyoxal (Figure 24) is of interest since analysis of the dependence of reaction rate on reagent concentration suggests the formation of a protein-phenylglyoxal complex prior to the modification of arginine. Note also that a stoichiometry of 1:1 is suggested based on [14C] phenylglyoxal incorporation while the original studies with free arginine[2] suggested 2:1 stoichiometry. The reaction of phenylglyoxal with arginyl residues in a myosin fragment[44] (Figures 25 and 26) also suggests "saturation kinetics" with the formation of a reagent-protein complex prior to modification of an arginine residue. The effect of bicarbonate on the reaction of phenylglyoxal with arginine has been discussed above. Fonda and co-workers[45] have extended these observations to a consideration of the modification of arginyl residues in glutamate decarboxylase. The holoenzyme is resistant to inactivation by a variety of reagents specific for arginine while the apoenzyme is susceptible. Phenylglyoxal was the most effective (k_2 = 107.68 M^{-1} min^{-1} in 0.125 M bicarbonate, pH 7.5) of the reagents tested. Figure 27 shows the time course of inactivation as a function of pH. The comparison of different buffers for this reaction is shown in Figure 28 while the effect of bicarbonate concentration is shown in Figure 29. As discussed by

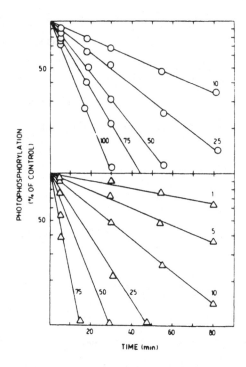

FIGURE 22.   Effect of 2,3-butanedione and phenylglyoxal on photophosphorylation in *Rhodospirillum rubrum* chromatophores. The experiments were performed in 50 mM borate buffer (pH 7.8) at 25°C with either 2,3-butanedione (o———o) or phenylglyoxal (△———△) at the concentrations indicated in the figure. The reactions were performed in the dark. (From Vallejos, R. H., Lescano, W. I. M., and Lucero, H. A., *Arch. Biochem. Biophys., 190,* 578, 1978. With permission.)

these investigators, the bicarbonate effect may be a *general* effect but it is our experience that the modification of arginyl residues in proteins proceeds more rapidly in this buffer system.

The studies of Davidson and Flynn[46] on the modification of an arginyl residue in an aldehyde reductase provided another evaluation of several different reagents. Figure 30 shows the results of an experiment performed in 0.050 M sodium borate, pH 7.0, at 25°C in which 1,2-cyclohexanedione, methylglyoxal, phenylglyoxal, and 2,3-butanedione are compared. 2,3-Butanedione is the most potent inactivator with phenylglyoxal being somewhat less effective while 1,2-cyclohexanedione is least effective. Another comparison of phenylglyoxal and 2,3-butanedione is provided from the studies of Poulose and Kolattukudy[47] on the participation of arginyl residues in fatty acid synthetase. Figure 31 contains a comparison of the effect of these two reagents on the various catalytic activities of this multifunctional enzyme. These experiments with phenylglyoxal were performed in 0.1 M sodium phosphate, pH 7.6, containing 1.0 M EDTA and 0.5 mM dithioerythritol, while those with 2,3-butane-dione were performed in 0.020 M borate, 0.200 M KCl, pH 7.6, containing 1.0 mM EDTA and 1.0 mM dithioerythritol. Phenylglyoxal was more potent than 2,3-butanedione in the inactivation of the three catalytic activities. Figure 32 provides a further analysis of the reaction of fatty acid synthetase with phenylglyoxal. It is noted that only four arginyl residues out of a total of 106 arginyl residues per subunit are modified under these reaction conditions.

The investigation of the reaction of *Lactobacillus casei* thymidylate synthetase with phen-ylglyoxal is an interesting example of the use of this reagent.[58] Figure 33 describes the pH dependence (*N*-ethylmorpholine buffers) for the inactivation. A time-course study for the modification of arginyl residues by phenylglyoxal (350–fold molar excess, 0.200 M

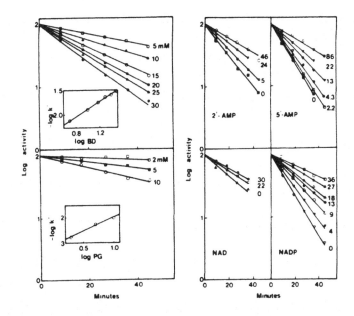

FIGURE 23. Comparison of the modification of an energy-dependent transhydrogenase from *Escherichia coli* cell membranes with 2,3-butanedione and phenylglyoxal. On the left is shown the kinetics of inactivation of the energy-dependent transhydrogenase by 2,3-butanedione (BD) (upper panel) and phenylglyoxal (PG) (lower panel). The membranes were prepared in 50 mM sodium borate, pH 7.8, and incubated at 23°C at a concentration of 1.1 mg and 1.96 mg protein/ml with the indicated concentration of 2,3-butanedione and phenylglyoxal, respectively. Samples were withdrawn and assayed at timed intervals. Activity is expressed as a percentage of the control activity taken at the onset of incubation. The insets show the relationship between the pseudo-first-order rate constant of inactivation (k^1, expressed as min^{-1}) and the inhibitor concentration (expressed as mM). The effect of substrates and substrate analogs on the inactivation of the energy-dependent transhydrogenase by 2,3-butanedione is shown on the right. Membranes at a concentration of 1.0 (top panels) and 1.4 (bottom panels) mg protein/ml in 50 mM sodium borate, pH 7.8, were incubated at 22°C with 53.7 mM 2,3-butanedione, in the absence or presence of the indicated millimolar concentrations of substrates and substrate analogs. Samples were withdrawn at timed intervals for assay. Activity is expressed as a percentage of the control activity taken at the onset of incubation. (From Homyk, M. and Bragg, P. D., *Biochim. Biophys. Acta*, 571, 201, 1979. With permission.)

N-ethylmorpholine, pH 8.2, 25°C) in the presence and absence of a competitive inhibitor (2′-deoxyuridylate) is shown in Figure 34.

Studies from Cooperman's laboratory[48] on the modification of yeast inorganic pyrophosphatase presented some interesting data on the stability of the reaction product between arginine and phenylglyoxal. Figure 35 shows the change in the UV spectrum of the adduct between 2 molecules of phenylglyoxal and 1 molecule of arginine on incubation in 0.1 M sodium phosphate, pH 8.0. These data are consistent with a model for reaction where there is a rapid dissociation to form free arginine and reagent followed by the formation of a new reaction product with undefined stoichiometry.

Studies[49] on the modification of arginyl residues in choline acetyltransferase provide a further comparison of 2,3-butanedione and phenylglyoxal as well as a study of camphorquinone-10-sulfonic acid. Figure 36 compares the rate of inactivation of choline acetyltransferase by the three reagents. Phenylglyoxal is the most effective inactivator but it must be noted that the studies were performed in 0.040 M HEPES, pH 7.8 (25°C) in the *absence* of borate which is critical[36] for reaction of arginyl residues with 2,3-butanedione.

Hayman and Colman[50] have studied the modification of arginyl residues in isocitrate dehydrogenase. Figure 37 shows the dependence of first-order rate constant for inactivation of catalytic activity as a function of 2,3-butanedione concentration (0.050 M MES, pH 6.2 containing 20% glycerol and 2.1 mM MnSO$_4$, 30°C). A second-order rate constant of

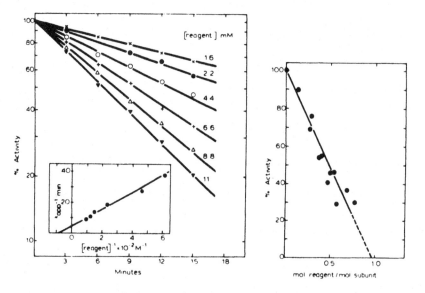

FIGURE 24.   The inactivation of yeast hexokinase by phenylglyoxal. On the left is shown a semilogarithmic plot of the time course of hexokinase inactivation by different concentrations of phenylglyoxal. Hexokinase (20 μM) was incubated in 35 mM Veronal buffer, pH 7.5, at 25°C at the concentration of phenylglyoxal indicated in the figure. The inset shows a double reciprocal plot of k_{app} vs. reagent concentration showing saturation kinetics. On the right is shown the stoichiometry of the inactivation of hexokinase by phenylglyoxal as determined by the incorporation of [^{14}C]phenylglyoxal into the protein. Hexokinase (20 μM) was incubated with 2 mM phenylglyoxal in 35 mM Veronal buffer, pH 7.5 at 30°C. (From Philips, M., Pho, D. B., and Pradel, L.-A., *Biochim. Biophys. Acta*, 566, 296, 1979. With permission.)

0.21 min^{-1} M^{-1} was obtained. The stoichiometry of the reaction is shown in Figure 38. The study[19] from Strittmatter's laboratory on the modification of arginine in rat liver microsomal stearylcoenzyme A desaturase provides an excellent example of the effect of borate on the 2,3-butanedione modification. Figure 39 shows the reversibility of enzyme inactivation by 2,3-butanedione on transfer from borate into Tris buffer and Figure 40 describes the correlation between inactivation, reactivation, and the extent of arginine modification. Another example of the effect of borate buffer on the reaction of 2,3-butanedione with protein is provided by the work of Varimo and Londesborough.[51] Figure 41 shows the pH dependence for the inactivation of yeast adenylate cyclase in borate buffer and HEPES buffer. Phenylborate or *m*-aminophenylborate buffers are also effective with 2,3-butanedione as demonstrated by studies on the modification of arginyl residues in bovine erythrocyte superoxide dismutase.[52] In general the modification of arginyl residues by 2,3-butanedione proceeds more effectively at alkaline pH as illustrated by results with an ATPase[53] (Figure 42) and saccharopine dehydrogenase[54] (Figure 43).

Studies by Aurebekk and Little[55] compared the rate of inactivation of phospholipase c (*Bacillus cereus*) by 2,3-butanedione, 1,2-cyclohexanedione, and phenylglyoxal in 0.020 M sodium borate, pH 7.0, as shown in Figure 44. The rate of reaction with 1,2-cyclohexanedione was intermediate between the other two reagents and was examined in further detail. The pseudo-first-order rate constant for the inactivation (in 0.2 M sodium borate, pH 8.0, 37°C) was plotted vs. 1,2-cyclohexanedione concentration; a straight line through the origin was obtained. A second-order rate constant (0.42 M^{-1} min^{-1}) was obtained for these reaction conditions. Although neutral hydroxylamine will reverse the 1,2-cyclohexanedione-arginine adduct,[8] it was not possible to use this observation in these studies on phospholipase c since the activity was lost in the presence of hydroxylamine. Only partial reactivation with neutral hydroxylamine is observed with 1,2-cyclohexanedione-modified prostatic acid phosphatase[56] (Figure 45).

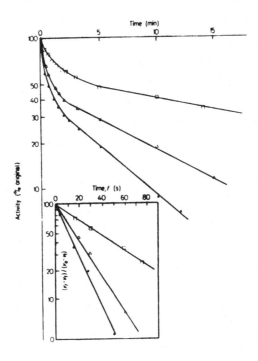

FIGURE 25. Rates of inactivation of K$^+$ EDTA-ATPase of myosin subfragment 1 as a function of phenylglyoxal concentration. Myosin subfragment 1 (obtained by the limited proteolysis of rabbit skeletal muscle myosin filaments by chymotrypsin) (1 mg/ml) was allowed to react with 1 mM (□), 2 mM (△), or 3 mM (●) phenylglyoxal in 0.1 M potassium bicarbonate, pH 8, at 25°C. ATPase tests were performed at pH 7.5 on 50-μl portions at the indicated times. The biphasic reaction is described in terms of K$_1$, the faster rate constant for partial inactivation and K$_2$, the slower rate constant for total inactivation. Inset: determination of the pseudo-first-order rate constants K$_1$ for the rapid phase of inactivation. V$_o$ = original activity, V$_t$ = activity at time t; for each phenylglyoxal concentration, V$_F$ is the velocity at the end of the faster phase of the reaction. (From Mornet, D., Pantel, P., Audemard, E., and Kassab, R., *Eur. J. Biochem.*, 100, 421, 1979. With permission.)

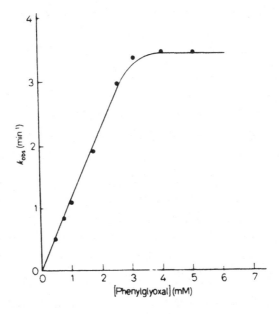

FIGURE 26. Dependence of the pseudo-first-order rate constants for K$^+$ EDTA-ATPase inactivation on the concentration of phenylglyoxal. The rate constants were calculated from the inset in Figure 28. (From Mornet, D., Pantel, P., Audemard, E., and Kassab, R., *Eur. J. Biochem.*, 100, 421, 1979. With permission.)

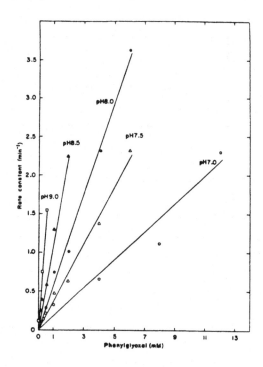

FIGURE 27.   The effect of pH on the apparent first-order rate constants of glutamate apodecarboxylase inactivation by phenylglyoxal. Apoenzyme (33 μM) was incubated with varying concentrations of phenylglyoxal in 83 mM bicarbonate buffer. The pH of each solution was determined after the addition of apoenzyme in 10 mM pyridine-Cl, pH 4.6. (From Cheung, S.-T. and Fonda, M. L., *Arch. Biochem. Biophys.*, 198, 541, 1979. With permission.)

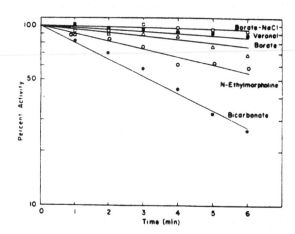

FIGURE 28.   The effect of buffer on the inactivation of glutamate apodecarboxylase by phenylglyoxal at pH 7.5. The apoenzyme was incubated with 2 mM phenylglyoxal in 35 mM borate buffer (with or without 1 M NaCl), 50 mM Veronal buffer, 140 mM N-ethylmorpholine-Cl buffer, or 83 mM sodium bicarbonate buffer. (From Cheung, S.-T. and Fonda, M. L., *Arch. Biochem. Biophys.*, 199, 457, 1980. With permission.)

Lanzillo et al.[57] have described the reaction of arginine residues in bacterial dipeptidase-4 with either *p*-hydroxyphenylglyoxal or 2,3-butanedione. The inactivation with *p*-hydroxyphenylglyoxal followed pseudo-first-order kinetics (0.2 M N-ethylmorpholine, pH 8.0). The reaction with 2,3-butanedione was biphasic in nature either in the presence or absence of 50 mM sodium borate. It was suggested that the two reagents were reacting with different populations of arginine residues.

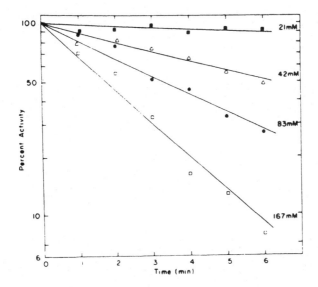

FIGURE 29. The effect of bicarbonate concentration on the inactivation of glutamate apodecarboxylase by 2 mM phenylglyoxal at pH 7.5. The final concentrations of bicarbonate are indicated. (From Cheung, S.-T. and Fonda, M. L., *Arch. Biochem. Biophys.*, 198, 541, 1979. With permission.)

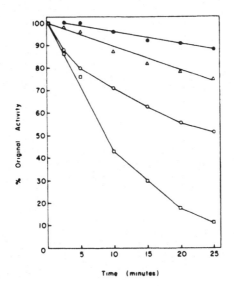

FIGURE 30. Modification of an aldehyde reductase by several reagents specific for reaction with arginine. Shown is the inactivation of pig kidney aldehyde reductase by 10 mM 1,2-cyclohexanedione (●), 10 mM methylglyoxal (△), 10 mM phenylglyoxal (○), and 10 mM 2,3-butanedione (□). The enzyme (0.1 mg/ml) was incubated with the various reagents in 50 mM borate buffer, pH 7.0, at 25°C. Portions were removed at the indicated times, diluted into ice cold 0.1 M sodium phosphate, pH 7.0, and assayed for catalytic activity. (From Davidson, W. S. and Flynn, T. G., *J. Biol. Chem.*, 254, 3724, 1979. With permission.)

Several additional studies have appeared which compared the relative effectiveness of phenylglyoxal, 1,2-cyclohexanedione, and 2,3-butanedione. Cheng and Nowak[58] examined the rate of irreversible inactivation of chicken liver phosphoenol carboxykinase by these three reagents. The reactions were performed in 65 mM Tris-Cl, pH 7.5 at 22°C. Phenylglyoxal was the most effective reagent (3.42 M^{-1} min^{-1}) with 2,3-butanedione somewhat

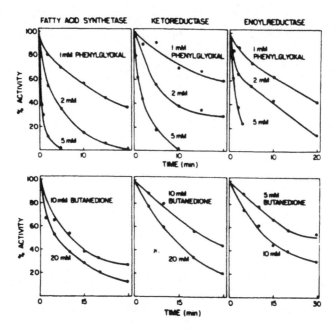

FIGURE 31.   Time course of inactivation of ketoacyl reductase, enoyl reductase, and the overall activity of fatty acid synthetase by phenylglyoxal and 2,3-butanedione. Incubation with phenylglyoxal was carried out at a protein concentration of 4.1, 4.3, and 3.3 mg/ml for fatty acid synthetase, ketoacyl reductase, and enoyl reductase, respectively; incubations with 2,3-butanedione were done at 0.33, 0.165, and 1.63 mg/ml, respectively. The modification with phenylglyoxal was performed in 100 m*M* sodium phosphate, pH 7.6, containing 0.5 m*M* dithiothreitol and 1.0 m*M* EDTA at 30°C. The modification with 2,3-butanedione was performed in 20 m*M* borate containing 200 m*M* KCl, 1.0 m*M* dithiothreitol, and 1.0 m*M* EDTA at pH 7.6 at 30. (From Poulose, A. J. and Kolattukudy, P. E., *Arch. Biochem. Biophys.*, 199, 457, 1980. With permission.)

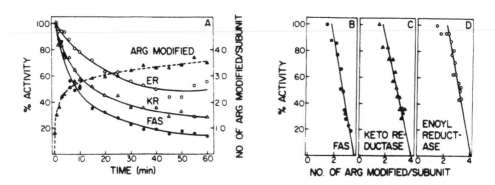

FIGURE 32.   Analysis of the modification of arginine residues in fatty acid synthetase by phenylglyoxal. Shown in panel A is the time course of inactivation of the three enzymatic activities and the number of arginine residues modified with 1 m*M* [2-^{14}C]phenylglyoxal in 100 m*M* sodium phosphate buffer (pH 7.0) containing 0.5 m*M* dithiothreitol and 1.0 m*M* EDTA. The reactions were performed at a protein concentration of 8.8 mg/ml at 30°C. Panels B to D show the stoichiometry of modification for overall fatty acid synthetase (FAS), keto reductase, and enoyl reductase. (From Poulose, A. J. and Kolattukudy, P. E., *Arch. Biochem. Biophys.*, 199, 457, 1980. With permission.)

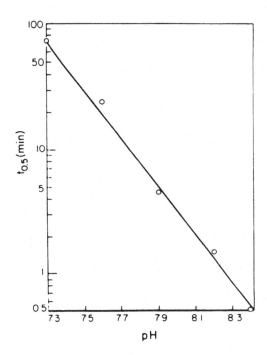

FIGURE 33.   pH Dependence of inactivation of thymidylate synthetase by phenylglyoxal. Enzyme (7.1 μ*M*) was incubated under argon at 25°C in 200 m*M* *N*-ethylmorpholine at the pH indicated in the presence of 5 m*M* phenylglyoxal. The $t_{0.5}$ at each of the indicated pH values was determined from a series of semilog plots of inactivation vs. time. (From Belfort, M., Maley, G. F., and Maley, F., *Arch. Biochem. Biophys.*, 204, 340, 1980. With permission.)

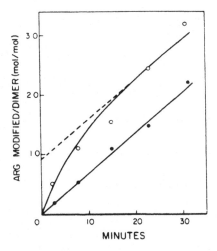

FIGURE 34.   The rate of modification of arginine in thymidylate synthetase by phenylglyoxal. Enzyme (14.3 μ*M*) in 200 m*M* *N*-ethylmaleimide (pH 8.2) was preincubated for 30 min at 25°C in the absence (○) and presence (●) of a 200-fold molar excess of deoxyuridylate (2.86 m*M*). At 0 min, phenylglyoxal was added to a concentration of 5 m*M* (350-fold molar excess over enzyme). At the times indicated, 100-μl portions were added to 1 ml of cold 0.1 *N* HCl in acetone to halt arginine modification and to precipitate the enzyme. The number of arginine residues modified was calculated by comparison with an unmodified control. (From Belfort, M., Maley, G. F., and Maley, F., *Arch. Biochem. Biophys.*, 204, 340, 1980. With permission.)

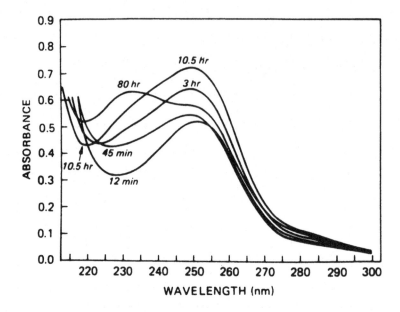

FIGURE 35.   Ultraviolet absorption spectral changes on hydrolysis of the reaction product of phenylglyoxal and arginine. Shown are the ultraviolet spectral changes on hydrolysis of Nα–acetyl-L-(diphenylglyoxal)arginine (NAcArg(PhGx)₂) in 0.1 *M* sodium phosphate buffer, pH 8.0, at 25°C. Spectra were obtained at the times indicated in the figure. (From Bond, M. W., Chiu, N. Y., and Cooperman, B. S., *Biochemistry*, 19, 94, 1980. With permission.)

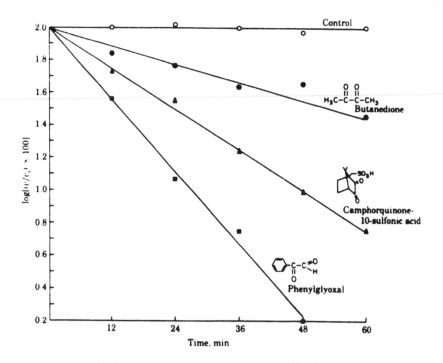

FIGURE 36.   The inactivation of choline acetyltransferase (ChoAcTase) by several reagents specific for the modification of arginine. The reagents indicated in the figure were present at a concentration of 10 m*M* in 50 m*M* HEPES, pH 7.8, at 25°C; v_i and v, initial enzyme activity and enzyme activity at any time point. (From Mautner, H. G., Pakula, A. A., and Merrill, R. E., *Proc. Natl. Acad. Sci. U.S.A.*, 78, 7449, 1981. With permission.)

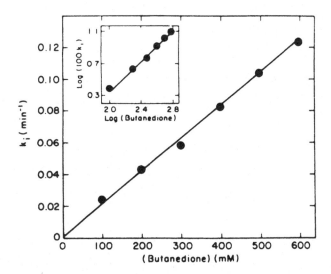

FIGURE 37. The loss of catalytic activity in porcine diphosphopyridine nucleotide-specific isocitrate dehydrogenase on modification with 2,3-butanedione. Shown is the dependence of k_i (pseudo-first-order rate constant) on reagent concentration. The reactions were 50 mM in MES (pH 6.2), 20% in glycerol, and contained 2.1 mM MnSO$_4$ at 30°C. The 2,3-butanedione concentration is indicated in the figure. The rate constant for each reagent concentration was determined from a semilogarithmic plot of the loss of catalytic activity as a function of time. The second-order rate constant is 0.21 M^{-1} min^{-1}. The inset shows a plot of log k_i vs. log [2,3-butanedione], with a slope of 0.95. (From Hayman, S. and Colman, R. F., *Biochemistry*, 17, 4161, 1978. With permission.)

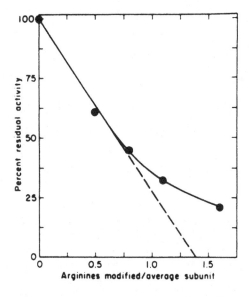

FIGURE 38. Stoichiometry for the modification of DPN-dependent isocitrate dehydrogenase with 2,3-butanedione. The enzyme was incubated for various times up to 73 min at 30°C in 50 mM MES (pH 6.2) containing 2.1 mM MnSO$_4$ and 0.1 M 2,3-butanedione. Portions of the reacted enzyme containing 0.2 mg protein were diluted with an equal volume of 2 N HCl at 0°C to both stop the reaction and prevent the regeneration of free arginine. The modified enzyme was then dialyzed overnight at 4°C against 1 N HCl. The samples were dried *in vacuo* over solid NaOH and subjected to acid hydrolysis. Unmodified enzyme had an arginine content of 13.4 residues per average subunit of 40,000 molecular weight. (From Hayman, S. and Colman, R. F., *Biochemistry*, 17, 4161, 1978. With permission.)

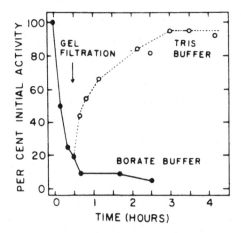

FIGURE 39.   The reversal of 2,3-butanedione inactivation of stearylcoenzyme A desaturase. Shown is the reversibility of desaturase inactivation by removal of borate. Desaturase (16 μ*M*, specific activity = 190 units/mg) was treated with 2,3-butanedione (40 m*M* in 50 m*M* sodium borate (pH 8.1); after 30 min at 25°C, 1 ml of this mixture was filtered through Sephadex G-25 (20 × 1 cm) equilibrated either with the same borate buffer or 20 m*M* Tris-acetate/100 m*M* NaCl (pH 8.1). The enzyme, which eluted in the void volume within 3 to 4 min, was incubated at 25°C, and portions were withdrawn at the times indicated for measurement of desaturase activity: (●) borate buffer; (○) Tris buffer. (From Enoch, H. G. and Strittmatter, P., *Biochemistry*, 17, 4927, 1978. With permission.)

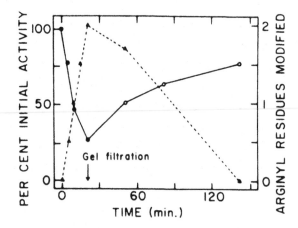

FIGURE 40.   The correlation of the reversible modification of stearylcoenzyme A desaturase activity with the modification of arginyl residues. The treatment of desaturase with 2,3-butanedione and the removal of reagent and borate by gel filtration were carried out as described under Figure 39. At various times, samples of the reaction mixture were chilled rapidly to 0°C and used immediately for the measurement of desaturase activity (●) before and (○) after gel filtration, and arginine, (▲) before and (△) after gel filtration. (From Enoch, H. G. and Strittmatter, P., *Biochemistry*, 17, 4927, 1978. With permission.)

less effective (3.13 M^{-1} min^{-1}) while 1,2-cyclohexanedione was much less effective (0.313 M^{-1} min^{-1}). In studies with *E. coli* threonine dehydrogenase[59] (25 μ*M* triethanolamine-25 μ*M* sodium borate-2.5 μ*M* 2-mercaptoethanol, pH 7.4), 2,3-butanedione and 2,3-pentanedione were the most effective reagents with phenylglyoxal considerably less effective but still markedly better than 1,2-cyclohexanedione.

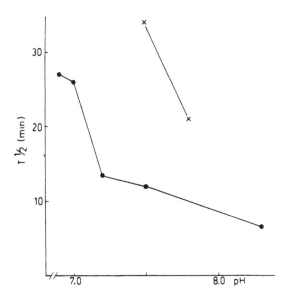

FIGURE 41.   pH Dependence for the inactivation of adenyl cyclase by 2,3-butanedione in two different buffers. Shown are the half-inactivation times for adenylate cyclase at 30°C with 20 mM 2,3-butanedione in 25 mM borate (●) and 25 mM HEPES (x) as a function of pH. Protein concentration during the incubation was 30 mg/ml. (From Varimo, K. and Londesborough, S., *FEBS Lett.*, 106, 153, 1979. With permission.)

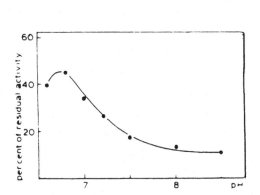

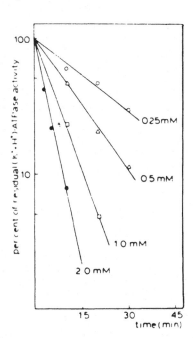

FIGURE 42.   The inactivation of (K$^+$ + H$^+$)-ATPase by 2,3-butanedione. On the left is shown the inactivation by 2,3-butanedione as a function of pH. (K$^+$ + H$^+$)-ATPase preparation (0.5 mg/ml) was incubated for 20 min at 37°C with 0.5 mM 2,3-butanedione in 125 mM borate buffer containing 5 mM MgCl$_2$, previously brought to the indicated pH values with 5 M NaOH. (K$^+$ + H$^+$)-ATPase activity is expressed as percent of a control preparation without 2,3-butanedione. On the right is shown the inactivation by 2,3-butanedione as a function of time. (K$^+$ + H$^+$)-ATPase preparation (0.5 mg protein/ml) was incubated at 37°C with the indicated concentrations of 2,3-butanedione in 125 mM sodium borate (pH 7.0), 5 mM MgCl$_2$. Enzyme activity is expressed as percent of control activity without butanedione. (From Schrijen, J. J., Luyben, W. A. H. M., DePont, J. J. H. M., and Bonting, S. L., *Biochim. Biophys. Acta*, 597, 331, 1980. With permission.)

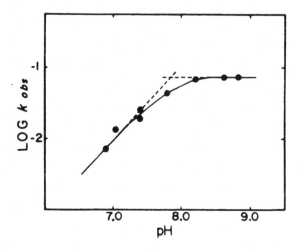

FIGURE 43. The effect of pH on the apparent first-order rate constant for the inactivation of saccharopine dehydrogenase by 2,3-butanedione. The enzyme (0.7 nmol) was incubated with 11.4 mM 2,3-butanedione in 0.1 ml of 0.08 M HEPES buffer at the pH values indicated. The buffers contained 0.2 M KCl and 10 mM borate in addition. Values of the apparent first-order rate constants (k_{obsd}) were obtained from the pseudo-first-order kinetic plots. (From Fujioka, M. and Takata, Y., *Biochemistry*, 20, 468, 1981. With permission.)

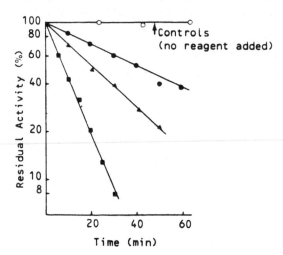

FIGURE 44. The inactivation of phospholipase C by arginine reagents. Enzyme (0.25 mg/ml) incubated with phenylglyoxal (32 mM) in 0.02 M sodium borate buffer (pH 7.0) at 22°C (●). Enzyme (0.22 mg/ml) incubated with 2,3-butanedione (50 mM) in 0.06 M sodium borate buffer (pH 7.5) at 22°C (■). Enzyme incubated with 1,2-cyclohexanedione (85 mM) in 0.2 M sodium borate buffer (pH 8.0) at 37°C (▲). (From Aurebekk, B. and Little, C., *Int. J. Biochem.*, 8, 757, 1977. With permission.)

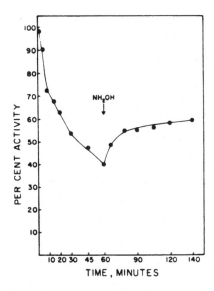

FIGURE 45. Reversibility of the inactivation of an acid phosphatase by 1,2-cyclohexane-dione. Acid phosphatase in 50 mM borate buffer (pH 8.1) was modified at 30°C by 50 mM 1,2-cyclohexanedione. At the time indicated by the arrow, neutral hydroxylamine solution was added to a final concentration of 0.2 M. (From McTigue, J. J. and Van Etten, R. L., *Biochim. Biophys. Acta*, 523, 422, 1978. With permission.)

REFERENCES

1. **Yankeelov, J. A., Jr.,** Modification of arginine by diketones, *Meth. Enzymol.*, 25, 566, 1972.
2. **Takahashi, K.,** The reaction of phenylglyoxal with arginine residues in proteins, *J. Biol. Chem.*, 243, 6171, 1968.
3. **Yankeelov, J. A., Jr., Mitchell, C. D., and Crawford, T. H.,** A simple trimerization of 2,3-butanedione yielding a selective reagent for the modification of arginine in proteins, *J. Am. Chem. Soc.*, 90, 1664, 1968.
4. **Nakaya, K., Horinishi, H., and Shibata, K.,** States of amino acid residues in proteins. XIV. Glyoxal as a reagent for discrimination of arginine residues, *J. Biochem.*, 61, 345, 1967.
5. **Riordan, J. F., McElvany, K. D., and Borders, C. L., Jr.,** Arginyl residues: anion recognition sites in enzymes, *Science*, 195, 884, 1977.
6. **Patthy, L. and Thész, J.,** Origin of the selectivity of α-dicarbonyl reagents for arginyl residues of anion-binding sites, *Eur. J. Biochem.*, 105, 387, 1980.
7. **Takahashi, K.,** Specific modification of arginine residues in proteins with ninhydrin, *J. Biochem.*, 80, 1173, 1976.
8. **Patthy, L. and Smith, E. L.,** Reversible modification of arginine residues. Application to sequence studies by restriction of tryptic hydrolysis to lysine residues, *J. Biol. Chem.*, 250, 557, 1975.
9. **Chaplin, M. F.,** The use of ninhydrin as a reagent for the reversible modification of arginine residues in proteins, *Biochem. J.*, 155, 457, 1976.
10. **Hiraga, Y. and Kinoshita, T.,** Post-column derivatization of guanidino compounds in high-performance liquid chromatography using ninhydrin, *J. Chromatogr.*, 226, 43, 1981.
11. **Jonas, A. and Weber, G.,** Presence of arginine residues at the strong, hydrophobic anion binding sites of bovine serum albumin, *Biochemistry*, 10, 1335, 1971.
12. **Glass, J. D. and Pelzig, M.,** Reversible modification of arginine residues with glyoxal, *Biochem. Biophys. Res. Commun.*, 81, 527, 1978.
13. **Pande, C. S., Pelzig, M., and Glass, J. D.,** Camphorquinone-10-sulfonic acid and derivatives: convenient reagents for reversible modification of arginine residues, *Proc. Natl. Acad. Sci. U.S.A.*, 77, 895, 1980.
14. **Rajagopalan, T. G., Stein, W. H., and Moore, S.,** The inactivation of pepsin by diazoacetylnorleucine methyl ester, *J. Biol. Chem.*, 241, 4295, 1966.
15. **Honegger, A., Hughes, G. J., and Wilson, K. J.,** Chemical modification of peptides by hydrazine, *Biochem. J.*, 199, 53, 1981.

16. **Sakaguchi, S.,** A new color reaction of protein and arginine, *J. Biochem.,* 5, 25, 1925.

17. **Izumi, Y.,** New Sakaguchi reaction, *Anal. Biochem.,* 10, 218, 1965.

18. **Izumi, Y.,** New Sakaguchi reaction. II, *Anal. Biochem.,* 12, 1, 1965.

19. **Enoch, H. G. and Strittmatter, P.,** Role of tyrosyl and arginyl residues in rat liver microsomal stearyl-coenzyme A desaturase, *Biochemistry,* 17, 4927, 1978.

20. **Smith, R. E. and MacQuarrie, R.,** A sensitive fluorometric method for the determination of arginine using 9,10-phenanthrenequinone, *Anal. Biochem.,* 90, 246, 1978.

21. **Fliss, H. and Viswanatha, T.,** 2,3-Butanedione as a photosensitizing agent: application to α-amino acids and α-chymotrypsin, *Can. J. Biochem.,* 57, 1267, 1979.

22. **Gripon, J.-C. and Hofmann, T.,** Inactivation of aspartyl proteinases by butane-2,3-dione. Modification of tryptophan and tyrosine residues and evidence against reaction of arginine residues, *Biochem. J.,* 193, 55, 1981.

23. **Mäkinen, K. K., Mäkinen, P.-L., Wilkes, S. H., Bayliss, M. E., and Prescott, J. M.,** Photochemical inactivation of *Aeromonas* aminopeptidase by 2,3-butanedione, *J. Biol. Chem.,* 257, 1765, 1982.

24. **Riley, H. A. and Gray, A. R.,** Phenylglyoxal, in *Organic Syntheses,* Collective Vol. 2, Blatt, A. H., Ed., John Wiley & Sons, New York, 1943, 509.

25. **Schloss, J. V., Norton, I. L., Stringer, C. D., and Hartman, F. C.,** Inactivation of ribulosebisphosphate carboxylase by modification of arginyl residues with phenylglyoxal, *Biochemistry,* 17, 5626, 1978.

26. **Augustus, B. W. and Hutchinson, D. W.,** The synthesis of phenyl[2-³H]glyoxal, *Biochem. J.,* 177, 377, 1979.

27. **Borders, C. L., Jr., Pearson, L. J., McLaughlin, A. E., Gustafson, M. E., Vasiloff, J., An, F. Y., and Morgan, D. J.,** 4-Hydroxy-3-nitrophenylglyoxal. A chromophoric reagent for arginyl residues in proteins, *Biochim. Biophys. Acta,* 568, 491, 1979.

28. **Yamasaki, R. B., Vega, A., and Feeney, R. E.,** Modification of available arginine residues in proteins by *p*-hydroxyphenylglyoxal, *Anal. Biochem.,* 109, 32, 1980.

29. **Cheung, S.-T. and Fonda, M. L.,** Reaction of phenylglyoxal with arginine. The effect of buffers and pH, *Biochem. Biophys. Res. Commun.,* 90, 940, 1979.

30. **Yamasaki, R. B., Shimer, D. A., and Feeney, R. E.,** Colorimetric determination of arginine residues in proteins by *p*-nitrophenylglyoxal, *Anal. Biochem.,* 111, 220, 1981.

31. **Steinbach, L. and Becker, E. I.,** A synthesis for β-aroylacrylic acids substituted with electron-withdrawing groups, *J. Am. Chem. Soc.,* 76, 5808, 1954.

32. **Branlant, G., Tritsch, D., and Biellmann, J.-F.,** Evidence for the presence of anion-recognition sites in pig-liver aldehyde reductase. Modification by phenylglyoxal and *p*-carboxyphenyl glyoxal of an arginyl residue located close to the substrate-binding site, *Eur. J. Biochem.,* 116, 505, 1981.

33. **Eun, H.-M.,** Arginine modification by phenyglyoxal and (p-hydroxyphenyl)glyoxal: reaction rates and intermediates, *Biochem. Int.,* 17, 719, 1988.

34. **Meves, H., Rubly, N., and Stämpfli, R.,** The action of arginine-specific reagents on ionic and gating currents in frog myelinated nerve, *Biochim. Biophys. Acta,* 943, 1, 1988.

35. **Yankeelov, J. A., Jr.,** Modification of arginine in proteins by oligomers of 2,3-butanedione, *Biochemistry,* 9, 2433, 1970.

36. **Riordan, J. F.,** Functional arginyl residues in carboxypeptidase A. Modification with butanedione, *Biochemistry,* 12, 3915, 1973.

37. **Toi, K., Bynum, E., Norris, E., and Itano, H. A.,** Studies on the chemical modification of arginine. I. The reaction of 1,2-cyclohexanedione with arginine and arginyl residues of proteins, *J. Biol. Chem.,* 242, 1036, 1967.

38. **Patthy, L. and Smith, E. L.,** Identification of functional arginine residues in ribonuclease A and lysozyme, *J. Biol. Chem.,* 250, 565, 1975.

39. **Vallejos, R. H., Lescano, W. I. M., and Lucero, H. A.,** Involvement of an essential arginyl residue in the coupling activity of *Rhodospirillum rubrum* chromatophores, *Arch. Biochem. Biophys.,* 190, 578, 1978.

40. **Homyk, M. and Bragg, P. D.,** Steady-state kinetics and the inactivation by 2,3-butanedione of the energy-independent transhydrogenase of *Escherichia coli* cell membranes, *Biochim. Biophys. Acta,* 57, 201, 1979.

41. **Levy, H. M., Leber, P. D., and Ryan, E. M.,** Inactivation of myosin by 2,4-dinitrophenol and protection by adenosine triphosphate and other phosphate compounds, *J. Biol. Chem.,* 238, 3654, 1963.

42. **Bhagwat, A. S. and Ramakrishna, J.,** Essential histidine residues of ribulosebisphosphate carboxylase indicated by reaction with diethylpyrocarbonate and rose bengal, *Biochim. Biophys. Acta,* 662, 181, 1981.

43. **Philips, M., Pho, D. B., and Pradel, L.-A.,** An essential arginyl residue in yeast hexokinase, *Biochim. Biophys. Acta,* 566, 296, 1979.

44. **Mornet, D., Pantel, P., Audemard, E., and Kassab, R.,** Involvement of an arginyl residue in the catalytic activity of myosin heads, *Eur. J. Biochem.,* 100, 421, 1979.

45. **Cheung, S.-T. and Fonda, M. L.,** Kinetics of the inactivation of *Escherichia coli* glutamate apodecarboxylase by phenylglyoxal, *Arch. Biochem. Biophys.,* 198, 541, 1979.

46. **Davidson, W. S. and Flynn, T. G.**, A functional arginine residue in NADPH-dependent aldehyde reductase from pig kidney, *J. Biol. Chem.*, 254, 3724, 1979.

47. **Poulose, A. J. and Kolattukudy, P. E.**, Presence of one essential arginine that specifically binds the 2'-phosphate of NADPH on each of the ketoacyl reductase and enoyl reductase active sites of fatty acid synthetase, *Arch. Biochem. Biophys.*, 199, 457, 1980.

48. **Bond, M. W., Chiu, N. Y., and Cooperman, B. S.**, Identification of an arginine important for enzymatic activity within the covalent structure of yeast inorganic pyrophosphatase, *Biochemistry*, 19, 94, 1980.

49. **Mautner, H. G., Pakula, A. A., and Merrill, R. E.**, Evidence for presence of an arginine residue in the coenzyme A binding site of choline acetyltransferase, *Proc. Natl. Acad. Sci. U.S.A.*, 78, 7449, 1981.

50. **Hayman, S. and Colman, R. F.**, Effect of arginine modification on the catalytic activity and allosteric activation by adenosine diphosphate of the diphosphopyridine nucleotide specific isocitrate dehydrogenase of pig heart, *Biochemistry*, 17, 4161, 1978.

51. **Varimo, K. and Londesborough, S.**, Evidence for essential arginine in yeast adenylate cyclase, *FEBS Lett.*, 106, 153, 1979.

52. **Malinowski, D. P. and Fridovich, I.**, Chemical modification of arginine at the active site of the bovine erythrocyte superoxide dismutase, *Biochemistry*, 18, 5909, 1979.

53. **Schrijen, J. J., Luyben, W. A. H. M., DePont, J. J. H. M., and Bonting, S. L.**, Studies on (K$^+$ + H$^+$)-ATPase. I. Essential arginine residue in its substrate binding center, *Biochim. Biophys. Acta*, 597, 331, 1980.

54. **Fujioka, M. and Takata, Y.**, Role of arginine residue in saccharopine dehydrogenase (L-lysine forming) from baker's yeast, *Biochemistry*, 20, 468, 1981.

55. **Aurebekk, B. and Little, C.**, Functional arginine in phospholipase C of *Bacillus cereus*, *Int. J. Biochem.*, 8, 757, 1977.

56. **McTigue, J. J. and Van Etten, R. L.**, An essential arginine residue in human prostatic acid phosphatase, *Biochim. Biophys. Acta*, 523, 422, 1978.

57. **Lanzillo, J. J., Dasarathy, Y., and Fanburg, B. L.**, Detection of essential arginine in bacterial peptidyl dipeptidase-4: arginine is not the anion binding site, *Biochem. Biophys. Res. Commun.*, 160, 243, 1989.

58. **Cheng, K.-C. and Nowak, T.**, Arginine residues at the active site of avian liver phosphoenolpyruvate carboxykinase, *J. Biol. Chem.*, 264, 3317, 1989.

59. **Epperly, B. R. and Dekker, E. E.**, Inactivation of *Escherichia coli* L-threonine dehydrogenase by 2,3-butanedione. Evidence for a catalytically essential arginine residue, *J. Biol. Chem.*, 264, 18296, 1989.

Chapter 12

CHEMICAL MODIFICATION OF TRYPTOPHAN

The specific chemical modification of tryptophan (Figure 1) in protein is one of the more challenging problems in protein chemistry. First, as will be apparent, the solvent conditions for providing specificity of modification are, in general, somewhat harsh. Secondly, there is the considerable possibility of either the concomitant or separate modification of a different amino acid residue. Thirdly, the analysis for the determination of the exact extent of modification requires a rigorous approach combining spectral analysis and amino acid analysis[1,2] after hydrolysis in a solvent which will not destroy tryptophan.

Treatment of tryptophan with hydrogen peroxide results in the oxidation of the indole ring.[3-6] Usually the reaction is performed at alkaline pH (1.0 M sodium bicarbonate, pH 8.4) with the H_2O_2 dioxane mixture prepared as described by Hachimori and co-workers.[3] The loss of tryptophan is monitored by the change in absorbance at 280 nm.[3,5,6] The difference in the molar extinction coefficient between tryptophan and the fully oxidized derivative is 3490 M^{-1} cm^{-1}.

The reaction of N-bromosuccinimide (NBS) with protein has been studied in some detail (Figure 2). This reagent was introduced for use in protein chemistry in 1958.[7] The early work with this reagent was summarized in 1967.[8-10]

The use of oxidation with N-bromosuccinimide to determine the tryptophan content of proteins is of value. One adds small increments of a freshly prepared solution of N-bromosuccinimide until there is no further decrease in absorbance at 280 nm. The change in the molar extinction coefficient of tryptophan on conversion to the oxindole derivative is taken to be 4×10^3 M^{-1} cm^{-1}.[11] It has been our experience that one must either perform the reaction in 8.0 M urea (pH adjusted to 4.0) or with the reduced, carboxymethylated derivative.[12] The spectra must be obtained as soon as possible after the addition of the N-bromosuccinimide since, unless the excess reagent and low molecular weight products of the reaction are rapidly removed, there is a reversal of the decrease in absorbance.[13] This is not a trivial consideration since there is at least one study[14] where there is a real difference in the extent of modification as determined by spectroscopy or amino acid analysis. The rigorous evaluation[13] of the reaction of N-bromosuccinimide with model tryptophanyl and tyrosyl compounds reported from Keitaro Hiromi's laboratory provides considerable insight into the problems to be encountered with the study of intact proteins. Figure 3 shows the changes in the UV spectrum of N-acetyltryptophan ethyl ester (ATEE) upon reaction with N-bromosuccinimide. These spectra were obtained within 5 min after the initiation of the reaction. At ratios of N-bromosuccinimide to N-acetyltryptophan ethyl ester of greater than 2 there is an apparent reversal of the decrease in absorbance at 280 nm as shown in Figure 4. Figure 5 shows the spectral changes occurring upon the reaction of N-bromosuccinimide with N-acetyltryptophan ethyl ester as a function of time and molar excess of N-bromosuccinimide. The maximal decrease in absorbance occurs at a ratio of N-bromosuccinimide to tryptophan of 2. If the data are obtained by stopped-flow spectroscopy, the molar excess of N-bromosuccinimide does not have an effect on the maximum decrease observed, but when the spectrum is obtained 5 min after the initiation of the reaction, there is a decrease in the observed magnitude of change in absorbance at 280 nm. The evaluation of spectral changes in a protein is further complicated by the reaction of N-bromosuccinimide with tyrosine. This is demonstrated in Figure 6 which shows the spectral changes occurring as a result of reaction of N-bromosuccinimide with N-acetyltyrosine ethyl ester. Here an increase in absorbance at 280 nm can be observed. Figure 7 shows that the increase in absorbance of N-acetyltyrosine ethyl ester on reaction with N-bromosuccinimide is dependent on the molar excess of N-bromosuccinimide. The use of this procedure for the analysis of tryptophan

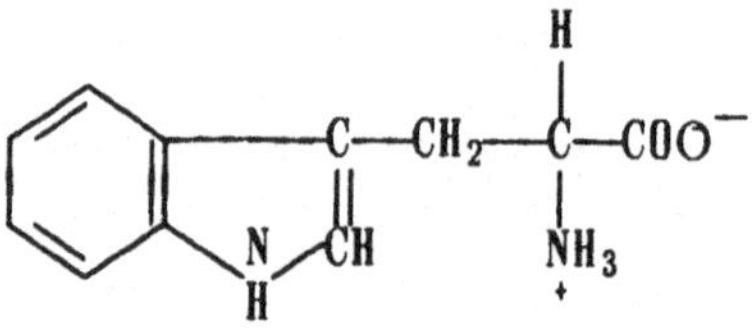

FIGURE 1.   The structure of tryptophan.

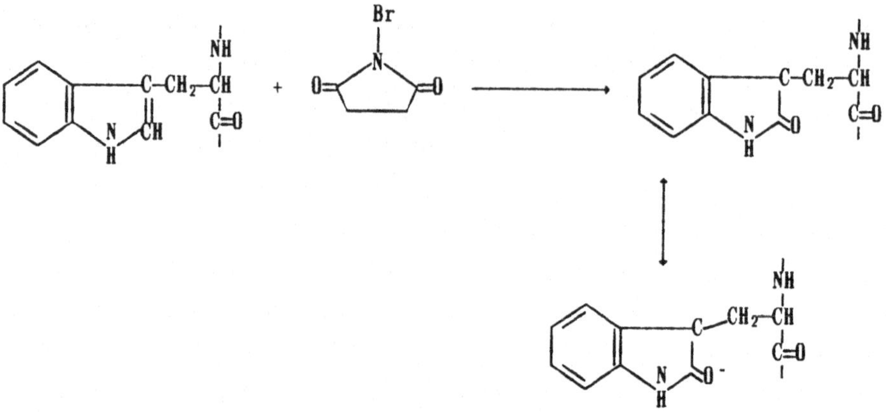

FIGURE 2.   The reaction of tryptophan with *N*-bromosuccinimide.

content in proteins has been largely supplanted by ion-exchange analysis following modified hydrolytic procedures.[1,2,14]

The primary use of the *N*-bromosuccinimide modification of proteins during the past decade has been in studies on the effect of such modification on biological (catalytic) activity. In general, the modification reaction is performed in 0.1 *M* sodium acetate, pH 4 to 5. The *N*-bromosuccinimide should be recrystallized from water before use. The presence of halides such as chloride or bromide in the solvent must be avoided since the addition of *N*-bromosuccinimide will oxidize these ions to the elemental form with disastrous and irreproducible effects on the proteins under study. In general, a twofold molar excess of *N*-bromosuccinimide per mole of tryptophan is necessary to achieve modification. Daniel and Trowbridge[15] found that (at pH 4.0) the reaction of *N*-bromosuccinimide with acetyl-L-tryptophan ethyl ester required 1.5 mol of *N*-bromosuccinimide per mole of the acetyl-L-tryptophan ethyl ester, while trypsinogen required 2.0 to 2.3 mol *N*-bromosuccinimide per mole of tryptophan oxidized, and trypsin required 1.5 to 2.0 mol *N*-bromosuccinimide per mole tryptophan oxidized. An interesting phenomenon was reported by Freisheim and Huennekens.[16] At pH 4.0, only tryptophan in dihydrofolate reductase reacts with NBS while at pH 6.0, a sulfhydryl group apparently is preferentially oxidized by the reagent prior to the reaction of tryptophan. This observation was pursued in greater detail by Freisheim et al.[17] Figure 8 shows the relationship between the decrease in absorbance at 280 nm and the catalytic activity of dihydrofolate reductase as a function of the molar excess of *N*-bromosuccinimide at pH 6.5 (0.1 *M* phosphate). The initial increase in activity reflects oxidation of a cysteinyl residue while the decrease in activity seen at a higher molar excess of reagent appears to be related to the oxidation of tryptophanyl residues in the protein (Figure 9). Poulos and Price have reported on the reaction of a tryptophanyl residue in bovine pancreatic DNase with *N*-bromosuccinimide.[18] Prior reaction of the DNase with another "tryptophan" reagent, 2-hydroxy-5-nitrobenzyl bromide, modified a different residue from the one modified by *N*-bromosuccinimide. These investigators used spectral analysis to determine the

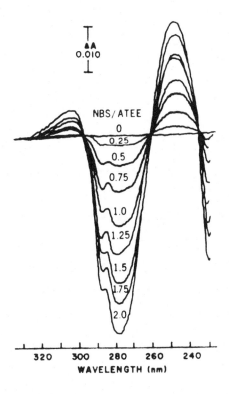

FIGURE 3. Difference UV absorption spectra of *N*-acetyltryptophan ethyl ester caused by reaction with *N*-bromosuccinimide. *N*-acetyltryptophan ethyl ester 19 μ*M*, numbers indicate the molar ratios of *N*-bromosuccinimide to *N*-acetyltryptophan ethyl ester. The reactions were performed in 0.1 *M* acetate buffer, pH 4.5 at 25°C. The difference spectra were obtained within 5 min of the start of the reaction. (From Ohnishi, M., Kawagishi, T., Abe, T., and Hiromi, K., *J. Biochem.*, 87, 273, 1980. With permission.)

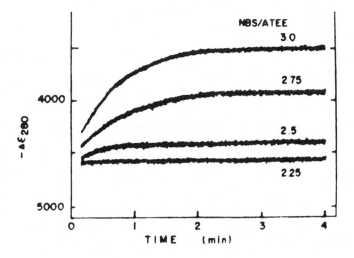

FIGURE 4. Time course of the difference absorbance change of *N*-acetyltryptophan ethyl ester at 280 nm caused by *N*-bromosuccinimide. *N*-acetyltryptophan ethyl ester, 49 μ*M;* 0.1 *M* acetate buffer, pH 4.5; 25°C. The numbers in the figure indicate the molar ratios of *N*-bromosuccinimide to *N*-acetyltryptophan ethyl ester. (From Ohnishi, M., Kawagishi, T., Abe, T., and Hiromi, K., *J. Biochem.*, 87, 273, 1980. With permission.)

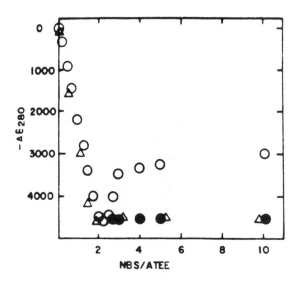

FIGURE 5. Dependence of the difference UV absorption change (decrease) at 280 nm of *N*-acetyltryptophan ethyl ester (ATEE) on time and molar excess of *N*-bromosuccinimide (NBS). The open circles show the difference at 5 min after the addition of *N*-bromosuccinimide and the closed circles the change at 0 min (obtained by extrapolation of the time curves). The triangles represent data obtained by the stopped-flow method. The concentration of *N*-acetyltryptophan ethyl ester was 49 μ*M* in 0.1 *M* acetate buffer, pH 4.5, at 25°C. (From Ohnishi, M., Kawagishi, T., Abe, T., and Hiromi, K., *J. Biochem.*, 87, 273, 1980. With permission.)

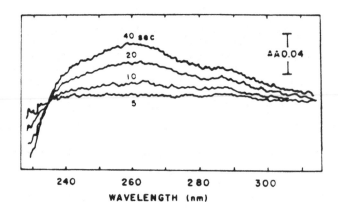

FIGURE 6. The difference UV absorption spectra of *N*-acetyltyrosine ethyl ester on reaction with *N*-bromosuccinimide. *N*-acetyltyrosine ethyl ester, 25 μ*M;* *N*-bromosuccinimide, 100 μ*M;* 0.1 *M* acetate buffer, pH 4.5; 25°C. The data were obtained with a stopped-flow spectrophotometer in a rapid scanning mode. The spectra were recorded at 5, 10, 20, and 40 s after the start of the reaction. A spectrum was obtained within 10 msec (scan speed). (From Ohnishi, M., Kawagishi, T., Abe, T., and Hiromi, K., *J. Biochem.*, 87, 273, 1980. With permission.)

extent of tryptophan modification. Subsequent studies from another laboratory[14] on the modification of DNase with *N*-bromosuccinimide suggested that apparently 2 mol of tryptophan are modified per mole of enzyme at 100% inactivation with a sixfold molar excess of *N*-bromosuccinimide in 0.01 *M* CaCl$_2$ at pH 4.0. Using amino acid analysis (after hydrolysis in 6 *N* HCl containing mercaptoacetic acid, phenol, and 3-(2-aminoethyl) indole for 24 h at 110°C), these investigators showed that all three tryptophanyl residues are modified under the above experimental conditions. The study on the modification of tryptophan in galactose oxidase[19] is worth comment in that these investigators report the amino acid composition of the modified protein after hydrolysis in 3 *N* *p*-toluenesulfonic acid. There

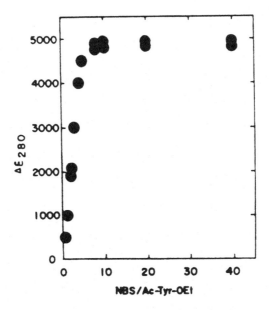

FIGURE 7. Dependence of the difference UV absorption change (increase) of *N*-acetyltyrosine ethyl ester (Ac-Tyr-OET) caused by reaction with *N*-bromosuccinimide on the *N*-bromosuccinimide (NBS)/*N*-acetyltyrosine ethyl ester ratio. *N*-acetyltyrosine ethyl ester, 25 μ*M*; 0.1 *M* acetate, pH 4.5; 25°C. The spectra were obtained 5 min after the start of the reaction. (From Ohnishi, M., Kawagishi, T., Abe, T., and Hiromi, K., *J. Biochem.*, 87, 273, 1980. With permission.)

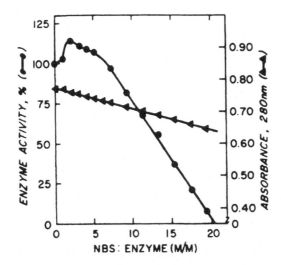

FIGURE 8. Activity and UV absorbance changes of dihydrofolate reductase as a function of the molar excess of *N*-bromosuccinimide. The enzyme concentration was 9.8 μ*M* in 0.05 *M* potassium phosphate, pH 6.5, at 25°C. The maximum changes in enzyme activity or absorbance at 280 nm occurred in the first 2 to 3 min following the addition of *N*-bromosuccinimide. Enzyme activity is expressed as a percent of an untreated control. (From Warwick, P. E., D'Souza, L., and Freisheim, J. H., *Biochemistry*, 11, 3775, 1972. With permission.)

was excellent agreement between the extent of tryptophan modification as judged by direct amino acid analysis and the value observed by spectral analyses. This study shows one of the consequences of the conversion of tryptophan from the indole to the oxindole. Tryptophan is responsible for the majority of the innate fluorescence of proteins and oxidation by *N*-bromosuccinimide obviates this property as shown in Figure 10. Although the reaction

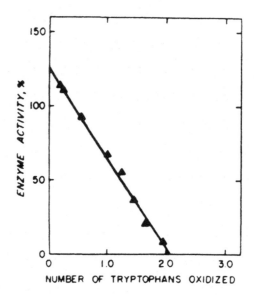

FIGURE 9. Stoichiometry for the inactivation of dihydrofolate reductase by *N*-bromosuccinimide. Shown is the activity of dihydrofolate reductase as a function of the number of tryptophanyl residues oxidized. The experimental conditions were as described in Figure 8. (From Warwick, P. E., D'Souza, L., and Freisheim, J. H., *Biochemistry*, 11, 3775, 1972. With permission.)

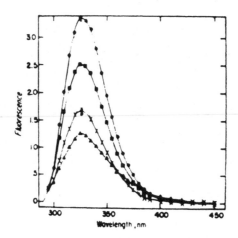

FIGURE 10. Corrected fluorescence emission spectra of deoxygenated solutions of galactose oxidase: unmodified (●); with 0.85 oxidized tryptophans (■); with 2.0 oxidized tryptophans (×); and with 3.0 oxidized tryptophans (▲). The spectra were recorded in 100 m*M* sodium acetate, pH 4.15, after the modification with *N*-bromosuccinimide was performed in 5 m*M* sodium acetate, pH 4.15. The protein concentration was 0.14 mg/ml. The error bars represent the standard deviation of time-averaged recordings. (From Kosman, D. J., Ettinger, M. J., Bereman, R. D., and Giordano, R. S., *Biochemistry*, 16, 1597, 1977. With permission.)

between *N*-bromosuccinimide and tryptophan residues in protein is quite rapid, Fujimori and co-workers,[20] using stopped-flow kinetics, were able to determine kinetically different tryptophanyl residues in *Bacillus subtilis* α-amylase. Figure 11 shows the change in the absorbance spectrum of the protein on reaction with *N*-bromosuccinimide, obtained 5 min after the addition of reagent. Figure 12 compares the extent of reaction after 5 min with that obtained using stopped-flow techniques. Four of the eleven tryptophan residues were mod-

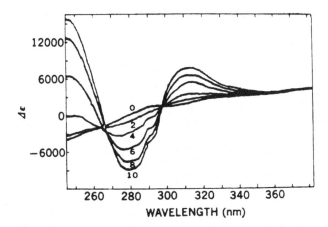

FIGURE 11. Changes in the UV absorption spectrum of *Bacillus subtilis* α-amylase on reaction with *N*-bromosuccinimide. Shown are the difference spectra of the enzyme caused by modification with *N*-bromosuccinimide at pH 7.0 (0.01 *M* phosphate buffer) at 25°C. The numbers in the figure indicate the molar ratio of *N*-bromosuccinimide to the enzyme (0, base line, no reagent added). The spectra were taken at 5 min after mixing. The enzyme concentration was 2.8 μ*M*. ΔE, Difference absorbance per mole of the enzyme. (From Fujimori, H., Ohnishi, M., and Hiromi, K., *J. Biochem.*, 83, 1503, 1978. With permission.)

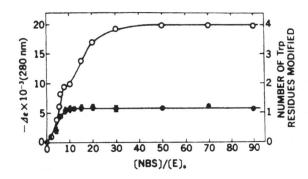

FIGURE 12. Spectrophotometric titration of *Bacillus subtilis* α-amylase with *N*-bromosuccinimide (NBS) at pH 7.0. The enzyme concentration was fixed at 2.8 μ*M*. (○), The value of $- \Delta E_{280}$ was measured with a spectrophotometer at 5 min after mixing the enzyme and *N*-bromosuccinimide solutions in a quartz cuvette. (●), The most rapid decrease in absorbance at 280 nm observed by the stopped-flow method within 0.3 s. The number of modified tryptophan residues was calculated from ΔE_{280} using a molar difference absorption per mol of tryptophan residue at 280 nm (ΔE_{280}) of 5,000 cm^{-1}. (From Fujimori, H., Ohnishi, M., and Hiromi, K., *J. Biochem*, 83, 1503, 1978. With permission.)

ified at the maximum extent of reaction but one of these clearly reacted more rapidly than the other residues. Similar results were obtained when changes in the intrinsic fluorescence of the protein were used to monitor the reaction as shown in Figure 13. These investigators were able to determine a second-order rate constant of $3.5 \times 10^5 \, M^{-1} \, s^{-1}$ for the tryptophanyl residue reacting most rapidly.

There are several other facets of the use of *N*-bromosuccinimide for the modification of tryptophanyl residue in proteins which should be considered. The use of the reagent at mildly acidic pH has been mentioned above. Not only does increasing pH decrease specificity in terms of reaction with amino acid residues other than tryptophan but there is a decrease in the modification of tryptophan. This is shown by the studies[21] on the modification of a glucoamylase from *Aspergillus saitoi*. As shown in Figure 14 there is a modest decrease in modification as the pH is increased from 4.0 to 6.0 with a dramatic decrease at pH 7.0. At

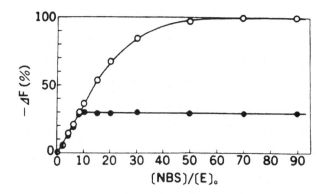

FIGURE 13. The fluorescence titration curve of *Bacillus subtilis* α-amylase with *N*-bromosuccinimide (NBS) at pH 7.0. The enzyme concentration was fixed at 2.8 μ*M* in 0.01 *M* sodium phosphate, pH 7.0. The decrease in fluorescence intensity at 340 nm ($-\Delta F$) of the enzyme excited at 280 nm caused by the addition of *N*-bromosuccinimide is expressed in terms of the percentage fluorescence intensity change with respect to the fluorescence intensity of the native enzyme and plotted against the molar ratio of *N*-bromosuccinimide to the enzyme. (●), The most rapid decrease in fluorescence intensity observed by the stopped-flow method within 0.3 s. (○), The value obtained with a spectrofluorometer at 5 min after mixing. (From Fujimori, H., Ohnishi, M., and Hiromi, K., *J. Biochem.*, 83, 1503, 1978. With permission.)

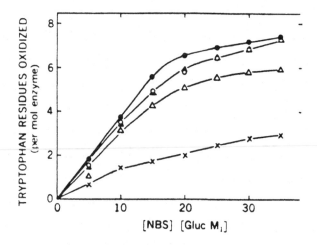

FIGURE 14. *N*-bromosuccinimide oxidation of a glucoamylase (Gluc M₁) as a function of pH. *N*-Bromosuccinimide (6.6 m*M*) was added in 1- to 10-μl portions at 5 min intervals to 1 ml of 6.67 μ*M* Gluc M₁ in 0.1 *M* acetate buffer at pH 4.0 (●), pH 4.5 (○), pH 5.0 (▲), pH 6.0 (△), and pH 7.0 (×). The decrease in absorbance at 280 nm was measured after each addition of *N*-bromosuccinimide at 25°C. The amount of tryptophan residues oxidized was calculated according to the method of Spande and Witkop. (From Inokuchi, N., Takahashi, T., Yoshimoto, A., and Irie, M., *J. Biochem.*, 91, 1661, 1982. With permission.)

pH values close to neutrality there is the increased possibility of modification of amino residues other than tryptophan. The pH dependence of *N*-bromosuccinimide tryptophan modification may well reflect local conformational effects rather than intrinsic chemistry. Stopped-flow studies[22] of the *N*-bromosuccinimide modification of tryptophan-62 in lysozyme shows a marked pH dependence with an observed pKa of 6.2 while there is no pH dependence (3.5 to 8.5) for the modification of *N*-acetyltryptophan ethyl ester. In studies[23] on the reaction on *Escherichia coli* lac repressor protein with *N*-bromosuccinimide at pH 7.8 (1.0 *M* Tris), cysteine was modified as readily as tryptophan with lesser modification of methionine and tyrosine (Figure 15). Although the great majority of *N*-bromosuccinimide modifications of proteins are performed at pH values less than 5.0 to avoid modification of

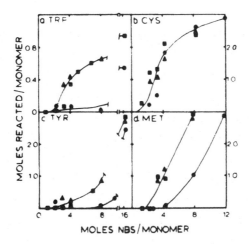

MOLES NBS/MONOMER

FIGURE 15. The modification of *Escherichia coli* lac repressor protein with *N*-bromosuccinimide. Shown are the moles of amino acid reacted with *N*-bromosuccinimide per monomer of repressor protein. The modification was performed in 1.0 *M* Tris/Cl, pH 7.8, for 15 min at ambient temperature in the dark. The reactions were terminated by the addition of dithiothreitol and the modified protein preparations dialyzed vs. water for subsequent analysis. The amount of tryptophan, tyrosine, and methionine were determined by amino acid analysis after hydrolysis in methanesulfonic acid. Cysteine was determined by titration with 2-chloromercuri-4-nitrophenol in 8 *M* urea. ■——■, Repressor reacted with *N*-bromosuccinimide alone; ●——●, repressor reacted with *N*-bromosuccinimide in the presence of isopropyl-l-thio-β-D-galactoside; ▲——▲, repressor reacted with *N*-bromosuccinimide in the presence of *o*-nitrophenyl-β-D-fucoside. (From O'Gorman, R. B. and Matthews, K. S., *J. Biol. Chem.*, 252, 3565, 1977. With permission.)

other functional groups, success can be achieved under less acidic conditions. Kumar et al.[24] modified tryptophanyl residues in transcarboxylase in 0.25 *M* potassium phosphate, pH 6.5, containing 0.1 *M* dithiothreitol and 0.1 m*M* phenylmethylsulfonyl fluoride. These investigators also demonstrated that the loss of activity upon modification was not a reflection of gross conformational change by examination of the quenching of intrinsic fluorescence and changes in the susceptibility to tryptic cleavage. In general, modification should occur at a 4 to 6 molar excess (with respect to total tryptophan) of *N*-bromosuccinimide. Under most reaction conditions, the modification of tryptophanyl residues with *N*-bromosuccinimide is quite rapid. Time-dependent reactions have, however, been observed such as that reported for xylanase.[25] Reaction with 2-hydroxy-5-nitrobenzyl bromide was also time dependent under these reaction conditions. The use of *N*-bromosuccinimide in the study of proteins is summarized in Table 1.

The reaction of *N*-bromosuccinimide with proteins can also result in the cleavage of peptide bonds at tryptophan, tyrosine, and histidine.[26] Thus, the careful investigator will also evaluate the integrity of the polypeptide chain(s) of the protein of interest. Whereas peptide bond cleavage is usually an unwanted side reaction, Feldhoff and Peters[27] have devised a procedure which has enhanced specificity for tryptophan. Their procedure uses 8.0 *M* urea, 2.0 *M* acetic acid as the solvent with a 20-fold molar excess of *N*-bromosuccinimide. Their approach offers at least two advantages; first, the protein is denatured so that all residues should be equally available and, second, the *N*-bromosuccinimide reacts with urea to yield *N*-bromourea, a less severe oxidizing agent which should have increased specificity for tryptophanyl residues. The use of *N*-chlorosuccinimide for peptide bond cleavage of tryptophanyl residues is considered a superior approach[28] (see Chapter 5). A direct comparison of *N*-bromosuccinimide and *N*-chlorosuccinimide in the modification of the single tryptophanyl residue in *Clostridum perfringes* epsilon toxin has been performed.[29] Modification with *N*-bromosuccinimide (50 m*M* sodium acetate, pH 5.0) resulted in the total loss of tryptophan and marked reduction in tyrosine (71% decrease) and methionine

Table 1
EXAMPLES OF THE MODIFICATION OF PROTEINS WITH
N-BROMOSUCCINIMIDE

Protein	Solvent	Molar excess[a]	Extent of modification	Ref.
Trypsinogen	pH 7.0[b]	1—4	1—2	1
Trypsin	pH 4.0[b]	1—4	1—2	1
Dihydrofolate reductase	0.1 *M* sodium phosphate, pH 6.0	15	2.0	2
		15	2.7	2
	0.1 *M* sodium acetate, pH 4.0	12	3.8	2
	0.13 *M* sodium acetate formate, 5.3 *M* urea, pH 4.0			
Bovine pancreatic DNAse	0.1 *M* sodium acetate, pH 4.0 containing 0.033 *M* CaCl$_2$	6	1.0	3
Bovine pancreatic DNAse	pH 4.0, 0.010 *M* CaCl$_2$	1—6	3[c]	4[c]
Dihydrofolate reductase	0.05 *M* potassium phosphate, pH 6.5	20	2.0	5
Pyrocatechase *(B. fuscum)*[d]	0.1 *M* phosphate, pH 7.0	—	2	6
Relaxin	0.2 *M* sodium acetate, pH 4.7	—		7
Rhodopsin	0.1 *M* Tris acetate, pH 7.4	50	6	8
	containing 1% emulphogene	100	9	8
Pig kidney amino acylase	0.1 *M* sodium acetate, pH 5.0—1.0 *M* urea	50	6	9
Galactose oxidase	0.005 *M* sodium acetate, pH 4.15	7	2	10
Bovine thrombin	0.1 sodium acetate, pH 4.0	1	0.5	11
		2	1.1	11
Papain[e]	0.05 *M* sodium acetate, pH 4.75	6[f]	1.4	12
Lac repressor protein	1.0 *M* Tris HCl, pH 7.8	8	0.7[g]	13
α-Mannosidase *(P. vulgaris)*	1.0 *M* sodium acetate, pH 4.0	35	10	14
α-Amylase *(B. subtilis)*	0.01 *M* sodium phosphate, pH 7.0	8	2	15
		50	4	15
Dihydrofolate reductase	0.015 *M* bis Tris HCl, pH 6.5			16
	0.5 *M* KCl	4	1.2	
Xylanase	50 m*M* NaOAc, pH 4.5	—	—[h]	17
Transcarboxylase	250 m*M* potassium phosphate, pH 6.5[j]	—	10/90[i]	18
Cellulase	50 m*M* NaOAc, pH 5.0	30	8/12	19
Winged bean	0.1 *M* sodium citrate, pH 6.0	10	2/4	20

[a] Reagent to protein.

[b] pH maintained at 4.0 by addition of KOH.

[c] Spectral analysis suggested 2 mol tryptophan oxidized while amino acid analysis demonstrates that all three tryptophan residues modified.

[d] Thiophenylated apoenzyme [apoenzyme modified with 5,5′-dithiobis (2-nitrobenzoic acid)].

[e] Not activated.

[f] Also modified tyrosine at this concentration.

[g] Also had substantial modification of tyrosine, cysteine, and methionine.

[h] There is an apparent time-dependent reaction with both *N*-bromosuccinimide and 2-hydroxy-5-nitrobenzyl bromide.

Table 1 (continued)
EXAMPLES OF THE MODIFICATION OF PROTEINS WITH
N-BROMOSUCCINIMIDE

ı Containing 0.1 mM dithiothreitol and 0.1 M phenylmethylsulfonyl fluoride. The reaction was terminated by the addition of a 10-fold molar excess of N-acetyltryptophanamide.

ɪ At maximum inactivation. A total of 40 tryptophanyl residues were available for oxidation in the native state.

References for Table 1

1. **Daniel, V. W., III and Trowbridge, C. G.,** The effect of N-bromosuccinimide upon trypsinogen activation and trypsin catalysis, *Arch. Biochem. Biophys.,* 134, 506, 1969.
2. **Freisheim, J. H. and Huennekens, F. M.,** Effect of N-bromosuccinimide on dihydrofolate reductase, *Biochemistry,* 8, 2271, 1969.
3. **Poulos, T. L. and Price, P. A.,** The identification of a tryptophan residue essential to the catalytic activity of bovine pancreatic deoxyribonuclease, *J. Biol. Chem.,* 246, 4041, 1971.
4. **Sartin, J. L., Hugli, T. E., and Liao, T.-H.,** Reactivity of the tryptophan residues in bovine pancreatic deoxyribonuclease with N-bromosuccinimide, *J. Biol. Chem.,* 255, 8633, 1980.
5. **Warwick, P. E., D'Souza, L., and Freisheim, J. H.,** Role of tryptophan in dihydrofolate reductase, *Biochemistry,* 11, 3775, 1972.
6. **Nagami, K.,** The participation of a tryptophan residue in the binding of ferric iron to pyrocatechase, *Biochem. Biophys. Res. Commun.,* 51, 364, 1973.
7. **Schwabe, C. and Braddon, S. A.,** Evidence for the essential tryptophan residue at the active site of relaxin, *Biochem. Biophys. Res. Commun.,* 68, 1126, 1976.
8. **Cooper, A. and Hogan, M. E.,** Reactivity of tryptophans in rhodopsin, *Biochem. Biophys. Res. Commun.,* 68, 178, 1976.
9. **Kördel, W. and Schneider, F.,** Chemical modification of two tryptophan residues abolishes the catalytic activity of aminoacylase, *Hoppe Seyler's Z. Physiol. Chem.,* 357, 1109, 1976.
10. **Kosman, D. J., Ettinger, M. J., Bereman, R. D., and Giordano, R. S.,** Role of tryptophan in the spectral and catalytic properties of the copper enzyme, galactose oxidase, *Biochemistry,* 16, 1597, 1977.
11. **Uhteg, L. C. and Lundblad, R. L.,** The modification of tryptophan in bovine thrombin, *Biochim. Biophys. Acta,* 491, 551, 1977.
12. **Glick, B. R. and Brubacher, L. S.,** The chemical and kinetic consequences of the modification of papain by N-bromosuccinimide, *Can. J. Biochem.,* 55, 424, 1977.
13. **O'Gorman, R. B. and Matthews, K. S.,** N-bromosuccinimide modification of *lac* repressor protein, *J. Biol. Chem.,* 252, 3565, 1977.
14. **Paus, E.,** The chemical modification of tryptophan residues of α-mannosidase from *Phaseolus vulgaris,* *Biochim. Biophys. Acta,* 533, 446, 1978.
15. **Fujimori, H., Ohnishi, M., and Hiromi, K.,** Tryptophan residues of saccharifying α-amylase from *Bacillus subtilis.* A kinetic discrimination of states of tryptophan residues using N-bromosuccinimide, *J. Biochem.,* 83, 1503, 1978.
16. **Thomson, J. W., Roberts, G. C. K., and Burgen, A. S. V.,** The effects of modification with N-bromosuccinimide on the binding of ligands to dihydrofolate reductase, *Biochem. J.,* 187, 501, 1980.
17. **Keskar, S. S., Srinivasan, M. C., and Deshpande, V. V.,** Chemical modification of a xylanase from a thermotolerant *Streptomyces.* Evidence for essential tryptophan and cysteine residues at the active site, *Biochem. J.,* 261, 49, 1989.
18. **Kumar, G. K., Beegen, H., and Wood, H. G.,** Involvement of tryptophans at the catalytic and subunit-binding domains of transcarboxylase, *Biochemistry,* 27, 5972, 1988.
19. **Clarke, A. J.,** Essential tryptophan residues in the function of cellulase from Schizophyllum commune, *Biochim. Biophys. Acta,* 912, 424, 1987.
20. **Higuchi, M., Inoue, K., and Iwai, K.,** A tryptophan residue is essential to the sugar-binding site of winged bean basis lectin, *Biochim. Biophys. Acta,* 829, 51, 1985.

(79% decrease). Reaction with N-chlorosuccinimide (50 mM Tris, pH 8.5) resulted in the total loss of both tryptophan and methionine but no significant change in tyrosine. Reaction with chloroamine T (50 mM Tris, pH 8.5) resulted only in the loss of methionine. Activity was lost only with the modification of tryptophan. Peptide bond cleavage was not observed under these reaction conditions.

The conversion of tryptophanyl residues to 1-formyltryptophanyl residues has been re-

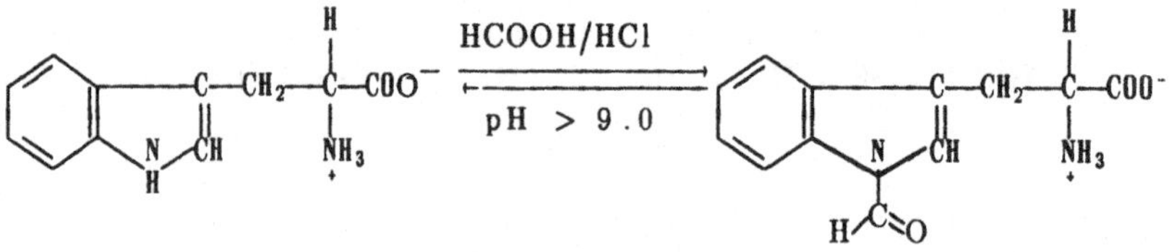

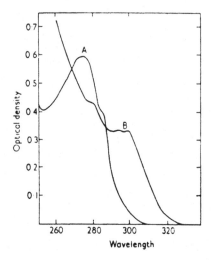

FIGURE 16.   A scheme for the reversible formylation of tryptophan residues.

FIGURE 17.   Changes in the UV absorption spectrum of trypsin occurring as a result of formylation of tryptophan residues. Shown is the spectrum of trypsin (18 μM in 8.0 M urea, pH 4.0) before (curve A) and after (curve B) 1-formylation of tryptophanyl residues. Formylation of trypsin was accomplished by dissolving trypsin in formic acid saturated with gaseous HCl at 20°C (2.5 mg/ml). At suitable time intervals, 0.4 ml samples of the solution were diluted with 2 ml of 8 M urea, pH 4.0 for recording the UV spectra. When the maximum increase in absorbance at 298 nm was reached (about 60 min), the solvent was partially removed under vacuum over KOH pellets for 15 min in order to eliminate most of the HCl and the sample was subsequently lyophilized. (From Coletti-Previero, M.-A., Previero, A., and Zuckerkandl, E., *J. Mol. Biol.*, 39, 493, 1969. With permission.)

ported. The reaction conditions are somewhat harsh, but the procedure is reversible (Figure 16) and should prove quite useful for small peptides and has been applied to several proteins. Coletti-Previero and co-workers[30] have successfully applied this procedure to bovine pancreatic trypsin. Trypsin was dissolved in formic acid saturated with HCl at a concentration of 2.5 mg/ml at 20°C. The formylation reaction is associated with an increase in absorbance at 298 nm[31] (Figure 17). It therefore is possible to follow the reaction spectrophotometrically. The reaction is judged complete when there is no further increase in absorbance at 298 nm. The above reaction with trypsin was complete after an incubation period of 1 h. The solvent was partially removed *in vacuo* over KOH pellets followed by lyophilization. The formyl-tryptophan derivative is unstable at alkaline pH. At pH 9.5 (pH-stat), conversion back to tryptophan is complete after 200 min incubation at 20°C as shown in Figure 18. Holmgren has successfully applied this procedure to thioredoxin.[32] A procedure for the acylation of the carbon at position 2 on the indole ring has also been reported.[33] A more recent study on N-formylation of tryptophanyl residues in proteins involved the study of epitopes in horse heart cytochrome c.[34] The single tryptophanyl residue was formylated with formic acid saturated with HCl. The modified protein had markedly reduced affinity for a monoclonal antibody resulting from local conformational change.

One of the most useful modification procedures for tryptophanyl residues in proteins

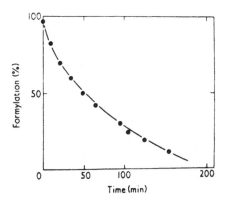

FIGURE 18. Deformylation of tryptophanyl residues in trypsin by incubation at alkaline pH. Shown is the hydrolysis of 1-formyltryptophan in trypsin during incubation at pH 9.5, as measured spectrophotometrically at 298 nm (ϵ = 4880) at 20°C. The solution of formylated trypsin after incubation at pH 8.0 was allowed to stand in the reaction chamber of a pH stat at pH 9.5, 25°C and maintained at this value by the addition of 0.1 M NaOH. (From Coletti-Previero, M.-A., Previero, A., and Zuckerkandl, E., *J. Mol. Biol.*, 39, 493, 1969. With permission.)

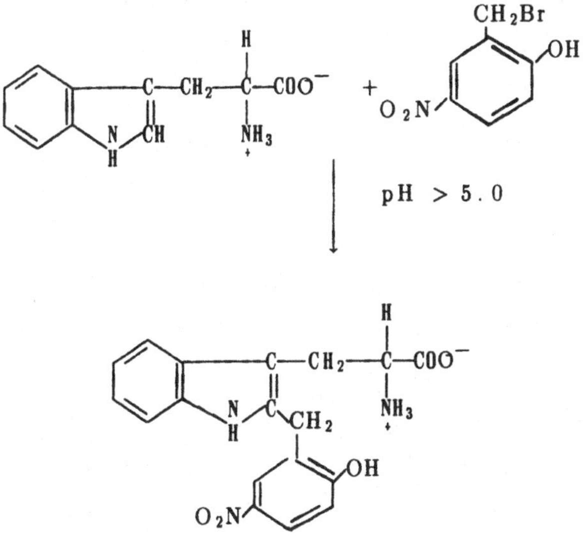

FIGURE 19. A scheme for the reaction of 2-hydroxy-5-nitrobenzyl bromide with tryptophan.

involves the use of 2-hydroxy-5-nitrobenzyl bromide and its various derivatives (Figure 19). 2-Hydroxy-5-nitrobenzyl bromide, frequently referred to as Koshland's reagent, was introduced by Koshland and co-workers.[35,36] Barman and Koshland[37] have reported the use of 2-hydroxy-5-nitrobenzyl bromide for the quantitative determination of tryptophanyl residues in proteins. Although this approach to the quantitative determination of tryptophanyl residues in proteins has been largely replaced by the development of new methods for the hydrolysis of proteins, it can still be useful in certain instances. For this procedure the sample is incubated for 16 to 20 h at 37°C in 1.0 ml 10 M urea (the urea should be recrystallized (EtOH/H$_2$O) prior to use), pH 2.7 (pH adjusted with concentrated HCl). This solution is cooled to ambient temperature and approximately 5.0 mg of 2-hydroxy-5-nitrobenzyl bromide (in 0.1 ml acetone) is added followed by vigorous stirring (we have found the Pierce Reacti-Vials® very useful for this purpose). Occasionally a precipitate of 2-hydroxy-5-nitrobenzyl alcohol (the hydrolytic product of 2-hydroxy-5-nitrobenzyl bromide) forms which can be

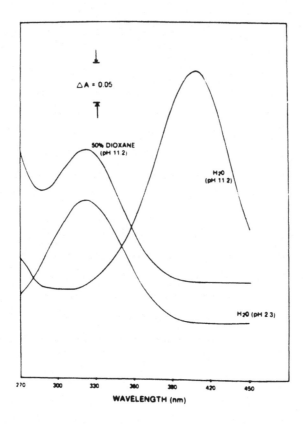

FIGURE 20.   The UV absorption spectra of 2-hydroxy-5-nitro-benzyl alcohol (HNB-OH) in different solvents. The concentration of HNB-OH was 33.2 μM. (From Clemmer, J. D., Carr, J., Knaff, D. B., and Holwerda, R. A., *FEBS Lett.*, 91, 346, 1978. With permission.)

removed by centrifugation. The labeled protein is obtained free of reagent by gel filtration. This step is generally performed under acidic condition (e.g., 0.18 M acetic acid, 10% acetic acid, or 10% formic acid).* Depending upon the protein under study, it might be necessary to perform this step in 10 M urea (pH 2.7) to maintain the solubility of the modified protein. A portion of the modified protein is taken to a pH greater than 12 with NaOH. The extent of incorporation is determined at 410 nm using an extinction coefficient of 18,000 M^{-1} cm^{-1}. It is necessary to determine the concentration of protein by a technique other than absorbance at 280 nm because of the modification of tryptophan. We have found it convenient to either use amino acid analysis after acid hydrolysis or the ninhydrin reaction[38] after alkaline hydrolysis.[39]

The most frequent use of 2-hydroxy-5-nitrobenzyl bromide has been in the specific modification of tryptophan in peptides and proteins. Under appropriate reaction conditions (pH 4.0 or below), the reagent is highly specific for reaction with tryptophan. We have, on occasion, seen the modification of methionine residues under these conditions. This reagent also has the advantage of being a "reporter" group in the sense that the spectrum of the hydroxynitrobenzyl derivative is sensitive to changes in the microenvironment as shown in Figure 20. This decrease observed in absorbance at 410 nm associated with an increase in

---

*   Despite its wide use as a solvent for peptides and proteins, the use of formic acid is not recommended because of the potential of side reactions at amino functional groups; see Shively, J. E., Hawke, D., and Jones, B. N., Microsequence analysis of peptides and protein. III. Artifacts and effects of impurities on analysis, *Anal. Biochem.*, 120, 312, 1982.

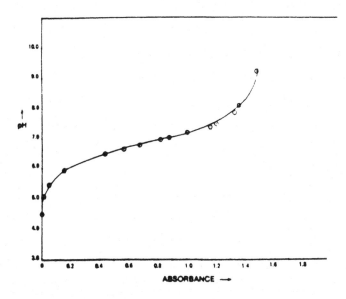

FIGURE 21. Spectrophotometric titration curve for 2-hydroxy-5-nitrobenzyl alcohol (HNB-OH). Shown is the absorbance of HNB-OH (76.4 μM) at 410 nm as a function of pH (phosphate buffers). (From Clemmer, J. D., Carr, J., Knaff, D. B., and Holwerda, R. A., *FEBS Lett.*, 91, 346, 1978. With permission.)

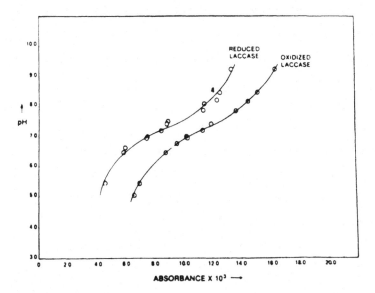

FIGURE 22. Effect of pH on the absorbance (410 nm) of two forms of laccase modified with 2-hydroxy-5-nitrobenzyl bromide (HNB-laccase). Shown are spectrophotometric titration curves for oxidized and reduced HNB-laccase (2.5 μM; 0.38 mol HNB/mole laccase). The absorbance at 410 nm is shown as a function of pH (phosphate buffers). (From Clemmer, J. D., Carr, J., Knaff, D. B., and Holwerda, R. A., *FEBS Lett.*, 91, 346, 1978. With permission.)

absorbance at 320 nm upon the addition of dioxane is similar to that seen with acidification and reflects the increase in the pKa of the phenolic hydroxyl group. The spectrophotometric titration curve for 2-hydroxy-5-nitrobenzyl alcohol is shown in Figure 21. Titration curves of oxidized and reduced laccase[40] which had been modified with 2-hydroxy-5-nitrobenzyl bromide are shown in Figure 22. From this experiment it was concluded that the tryptophanyl

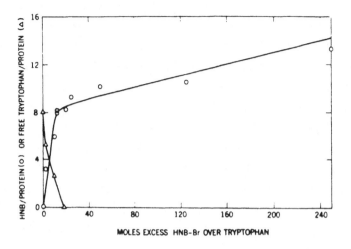

FIGURE 23.   The titration of the tryptophanyl residues of carboxymethyl chymotrypsinogen with 2-hydroxy-5-nitrobenzyl bromide. Carboxymethyl chymotrypsinogen (reduced and S-carboxymethylated with iodoacetic acid) was incubated in 10 M urea, pH 2.7, for 16 to 18 h at which point 1-ml portions (5 mg of protein) were reacted with increasing amounts of 2-hydroxy-5-nitrobenzyl bromide dissolved in 0.1 ml acetone. The modified protein was separated from excess reagent by gel filtration (G-25 Sephadex) and subsequently analyzed for tryptophan (amino acid analysis after alkaline hydrolysis) and for the incorporation of the 2-hydroxy-5-nitrobenzyl group. (From Barman, T. E. and Koshland, D. E., Jr., *J. Biol. Chem.*, 242, 5771, 1967. With permission.)

residues in laccase modified with 2-hydroxy-5-nitrobenzyl bromide are in an essentially aqueous microenvironment. The chemistry of the reaction of 2-hydroxy-5-nitrobenzyl bromide with tryptophan has been studied in some detail.[41] Disubstitution on the indole ring is a possibility and is usually seen as a sudden "break" in the plot of extent of modification vs. reagent excess (see Figure 23).

In our hands, the following procedure has been found useful. The protein or peptide to be modified is taken into 0.1 to 0.2 M sodium acetate buffer, pH 4 to 5. Reaction with other nucleophilic centers on the protein will become more of a problem as one approaches neutral pH. A 100-fold molar excess of 2-hydroxy-5-nitrobenzyl bromide (dissolved in a suitable water-miscible organic solvent such as acetone or dimethyl sulfoxide) is added in the dark. After 5 min (this time period was arbitrarily selected; the reaction can be considered to be essentially instantaneous to either modify tryptophan or undergo hydrolysis) the reaction mixture is taken by gel filtration into a solvent suitable for subsequent analysis. The extent of modification is determined under basic conditions as described above for the use of this reagent in the quantitative determination of tryptophan.

The use of 2-hydroxy-5-nitrobenzyl bromide does present problems in that the reagent is extremely sensitive to hydrolysis and is not very soluble under aqueous conditions. These difficulties are avoided and the characteristics of the reaction preserved by the use of the dimethyl sulfonium salt obtained from the reaction of 2-hydroxy-5-nitrobenzyl bromide with dimethyl sulfide.[43] This compound is easily synthesized or can be obtained from various commercial sources. This water-soluble sulfonium salt derivative has recently been used to modify a tryptophanyl residue in rabbit skeletal myosin subfragment-1.[44] Purification of peptide-containing modified tryptophanyl residues was achieved by immunoaffinity chromatography using rabbit antibody to bovine serum albumin previously modified with dimethyl(2-hydroxy-5-nitrobenzyl) sulfonium bromide.

Horton and Koshland[45] have also developed a clever approach for modification of hydrolytic enzymes such as the serine proteases which catalyze the reaction shown in Figure 24. If 2-hydroxy-5-nitrobenzyl bromide is substituted at the phenolic hydroxyl, it is essentially unreactive as originally shown for the methoxy derivative. Horton and Young[46] prepared

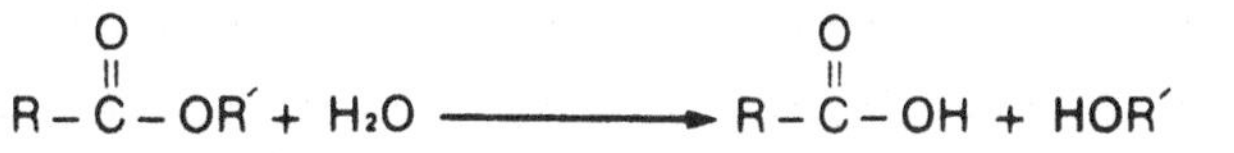

FIGURE 24. The hydrolysis of an ester catalyzed by a serine protease.

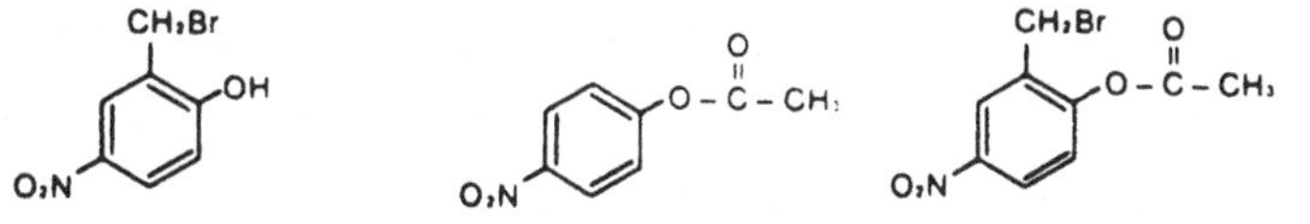

FIGURE 25. The structures of 2-hydroxy-5-nitrobenzyl bromide (left), p-nitrophenyl acetate (center), and 2-acetoxy-5-nitrobenzyl bromide.

2-acetoxy-5-nitrobenzyl bromide. This derivative, like the methoxy derivative, is essentially unreactive. There is considerable structural identity between 2-acetoxy-5-nitrobenzyl bromide and p-nitrophenyl acetate, which is a nonspecific substrate for chymotrypsin (Figure 25). α-Chymotrypsin removes the acetyl group from 2-acetoxy-5-nitrobenzyl bromide, thus generating 2-hydroxy-5-nitrobenzyl bromide at the active site which then either rapidly reacts with a neighboring nucleophile or undergoes hydrolysis. Uhteg and Lundblad[47] have used both the acetoxy and butyroxy derivatives in the study of thrombin. A similar approach has been used in the study of papain with 2-chloromethyl-4-nitrophenyl N-carbobenzoxy-glycinate.[48] It has been subsequently shown that this modification occurs at a specific tryptophan residue in papain.[49]

2-Hydroxy-5-nitrobenzyl bromide has been proved to be of use in the study of the functional role of tryptophan in the enzymes, as shown in Table 2.

Reagents with reaction characteristics similar to 2-hydroxy-5-nitrobenzyl bromide are the o-nitrophenylsulfenyl derivatives.[50] The reaction product resulting from the sulfonylation of lysozyme[51] in o-nitrobenzenesulfenyl chloride (2-nitrophenylsulfenyl chloride) (40-fold molar excess) pH 3.5 (0.1 M sodium acetate) has spectral characteristics which can be used to determine the extent of reagent incorporation (at 365 nm $\epsilon = 4 \times 10^{-3} M^{-1} cm^{-1}$) (Figure 26). These reagents show considerable specificity for the modification of tryptophan at pH ≤4.0 (Figure 27). Possible side reactions with other nucleophiles such as amino groups need to be considered. In the case of human chorionic somatomammotropin and human pituitary growth hormone,[52] reaction with o-nitrophenylsulfenyl chloride (2-nitrophenylsulfenyl chloride) was achieved in 50% acetic acid but not in 0.1 sodium acetate, pH 4.0. Wilchek and Miron[53] have reported on the reaction of 2,4-dinitrophenylsulfenyl chloride with tryptophan in peptides and protein and subsequent conversion of the modified tryptophan to 2-thiotryptophan by reaction with β-mercaptoethanol at pH 8.0 (see Figure 28). The thiolysis of the modified tryptophan is responsible for changes in the spectral properties of the derivative (Figure 29). The characteristics of the modified tryptophan have resulted in the development of a facile purification scheme for peptides containing the modified tryptophan residues.[54,55] Mollier et al.[56] examined the reaction of o-nitrophenylsulfenyl chloride (2-nitrophenylsulfenyl chloride) with notexin (a phospholipase obtained from Notechis scutalatus scutalatus venom which contains two tryptophanyl residues). Reaction with 2-nitrophenylsulfenyl chloride (2-fold molar excess) in 50% (v/v) acetic acid resulted in two derivative proteins on HPLC analysis. One derivative contained two modified tryptophanyl residues (20 and 110) while the other derivative was modified only at position 20.

Table 2
EXAMPLES OF THE MODIFICATION OF PROTEINS WITH 2-HYDROXY-5-NITROBENZYL BROMIDE

Protein	Solvent	Molar excess	Residues modified	Ref.
Pepsin	0.1 M NaCl[a]	300	2/4	1
Streptococcal proteinase	0.46 M sodium phosphate, pH 3.1	200	1.8/4	2
Pancreatic deoxyribonuclease	0.050 M CaCl$_2$[b]	100	1/3	3
Carbonic anhydrase	0.1 M phosphate, pH 6.8	100	—[c]	4
Trypsin	0.1 M NaCl, 0.02 M CaCl$_2$[d] pH 4.2 (pH-Stat)	ca. 100	1/4	5
Human chorionic somato-mammotropin	0.05 M glycine, pH 2.8	—	—	6
Naja naja neurotoxin	0.2 M acetic acid[e]	40	—[f]	7
Glyceraldehyde-3-phosphate dehydrogenase	pH 6.75[g]	30[h]	1/3	8
α-Mannosidase *(Phaseolus vulgaris)*	0.1 M sodium acetate, pH 3.7	100	5/28	9
Thrombin	0.2 M acetate, pH 4.0	100	1/8	10
Laccase	pH 6.95[i]	50	0.30/6	11
	pH 4.00[i]	50	0.58/6	11
	pH 3.30[i]	110	2.39/6	11
Human serum albumin	10 M urea, pH 4.4	1000	1.1/1[j]	12
Xylanase	50 mM NaOAc, pH 5.0	—	—[k]	13
Winged bean	0.1 M sodium citrate, pH 3.1	100	0.9/4	14
		200	1.7/4	
		400	1.8/4	

[a]   pH Adjusted with 50% acetic acid.
[b]   pH Remained between 4.0 an 4.5 without need for buffer.
[c]   Variation with respect to enzyme source.
[d]   pH Maintained at 4.2 by addition of NaOH (pH Stat).
[e]   pH 2.7.
[f]   Polymerization occurred.
[g]   pH Maintained at 6.75 by the addition of 0.1 M NaOH.
[h]   Dimethyl (2-hydroxy-5-nitrobenzyl) sulfonium bromide was used in the experiments. Prior to reaction, the active site sulfhydryl was blocked by reaction with 5,5'-dithiobis(2-nitrobenzoate).
[i]   Unbuffered, pH maintained by titration with NaOH.
[j]   Incorporation determined at pH 7.4 after the following relationship:[55] moles 2-hydroxy-5-nitrobenzyl bromide per mole albumin = $(A_{410} \times 69,000 \times 0.498)/13,800 \times (A_{280} - 0.167) \times A_{410}$.
[k]   A time-dependent inactivation reaction was observed.

References for Table 2

1. **Dopheide, T. A. A. and Jones, W. M.,** Studies on the tryptophan residues in porcine pepsin, *J. Biol. Chem.*, 243, 3906, 1968.
2. **Robinson, G. W.,** Reaction of a specific tryptophan residue in streptococcal proteinase with 2-hydroxy-5-nitrobenzyl bromide, *J. Biol. Chem.*, 245, 4832, 1970.
3. **Poulos, T. L. and Price, P. A.,** The identification of a tryptophan residue essential to the catalytic activity of bovine pancreatic deoxyribonuclease, *J. Biol. Chem.*, 246, 4041, 1971.
4. **Lindskog, S. and Nilsson, A.,** The location of tryptophanyl groups in human and bovine carbonic anhydrases. Ultraviolet difference spectra and chemical modification, *Biochim. Biophys. Acta*, 295, 117, 1973.
5. **Imhoff, J. M., Keil-Dlouha, V., and Keil, B.,** Functional changes in bovine α- and β-trypsins caused by the substitution of tryptophan-199, *Biochimie*, 55, 521, 1973.
6. **Neri, P., Arezzini, C., Botti, R., Cocola, F., and Tarli, P.,** Modification of the tryptophanyl residue and its effect on the immunological and biological activity of human chorionic somatomammotropin, *Biochim. Biophys. Acta*, 322, 88, 1973.

References for Table 2 (continued)

7. **Karlsson, E., Eaker, D., and Drevin, H.,** Modification of the invariant tryptophan residue of two *Naja naja* neurotoxins, *Biochim. Biophys. Acta,* 328, 510, 1973.
8. **Heilman, H. D. and Pfleiderer, G.,** On the role of tryptophan residues in the mechanism of action of glyceraldehyde-3-phosphate dehydrogenase as tested by specific modification, *Biochim. Biophys. Acta,* 384, 331, 1975.
9. **Paus, E.,** The chemical modification of tryptophan residues of α-mannosidase from *Phaseolus vulgaris, Biochim. Biophys. Acta,* 533, 446, 1978.
10. **Uhteg, L. C. and Lundblad, R. L.,** The modification of tryptophan in bovine thrombin, *Biochem. Biophys. Acta,* 491, 551, 1977.
11. **Clemmer, J. D., Carr, J., Knaff, D. B., and Holwerda, R. A.,** Modification of laccase tryptophan residues with 2-hydroxy-5-nitrobenzyl bromide, *FEBS Lett.,* 91, 346, 1978.
12. **Fehske, K. J., Müller, W. E., and Wollert, U.,** The modification of the lone tryptophan residue in human serum albumin by 2-hydroxy-5-nitrobenzyl bromide. Characterization of the modified protein and the binding of L-tryptophan and benzodiazepines to the tryptophan-modifed albumin, *Hoppe Seyler's Z. Physiol. Chem.,* 359, 709, 1978.
13. **Keskar, S. S., Srinivasan, M. C., and Deshpande, V. V.,** Chemical modification of a xylanase from a thermotolerant *Streptomyces.* Evidence for essential tryptophan and cysteine residues at the active site, *Biochem. J.,* 261, 49, 1989.
14. **Higuchi, M., Inoue, K., and Iwai, K.,** A tryptophan residue is essential to the sugar-binding site of winged bean basis lectin, *Biochim. Biophys. Acta,* 829, 51, 1985.

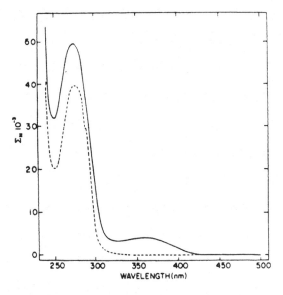

FIGURE 26. The UV absorbance spectrum of egg white lysozyme after modification of tryptophan-62 with 2-nitrophenylsulfenyl chloride (*o*-nitrobenzenesulfenyl chloride). Shown is the UV absorption spectrum of 1-NPS-lysozyme (——), and native lysozyme (——). The measurements were performed in water at pH 7.0.

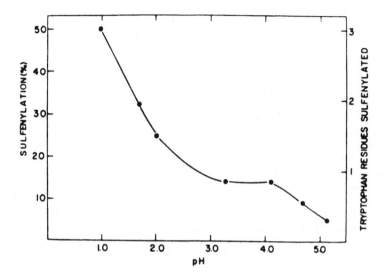

FIGURE 27. The extent of sulfenylation of tryptophanyl residues in egg white lysozyme by 2-nitrophenylsulfenyl chloride as a function of the pH. Sulfenylation was carried out at protein concentration of 0.5 μmol in 1 ml of 0.1 M buffered solutions (HCl-KCl at pH 1 to 2; sodium acetate at pH 3 to 5) with 20 μmol of 2-nitrophenylsulfenyl chloride for 5 h. (From Shechter, Y., Burstein, Y., and Patchornik, A., *Biochemistry*, 11, 653, 1972. With permission.)

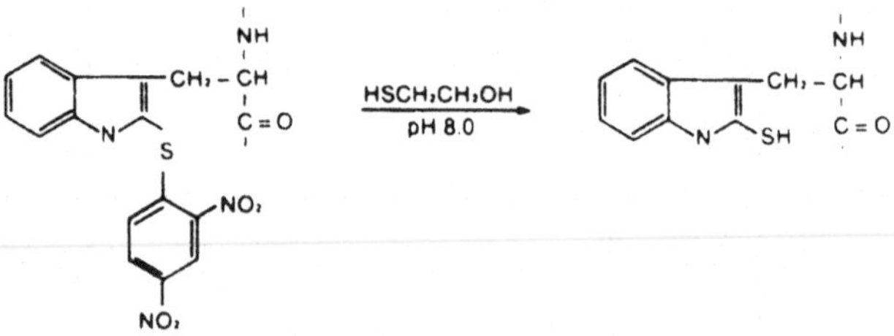

FIGURE 28. Thiolysis of the tryptophan derivative formed on reaction with 2,4-dinitrophenylsulfenyl chloride.

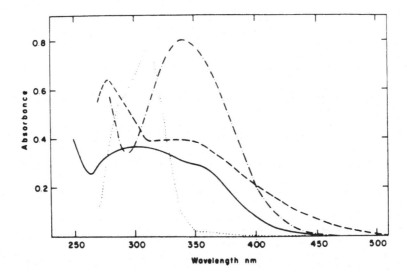

FIGURE 29.   UV absorption spectra of the derivatives formed by the thiolysis of 2-(2,4-dinitrophenylsulfenyl) tryptophan. Shown are the UV absorption spectra of 2,4-dinitrophenylsulfenyltryptophan (- - - -), 2-thioltryptophan (····), ditryptophanyl-2-disulfide (———), and S-2,4-dinitrophenyl-2-mercaptoethanol (—·—). The spectral studies were performed in 0.1 M ammonium bicarbonate. (From Wilchek, M. and Miron, T., *Biochem. Biophys. Res. Commun.*, 47, 1015, 1972. With permission.)

REFERENCES

1.   **Liu, T.-Y. and Chang, Y. H.,** Hydrolysis of proteins with *p*-toluenesulfonic acid. Determination of tryptophan, *J. Biol. Chem.*, 246, 2842, 1971.
2.   **Simpson, R. J., Neuberger, M. R., and Liu, T.-Y.,** Complete amino acid analysis of proteins from a single hydrolysate, *J. Biol. Chem.*, 251, 1936, 1976.
3.   **Hachimori, Y., Horinishi, H., Kurihara, K., and Shibata,K.,** States of amino residues in proteins. V. Different reactivities with H_2O_2 of tryptophan residues in lysozyme, proteinases and zymogens, *Biochim. Biophys. Acta*, 93, 346, 1964.
4.   **Kotoku, I., Matsushima, A., Bando, M., and Inada, Y.,** Tyrosine and tryptophan residues and amino groups in thrombin related to enzymic activities, *Biochim. Biophys. Acta*, 214, 490, 1970.
5.   **Sanda, A. and Irie, M.,** Chemical modification of tryptophan residues in ribonuclease from a *Rhizopus* sp., *J. Biochem.*, 87, 1079, 1980.
6.   **Matsushima, A., Takiuchi, H., Saito, Y., and Inada, Y.,** Significance of tryptophan residues in the D-domain of the fibrin molecule in fibrin polymer formation, *Biochim. Biophys. Acta*, 625, 230, 1980.
7.   **Patchornik, A., Lawson, W. B., and Witkop, B.,** Selective cleavage of peptide bonds. I. Mechanism of oxidation of β-substituted indoles with *N*-bromosuccinimide, *J. Am. Chem. Soc.*, 80, 4747, 1958.
8.   **Spande, T. F. and Witkop, B.,** Determination of the tryptophan content of protein with *N*-bromosuccinimide, *Meth. Enzymol.*, 11, 498, 1967.
9.   **Spande, T. F. and Witkop, B.,** Tryptophan involvement in the function of enzymes and protein hormones as determined by selective oxidation with *N*-bromosuccinimide, *Meth. Enzymol.*, 11, 506, 1967.
10.   **Spande, T. F. and Witkop, B.,** Tryptophan involvement in binding sites of proteins and in enzyme-inhibitor complexes as determined by oxidation with *N*-bromosuccinimide, *Meth. Enzymol.*, 11, 522, 1967.
11.   **Green, N. M.,** Avidin. 3. The nature of the biotin binding site, *Biochem. J.*, 89, 599, 1963.
12.   **Crestfield, A. M., Moore, S., and Stein, W. H.,** The preparation and enzymatic hydrolysis of reduced and *S*-carboxymethylated proteins, *J. Biol. Chem.*, 238, 622, 1963.
13.   **Ohnishi, M., Kawagishi, T., Abe, T., and Hiromi, K.,** Stopped-flow studies on the chemical modification with *N*-bromosuccinimide of model compounds of tryptophan residues, *J. Biochem.*, 87, 273, 1980.
14.   **Sartin, J. L., Hugli, T. E., and Liao, T.-H.,** Reactivity of the tryptophan residues in bovine pancreatic deoxyribonuclease with *N*-bromosuccinimide, *J. Biol. Chem.*, 255, 8633, 1980.

15. **Daniel, V. W., III and Trowbridge, C. G.,** The effect of *N*-bromosuccinimide upon trypsinogen activation and trypsin catalysis, *Arch. Biochem. Biophys.*, 134, 506, 1969.

16. **Freisheim, J. H. and Huennekens, F. M.,** Effect of *N*-bromosuccinimide on dihydrofolate reductase, *Biochemistry*, 8, 2271, 1969.

17. **Warwick, P. E., D'Souza, L., and Freisheim, J. H.,** Role of tryptophan in dihydrofolate reductase, *Biochemistry*, 11, 3775, 1972.

18. **Poulos, T. L. and Price, P. A.,** The identification of a tryptophan residue essential to the catalytic activity of bovine pancreatic deoxyribonuclease, *J. Biol. Chem.*, 246, 4041, 1971.

19. **Kosman, D. J., Ettinger, M. J., Bereman, R. D., and Giordano, R. S.,** Role of tryptophan in the spectral and catalytic properties of the copper enzyme, galactose oxidase, *Biochemistry*, 16, 1597, 1977.

20. **Fujimori, H., Ohnishi, M., and Hiromi, K.,** Tryptophan residues of saccharifying α-amylase from *Bacillus subtilis*. A kinetic discrimination of states of tryptophan residues using *N*-bromosuccinimide, *J. Biochem.*, 83, 1503, 1978.

21. **Inokuchi, N., Takahashi, T., Yoshimoto, A., and Irie, M.,** *N*-Bromosuccinimide oxidation of a glucoamylase from *Aspergillus saitoi*, *J. Biochem.*, 91, 1661, 1982.

22. **Ohnishi, M., Kawagishi, T., and Hiromi, K.,** Stopped-flow chemical modification with *N*-bromosuccinimide: a good probe for changes in the microenvironment of the Trp 62 residue of chicken egg white lysozyme, *Arch. Biochem. Biophys.*, 272, 46, 1989.

23. **O'Gorman, R. B. and Matthews, K. S.,** *N*-Bromosuccinimide modification of lac repressor protein, *J. Biol. Chem.*, 252, 3565, 1977.

24. **Kumar, G. K., Beegen, H., and Wood, H. G.,** Involvement of tryptophans at the catalytic and subunit-binding domains of transcarboxylase, *Biochemistry*, 27, 5972, 1988.

25. **Keskar, S. S., Srinivasan, M. C., and Deshpande, V. V.,** Chemical modification of a xylanase from a thermotolerant *Streptomyces*. Evidence for essential tryptophan and cysteine residues at the active site, *Biochem. J.*, 261, 49, 1989.

26. **Ramachandran, L. K. and Witkop, B.,** *N*-Bromosuccinimide cleavage of peptides, *Meth. Enzymol.*, 11, 283, 1967.

27. **Feldhoff, R. C. and Peters, T., Jr.,** Determination of the number and relative position of tryptophan residues in various albumins, *Biochem. J.*, 159, 529, 1976.

28. **Shechter, Y., Patchornik, A., and Burstein, Y.,** Selective chemical cleavage of tryptophanyl peptide bonds by oxidative chlorination with *N*-chlorosuccinimide, *Biochemistry*, 15, 5071, 1976.

29. **Sakurai, J. and Nagahama, M.,** Role of one tryptophan residue in the lethal activity of Clostridium perfringens epsilon toxin, *Biochem. Biophys. Res. Commun.*, 128, 760, 1985.

30. **Coletti-Previero, M.-A., Previero, A., and Zuckerkandl, E.,** Separation of the proteolytic and esteratic activities of trypsin by reversible structural modifications, *J. Mol. Biol.*, 39, 493, 1969.

31. **Previero, A., Coletti-Previero, M.-A., and Cavadore, J. C.,** A reversible chemical modification of the tryptophan residue, *Biochim. Biophys. Acta*, 147, 453, 1967.

32. **Holmgren, A.,** Reversible chemical modification of the tryptophan residues of thioredoxin from *Eschericia coli* B., *Eur. J. Biochem.*, 26, 528, 1972.

33. **Previero, A., Prota, G., and Coletti-Previero, M.-A.,** C-Acylation of the tryptophan indole ring and its usefulness in protein chemistry, *Biochim. Biophys. Acta*, 285, 269, 1972.

34. **Cooper, H. M., Jemmerson, R., Hunt, D. F., Griffin, P. R., Yates, J. R., III, Shabanowitz, J., Zhu, N.-Z., and Paterson, Y.,** Site-directed chemical modification of horse cytochrome c results in changes in antigenicity due to local and long-range conformation perturbations, *J. Biol. Chem.*, 262, 11591, 1987.

35. **Koshland, D. E., Jr., Karkhanis, Y. D., and Latham, H. G.,** An environmentally-sensitive reagent with selectivity for the tryptophan residue in proteins, *J. Am. Chem. Soc.*, 86, 1448, 1964.

36. **Horton, H. R. and Koshland, D. E., Jr.,** A highly reactive colored reagent with selectivity for the tryptophanyl residue in proteins, 2-Hydroxy-5-nitrobenzyl bromide, *J. Am. Chem. Soc.*, 87, 1126, 1965.

37. **Barman, T. E. and Koshland, D. E., Jr.,** A colorimetric procedure for the quantitative determination of tryptophan residues in proteins, *J. Biol. Chem.*, 242, 5771, 1967.

38. **Moore, S.,** Amino acid analysis: aqueous dimethyl sulfoxide as solvent for the ninhydrin reaction, *J. Biol. Chem.*, 243, 6281, 1968.

39. **Fruchter, R. G. and Crestfield, A. M.,** Preparation and properties of two active forms of ribonuclease dimer, *J. Biol. Chem.*, 240, 3868, 1965.

40. **Clemmer, J. D., Carr, J., Knaff, D. B., and Holwerda, R. A.,** Modification of laccase tryptophan residues with 2-hydroxy-5-nitrobenzyl bromide, *FEBS Lett.*, 91, 346, 1978.

41. **Loudon, G. M. and Koshland, D. E., Jr.,** The chemistry of a reporter group: 2-hydroxy-5-nitrobenzyl bromide, *J. Biol. Chem.*, 245, 2247, 1970.

42. **Lundblad, R. L. and Noyes, C. M.,** Observations on the reaction of 2-hydroxy-5-nitrobenzyl bromide with a peptide-bound tryptophanyl residue, *Anal. Biochem.*, 136, 93, 1984.

43. **Horton, H. R. and Tucker, W. P.,** Dimethyl (2-hydroxy-5-nitrobenzyl) sulfonium salts. Water-soluble environmentally sensitive protein reagents, *J. Biol. Chem.*, 245, 3397, 1970.

44. **Peyser, Y. M., Muhlrad, A., and Werber, M. M.,** Tryptophan-130 is the most reactive tryptophan residue in rabbit skeletal myosin subfragment-1, *FEBS Lett.,* 259, 346, 1990.
45. **Horton, H. R. and Koshland, D. E., Jr.,** Reactions with reactive alkyl halides, *Meth. Enzymol.,* 11, 556, 1967.
46. **Horton, H. R. and Young, G.,** 2-Acetoxy-5-nitrobenzyl chloride. A reagent designed to introduce a reporter group near the active site of chymotrypsin, *Biochim. Biophys. Acta,* 194, 272, 1969.
47. **Uhteg, L. C. and Lundblad, R. L.,** The modification of tryptophan in bovine thrombin, *Biochim. Biophys. Acta,* 491, 551, 1977.
48. **Mole, J. E. and Horton, H. R.,** A kinetic analysis of the enhanced catalytic efficiency of papain modified by 2-hydroxy-5-nitrobenzylation, *Biochemistry,* 12, 5285, 1973.
49. **Chang, S.-M. T. and Horton, H. R.,** Structure of papain modified by reaction with 2-chloromethyl-4-nitrophenyl *N*-carbobenzoxylglycinate, *Biochemistry,* 18, 1559, 1979.
50. **Fontana, A. and Scoffone, E.,** Sulfenyl halides as modifying reagents for polypeptides and proteins, *Meth. Enzymol.,* 25, 482, 1972.
51. **Shechter, Y., Burstein, Y., and Patchornik, A.,** Sulfenylation of tryptophan-62 in hen egg-white lysozyme, *Biochemistry,* 11, 653, 1972.
52. **Bewley, T. A., Kawauchi, H., and Li, C. H.,** Comparative studies of the single tryptophan residue in human chorionic somatomammotropin and human pituitary growth hormone, *Biochemistry,* 11, 4179, 1972.
53. **Wilchek, M. and Miron, T.,** The conversion of tryptophan to 2-thioltryptophan in peptides and proteins, *Biochem. Biophys. Res. Commun.,* 47, 1015, 1972.
54. **Chersi, A. and Zito, R.,** Isolation of tryptophan-containing peptides by adsorption chromatography, *Anal. Biochem.,* 73, 471, 1976.
55. **Rubinstein, M., Schechter, Y., and Patchornik, A.,** Covalent chromatography — the isolation of tryptophanyl containing peptides by novel polymeric reagents, *Biochem. Biophys. Res. Commun.,* 70, 1257, 1976.
56. **Mollier, P., Chwetzoff, S., Bouet, F., Harvey, A. L., and Ménez, A.,** Tryptophan 110, a residue involved in the toxic activity but not in the enzymatic activity of notexin, *Eur. J. Biochem.,* 185, 263, 1989.

Chapter 13

THE MODIFICATION OF TYROSINE

The specific modification of tyrosyl residues (Figure 1) in proteins has provided considerable information regarding the participation of these residues in the catalytic processes of enzymes as well as specific binding processes of proteins. There has also been considerable interest in the modification of tyrosyl residues to introduce spectral probes into proteins such as the modification of tyrosyl residues with aromatic diazonium compounds or tetranitromethane.

There are a number of reagents which may result in the modification of tyrosyl residues. The two most frequently used modifications of tyrosyl residues in proteins are reaction with *N*-acetylimidizole to form the *O*-acetyl derivative and nitration with tetranitromethane to form the 3-nitro derivative. Each of these modifications is considered in some detail later in this chapter.

There is considerable literature concerning the reaction of tyrosyl residues with aromatic diazonium compounds.[1-3] Diazonium salts readily couple with proteins to form colored derivatives with interesting spectral properties. Reaction with diazonium salts is accomplished at alkaline pH (pH 8 to 9, bicarbonate/carbonate or borate buffers). It is relatively difficult to obtain specific residue class modification with the aromatic diazonium salts but tyrosine, lysine, and histidine are rapidly modified.[4,5] Largely as a result of this lack of specificity, the use of this class of reagents has been somewhat limited. The reaction of tyrosyl residues with diazotized arsanilic acid is shown in Figure 2.

The reaction of chymotrypsinogen A with diazotized arsanilic acid has been investigated.[6] Diazotization of arsanilic acid is accomplished by treatment of *p*-arsanilic acid with nitrous acid (0.55 mM sodium nitrite in 0.15 M HCl at 0°C). After adjustment of the pH to 5.5 with NaOH the reagent is diluted to a final concentration of 0.02 M. Reaction with chymotrypsinogen is accomplished in 0.5 M sodium bicarbonate buffer, pH 8.5 with a 20-fold excess of reagent at 0°C. The reaction is terminated by the addition of a sufficient quantity of aqueous phenol (0.1 M) to react with excess reagent. The extent of the formation of monoazotyrosyl and monoazohistidyl derivatives is determined by spectral analysis.[4,5] The extent of reagent incorporation is determined by atomic absorption analysis for arsenic. Tyrosine ($\sim$ 1.0 mol/mol) and lysine ($\sim$ 4 mol/mol) were the only amino acid residues modified to any significant extent under these reaction conditions. The arsaniloazo functional group provides a spectral probe that can be used to study conformational change in proteins. In this particular study, there was a substantial change in the circular dichroism spectrum during the activation of the modified chymotrypsinogen preparation by trypsin. It is of interest that the modification of chymotrypsinogen by diazotized arsanilic acid does not apparently affect either the rate of activation or amount of potential catalytic activity as judged by the hydrolysis of *N*-benzoyl-L-tyrosine ethyl ester.

The reaction of α-chymotrypsin with three diazonium salt derivatives (analogs) of *N*-acetyl-D-phenylanine methyl ester[7] has been studied. The corresponding aromatic amine was converted to the diazonium salt by the action of nitrous acid (sodium nitrite per 0.6 M HCl at 0°C) and, after neutralization (NaOH) and dilution with 0.2 M sodium borate, pH 8.4, was used immediately for the modification of α-chymotrypsin (diazonium salt at a tenfold molar excess) in 0.2 M sodium borate, pH 8.4 at ambient temperature for 1 h. The reaction was terminated by gel filtration (G-25 Sephadex) in 0.001 M HCl. Amino acid analysis showed that only tyrosine is modified under these reaction conditions. Subsequent analysis showed that Tyr[146] is modified by each of the three reagents. The peptide with the modified tyrosine residue (possessing a yellow color) absorbs to the gel filtration matrix (G-10 equilibrated with 0.001 M HCl) and is eluted with 50% acetic acid. (This phenomenon is

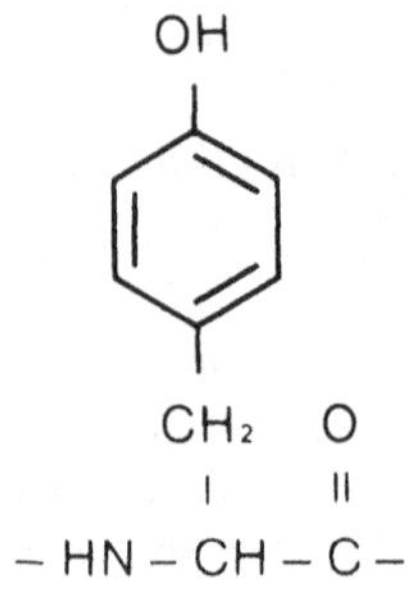

FIGURE 1.   The structure of tyrosine.

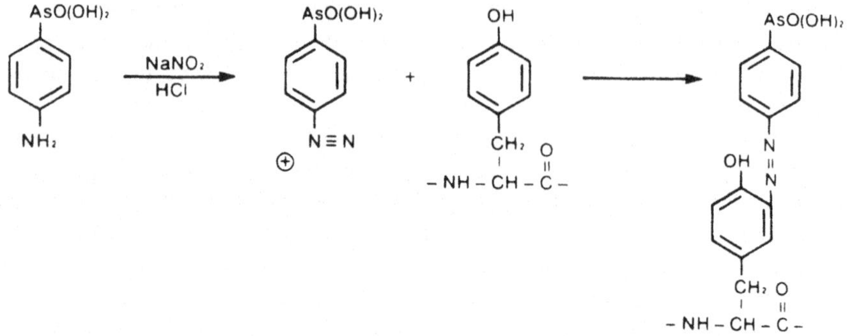

FIGURE 2.   The formation of diazotized arsanilic acid and the modification of tyrosine with this reagent.

somewhat similar to that observed with tryptophan-containing peptides which have been modified with 2-hydroxy-5-nitrobenzyl bromide.[8])

Pancreatic ribonuclease has been modified by a diazonium salt derivative of uridine 2′(3′)5′-diphosphate.[9] Modification occurs at a specific tyrosine residue (Tyr[73]). Modification of ribonuclease with 5′-(4-diazophenyl phosphoryl)–uridine 2′(3′)-phosphate was accomplished by *in situ* generation of the diazonium salt from the corresponding amine by $NaNO_2$/ HCl in the cold. The pH was then adjusted to pH 8.4 (NaOH); the solution was added to ribonuclease in 0.1 M borate, pH 8.4 and the reaction allowed to proceed for 1 h at ambient temperature. The reaction was terminated by gel filtration (G-25 Sephadex) in 0.1 M acetic acid. The extent of modification was determined by spectral analysis and by amino acid analysis. Tyrosine was the only amino acid residue modified. Although it is relatively easy to assess the loss of tyrosyl residues, precise determination of diazotization can be obtained only after reduction to the corresponding amine with sodium sulfite. These investigators also examined the reaction of ribonuclease with *p*-diazophenylphosphate under the same conditions of solvent and temperature. Reaction with this reagent was far less specific, with losses of lysine, histidine, and tyrosine (3 mol/mol ribonuclease).

Reaction of bovine carboxypeptidase A with various diazonium salts has been explored in greater detail than that of the above proteins. Vallee and co-workers[10,11] reported on the reaction of bovine carboxypeptidase A crystals with diazotized *p*-arsanilic acid (conditions not specified) and obtained specific modification of Tyr[248]. Purification of the peptide containing the modified tyrosine residue was achieved by using antibody directed against the arsaniloazotyrosyl group. The antibodies were obtained from rabbits using arsaniloazovalbumin and arsaniloazobovine γ-globulin as antigen. The reaction of bovine carboxypeptidase A with diazotized 5-amino-1H-tetrazole has been reported.[12] Diazotized 5-amino-1H-tetra-

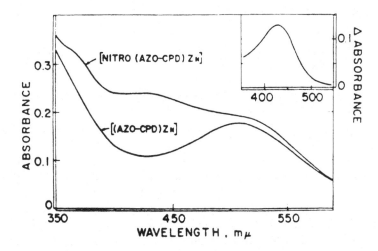

FIGURE 3. The UV absorption spectra of azocarboxypeptidase and nitroazocarboxypeptidase. Azocarboxypeptidase was obtained by the reaction of carboxypeptidase A with a sevenfold molar excess of diazonium-1H-tetrazole in 1.0 M NaCl - 0.067 M potassium bicarbonate/carbonate, pH 8.8, at 0 to 4°C; the reaction was quenched after 30 min by the addition of excess Tris-Cl, pH 8.0 and excess reagent removed by dialysis. Nitroazocarboxypeptidase was obtained by the reaction of tetranitromethane with carboxypeptidase previously modified with a sevenfold molar excess of diazonium-1H-tetrazole as described above. Shown is the absorption spectra of azocarboxypeptidase ((AZO CPD)ZN) and nitroazocarboxypeptidase (NITRO (AZO CPN)ZN) in 0.1 N NaOH both at 100 μM. The inset represents the difference spectrum of nitroazocarboxypeptidase minus azocarboxypeptidase. (From Riordan, J. F., Sokolovsky, M., and Vallee, B. L., *Biochemistry*, 6, 3609, 1967. With permission.)

zole also specifically reacts with Tyr[248] in bovine carboxypeptidase A (in 0.67 M potassium bicarbonate/carbonate, 1.0 M NaCl, pH 8.8). A sevenfold molar excess of reagent was used and the reaction terminated after 30 min by the addition of Tris buffer. The extent of modification of tyrosine to tetrazolylazotyrosine is determined by absorbance at 483 nm (Figure 3) ($\epsilon = 8.7 \times 10^3$ M^{-1} cm^{-1}). Modification of Tyr[248] in carboxypeptidase A by this reagent permits the subsequent modification of Tyr[198] by tetranitromethane.

More recently, Bagert and Rohm[13] have demonstrated that tyrosine residues in *E. coli* asparaginase can be selectively modified with *N*-bromosuccinimide (50 mM sodium borate, pH 8.5 at 0°C). Under these conditions, *N*-bromosuccinimide appears to act as an affinity label. Diazonium-1H-tetrazole modified the same tyrosyl residue.

Iodination is somewhat infrequently used for the modification of tyrosyl residues in protein.[14] The reaction is still of considerable value since the process of the radiolabeling of proteins with either of the iodine radioisotopes (^{125}I, ^{131}I) primarily involves the modification of tyrosine residues in proteins. It is, of course, of critical importance to appreciate the strength of the elemental halides as oxidizing agents.

Iodination has been utilized to study the reactivity of tyrosyl residues in cytochrome b$_5$.[15] Iodination is accomplished with a tenfold molar excess of I$_2$ (15 mM I$_2$ in 30 mM KI) in 0.025 M sodium borate, pH 9.8. Iodination with limiting amounts of iodine is accomplished with a two- to six-fold molar excess of iodine in 0.020 M potassium phosphate, pH 7.5 at 0°C. Monoiodination and diiodination of tyrosyl residues is observed. Iodination with a tenfold molar excess of I$_2$ results in the formation of 3 mol of diiodotyrosine per mole of cytochrome c.[16] The fourth tyrosyl residue is modified only in the presence of 4.0 M urea. Iodination of tyrosine results in a decrease in the pKa of the phenolic hydroxyl groups. Iodination with a limiting amount of iodine as described above results first in the formation of 2 mol of monoiodotyrosine, and then 1 mol of diiodotyrosine, and 1 mol of monoiodotyrosine. Tyrosyl residues which can be iodinated are also available for *O*-acetylation with acetic anhydride (0.1 M potassium phosphate, pH 7.5; acetic anhydride added in two portions over 1 h at 0°C; maintained at pH 7.8 with NaOH (1 M) addition).

The modification of tyrosyl residues in phosphoglucomutase by iodination has been reported.[17] Modification is achieved by reaction in $0.1\ M$ borate, pH 9.5 with 1 mM I_2 (obtained by an appropriate dilution of a stock iodine/iodide solution, $0.05\ M$ I_2 in $0.24\ M$ KI) at 0°C for 10 min. Complete loss of enzymatic activity was observed with these reaction conditions, but the stoichiometry of modification was not established. Nitration of 7/20 tyrosyl residues resulted in 83% loss of catalytic activity. These investigators also studied the reaction of phosphoglucomutase with diazotized sulfanilic acid and *N*-acetylimidazole.

The above modifications utilize reaction of tyrosyl residues in proteins with iodine/iodide solutions at alkaline pH. Iodination of tyrosyl residues can also be accomplished with iodine monochloride (ICl) at mildly alkaline pH. One such study explores the modification of galactosyltransferase.[18] The modification is accomplished by reaction in $0.2\ M$ sodium borate, pH 8.0. The reaction is initiated by desired amount of a stock solution of ICl.[19] A stock solution of $0.02\ M$ ICl is prepared by adding 21 ml $11.8\ M$ HCl (stock concentrated HCl) to approximately 150 ml of H_2O containing 0.555 g KCl, 0.3567 g KIO_3, and 29.23 g NaCl. The solvent is taken to a final volume of 250 ml with H_2O. Free iodine is then extracted with CCl_4, if necessary, and the solution aerated to remove trace amounts of CCl_4. The resulting solution of ICl is stable for an indefinite period of time under ambient conditions. Reaction proceeds for 1 min at ambient temperature and is terminated by the addition of a 1/6 volume of $0.5\ M$ $Na_2S_2O_3$ (50 µl for a 0.300-ml reaction mixture). Radiolabeled sodium iodide ($Na^{125}I$) is included to provide a mechanism for establishing the stoichiometry of the reaction. The reaction mixture, after the addition of $Na_2S_2O_3$, is subjected to gel filtration on Bio-Gel P-10 in $0.1\ M$ Tris, pH 7.4. In experiments designed to assess the relationships between reagent (ICl) concentration and the extent of modification, a maximum of 10 g-atom of iodine were incorporated into galactosyltransferase at a 40-fold molar excess of reagent. Incorporation of iodine is linear up to this excess of reagent and slowly declines at higher concentration of ICl. Modification of tryptophanyl residues was excluded by direct analysis, and the only iodinated amino acids obtained from the modified protein were monoiodotyrosine and diiodotyrosine. Modification of other residues such as histidine and methionine by oxidation without incorporation of iodine was not excluded.

Iodination can also be accomplished by peroxidase per H_2O_2 per NaI. A recent procedure was described for the modification of tyrosyl residues in insulin.[20] In these studies 20 mg of porcine insulin in 20 ml $0.4\ M$ sodium phosphate, $6.0\ M$ urea, pH 7.8 was combined with 10 ml $Na^{125}I$ (1 mCi) and 3.6 mg urea, and H_2O_2 (5 µl 0.3 mM solution) and peroxidase (Sigma, 0.2 mg/ml; 5 µl) added. The preparative reaction was terminated by dilution with an equal volume of 40% (w/v) sucrose. It is of interest to note that the enzyme-catalyzed iodination proceeds with efficiency in $6.0\ M$ urea. Iodination of tyrosyl residues in peptides and proteins can also be accomplished with chloramine T.[21,22] In a recent study,[23] the solution structure of insulin-like growth factor was investigated by iodination of tyrosyl residues mediated by either chloramine T or lactoperoxidase. Chloramine T was more effective than lactoperoxidase.

Tyrosyl residues in proteins are also modified by reaction with cyanuric fluoride (Figure 4).[24,25] The reaction proceeds at alkaline pH (9.1) via modification of the phenolic hydroxyl group with a change in the spectral properties of tyrosine. The phenolic hydroxyl groups must be ionized (phenoxide ion) for reaction with cyanuric fluoride. The modification of tyrosyl residues in elastase[26] and yeast hexokinase[27] with cyanuric fluoride has been reported.

Modification of tyrosyl residues can occur as an interesting side reaction with other residue-specific reagents such as 7-chloro-4-nitrobenzo-2-oxa-1,3-diazole.[28,29] Nbf-Cl reacts primarily with amino groups and sulfydryl groups in proteins. A scheme for the reaction of Nbf-Cl with tyrosine and subsequent reversal by a thiol compound is shown in Figure 5. The reaction product obtained with tyrosine, unlike that obtained with either amino groups or sulfydryl groups, is not fluorescent and has an absorption maximum at 385 nm compared to 475 nm for amino derivatives and 425 nm for sulfydryl derivatives.[28] Transfer of the Nbf

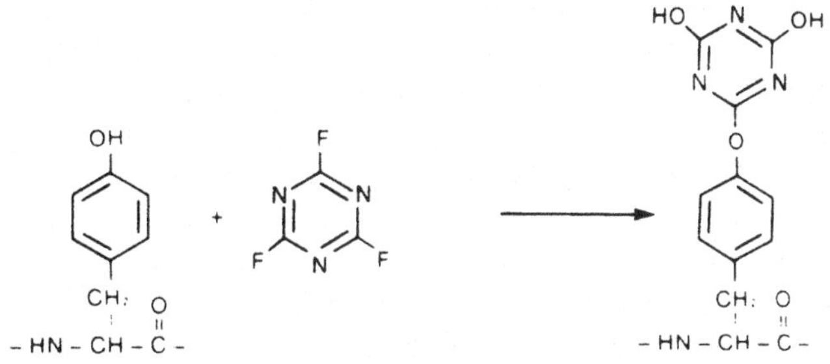

FIGURE 4. A scheme for the modification of tyrosyl residues with cyanuric fluoride.

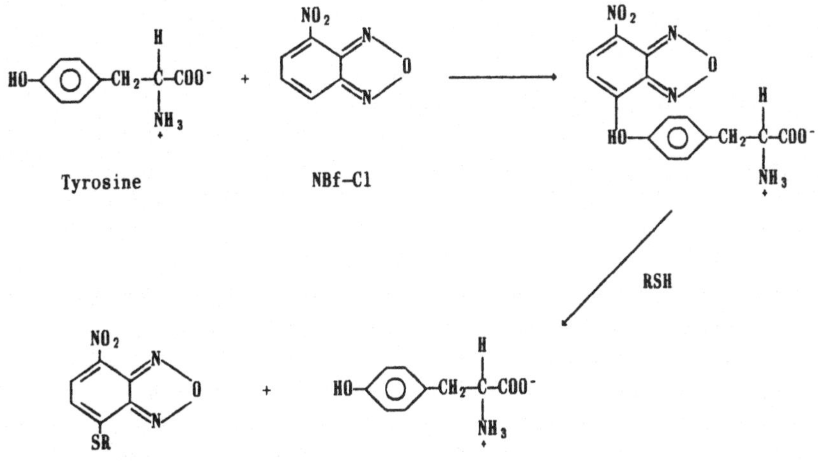

FIGURE 5. The structure of 7-chloro-4-nitrobenzo-2-oxa-1,3-diazole (Nbf-Cl) including a scheme for reaction with tyrosine and reversal with a thiol.

moiety from the phenolic hydroxyl group of tyrosine to a nitrogen nucleophile in a protein has been observed.[29] Modification of the phenolic hydroxyl group with 2,4-dinitrofluorobenzene has also been reported.[30]

Although the above reagents have proved useful for the selective modification of tyrosyl residues in proteins, the majority of the studies in this area have utilized reaction with either N-acetylimidazole and/or tetranitromethane.

The development of N-acetylimidazole as a reagent (Figure 6) for the selective modification of tyrosyl residues can, in part, be traced to the early observations[31-33] that N-acetylimidazole is, in fact, an energy-rich compound. The preparation of O-acyl derivatives via the action of carboxylic acid anhydrides (i.e., acetic anhydride) has been used for some time, but it is very difficult to obtain selective modification of tyrosine as these reagents readily react with primary amines to form stable N-acyl derivatives.[34,35] It is, however, possible to obtain the selective modification of tyrosine with acetic anhydride by reaction at mildly acidic pH (1.0 M acetate, pH 5.8, 25°C); approximately 20,000-fold molar excess of acetic anhydride (5.1 × 10^{-2} M acetic anhydride, 2.9 × 10^{-6} M enzyme).[36] Bernad and colleagues[37] have reported on an extensive study comparing the modification of lysyl residues and tyrosyl residues in lysozyme with dicarboxylic acid anhydrides. In 50 mM HEPES-1.25 M NaCl, pH 8.2, amino groups (primarily lysine residues) were far more reactive than hydroxyl groups (including tyrosine, serine, and threonine).

A related reaction is the trimesylation of tyrosyl with di(trimethylsilylethyl) trimesic acid.[38]

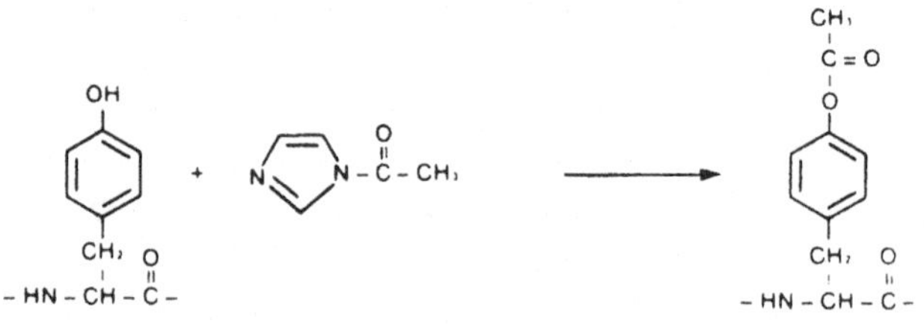

FIGURE 6.   A scheme for the reaction of tyrosyl residues with *N*-acetylimidazole.

This reaction has been used to solubilize membrane proteins and modification occurs at other hydroxyl groups (i.e., serine and threonine) as well as at amino functional groups.

N-acetylimidazole was first used as a reagent for the modification of tyrosyl residues in bovine pancreatic carboxypeptidase A.[39] This same group of investigators subsequently reported on the use of *N*-acetylimidazole for the determination of "free" tyrosyl residues in proteins[40] as opposed to "buried" residues. This has not necessarily proved to be the case.[41] The reaction of *N*-acetylimidazole with proteins has been well characterized.[42] *N*-acetylimidazole is commercially available but also can be easily synthesized.[33] Our laboratory generally synthesizes the reagent and always subjects reagent obtained from a commercial source to recrystallization from benzene after drying with sodium sulfate. It should be noted that, as with many reagents, *N*-acetylimidazole is hygroscopic and should be stored in a container, preferably a vacuum desiccator, over a suitable desiccant. A partial listing of proteins which have been modified with *N*-acetylimidazole is presented in Table 1. A stock solution of reagent is prepared in *dry* benzene (this stock solution is relatively stable for 2 to 4 weeks at 4°C) and a portion containing the desired amount of reagent introduced to the reaction vessel. The solvent (benzene) is removed by a stream of *dry* air or *dry* nitrogen. The reaction is initiated by the addition of the protein solution to be modified to the residue of reagent. The reaction is usually performed at pH 7.0 to 7.5. A wide variety of buffers has been used for the study of the reaction of *N*-acetylimidazole. A high concentration of nucleophilic species such as Tris should be avoided because of reagent instability.[39] Likewise, although the modification occurs more rapidly at pH values more alkaline than 7.5, reagent and product (*O*-acetyl tyrosine) stability become a significant problem.

There are several approaches to the determination of the extent of tyrosine modification by *N*-acetylimidazole. The amount of acetylhydroxamate produced by the reaction of hydroxylamine can be determined.[43] The procedure described by these investigators involves the addition of 0.25 ml of a hydroxylamine solution (4 M $NH_2OH \cdot HCl$/3.5 M NaOH/0.001 M EDTA; 1/2/1) to 1.0 ml of the acetylated protein sample. After 1 min, 0.5 ml 25% trichloroacetic acid and 0.5 ml 20% $FeCl_2$, 6 H_2O in 2.5 M HCl is added and the absorbance of the supernatant fraction determined at 540 nm. We have found it convenient to use *p*-nitrophenyl acetate as the standard for this reaction. Secondly, *O*-acetylation of tyrosine produced a decrease in absorption at 278 nm. A $\Delta\epsilon = 1160\ M^{-1}\ cm^{-1}$ has been reported[42] while a subsequent study reported a $\Delta\epsilon = 1210\ M^{-1}\ cm^{-1}$.[41] We have had more reliable results with the latter value in this laboratory. We have also found it more accurate to determine changes in absorbance at 278 nm as a function of time taking into account spectral changes introduced by the addition of reagent to a solvent blank.[41] One of the major advantages of reaction with *N*-acetylimidazole is the ease of reversal of the reaction. The *O*-acetyl derivative of tyrosine is unstable under mildly alkaline conditions, and presence of a nucleophile such as Tris greatly decreases the stability of the *O*-acetyl derivative. Quantitative deacetylation occurs with hydroxylamine at pH 7.5. As would be expected the rate of regeneration of free tyrosine is a function of hydroxylamine concentration. It should be noted that the primary side-reaction products of the reaction of *N*-acetylimidazole with

Table 1
REACTION OF PROTEINS WITH *N*-ACETYLIMIDAZOLE

Protein	Solvent/temp	Reagent excess[a]	*O*–AcTyr/ Tyr[b]	Ref.
Carboxypeptidase[c]	0.02 *M* sodium barbital, 2.0 *M* NaCl, pH 7.5/23°C	60	4.3/19[d]	1
Pepsinogen	0.02 *M* sodium Veronal, 2.0 *M* NaCl, pH 7.5/25°C	60	7/16[e]	2
Pepsin	2.0 *M* NaCl, pH 5.8/25°C[f]	60	9/15[g]	2
Trypsin	0.01 *M* sodium borate, 0.01 *M* CaCl$_2$, pH 7.6/0°C	30	1.7/10[h]	3
Trypsin	0.01 *M* sodium borate,[i] 0.01 *M* CaCl$_2$, pH 7.6/0°C	465	3.0/10[j]	3
α-Amylase[k]	0.02 *M* Tris·Cl, pH 7.5/25°C	500	3.5/12[l]	4
Subtilisin novo	0.016 *M* barbital, pH 7.5/	100	7/10[m]	5
Subtilisin carlsberg	0.016 *M* barbital, pH 7.5/	130	8.4/13[m]	5
Hemerythrin	0.05 *M* sodium borate, 0.05 *M* Tris, pH 7.5/0°C	800	—[n]	6
Thrombin	0.02 *M* Tris, 0.02 *M* imida-zole, 0.02 *M* acetate, pH 7.5/23°C	300	4.4/12	7
Fructose diphosphatase	0.050 *M* sodium borate, pH 7.5	—	—	8
Erythrocyte ATPase				
Stroma	0.010 *M* Tris, pH 7.4/23°C[o]	—	—	9
Intact cells	0.010 *M* Tris, 0.140 *M* NaCl, pH 7.4/23°C[p]	—	—	9
α-Lactalbumin		200	2/5[q]	10,11
Pancreatic colipase	—	—	—	12,13
Pancreatic α-amylase	0.01 *M* phosphate, pH 7.5[r], 0.1 m*M* CaCl/25°C	120	5.9/18	14
Sweet potato α-amylase	0.01 *M* acetate, pH 7.5/ 25°C[r]	120	5.3/17	14
Aspergillus niger glucamy-lase	0.01 *M* acetate, pH 7.5/25°C	120	11.3/33	14
Emulsin β-D-glucosidase	0.01 *M* phosphate, pH 6.1/ 25°C[r]	300	—	15
Human placental taurine transporter	10 m*M* HEPES-Tris, pH 7.4 with 100 m*M* K$_2$SO$_4$ at 22°C	—	—	16
Renal Na,K ATPase	50 m*M* sodium borate with 2 m*M* EDTA, pH 7.5 at 20°C	—	—	17

[a] Moles *N*-acetylimidazole/mole protein.

[b] Moles *O*-acetyltyrosine/moles tyrosine in modified protein.

[c] Bovine pancreatic carboxypeptidase A-Anson.

[d] Changes in catalytic activity reversed by treatment with 0.01 *M* hydroxylamine, pH 7.5 at 23°C. Primary amino groups were not acetylated under those reaction conditions.

[e] Five out of ten lysine residues modified.

[f] pH Maintained by NaOH from pH stat.

[g] Lysine not acetylated under these conditions. Reaction with 1.0 *M* hydroxylamine at pH 5.8 (60 min; 37°C) reversed changes in catalytic activity produced on reaction with *N*-acetylimidazole and presumably deacety-lated *O*-acetyl tyrosyl residues.

[h] Also 1.0 serine and 0.3 lysine.

[i] Also used Tris, TES, HEPES, and barbital buffers without any significant difference in nature of the reac-tion.

[j] Also 1.7 (probably serine and histidine) and 2.5 lysine residues modified.

[k] From *Bacillus subtilis*.

Table 1 (continued)
REACTION OF PROTEINS WITH *N*-ACETYLIMIDAZOLE

[l]   Approximately 2 lysine residues modified under these conditions. Only a single tyrosine residue is modified with tetranitromethane. Either reagent (tetranitromethane or *N*-acetylimidazole) led to a 70 to 80% loss of catalytic activity.

[m]   The reaction with *N*-acetylimidazole was performed with subtilisin preparation previously treated with phenylmethanesulfonyl fluoride. The active enzyme catalyzes the rapid hydrolysis of *N*-acetylimidazole under reaction conditions.

[n]   Reaction performed on protein where lysine residue had been previously blocked by reaction with ethyl acetimidate. *N*-acetylimidazole was added in 4 200-fold molar excess portion at 2-h intervals.

[o]   Reaction for 1 h at ambient temperature with amount of *N*-acetylimidazole equivalent (weight/weight basis) to stroma. The reaction mixture was washed with distilled water to remove *N*-acetylimidazole.

[p]   Reaction for 1 h at ambient temperature. The quantity of *N*-acetylimidazole used is not given. It is stated that this reagent should readily pass across the cell membrane but this conclusion is based on analogy with acetic anhydride.

[q]   Extensive modification of amino groups was reported.

[r]   *N*-acetylimidazole added as a solid; pH maintained at 7.5 with pH stat.

References for Table 1

1. **Simpson, R. T., Riordan, J. F., and Vallee, B. L.,** Functional tyrosyl residues in the active center of bovine pancreatic carboxypeptidase A, *Biochemistry,* 2, 616, 1963.
2. **Perlmann, G. E.,** Acetylation of pepsin and pepsinogen, *J. Biol. Chem.,* 241, 153, 1966.
3. **Houston, L. L. and Walsh, K. A.,** The transient inactivation of trypsin by mild acetylation with *N*-acetylimidazole, *Biochemistry,* 9, 156, 1970.
4. **Connellan, J. M. and Shaw, D. C.,** The inactivation of *Bacillus subtilis* α-amylase by *N*-acetylimidazole and tetranitromethane. Reaction of tyrosyl residues, *J. Biol. Chem.,* 245, 2845, 1970.
5. **Myers, B., II and Glazer, A. N.,** Spectroscopic studies of the exposure of tyrosine residues in proteins with special reference to the subtilisins, *J. Biol. Chem.,* 246, 412, 1971.
6. **Fan, C. C. and York, J. L.,** The role of tyrosine in the hemerythrin active site, *Biochem. Biophys. Res. Commun.,* 47, 472, 1972.
7. **Lundblad, R. L., Harrison, J. H., and Mann, K. G.,** On the reaction of purified bovine thrombin with *N*-acetylimidazole, *Biochemistry,* 12, 409, 1973.
8. **Kirtley, M. E. and Dix, J. C.,** Effects of acetylimidazole on the hydrolysis of fructose diphosphate and *p*-nitrophenyl phosphate by liver fructose diphosphatase, *Biochemistry,* 13, 4469, 1974.
9. **Masiak, S. J. and D'Angelo, G.,** Effects of *N*-acetylimidazole on human erythrocyte ATPase activity. Evidence for a tyrosyl residue at the ATP binding site of the (Na$^+$, K$^+$)-dependent ATPase, *Biochim. Biophys. Acta,* 382, 83, 1975.
10. **Kronman, M. J., Hoffman, W. B., Jeroszko, J., and Sage, G. W.,** Inter and intramolecular interactions of α-lactalbumin. XI. Comparison of the ''exposure'' of tyrosyl, tryptophyl and lysyl side chains in the goat and bovine proteins, *Biochim. Biophys. Acta,* 285, 124, 1972.
11. **Holohan, P., Hoffman, W. B., and Kronman, M. J.,** Chemical modification of tyrosyl and lysyl residues in goat alpha lactalbumin and the effect on the interaction with the galactosyl transferase, *Biochim. Biophys. Acta,* 621, 333, 1980.
12. **Erlanson, C., Barrowman, J. A., and Borgström, B.,** Chemical modifications of pancreatic colipase, *Biochim. Biophys. Acta,* 489, 150, 1977.
13. **Erlanson-Albertsson, C.,** The importance of the tyrosine residues in pancreatic colipase for its activity, *FEBS Lett.,* 117, 295, 1980.
14. **Hoschke, A., Laszlo, E., and Hollo, J.,** A study of the role of tyrosine groups at the active centre of amylolytic enzymes, *Carbohydrate Res.,* 81, 157, 1980.
15. **Kiss, L., Korodi, I., and Nanasi, P.,** Study on the role of tyrosine side-chains at the active center of emulsin β-D-glucosidase, *Biochim. Biophys. Acta,* 662, 308, 1981.
16. **Kulanthaivel, P., Leibach, F. H., Mahesh, V. B., and Ganapathy, V.,** Tyrosine residues are essential for the activity of the human placental taurine transporter, *Biochim. Biophys. Acta,* 985, 139, 1989.
17. **Arguello, J. M. and Kaplan, J. H.,** N-acetylimidazole inactivates renal Na,K-ATPase by disrupting ATP binding at the catalytic site, *Biochemistry,* 29, 5775, 1990.

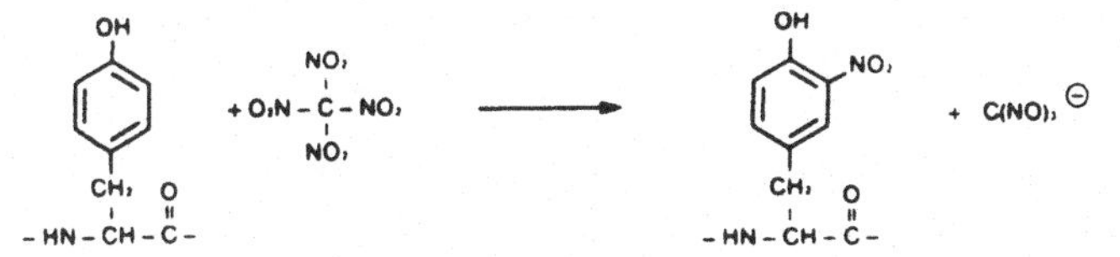

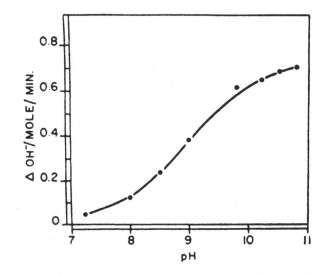

FIGURE 7. A scheme for the modification of tyrosyl residues with te-tranitromethane.

FIGURE 8. Dependence of the rate of nitration of N-acetylty-rosine on pH. Rates were calculated from the initial linear slope of the titration curves when nitrations were performed on the pH-stat. (From Sokolovsky, M., Riordan, J. F., and Vallee, B. L., *Biochemistry*, 5, 3582, 1966. With permission.)

proteins, ϵ-N-acetyllysines and N-acetyl amino terminal amino acids, are stable to neutral or alkaline hydroxylamine. Assignment of changes in the biological activity of a protein on reaction with N-acetylimidazole to the O-acetylation of tyrosine can be verified by the reversibility of such changes in the presence of hydroxylamine.

The possible use of tetranitromethane for the modification of tyrosyl residues in proteins was advanced over 30 years ago.[44] This reagent was used shortly after for the modification of several proteins including thrombin.[45] However, it was not until some 2 decades later that the studies of Vallee, Riordan, and Sokolovsky established the specificity and characteristics of the reaction of tetranitromethane with proteins.[46,47]

The modification (Figure 7) proceeds optimally at alkaline pH (see Figure 8). The rate of modification of N-acetyltyrosine is twice as rapid at pH 8.0 as at pH 7.0; it is approximately ten times as rapid at pH 9.5 as at pH 7.0. As shown above, the reaction of tetranitromethane with tyrosine produces 3-nitrotyrosine, nitroformate, and two protons. The spectral properties of nitroformate (ϵ at 350 nm $= 14,400$) suggested that monitoring the formation of this species would be a sensitive method for monitoring the time course of the reaction of tetranitromethane with tyrosyl residues.[46] Although determining the rate of nitroformate production appears to be effective in studying the reaction of tetranitromethane with model compounds such as N-acetyltyrosine (Figure 9), it has not proved useful with proteins.[48,49] Although the reaction of tetranitromethane with proteins is reasonably specific for tyrosine, oxidation of sulfhydryl groups (Figure 10) has been reported[48,49] as has reaction with his-

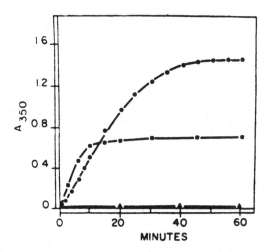

FIGURE 9.   Time course of formation of nitroformate on reaction of tetranitromethane with several amino acid derivatives. Shown is the increase in absorbance at 350 nm on the reaction of tetranitromethane with *N*-acetyltyrosine (●), glutathione (■), and *N*-carbobenzoxyglycyl-L-tryptophan, *N*-acetylhistidine, or *N*-carbobenzoxy-L-methionyl-glycine (▲), all 0.1 m*M*. Tetranitromethane (5 μl, 42 μmol) was added to 3 ml 0.05 *M* Tris, pH 8.0, containing the amino acid derivative at 20°C. The data are corrected for the absorbance due to *N*-acetyl-3-nitrotyrosine. (From Sokolovsky, M., Riordan, J. F., and Vallee, B. L., *Biochemistry, 5,* 3582, 1966. With permission.)

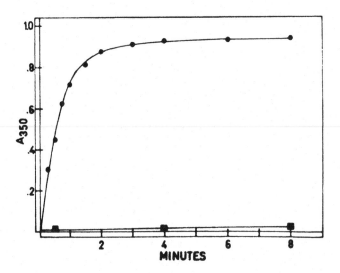

FIGURE 10.   The formation of nitroformate on the reaction of tetranitromethane with reduced or oxidized glutathione. Shown is the increase in A$_{350}$ on the addition of a tenfold molar excess of tetranitromethane to either 100 μ*M* reduced glutathione (●) or 100 μ*M* oxidized glutathione (■) in 0.1 *M* acetate, pH 5.5, at 20°C. (From Sokolovsky, M., Harrell, D., and Riordan, J. F., *Biochemistry, 8,* 4740, 1969. With permission.)

tidine,[48] methionine,[48] and tryptophan.[48,50] Reaction with histidine and tryptophan is, however, unusual and, in general, care need be taken only with respect to potential reaction with sulfhydryl groups. The reaction of tetranitromethane with 2-keto-4-hydroxyglutarate aldolase[51] provides a particularly good example of sulfhydryl modification. Figure 11 describes the inactivation of the enzyme as a function of tetranitromethane concentration in 0.05 *M* Tris, pH 8.0 at 20°C. Cysteinyl residues are lost as a result of this modification (Figure 12). Under conditions where 4 cysteinyl residues are modified in the enzyme, only 0.4 mol of 3-nitrotyrosine is formed per mole of enzyme (Figure 13). The relationship

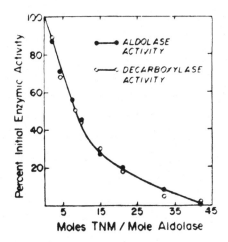

FIGURE 11.   The reaction of 2-keto-4-hydroxyglutarate aldolase (KHG-aldolase) with tetranitromethane. Shown is the inactivation of aldolase and β-decarboxylase activities by varying molar excesses of tetranitromethane. KHG-aldolase (0.24 mg) was incubated in 0.20 ml of 0.05 *M* Tris-HCl buffer (pH 8.0) for 30 min at 20°C with the indicated concentrations of tetranitromethane. Portions were withdrawn, diluted 50-fold with the same buffer at 0°C, and assayed for aldolase and β-decarboxylase activities. (From Lane, R. S. and Dekker, E. E., *Biochemistry*, 11, 3295, 1972. With permission.)

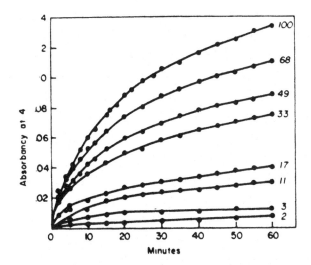

FIGURE 12.   Kinetics of the reaction of 5,5'-dithiobis(2-nitrobenzoic acid) with native and tetranitromethane-modified 2-keto-4-hydroxyglutarate aldolase (KHG-aldolase). Titrations were carried out at 25°C in 1.0 ml of 0.05 *M* Tris-HCl buffer (pH 8.0) with 0.5 m*M* 5,5'-dithiobis(2-nitrobenzoic acid). The protein concentration was approximately 0.4 mg/ml. The values listed in the right-hand margin represent the percent initial KHG-aldolase activity remaining after the enzyme (1.04 mg) was incubated in 0.8 ml of 0.05 *M* Tris-HCl buffer (pH 8.0) for 30 min at 20°C with increasing amounts of tetranitromethane (molar excess 2- to 39-fold). The protein solutions were exhaustively dialyzed against 0.05 *M* Tris-HCl buffer (pH 8.0) at 4°C prior to titration with 5,5'-dithiobis (2-nitrobenzoic acid). (From Lane, R. S. and Dekker, E. E., *Biochemistry*, 11, 3295, 1972. With permission.)

between cysteinyl residue modification and tetranitromethane concentration is shown in Figure 14. The loss of cysteine reflected *both* cystine formation and oxidation to cysteic acid. It is noted that significant reaction with model compounds containing histidine, methionine, or tryptophan was observed only at pH values greater than 8.[48]

The other potential problem associated with the use of tetranitromethane for the modifi-

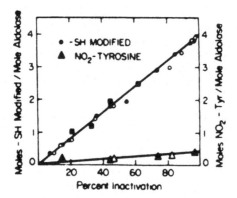

FIGURE 13.   Relationship of tyrosine and cysteine modification to the loss of catalytic activity of 2-keto-4-hydroxyglutarate aldolase (KHG-aldolase) on reaction with tetranitromethane. Shown is the extent of tetranitromethane inactivation as a function of the number of modified cysteinyl and tyrosyl residues. Experimental conditions for the attainment of different levels of inactivation were the same as outlined in the caption to Figure 12. After reaction for 30 min at 20°C, the protein solutions were exhaustively dialyzed against 0.05 M Tris-HCl buffer (pH 8.0) at 4°C. The dialyzed solutions were used to determine protein content, aldolase activity (closed symbols), β-decarboxylase activity (open symbols), sulfhydryl content (○,●), and nitrotyrosyl content (△,▲). The difference in sulfhydryl content between the native and tetranitromethane-inactivated KHG-aldolase was taken as the number of sulfhydryl groups modified; (■), the number of thiol groups modified when the reaction was carried out in the presence of 10 mM DL-2-keto-4-hydroxyglutarate(KHG). (From Lane, R. S. and Dekker, E. E., *Biochemistry*, 11, 3295, 1972. With permission.)

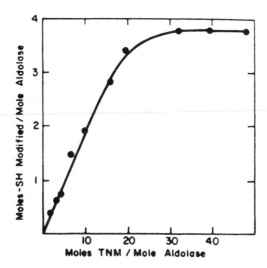

FIGURE 14.   Extent of sulfhydryl group modification in 2-keto-4-hydroxyglutarate aldolase as a function of tetranitromethane (TNM) concentration. Reaction conditions were as described in the caption to Figure 12. After incubation for 30 min at 20°C, the protein solutions were dialyzed exhaustively against 0.05 M Tris-HCl buffer (pH 8.0) at 4°C and sulfhydryl groups were determined by titration with 5,5'-dithiobis(2-nitrobenzoic acid). (From Lane, R. S. and Dekker, E. E., *Biochemistry*, 11,3295, 1972. With permission.)

cation of tyrosyl residues in proteins is the covalent cross-linkage of tyrosyl residues resulting in inter- and intramolecular association. The magnitude of this problem is dependent on variables such as protein concentration and solvent conditions (i.e., pH). With respect to this latter consideration it is noted that acidification of reaction mixtures tends to favor the cross-linkage reaction.[49] As would be expected, the extent of cross-linkage observed varies with the protein being studied. For example, reaction of pancreatic deoxyribonuclease with tetranitromethane results in extensive formation of dimer.[52] Polymerization of protein on treatment with tetranitromethane can be effectively evaluated by gel filtration (Figure 15).

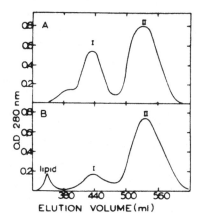

FIGURE 15. Gel filtration patterns of nitrated horse phospholipase A_2 in 1% ammonium bicarbonate, pH 8.0, from a column (3.5 × 300 cm) of Sephadex G-75. The following are the experimental conditions: equine phospholipase A_2 was nitrated in the (A) absence and (B) presence of egg yolk lysolecithin used as the sample. Peaks I represent dimeric enzymes; peaks II are monomeric enzymes. (From Meyer, H., Verhoef, H., Hendriks, F. F. A., Slotboom, A. J., and de Haas, G. H., *Biochemistry*, 18, 3582, 1979. With permission.)

The experiments described in Figure 15[53] deserve further comment. The modification of phospholipase A_2 by tetranitromethane is accomplished in 0.050 M Tris, 0.1 M NaCl, 0.010 M $CaCl_2$, pH 8.0 with a tenfold molar excess of tetranitromethane. The time course for the inactivation of enzyme obtained from either (A) equine, (B) porcine, or (C) bovine sources is shown in Figure 16. When the reaction is performed in the absence of substrate (egg yolk lysolecithin micelles shown in solid symbols in Figure 16), significant polymerization is observed (Figure 15, panel A). When substrate is included, the rate of inactivation is increased (open symbols in Figure 16) and the extent of polymerization decreases (Figure 15, panel B). It is suggested that the increased rate of inactivation reflects the increased solubility of tetranitromethane in the apolar interior of the substrate micelle enhancing reaction with enzyme bound to the micelle. The binding of phospholipase to the micelle reduces polymerization, which probably only occurs with enzyme in solution. Tetranitromethane-mediated cross-linking at tyrosyl residues is a type of zero-length cross-linking (see Chapter 5) and has been recently used to measure the self-association of neurophysin.[54] This technique has permitted the "synthesis" of neurophysin dimers and neurophysin-protein conjugates. A related reaction is the free radical induced cross-linking between tyrosyl residues and thymine providing a basis for the formation of nucleic acid-protein conjugates occurring as a result of ionizing radiation.[55] Finally, treatment of apoovotransferrin with periodate (50 mM HEPES, pH 7.4 with 5 mM sodium periodate) resulted in protein cross-linking via 3,3'-dityrosine.[56]

The extent of modification of tyrosyl residues by tetranitromethane in proteins can be assessed by either spectrophotometric means or by amino acid analysis. At alkaline pH (pH ≥8), 3-nitrotyrosine has an absorption maximum at 428 nm (Figure 17) with $\epsilon = 4100$ M^{-1} cm^{-1}; the absorption maximum of tyrosine at 275 nm increases from $\epsilon = 1360$ M^{-1} cm^{-1} to 4000 M^{-1} cm^{-1}. At acid pH (pH ≤6), the absorption maximum is shifted from 428 nm to 360 nm with an isosbestic point at 381 nm ($\epsilon = 2200$ M^{-1} cm^{-1}) (see Figure 18). We have found it convenient to determine the A_{428} in 0.1 M NaOH. Amino acid analysis after acid hydrolysis has also proved to be a convenient method of assessing the extent of 3-nitrotyrosine formation. 3-Nitrotyrosine is stable to acid hydrolysis (6 N HCl/105°C/24 h).[47] This approach has the added advantage that other modifications of tyrosine such as free radical-mediated cross-linkage can be either excluded or quantitatively determined. If nitration to form 3-nitrotyrosine is the only modification of tyrosyl residues in a protein

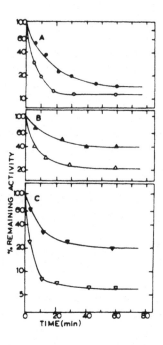

FIGURE 16. The modification of equine, porcine, and bovine phospholipase A$_2$ by tetranitromethane in the presence or absence of egg yolk lysolecithin. Shown is the loss of phospholipase A$_2$ activity as a function of time upon addition of tetranitromethane. The following are the experimental conditions. To a solution (2 ml) of (A) equine, (B) porcine, and (C) bovine phospholipase A$_2$ (1 mg/ml) in a buffer containing 0.1 M NaCl, 10 mM CaCl$_2$, and 50 mM Tris-HCl, pH 8.0, was added 20 μl of a solution of 1% tetranitromethane in ethanol. Incubation was performed at 30°C. At suitable time intervals, portions (25 to 200 μl) were withdrawn for the determination of enzymatic activity; (●) equine, (▲) porcine, and (▼) bovine phospholipases. Similar incubations were made in the presence of egg yolk lysolecithin (10 mg/ml): (○) equine, (△) porcine, and (▽) bovine phospholipases. For the bovine enzyme in the presence of lysolecithin, 50 mM CaCl$_2$ was used. (From Meyer, H., Verhoef, H., Hendriks, F. F. A., Slotboom, A. J., and de Haas, G. H., *Biochemistry*, 18, 3582, 1979. With permission.)

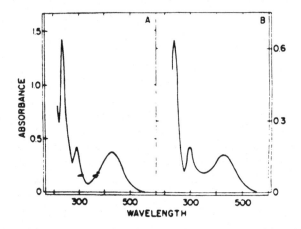

FIGURE 17. UV absorption spectra of *N*-acetyl-3-nitrotyrosine and nitrocarboxypeptidase. Shown is (A) the absorption spectrum of *N*-acetyl-3-nitrotyrosine minus *N*-acetyltyrosine, both at 0.100 mM; (B) the absorption spectrum of nitrocarboxypeptidase minus carboxypeptidase both at 17.6 μM. Both spectra were obtained in 0.05 M Tris-1 M NaCl, pH 8.0, at ambient temperature. (From Riordan, J. F., Sokolovsky, M., and Valiee, B. L., *Biochemistry*, 6, 3609, 1967. With permission.)

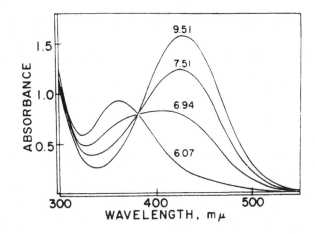

FIGURE 18. pH dependence of the UV absorption spectra of the 3-nitro derivative of tyrosine. Shown are the absorption spectra of *N*-acetyl-3-nitrotyrosine (250 μM) in 0.2 M Tris, 0.2 M acetate, 0.5 M NaCl at the pH indicated. (From Riordan, J. F., Sokolovsky, M., and Vallee, B. L., *Biochemistry*, 6, 358, 1967. With permission.)

occurring on reaction with tetranitromethane, the sum of 3-nitrotyrosine and tyrosine should be equivalent to the amount of tyrosine in the unmodified protein.

There are several consequences of the nitration of a tyrosyl residue. The most obvious is the placing of a somewhat bulky substituent (the nitro group) *ortho* to the phenolic hydroxyl function. The properties of the substituent nitro group "push" electrons into the benzene ring (inductive effect), lowering the pKa of the phenolic hydroxyl from approximately 10.3 to approximately 7.3. This of course means that the phenolic hydroxyl of the nitrated tyrosyl residue will be in a partially ionized state at physiological pH. The nitro function can be reduced to the corresponding amine under relatively mild conditions ($Na_2S_2O_4$, 0.05 M Tris, pH 8.0).[57] The conversion of 3-nitrotyrosine to 3-aminotyrosine is associated with loss of the absorption maximum at 428 nm (Figure 19) and the change in the pKa of the phenolic hydroxyl group from approximately 7.0 to 10.0. The resultant amine function can be subsequently modified.[58]

In addition to changing the properties of a given tyrosyl residue, nitration also introduces a spectral probe which can be used to detect conformational change in the protein. The concept of using reagents to introduce probes with unique spectral and fluorescent properties has been introduced in Chapter 1. 3-Nitrotyrosine has an absorption maximum at 428 nm at alkaline pH. This spectral property was first used by Riordan and co-workers with studies on nitrated carboxypeptidase A[59] to study changes in the microenvironment around the modified residue. Addition of β-phenylpropionate, a competitive inhibitor of carboxypeptidase and nitrated carboxypeptidase, decreased the absorbance of mononitrocarboxypeptidase at 428 nm (Figure 20). This change is consistent with an increase in the hydrophobic quality of the microenvironment surrounding the modified tyrosyl residue. There was a direct correlation between inhibition of esterase activity by β-phenylpropionate and the decrease in absorbance at 428 nm (Figure 21).

Other uses of tetranitromethane in the study of the relationship between structure and function in various proteins are presented in Table 2. The methods used in the various studies are closely related to those described above.

The study of the reaction of tetranitromethane with staphylococcal nuclease[50] is of particular interest for several reasons. First, this study demonstrated that tetranitromethane could modify a tryptophan residue in this protein following denaturation. There were distinctly

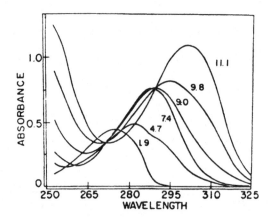

FIGURE 19.   pH Dependence of the UV absorption spectra of the 3-amino derivative of tyrosine. Shown are the absorption spectra of 267 μM 3-aminotyrosine in 0.2 M Tris, 0.2 M acetate, 0.5 M NaCl at the pH value indicated. 3-Aminotyrosine was prepared by the reaction of 3-nitrotyrosine with a 6-fold molar excess of sodium hydrosulfite ($Na_2S_2O_2$) in 0.05 M Tris, pH 8.0. (From Sokolovsky, M., Riordan, J. F., and Vallee, B. L., *Biochem. Biophys. Res. Commun.*, 27, 20, 1967. With permission.)

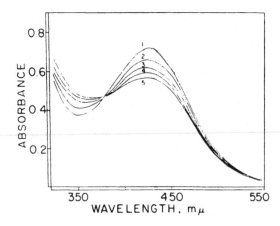

FIGURE 20.   The effect of β-phenylpropionate, a competitive inhibitor of carboxypeptidase, on the UV absorption spectrum of nitrocarboxypeptidase. Spectra were measured in 0.2 M Tris, 0.2 M acetate, 0.5 M NaCl, pH 8.0. The concentrations of β-phenylpropionate were as follows: 1(control), none; 2, 0.01 M; 3, 0.025 M; 4, 0.05 M; and 5, 0.1 M. (From Riordan, J. F., Sokolovsky, M., and Vallee, B. L., *Biochemistry*, 6, 358, 1967. With permission.)

different patterns of reaction (in terms of both extent of modification and residues modified) in the presence and absence of deoxythymidine 3′,5′-diphosphate, a competitive inhibitor, and the ribonuclease activity of the enzyme was affected to a greater degree than the deoxyribonuclease activity. Nitration of one tyrosine residue markedly affected the nitration of a second tyrosyl residue, and a substantial increase in the enzymatic activity of the modified enzyme was obtained by reduction with sodium dithionite under conditions similar to those described above. Selective substitution at the resulting amine group could be achieved, reflecting the low pKa (4.75). In this study, while reaction of dansyl chloride with the native

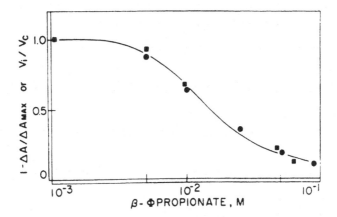

FIGURE 21. The effect of a competitive inhibitor on the catalytic and spectral properties of nitrocarboxypeptidase. Shown is the effect of β-phenylpropionate on the esterase activity (■) and on the absorbance at 428 nm (●) of nitrocarboxypeptidase. $\Delta A / \Delta A_{max}$ represents the fractional decrease in absorbance at 428 nm observed in the presence of the concentration of β-phenylpropionate indicated, while ΔA_{max} is the maximal decrease in absorbance at 428 nm calculated by extrapolation to infinite concentration of β-phenylpropionate. (From Riordan, J. F., Sokolovsky, M., and Vallee, B. L., *Biochemistry*, 6, 358, 1967. With permission.)

protein at pH 8.2 resulted in random modification at a number of lysine residues, reaction with the aminotyrosyl staphylococcal nuclease at pH 5.0 resulted in specific modification. The spectral studies of the two forms of the modified protein shown in Figures 22 and 23 provide an excellent example of the use of 3-nitrotyrosine as a "reporter" group in the protein. Also of interest was the separation of various forms of the modified enzyme by ion-exchange chromatography.

One of the early suggestions for the use of tetranitromethane concerned differentiation between "free" and "buried" tyrosyl residues.[47] Free residues were assumed to be readily accessible to solvent (e.g., on the surface of a globular protein) while buried residues were considered to be in the interior of the molecule (a more "hydrophobic" region). While this may be true in some cases, it is not likely to be a general occurrence. This argument has been addressed by Myers and Glazer.[41] The example of cytochrome c (horse) is worth consideration. Two of the four tyrosyl residues in this protein are converted to 3-nitrotyrosine on reaction with tetranitromethane at pH 8.0 (0.05 M Tris).[60] The two residues modified, Tyr-47 and Tyr-67, are located in the interior while the two residues on the surface of the protein, Tyr-74 and Tyr-97, are not modified. Myers and Glazer emphasize the importance of viewing tetranitromethane (for example) as an organic compound which is more soluble in organic solvents (hydrophobic) than in water. Thus, it is not unreasonable to suggest that reaction at a given residue might, in fact, reflect selective partitioning of the reagent, in this case tetranitromethane, into the microenvironment around the given residue. An analogous situation concerns this increased reaction of phospholipase with tetranitromethane in the presence of substrate (egg yolk lysolecithin).[53] In this case, tetranitromethane is considered to be concentrated in substrate micelles and therefore has an increased rate of reaction with residues involved in substrate binding.

An interesting effect of substrate on the reaction of an enzyme with tetranitromethane has been reported by Christen and Riordan.[61] Generally, protection of an enzyme from loss of activity secondary to chemical modification with the concomitant lack of modification of an amino acid residue is observed in the presence of substrate. Christen and Riordan, however, observed that aspartate aminotransferase was readily inactivated by tetranitromethane only in the presence of both substrates, glutamate and α-keto-glutarate ("syncatalytic" modification). This inactivation was associated with the modification of an additional tyrosyl residue.

Table 2
THE USE OF TETRANITROMETHANE TO MODIFY TYROSYL RESIDUES IN PROTEINS

Protein concentration	Solvent/temp	Molar excess TNM	Residues modified	Ref.
Carboxypeptidase A (10 mg/ml)	0.05 M Tris, 2 M NaCl/20°C	4	1.2/18	1
Staphylococcal nuclease (2 mg/ml)	0.05 M Tris, pH 8.1 (23°C)	2	1.1/7	2
		4	1.6/7	
		8	3.4/7	
		12	3.7/7	
		16	4.2/7	
		20	4.7/7	
		30	5.0/7	
		60	4.8/7	
	4 M guanidine	60	6.4/7	
Horse heart cytochrome c (1 mM)	0.05 M Tris, pH 8.0	16	2/4	3
Aspartate aminotransferase (5 mg/ml)	0.05 M Tris, pH 7.5 (22°C)	30	—	4
Thrombin (0.06 mg/ml)	0.03 M sodium phosphate, pH 8.0 (24°C)	1000	4.9/12	5
2-Keto-4-hydroxyglutarate aldolase (1.2 mg/ml)	0.05 M Tris, pH 8.0			6
Porcine carboxypeptidase-β (5—7 mg/ml)	0.05 M Tris, pH 8.0 (23°C)	8	1.2/21	7
Bovine pituitary growth hormone (4 mg/ml)	0.05 M Tris, pH 8.0 (0°C)	30	2.7/6	8
Ovine pituitary growth hormone (4 mg/ml)	0.05 M Tris, pH 8.0 (0°C)	30	3.0/6	8
Aspartate transcarbamylase (catalytic subunit, 4 mg/ml)	0.1 M potassium phosphate, pH 6.7 (23°C)	2/3/8		9
Mucor miehei protease (1 mg/ml)	0.1 M phosphate, pH 8.0 (15°C)	20	2.8/21	10
Turnip yellow mosaic virus capsids (1.75 mg/ml)	0.05 M Tris, pH 8.0 (22°C)	50	3/3	11
α_1-Antiprotease inhibitor (1 mg/ml)	0.05 M Tris, pH 8.0 (25°C)	120	3/7	12
	5 M guanidine (25°C)	60	7/7	12
α_1-Acid glycoprotein	0.1 M Tris, pH 8.0 (23°C)	10	2.7/12	13
Carboxypeptidase A crystals (5 mg/ml)	0.05 M Tris, pH 8.0 (20°C)		1/9	14
Bovine growth hormone (2 mg/ml)	0.03 M Ringer phosphate (25°C)	12	3/7	15
Equine growth hormone (2 mg/ml)	0.03 M Ringer phosphate (25°C)	12	3/7	15
Lactose repressor protein	0.1 M Tris, 0.1 M mannose, pH 7.8 (23°C)	800	2.4/8	16
Aspartate transcarbamylase (8.3 mg/ml)	0.1 M Tris, acetate (25°C)	750	2.2/10	17
Aspartate transcarbamylase (5 mg/ml)	0.1 M Tris, pH 8.0 (25°C)		2.2/10	18
Human serum albumin	pH 8.0	80	9/18 1.2/18	19,20
Prolactin (1 mg/ml)	0.05 M Tris, pH 8.0 (23°C)	175	1.9/7	21
Porcine pancreatic phospholipase (1 mg/ml)	0.05 M Tris, 0.1 M NaCl, 0.01 M CaCl$_2$, pH 8.0 (30°C)	10	—	22

Table 2 (continued)
THE USE OF TETRANITROMETHANE TO MODIFY TYROSYL RESIDUES IN PROTEINS

Protein concentration	Solvent/temp	Molar excess TNM	Residues modified	Ref.
Equine pancreatic phospholipase (1 mg/ml)	0.05 M Tris, 0.1 M NaCl, 0.01 M CaCl$_2$, pH 8.0 (30°C)	10	—	22
Bovine pancreatic phospholipase (1 mg/ml)	0.05 M Tris, 0.1 M NaCl, 0.01 M CaCl$_2$, pH 8.0 (30°C)	10	—	22
Troponin C (1 mg/ml)	0.05 M Tris, 0.002 M EGTA (23°C)	8	3/3	23
Mouse myeloma protein (5 × 10^{-5} M)	0.01 M Tris, pH 8.2 (23°C)	10		24
Escherichia coli elongation factor G (4—6 mg/ml)	0.1 M Tris, 0.01 M KCl, 5% glycerol, 0.2 mM EDTA, pH 8.0 (25°C)	250	4/20	25
Elapid venom cardiotoxins (7 mg/ml)	0.1 M Tris, pH 7.0 (25°C) or 0.05 M Tris, pH 8.0 (25°C)	—	—	26
Lactose repressor (0.1—1.0 mg/ml)	0.1 M Tris, pH 8.0 or 0.24 M potassium phosphate, 5% glucose, pH 8.0 (23°C)	50	—	27
L-Lactate monooxygenase (1.8 µM)	0.05 M Tris, pH 8.0, 7.5 (30°C)			28
Tryptophanase apoenzyme (0.1 µM)	0.05 M triethanolamine pH 8.0 (30°C)	—	—	29
β-Lactamase (1.3 mg/ml)	0.05 M Tris, pH 8.0 (25°C)	5.20		30
B. subtilis neutral protease	50 mM Tris-Cl, pH 8.0 with 5 mM CaCl$_2$/25°C	60	2	31
Fructose-1,6-bisphosphatase	50 mM Tris-Cl, pH 8.0	50	4	32
Alpha-1-anti-protease inhibitor	50 mM Tris-Cl, pH 8.0 at 22°C	105	3/6	33
Bovine thrombin	50 mM sodium phosphate, pH 8.0 with 100 mM NaCl or 50 mM Tris, pH 8.0 with 100 mM NaCl	50—200	1/12	34

References for Table 2

1. **Riordan, J. F., Sokolovsky, M., and Vallee, B. L.,** The functional tyrosyl residues of carboxypeptidase A. Nitration with tetranitromethane, *Biochemistry,* 6, 3609, 1967.
2. **Cuatrecasas, P., Fuchs, S., and Anfinsen, C. B.,** The tyrosyl residues at the active site of staphylococcal nuclease. Modifications by tetranitromethane, *J. Biol. Chem.,* 243, 4787, 1968.
3. **Skov, K., Hofmann, T., and Williams, G. R.,** The nitration of cytochrome c, *Can. J. Biochem.,* 47, 750, 1969.
4. **Christen, P. and Riordan, J. F.,** Syncatalytic modification of a functional tyrosyl residue in aspartate aminotransferase, *Biochemistry,* 9, 3025, 1970.
5. **Lundblad, R. L. and Harrison, J. H.,** The differential effect of tetranitromethane on the proteinase and esterase activity of bovine thrombin, *Biochem. Biophys. Res. Commun.,* 45, 1344, 1971.
6. **Lane, R. S. and Dekker, E. E.,** Oxidation of sulfhydryl groups of bovine liver 2-keto-4-hydroxyglutarate aldolase by tetranitromethane, *Biochemistry,* 11, 3295, 1972.
7. **Sokolovsky, M.,** Porcine carboxypeptidase B. Nitration of the functional tyrosyl residue with tetranitromethane, *Eur. J. Biochem.,* 25, 267, 1972.
8. **Glaser, C. B., Bewley, T. A., and Li, C. H.,** Reaction of bovine and ovine pituitary growth hormones with tetranitromethane, *Biochemistry,* 12, 3379, 1973.
9. **Kirschner, M. W. and Schachman, H. K.,** Conformational studies on the nitrated catalytic subunit of aspartate transcarbamylase, *Biochemistry,* 12, 2987, 1973.

References for Table 2 (continued)

10. **Rickert, W. S. and McBride-Warren, P. A.,** Structural and functional determinants of *Mucor miehei* protease. IV. Nitration and spectrophotometric titration of tyrosine residues, *Biochim. Biophys. Acta,* 371, 368, 1974.

11. **Re, G. G. and Kaper, J. M.,** Chemical accessibility of tyrosyl and lysyl residues in turnip yellow mosaic virus capsids, *Biochemistry,* 14, 4492, 1975.

12. **Busby, T. F. and Gan, J. C.,** The reaction of tetanitromethane with human plasma α_1-antitrypsin, *Int. J. Biochem.,* 6, 835, 1975.

13. **Kute, T. and Westphal, U.,** Steroid-protein interactions. XXXIV. Chemical modification of α_1-acid glycoprotein for characterization of the progesterone binding site, *Biochim. Biophys. Acta,* 420, 195, 1976.

14. **Muszynska, G. and Riordan, J. F.,** Chemical modification of carboxypeptidase A crystals. Nitration of tyrosine 248, *Biochemistry,* 15, 46, 1976.

15. **Daurat-Larroque, S. T., Portuguez, M. E. M., and Santome, J. A.,** Reaction of bovine and equine growth hormones with tetranitromethane, *Int. J. Peptide Protein Res.,* 9, 119, 1977.

16. **Alexander, M. E., Burgum, A. A., Noall, R. A., Shaw, M. D., and Matthews, K. S.,** Modification of tyrosine residues of the lactose repressor protein, *Biochim. Biophys. Acta,* 493, 367, 1977.

17. **Landfear, S. M., Lipscomb, W. N., and Evans, D. R.,** Functional modifications of aspartate transcarbamylase induced by nitration with tetranitromethane, *J. Biol. Chem.,* 253, 3988, 1978.

18. **Lauritzen, A. M., Landfear, S. M., and Lipscomb, W. N.,** Inactivation of the catalytic subunit of aspartate transcarbamylase by nitration with tetranitromethane, *J. Biol. Chem.,* 255, 602, 1980.

19. **Malan, P. G. and Edelhoch, H.,** Nitration of human serum albumin and bovine and human goiter thyroglobulins with tetranitromethane, *Biochemistry,* 9, 3205, 1970.

20. **Moravek, L., Saber, M. A., and Meloun, B.,** Steric accessibility of tyrosine residues in human serum albumin, *Collect. Czech. Chem. Commun.,* 44, 1657, 1979.

21. **Andersen, T. T., Zamierowski, M. M., and Ebner, K. E.,** Effect of nitration on prolactin activities, *Arch. Biochem. Biophys.,* 192, 112, 1979.

22. **Meyer, H., Verhoef, H., Hendriks, F. F. A., Slotboom, A. J., and de Haas, G. H.,** Comparative studies of tyrosine modification in pancreatic phospholipases. I. Reaction of tetranitromethane with pig, horse, and ox phospholipases A_2 and their zymogens, *Biochemistry,* 18, 3582, 1979.

23. **McCubbin, W. D., Hincke, M. T., and Kay, C. M.,** The utility of the nitrotyrosine chromophore as a spectroscopic probe in troponin C and modulator protein, *Can. J. Biochem.,* 57, 15, 1979.

24. **Gavish, M., Neriah, Y. B., Zakut, R., Givol, D., Dwek, R. A., and Jackson, W. R. C.,** On the role of Tyr 34_L in the antibody combining site of the dinitrophenyl binding protein 315, *Mol. Immunol.,* 16, 957, 1979.

25. **Alakhov, Y. B., Zalite, I. K., and Kashparov, I. A.,** Tyrosine residues in the C-terminal domain of the elongation factor G are essential for its interaction with the ribosome, *Eur. J. Biochem.,* 105, 531, 1980.

26. **Carlsson, F. H. H.,** The preparation of 3-nitrotyrosyl derivatives of three elapid venom cardiotoxins, *Biochim. Biophys. Acta,* 624, 460, 1980.

27. **Hsieh, W.-T. and Matthews, K. S.,** Tetranitromethane modification of the tyrosine residues of the lactose repressor, *J. Biol. Chem.,* 256, 4856, 1981.

28. **Durfor, C. N. and Cromartie, T. H.,** Inactivation of L-lactate monooxygenase by nitration with tetranitromethane, *Arch. Biochem. Biophys.,* 210, 710, 1981.

29. **Nihira, T., Toraya, T., and Fukui, S.,** Modification of tryptophanase with tetranitromethane, *Eur. J. Biochem.,* 119, 273, 1981.

30. **Wolozin, B. L., Myerowitz, R., and Pratt, R. F.,** Specific chemical modification of the readily nitrated tyrosine of the R_{TEM} β-lactamase and of *Bacillus cereus* β-lactamase. I. The role of this tyrosine in β-lactamase catalysis, *Biochim. Biophys. Acta,* 701, 153, 1982.

31. **Kobayashi, R., Kanatani, A., Yoshimoto, T., and Tsuru, D.,** Chemical modification of neutral protease from *Bacillus subtilis* var. *amylosacchariticus* with tetranitromethane: assignment of tyrosyl residues nitrated, *J. Biochem. (Tokyo),* 106, 1110, 1989.

32. **Liu, F. and Fromm, H. J.,** Investigation of the relationship between tyrosyl residues and the adenosine 5'-monophosphate binding site of rabbit liver fructose-1,6-bisphosphatase as studied by chemical modification and nuclear magnetic resonance spectroscopy, *J. Biol. Chem.,* 264, 18320, 1989.

33. **Mierzwa, S. and Chan, S. K.,** Chemical modification of human alpha-1-proteinase inhibitor by tetranitromethane. Structure-function relationship, *Biochem. J.,* 246, 37, 1987.

34. **Lundblad, R. L., Noyes, C. M., Featherstone, G. L., Harrison, J. H., and Jenzano, J. W.,** The reaction of bovine alpha-thrombin with tetranitromethane. Characterization of the modified protein, *J. Biol. Chem.,* 263, 3729, 1988.

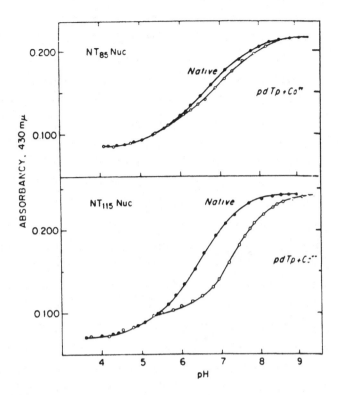

FIGURE 22. Spectrophotometric titrations of the single nitrotyrosyl hydroxyl group of mononitrotyrosyl 85-Staphylococcal nuclease(NT$_{85}$ Nuc) and mononitrotyrosyl-115-Staphylococcal nuclease(NT$_{115}$ Nuc). The upper panel represents the titration of NT$_{85}$ Nuc in the presence (pdTp + Ca^{++}) and absence (native) of 0.21 mM deoxythymidine 3′,5′-diphosphate (pdTp) and 10 mM CaCl$_2$ while the lower panel represents an identical experiment with NT$_{115}$ Nuc. Solution contained 0.05 mM protein in 0.1 N NaCl. (From Cuatrecasas, P., Fuchs, S., and Anfinsen, C. B., *J. Biol. Chem.*, 243, 4787, 1968. With permission.)

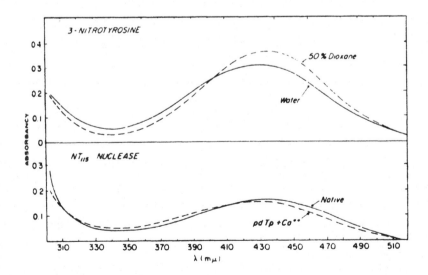

FIGURE 23. Comparison of the absorption spectra of 0.075 mM 3-nitrotyrosine in aqueous medium and in 50% dioxane with that of 0.04 mM NT$_{115}$ Nuc in the absence (native) and presence (pdTp + Ca^{++}) of 0.21 mM deoxythymidine 3′,5′-diphosphate and 10 mM CaCl$_2$. The spectra were determined in 0.05 M Tris-HCl buffer, pH 8.1. (From Cuatrecasas, P., Fuchs, S., and Anfinsen, C. B., *J. Biol. Chem.*, 243, 4787, 1968. With permission.)

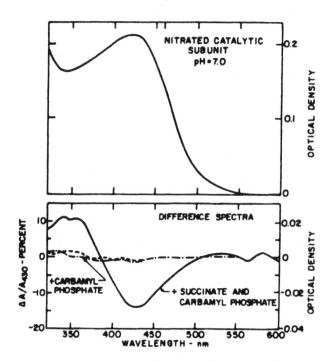

FIGURE 24.   UV absorption spectrum and difference spectrum of the catalytic subunit of aspartate transcarbamylase modified with tetranitromethane. The top panel represents the absorption spectrum of nitrated catalytic subunit containing 0.7 nitrotyrosine/polypeptide chain, at a concentration of 3.0 mg/ml in 0.04 M potassium phosphate buffer (pH 7.0). The bottom panel represents the difference spectra of the same sample. The protein vs. protein spectrum is represented by (- - -) which superimposes with the carbamyl phosphate (2 mM) difference spectrum represented by (—·—·—) above 450 nm. The solid line represents the difference spectrum obtained when succinate (2 mM) and carbamyl phosphate (4 mM) were added to one sample. (From Kirschner, M. W. and Schachman, H. K., *Biochemistry*, 12, 2987, 1973. With permission.)

Kirschner and Schachman[62] have reported some interesting spectral studies on the catalytic subunit of aspartate transcarbamylase modified by tetranitromethane (0.1 M potassium phosphate, pH 6.7). The addition of both substrates, carbamyl phosphate and succinate, resulted in a decrease in absorbance at 430 nm (Figure 24). This is consistent with the increase in the pKa of the phenolic hydroxyl (6.25 to 6.62). It should be noted that these investigators found that for the 3-nitrotyrosyl group in the modified aspartate transcarbamylase, $\epsilon_{430} = 4.0 \times 10^3$ cm^{-1} M^{-1} and $\epsilon_{390} = 2.8 \times 10^{-3}$ cm^{-1} M^{-1} (390 nm is the isosbestic point).

There are two other studies on the use of the spectral properties of proteins modified with tetranitromethane. The modification of pancreatic phospholipase[53] has been discussed above. The spectral properties of the modified enzymes have been reported in some detail.[63] Figure 25 shows a difference spectroscopy study of various nitrated derivatives. Curve A is the change in the UV spectrum of N-acetyl-3-nitrotyrosine ethyl ester accompanying an increase in pH from 6.0 to 8.0 while curve B shows a similar change in the spectra of equine NO$_2$Tyr^{69}-phospholipase A$_2$. Curve C shows the effect of 50% dioxane on the spectrum of the model compound. Curve D shows the effect of n-hexadecylphosphocholine on the UV spectrum of porcine NO$_2$Tyr^{69}-phospholipase A$_2$ while a similar experiment for equine NO$_2$Tyr-phospholipase A$_2$ is presented in curve E. Difference spectra of the dansylamino enzymes (prepared by reaction of dansyl chloride with 3-aminotyrosine obtained by reduction of 3-nitrotyrosine with sodium dithionite[61]) are presented in Figure 26. Difference spectra obtained from the interaction of various phospholipase preparations with n-dodecylphosphocholine below critical micellar concentration are shown in Figure 27.

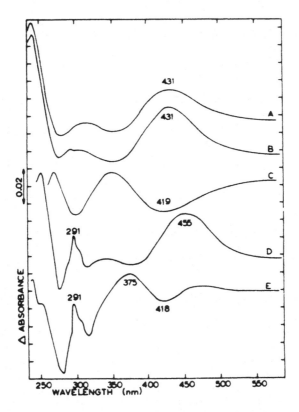

FIGURE 25. UV difference spectra produced by N-acetyl-3-nitrotyrosine ethyl ester and several nitrotyrosine phospholipases upon charge and solvent perturbation. The following are the experimental conditions. Curve A: N-acetyl-3-nitrotyrosine ethyl ester (25 µM) in 0.1 M NaCl and 50 mM sodium acetate, pH 6.0. After equilibration and base-line correction, the sample compartment only was brought to pH 8.0 with solid Tris, and the difference spectrum was recorded. Curve B: horse nitrotyrosine-69 phospholipase A$_2$ (40 µM) treated in the same way as described for curve A. Curve C: N-acetyl-3-nitrotyrosine ethyl ester (50 µM) in 0.2 M PIPES, pH 6.0; 50% dioxane (v/v) was present in the sample compartment and in the buffer solution of the reference compartment. Curve D: pig nitrotyrosine-69 phospholipase A$_2$ (40 µM) in 0.1 M NaCl and 50 mM sodium acetate, pH 6.0, in the presence of 5 mM n-hexadecylphosphocholine. Curve E: horse nitrotyrosine-19 phospholipase A$_2$ (40 µM) treated in the same way as described for curve D. (From Meyer, H., Puijk, W. C., Dijkman, R., Foda-van der Hoorn, M. M. E. L., Pattus, F., Slotboom, A. J., and de Haas, G. H., *Biochemistry*, 18, 3589, 1979. With permission.)

Moravek and co-workers have examined the reaction of human serum albumin with tetranitromethane.[64] This study is of particular interest because 3,5-dinitrotyrosyl residues were reported. While 8 of the 18 tyrosyl residues were readily converted to 3-nitrotyrosine, only 1 or 2 of these residues could be converted to the dinitro derivative.

p-Nitrobenzenesulfonyl fluoride (NBSF) is another environmentally sensitive reagent which can be used for the modification of tyrosyl residues in proteins. This reagent was developed by Liao and co-workers for the selective modification of tyrosyl residues pancreatic DNase.[65] The modification reaction with NBSF can be performed in solvents (i.e., 0.1 M Tris-Cl, pH 8.0; 0.1 M N-ethylmorpholine acetate, pH 8.0) typically used for the modification of tyrosine residues by other reagents such as tetranitromethane or N-acetylimidazole. The rate of reagent hydrolysis is substantial and increases with increasing pH. In a recent study, NBSF has been used to characterize tyrosyl residues in NAD(P)H:quinone reductase.[66] Analysis of the product of the reaction showed that NBSF-modified tyrosyl residues were located in hydrophobic regions of the protein. In another study,[67] the reaction of NBSF with tyrosyl residues in human placental taurine transporter was compared with modification observed with tetranitromethane, N-acetylimidazole, and Nbf-Cl. Tetranitromethane and Nbf-Cl were the most effective reagents. NBSF was an order of magnitude less effective while N-acetylimidazole was 500 times less potent.

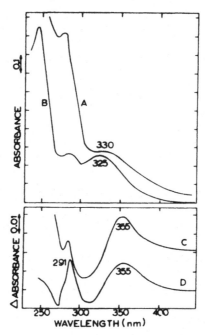

FIGURE 26.   UV (difference) absorbance spectra produced by *N*-acetyl-3-dansylaminotyrosine ethyl ester and horse dansylaminotyrosine-69 phospholipase A$_2$ upon interaction with *n*-hexadecylphosphocholine. The following are the experimental conditions. Absorbance spectra of the protein (45 μ*M;* curve A) and of the model compound (55 μ*M;* curve B) were measured in 0.1 *M* NaCl and 50 m*M* sodium acetate, pH 6.0. Difference absorbance spectra of the model compound (55 μ*M;* curve C) and of the protein (45 μ*M;* curve D) were recorded in the presence of 5 m*M* *n*-hexadecylphosphocholine. (From Meyer, H., Puijk, W. C., Dijkman, R., Foda-van der Hoorn, M. M. E. L., Pattus, F., Slotboom, A. J., and de Haas, G. H., *Biochemistry,* 18, 3589, 1979. With permission.)

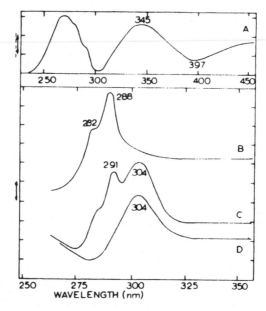

FIGURE 27.   UV difference absorption spectra produced by the interaction of pig nitrotyrosine-69 (A) phospholipase, (B) pig phospholipase, and (C) pig aminotyrosine-69 phospholipase with *n*-dodecylphosphocholine below the critical micellar concentration. The following are the experimental conditions. Protein concentrations were 40 μ*M* in 0.1 *M* NaCl and 50 m*M* sodium acetate, pH 6.0. Phospholipid was added up to 1.0 m*M*. Solvent perturbation of *N*-acetyl-3-aminotyrosine ethyl ester (curve D) was measured in 0.2 *M* PIPES, pH 6.0; 50% dioxane (v/v) was present in the sample compartment and in the buffer solution of the reference compartment. (From Meyer, H., Puijk, W. C., Dijkman, R., Foda-van der Hoorn, M. M. E. L., Pattus, F., Slotboom, A. J., and de Haas, G. H., *Biochemistry,* 18, 3589, 1979. With permission.)

REFERENCES

1. **Landsteiner, K.**, *The Specificity of Serological Reactions*, Harvard University Press, Cambridge, 1945.
2. **Fraenkel-Conrat, H., Bean, R. S., and Lineweaver, H.**, Essential groups for the interaction of ovomucoid (egg white trypsin inhibitor) and trypsin, and for tryptic activity, *J. Biol. Chem.*, 177, 385, 1949.
3. **Riordan, J. F. and Vallee, B. L.**, Diazonium salts as specific reagents and probes of protein conformation, *Meth. Enzymol.*, 25, 521, 1972.
4. **Tabachnick, M. and Sobotka, H.**, Azoproteins. I. Spectrophotometric studies of amino acid azo derivatives, *J. Biol. Chem.*, 234, 1726, 1959.
5. **Tabachnick, M. and Sobotka, H.**, Azoproteins. II. A spectrophotometric study of the coupling of diazotized arsanilic acid with proteins, *J. Biol. Chem.*, 235, 1051, 1960.
6. **Fairclough, G. F., Jr. and Vallee, B. L.**, Arsanilazochymotrypsinogen. The extrinsic Cotton effects of an arsanilazotyrosyl chromophore as a conformation probe of zymogen activation, *Biochemistry*, 10, 2470, 1971.
7. **Gorecki, M., Wilchek, M., and Blumberg, S.**, Modulation of the catalytic properties of α-chymotrypsin by chemical modification at Tyr 146, *Biochim. Biophys. Acta*, 535, 90, 1978.
8. **Robinson, G. W.**, Reaction of a specific tryptophan residue in streptococcal proteinase with 2-hydroxy-5-nitrobenzyl bromide, *J. Biol. Chem.*, 245, 4832, 1970.
9. **Gorecki, M. and Wilchek, M.**, Modification of a specific tyrosine residue of ribonuclease A with a diazonium inhibitor analog, *Biochim. Biophys. Acta*, 532, 81, 1978.
10. **Johansen, J. T., Livingston, D. M., and Vallee, B. L.**, Chemical modification of carboxypeptidase A crystals. Azo coupling with tyrosine-248, *Biochemistry*, 11, 2584, 1972.
11. **Harrison, L. W. and Vallee, B. L.**, Kinetics of substrate and product interactions with arsanilazotyrosine-248 carboxypeptidase A, *Biochemistry*, 17, 4359, 1978.
12. **Cueni, L. and Riordan, J. F.**, Functional tyrosyl residues of carboxypeptidase A. The effect of protein structure on the reactivity of tyrosine-198, *Biochemistry*, 17, 1834, 1978.
13. **Bagert, U. and Röhm, K.-H.**, On the role of histidine and tyrosine residues in *E. coli* asparaginase. Chemical modification and ¹[TH-nuclear magnetic resonance studies, *Biochim. Biophys. Acta*, 999, 36, 1989.
14. **Roholt, O. A. and Pressman, D.**, Iodination-isolation of peptides from the active site, *Meth. Enzymol.*, 25, 438, 1972.
15. **Huntley, T. E. and Strittmatter, P.**, The reactivity of the tyrosyl residues of cytochrome b_5, *J. Biol. Chem.*, 247, 4648, 1972.
16. **McGowan, E. B. and Stellwagen, E.**, Reactivity of individual tyrosyl residues of horse heart ferricytochrome c toward iodination, *Biochemistry*, 9, 3047, 1970.
17. **Layne, P. P. and Najjar, V. A.**, Evidence for a tyrosine residue at the active site of phosphoglucomutase and its interaction with vanadate, *Proc. Natl. Acad. Sci. U.S.A.*, 76, 5010, 1979.
18. **Silva, J. S. and Ebner, K. E.**, Protection by substrates and α-lactalbumin against inactivation of galactosyltransferase by iodine monochloride, *J. Biol. Chem.*, 255, 11262, 1980.
19. **Izzo, J. L., Bale, W. F., Izzo, M. J., and Roncone, A.**, High specific activity labeling of insulin with ¹³¹I, *J. Biol Chem.*, 239, 3743, 1964.
20. **Linde, S., Sonne, O., Hansen, B., and Gliemann, J.**, Monoiodoinsulin labelled in tyrosine residue 16 or 26 of the insulin B-chain. Preparation and characterization of some binding properties, *Hoppe-Seyler's Z. Physiol. Chem.*, 362, 573, 1981.
21. **Hunter, W. M. and Greenwood, F. C.**, Preparation of iodine-131 labelled human growth hormone of high specific activity, *Nature (London)*, 194, 495, 1962.
22. **Heber, D., Odell, W. D., Schedewie, H., and Wolfsen, A. R.**, Improved iodination of peptides for radioimmunoassay and membrane radioreceptor assay, *Clin. Chem.*, 24, 796, 1978.
23. **Maly, P. and Lüthi, C.**, The binding sites of insulin-like growth factor I (IGF I) to type I IGF receptor and to a monoclonal antibody. Mapping by chemical modification of tyrosine residues, *J. Biol. Chem.*, 263, 7068, 1988.
24. **Kurihara, K., Horinishi, H., and Shibata, K.**, Reaction of cyanuric halides with proteins. I. Bound tyrosine residues of insulin and lysozyme as identified with cyanuric fluoride, *Biochim. Biophys. Acta*, 74, 678, 1963.
25. **Gorbunoff, M. J.**, Cyanuration, *Meth. Enzymol.*, 25, 506, 1972.
26. **Gorbunoff, M. J. and Timasheff, S. N.**, The role of tyrosines in elastase, *Arch. Biochem. Biophys.*, 152, 413, 1972.
27. **Coffe, G. and Pudles, J.**, Chemical reactivity of the tyrosyl residues in yeast hexokinase. Properties of the nitroenzyme, *Biochim. Biophys. Acta*, 484, 322, 1977.
28. **Ferguson, S. J., Lloyd, W. J., Lyons, M. H., and Radda, G. K.**, The mitochondrial ATPase. Evidence for a single essential tyrosine residue, *Eur. J. Biochem.*, 54, 117, 1975.

29. **Ferguson, S. J., Lloyd, W. J., and Radda, G. K.,** The mitochondrial ATPase. Selective modification of a nitrogen residue in the β subunit, *Eur. J. Biochem.*, 54, 127, 1975.

30. **Andrews, W. W. and Allison, W. S.,** 1-Fluoro-2,4,-dinitrobenzene modifies a tyrosine residue when it inactivates the bovine mitochondrial F_1-ATPase, *Biochem. Biophys. Res. Commun.*, 99, 813, 1981.

31. **Wieland, T. and Schneider, G.,** *N*-acylimidazoles as acyl derivatives of high energy, *Ann. Chem. Justus Liebigs*, 580, 159, 1953.

32. **Stadtman, E. R. and White, F. H., Jr.,** The enzymic synthesis of *N*-acetylimidazole, *J. Am. Chem. Soc.*, 75, 2022, 1953.

33. **Stadtman, E. R.,** On the energy-rich nature of acetyl imidazole, an enzymatically active compound, in *A Symposium on the Mechanism of Enzyme Action*, McElroy, W. D. and Glass, B., Eds., Johns Hopkins Press, Baltimore, 1954, 581.

34. **Riordan, J. F. and Vallee, B. L.,** Acetylation, *Meth. Enzymol.*, 11, 565, 1967.

35. **Karibian, D., Jones, C., Gertler, A., Dorrington, K. J., and Hofmann, T.,** On the reaction of acetic and maleic anhydrides with elastase. Evidence for a role of the NH_2-terminal valine, *Biochemistry*, 13, 2891, 1974.

36. **Ohnishi, M., Suganuma, T., and Hiromi, K.,** The role of a tyrosine residue of bacterial liquefying α-amylase in the enzymatic hydrolysis of linear substrates as studied by chemical modification with acetic anhydride, *J. Biochem. (Tokyo)*, 76, 7, 1974.

37. **Bernad, A., Nieto, M. A., Vioque, A., and Palacian, E.,** Modification of the amino groups and hydroxyl groups of lysozyme with carboxylic acid anhydrides: a comparative study, *Biochim. Biophys. Acta*, 873, 350, 1986.

38. **Morton, R. C. and Gerber, G. E.,** Water solubilization of membrane proteins. Extensive derivatization with a novel polar derivatizing reagent, *J. Biol. Chem.*, 263, 7989, 1988.

39. **Simpson, R. T., Riordan, J. F., and Vallee, B. L.,** Functional tyrosyl residues in the active center of bovine pancreatic carboxypeptidase A, *Biochemistry*, 2, 616, 1963.

40. **Riordan, J. F., Wacker, W. E. C., and Vallee, B. L.,** *N*-Acetylimidazole: a reagent for determination of "free" tyrosyl residues of proteins, *Biochemistry*, 4, 1758, 1965.

41. **Myers, B. II and Glazer, A. N.,** Spectroscopic studies of the exposure of tyrosine residues in proteins with special reference to the subtilisins, *J. Biol. Chem.*, 246, 412, 1971.

42. **Riordan, J. F. and Vallee, B. L.,** *O*-Acetyltyrosine, *Meth. Enzymol.*, 25, 500, 1972.

43. **Tildon, J. T. and Ogilvie, J. W.,** The esterase activity of bovine mercaptalbumin. The reaction of the protein with *p*-nitrophenyl acetate, *J. Biol. Chem.*, 247, 1265, 1972.

44. **Herriott, R. M.,** Reactions of native proteins with chemical reagents, *Adv. Protein Chem.*, 3, 169, 1947.

45. **Astrup, T.,** Inactivation of thrombin by means of tetranitromethane, *Acta Chem. Scand.*, 1, 744, 1948.

46. **Riordan, J. F., Sokolovsky, M., and Vallee, B. L.,** Tetranitromethane. A reagent for the nitration of tyrosine and tyrosyl residues in proteins, *J. Am. Chem. Soc.*, 88, 4104, 1966.

47. **Sokolovsky, M., Riordan, J. F., and Vallee, B. L.,** Tetranitromethane. A reagent for the nitration of tyrosyl residues in proteins, *Biochemistry*, 5, 3582, 1966.

48. **Sokolovsky, M., Harell, D., and Riordan, J. F.,** Reaction of tetranitromethane with sulfhydryl groups in proteins, *Biochemistry*, 8, 4740, 1969.

49. **Riordan, J. F. and Vallee, B. L.,** Nitration with tetranitromethane, *Meth. Enzymol.*, 25, 515, 1972.

50. **Cuatrecasas, P., Fuchs, S., and Anfinsen, C. B.,** The tyrosyl residues at the active site of staphylococcal nuclease. Modifications by tetranitromethane, *J. Biol. Chem.*, 243, 4787, 1968.

51. **Lane, R. S. and Dekker, E. E.,** Oxidation of sulfhydryl groups of bovine liver 2-keto-4-hydroxyglutarate aldolase by tetranitromethane, *Biochemistry*, 11, 3295, 1972.

52. **Hugli, T. E. and Stein, W. H.,** Involvement of a tyrosine residue in the activity of bovine pancreatic deoxyribonuclease A, *J. Biol. Chem.*, 246, 7191, 1971.

53. **Meyer, H., Verhoef, H., Hendriks, F. F. A., Slotboom, A. J., and de Haas, G. H.,** Comparative studies of tyrosine modification in pancreatic phospholipases. I. Reaction of tetranitromethane with pig, horse and ox phospholipases A_2 and their zymogens, *Biochemistry*, 18, 3582, 1979.

54. **Sardana, V., Carlson, J. D., Breslow, E., and Peyton, D.,** Chemical modification and cross-linking of neurophysin tyrosine-49, *Biochemistry*, 26, 995, 1987.

55. **Margolis, S. A., Coxon, B., Gajewski, E., and Dizdaroglu, M.,** Structure of a hydroxyl radical induced cross-link of thymine and tyrosine, *Biochemistry*, 27, 6353, 1988.

56. **Hsuan, J. J.,** The cross-linking of tyrosine residues in apo-ovotransferrin by treatment with periodate anions, *Biochem. J.*, 247, 467, 1987.

57. **Sokolovsky, M., Riordan, J. F., and Vallee, B. L.,** Conversion of 3-nitrotyrosine to 3-aminotyrosine in peptides and proteins, *Biochem. Biophys. Res. Commun.*, 27, 20, 1967.

58. **Riordan, J. F., Sokolovsky, M., and Vallee, B. L.,** Environmentally sensitive tyrosyl residues. Nitration with tetranitromethane, *Biochemistry*, 6, 358, 1967.

59. **Riordan, J. F., Sokolovsky, M., and Vallee, B. L.,** The functional tyrosyl residues of carboxypeptidase A. Nitration with tetranitromethane, *Biochemistry*, 6, 3609, 1967.

60. **Skov, K., Hofmann, T., and Williams, G. R.,** The nitration of cytochrome c, *Can. J. Biochem.,* 47, 750, 1969.
61. **Christen, P. and Riordan, J. F.,** Syncatalytic modification of a functional tyrosyl residue in aspartate aminotransferase, *Biochemistry,* 9, 3025, 1970.
62. **Kirschner, M. W. and Schachman, H. K.,** Conformational studies on the nitrated catalytic subunit of aspartate transcarbamylase, *Biochemistry,* 12, 2987, 1973.
63. **Meyer, H., Puijk, W. C., Dijkman, R., Foda-van der Hoorn, M. M. E. L., Pattus, F., Slotboom, A. J., and de Haas, G. H.,** Comparative studies of tyrosine modification in pancreatic phospholipases. II. Properties of the nitrotyrosyl, aminotyrosyl, and dansylaminotyrosyl derivatives of pig, horse, and ox phospholipases A_2 and their zymogens, *Biochemistry,* 18, 3589, 1979.
64. **Moravek, L., Saber, M. A., and Meloun, B.,** Steric accessibility of tyrosine residues in human serum albumin, *Collect Czech. Chem. Commun.,* 44, 1657, 1979.
65. **Liao, T.-H., Ting, R. S., and Young, J. E.,** Reactivity of tyrosine in bovine pancreatic deoxyribonuclease with *p*-nitrobenzenesulfonyl fluoride, *J. Biol. Chem.,* 257, 5637.
66. **Haniu, M., Yuan, H., Chen, S., Iyanagi, T., Lee, T. D., and Shively, J. E.,** Structure-function relationship of NAD(P)H:quinone reductase: characterization of NH_2-terminal blocking group and essential tyrosine and lysine residues, *Biochemistry,* 27, 6877, 1988.
67. **Kulanthaivel, P., Leibach, F. H., Mahesh, V. B., and Ganapathy, V.,** Tyrosine residues are essential for the activity of the human placental taurine transporter, *Biochim. Biophys. Acta,* 985, 139, 1989.

Chapter 14

THE MODIFICATION OF CARBOXYL GROUPS

Diazo compounds have proved useful for some time in the esterification of the carboxyl groups of proteins. This is particularly true of diazomethane. The use of this compound was reviewed 20 years ago by the late Philip Wilcox,[1,2] and we are not aware of the extensive use of this compound during the past decade. Various α-keto diazo derivatives have proved particularly fruitful in the study of acid proteinases. Rajagopalan, Stein, and Moore[3] demonstrated that pepsin was inactivated by diazoacetyl-L-norleucine methyl ester. During the course of these studies, it was observed that cupric ions greatly enhanced both the rate and specificity of the modification. Originally it was suggested that cupric ions blocked nonspecific reaction with carboxyl groups not at the active site. Subsequently it was shown that cupric ions and diazoacetyl-norleucine methyl ester formed a highly reactive species, presumably a copper-complexed carbene, which then reacted with a specific *protonated* carboxyl group at the active site of pepsin.[4,5] The modification of carboxyl groups in a variety of acid proteinases with a variety of α-keto diazo compounds is shown in Table 1. These diazo compounds are by no means specific for carboxyl group modification in protein. Benzyloxycarbonyl-phenylalanyldiazomethylketone has been shown to modify cathepsin B_1, presumably by reaction with the active-site sulfhydryl group.[6] Other possible side reactions of α-keto diazo compounds have been reviewed by Widner and Viswanatha.[7] These side reactions result primarily from the oxidative modification of tryptophan, methionine, tyrosine, and cystine. These side reactions can be virtually obviated by vigorous exclusion of oxygen from the reaction and the addition of an oxygen scavenger (e.g., $Na_2S_2O_4$). These compounds are also precursors of carbenes via photoactivation (see Chapter 16).

Other approaches to the conversion of carboxylic acid functional groups to methyl or ethyl esters have been considered. Trialkyloxonium fluoroborate salts (Figure 1) have proved effective. Raftery and co-workers used triethyloxonium fluoroborate to modify the β-carboxyl groups of an aspartic residue essential for the enzymatic activity of lysozyme.[8,9] Paterson and Knowles[10] used trimethyloxonium fluoroborate to determine the number of carboxyl groups in pepsin which are essential for catalytic activity. This article discusses in some depth the rigorous precautions necessary for the preparation of this reagent. This reagent is highly reactive and considerable care is required for its introduction into the reaction mixture containing protein. The reaction is performed at pH 5.0 (0.020 M sodium citrate, pH maintained at 5.0 with 2.5 M NaOH). These investigators also report the preparation of the ^{14}C-labeled reagent from sodium methoxide and [^{14}C] methyliodide.

Woodward and co-workers[11,12] developed N-ethyl-5-phenylisoxazolium-3'-sulfonate (Woodward's Reagent K) and various other N-alkyl-5-phenylisoxazolium fluoroborates as reagents for the "activation" of carboxyl groups for synthetic purposes (Figure 2). Shaw and co-workers[13] used N-ethyl-5-phenylisoxazolium-3-sulfonate, the N-methyl and N-ethyl derivatives of 5-phenylisoxazolium fluoroborate or N-methylbenzisoxazolium fluoroborate (Figure 3) to activate carboxy groups on trypsin for subsequent modification with methylamine or ethylamine. The extent of modification obtained ranged from approximately 3 residues modified (N-methyl-5-phenylisoxazolium fluoroborate or N-ethyl-5-phenylisoxazolium fluoroborate, pH 3.80, 20°C, 80 min) to approximately 11 residues modified (N-methyl-5-phenylisoxazolium fluoroborate, pH 6.0, 20°C, 10 min). Reagent decomposition occurs quite rapidly, even at ice-bath temperature (2°C). The modification appears fairly selective for carboxyl groups although some modification of lysine was observed under conditions where extensive modification was obtained (250-fold molar excess of N-methyl-5-phenylisoxazolium fluoroborate, pH 4.75, 72 min, 20°C, methylamine as the attacking nucleophile).

Table 1
REACTION OF DIAZOACETYL COMPOUNDS WITH ACID PROTEINASES

Reagent	Solvent	Enzyme	Ref.
Diazoacetylnorleucine methyl ester	0.04 M sodium acetate, 0.1 M Cu (OAc)$_2$, pH 5.0	Pepsin	1
Tosyl-L-phenylalanyldiazomethane[a]	6.25 mM acetate, 1 mM CuCl$_2$, pH 5.4	Pepsin	2
α-Diazo-*p*-bromoacetophenone	6 mM acetate, 2 mM CuCl$_2$, pH 5.0	Pepsin	3
1-Diazo-3-(2,4-dinitrophenylamido)-propanone	0.1 M acetate, 1 mM CuSO$_4$, pH 5.6	Pepsin	4
Diazoacetyl-L-phenylalanine methyl ester	0.05 M sodium acetate, 2 mM Cu(OAc)$_2$, pH 5.0	Pepsin	5
Diazoacetylglycine[b] methyl ester	0.02 M sodium acetate, 1 mM Cu(OAc)$_2$, pH 5.6	Pepsin	6
Diazoacetic acid[b] methyl ester	0.02 M sodium acetate, 1 mM Cu(OAc)$_2$, pH 5.6	Pepsin	6
1-Diazo-4-phenyl-2-butanone	0.04 M sodium acetate, 0.1 mM CuSO$_4$, pH 5.5	Pepsin	7
N-Diazoacetyl-N′-2,4-dinitrophenylethylenediamine	0.04 M sodium acetate, 1 mM Cu(OAc)$_2$, pH 5.5	Awamorin[c]	8
Diazoacetylnorleucine methyl ester	0.02 M sodium acetate, Cu(OAc)$_2$[d], pH 5.0—5.6	*Rhizopus chinensis* acid proteinase	9
		Aspergillus saitoi acid proteinase	9
		Mucor pusillus acid proteinase	9
		Calf rennin	9
4-(3-diazo-2-oxopropylidene)-[e] 2,2,6,6-tetramethylpiperidine-1-oxyl	0.1 M sodium acetate, 0.05 mM Cu(OAc)$_2$, pH 5.5	Pepsin	10

[a]   L-1-diazo-4-phenyl-3-tosylamidobutanone.
[b]   Both of these compounds inhibited pepsin in the presence of cupric ions but there was a greater extent of carboxyl group modification than seen with diazoacetylnorleucine methyl ester.
[c]   An acid proteinase isolated from the mold *Aspergillus awamori*.
[d]   40– to 220-fold molar excess of cupric ions (as acetate salt) with respect to the individual enzyme is used with a 40- to 45-fold molar excess of diazoacetylnorleucine methyl ester.
[e]   Other spin-labeled compounds were prepared in this study including the cis and trans isomers of 3-(4-diazo-3-oxo-1-butenyl)-2,2,5,5-tetramethylpyrroline-1-oxyl.

References for Table 1

1. **Rajagopalan, T. G., Stein, W. H., and Moore, S.,** The inactivation of pepsin by diazoacetylnorleucine methyl ester, *J. Biol. Chem.,* 241, 4295, 1966.
2. **Delpierre, G. R. and Fruton, J. S.,** Specific inactivation of pepsin by a diazo ketone, *Proc. Natl. Acad. Sci. U.S.A.,* 56, 1817, 1966.
3. **Erlanger, B. F., Vratsanos, S. M., Wassermann, N., and Cooper, A. G.,** Stereochemical investigation of the active center of pepsin using a new inactivator, *Biochem. Biophys. Res. Commun.,* 28, 203, 1967.
4. **Kozlov, L. V., Ginodman, L. M., and Orekhovich, V. N.,** Inactivation of pepsin with aliphatic diazocarbonyl compounds, *Biokhimiya,* 32, 1011, 1967.
5. **Bayliss, R. S., Knowles, J. R., and Wybrandt, G. B.,** An aspartic acid residue at the active site of pepsin. The isolation and sequence of the heptapeptide, *Biochem. J.,* 113, 377, 1969.
6. **Lundblad, R. L. and Stein, W. H.,** On the reaction of diazoacetyl compounds with pepsin, *J. Biol. Chem.,* 244, 154, 1969.
7. **Fry, K. T., Kim, O.-K., Spona, J., and Hamilton, G. A.,** Site of reaction of a specific diazo inactivator of pepsin, *Biochemistry,* 9, 4624, 1970.

References for Table 1 (continued)

8. **Kovaleva, G. G., Shimanskaya, M. P., and Stepanov, V. M.,** The site of diazoacetyl inhibitor attachment to acid proteinase of *Aspergillus awamori* — An analog of penicillopepsin and pepsin, *Biochem. Biophys. Res. Commun.*, 49, 1075, 1972.
9. **Takahashi, K., Mizobe, F., and Chang, W.-J.,** Inactivation of acid proteases from *Rhizopus chinensis, Aspergillus saitoi* and *Mucor pusillus* and calf rennin by diazoacetyl norleucine methyl ester, *J. Biochem.*, 71, 161, 1972.
10. **Nakayama, S.-I., Nagashima, Y., Hoshino, M., Moriyama, A., Takahashi, K., Uematsu, Y., Watanabe, T., and Yoshida, M.,** Spin-labelling of porcine pepsin and *Rhizopus chinensis* acid protease by diazoketone reagents, *Biochem. Biophys. Res. Commun.*, 101, 658, 1981.

Structure	Nomenclature	Abbreviation
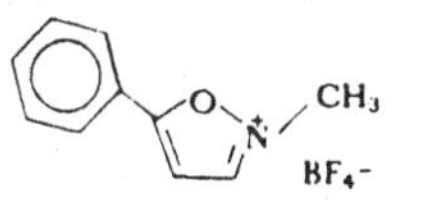	N-Methyl-5-phenylisoxazolium fluoroborate	MPI
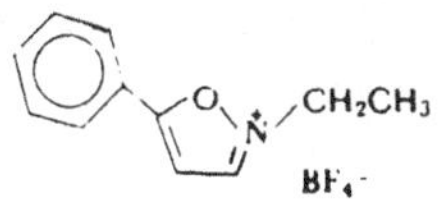	N-Ethyl-5-phenylisoxazolium fluoroborate	EPI
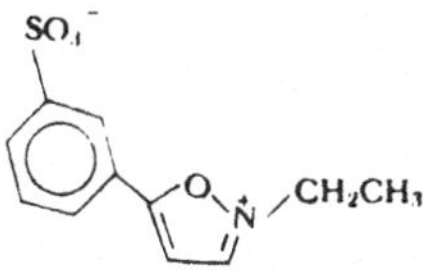	N-Ethyl-5-phenylisoxazolium-3'-sulfonate Woodwards K reagent)	K
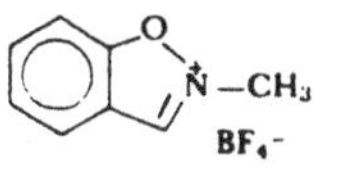	N-Methyl-benzisoxazolium fluoroborate	MBI

FIGURE 1. The structures of some isoxazolium salts. (From Bodlaender, P., Feinstein, G., and Shaw, E., *Biochemistry*, 8, 4941, 1969. With permission.)

Saini and Van Etten[14] reported on the reaction of N-ethyl-5-phenylisoxazolium-3'-sulfonate with human prostatic acid phosphatase. The modification was performed with a 4,000- to 10,000-fold molar excess of reagent in 0.020 M pyridinesulfonic acid, pH 3.6 at 25°C. Ethylamine was utilized as the attacking nucleophile to determine the extent of modification. A substantial number of carboxyl groups in the protein were modified under these experimental conditions. Arana and Vallejos[15] have compared the reaction of chloroplast coupling factor with N-ethyl-5-phenylisoxazolium-3'-sulfonate (Woodward's Reagent K) and dicyclohexylcarbodiimide. Reaction with Woodward's Reagent K was accomplished at 25°C in 0.040 M Tricine, pH 7.9 while reaction with dicyclohexylcarbodiimide was accomplished at 30°C in 0.040 M MOPS, pH 7.4. ATP and derivatives such as ADP and inorganic phosphate protect against the loss of activity occurring upon reaction with Woodward's Reagent K but do not have any effect on inactivation by dicyclohexylcarbodiimide. The reverse was seen with divalent cations such as Ca^{2+}. The modification of an essential carboxyl group in pancreatic phospholipase A_2 by 5-ethyl-5-phenylisoxazolium-3-sulfonate has been

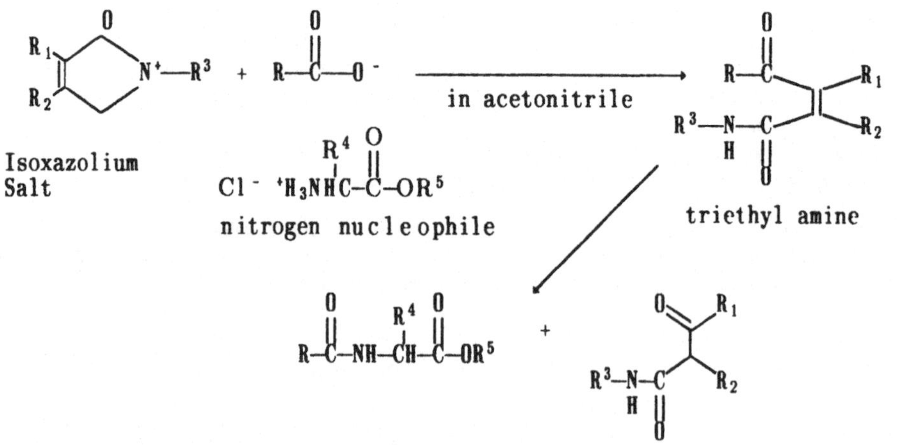

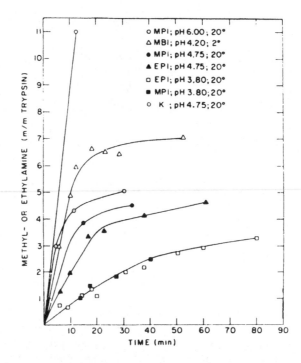

FIGURE 2. Modification of a protein carboxyl group with a nitrogen nucleophile mediated with an isoxazolium salt.

FIGURE 3. The reaction of isoxazolium salts with β-trypsin at various pH values. The isoxazolium salts were MPI, *N*-methyl-5-phenylisoxazolium fluoroborate; EPI, *N*-ethyl-5-phenylisoxazolium fluoroborate; K, *N*-ethyl-5-phenylisoxazolium-3'-sulfonate (Woodwards Reagent K); and MBI, *N*-methyl-benzisoxazolium fluoroborate. In all reactions, the initial reagent and protein concentrations were 10 and 5 mg/ml, respectively, except for the reaction with Reagent K in which the respective concentrations were 5 and 1.5 mg/ml. Each point was obtained by removing a portion from the reaction mixture and adjusting its pH to 2.5 with formic acid at the indicated times. Amino acid analyses were performed on the gel-filtered samples to determine methyl- or ethylamine content per mole of trypsin. (From Bodlaender, P., Feinstein, G., and Shaw, E., *Biochemistry*, 8, 4941, 1969. With permission.)

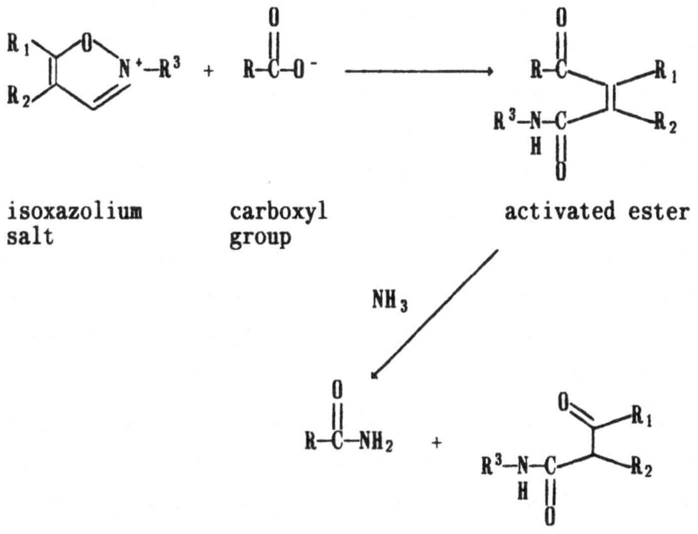

FIGURE 4. Isosteric modification of a carboxyl group.

reported.[16] The reaction was performed in 0.01 M sodium phosphate, pH 4.75 (pH stat) at 25°C. A second-order rate constant of $k_2 = 25.5$ M^{-1} min^{-1} was obtained for the loss of catalytic activity. This rate inactivation is increased more than twofold in the presence of 30 mM CaCl$_2$ (69.3 M^{-1} min^{-1}). Quantitative information on the extent of modification is obtained with [^{14}C] glycine ethyl ester. It is of interest that treatment with a water-soluble carbodiimide, 1-(3'-dimethyl-aminopropyl)-3-ethylcarbodiimide, results in the loss of catalytic activity in a reaction with characteristics different from those seen with Woodward's Reagent K. Koistra and Sluyterman[17] modified guanidated mercuripapain with N-ethylbenziosoxazolium tetrafluoroborate at pH 4.2/0°C to yield a protein modified with N-ethylsalicylamide esters. When the active ester groups on the protein were allowed to undergo amminolysis (2.0 M ammonium acetate, pH 9.2) and the esters were converted to the corresponding amides (an isosteric modification, see Figure 4). The conversion to the amides resulted in the loss of a bulky substituent group with an increase in activity.

The use of carbodiimide-mediated modification (Figure 5) of carboxyl functional groups in proteins is by far the most widely used method for the study of such functional groups (Figure 6). The most popular approach utilizes a water-soluble carbodiimide (Figure 7) as the activating agent as introduced by Hoare and Koshland.[18] These investigators show that virtually quantitative modification of the carboxyl groups in lysozyme (8.1/11), chymotrypsin (15.5/17), and trypsin (12.5/11) occurred with 0.1 M carbodiimide at pH 4.75 with 1.0 M glycine methyl ester in a pH stat at 25°C. The possibility of side reaction was discussed with reference to the possible modification of the phenolic hydroxyl of tyrosine to form the O-arylisourea. Modification of the active-site serine residue in α-chymotrypsin with 1-cyclohexyl-3-(2-morpholinyl-(4)-ethyl) carbodiimide metho-p-toluenesulfonate at neutral pH (Figure 8) has been reported.[19] Note in particular the increased rate at neutral or alkaline pH. This is not consistent with carboxyl group modification which *requires a protonated carboxyl group*. The modification of the active-site cysteinyl group in papain has been reported[20] as occurring under conditions (pH 4.75, 25°C) where 6/14 carboxyl groups are modified together with 9/19 tyrosyl residues. Modification of the tyrosyl residues is reversed by 0.5 M hydroxylamine, pH 7.0 (5 h at 25°C) as first demonstrated by Carraway and Koshland.[21] Despite the problems with side reaction, modification of carboxyl group in proteins with a water-soluble carbodiimide and an appropriate nucleophile (e.g., [^{14}C] glycine ethyl ester, norleucine methyl ester — easily detected by amino acid analysis, aminome-

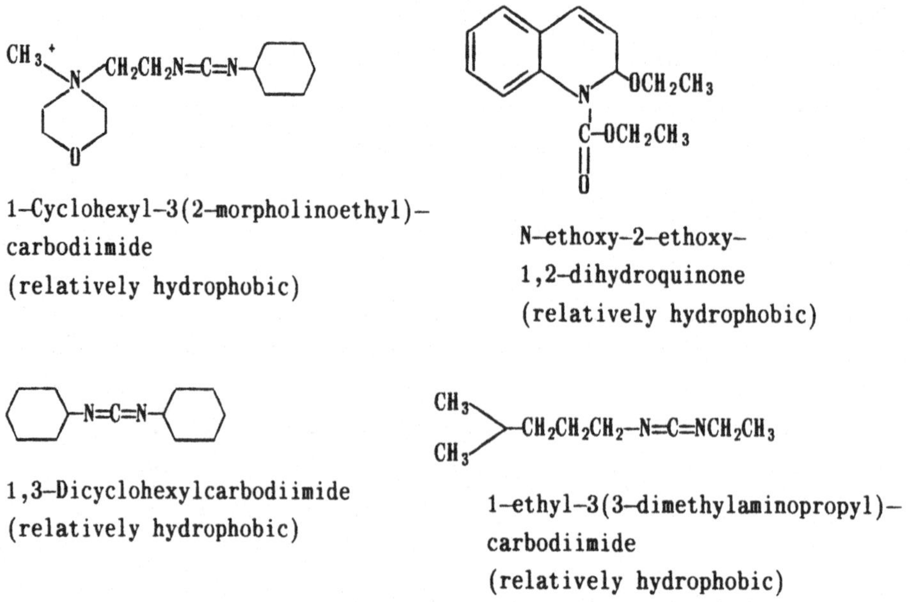

1-Cyclohexyl-3(2-morpholinoethyl)-
carbodiimide
(relatively hydrophobic)

N-ethoxy-2-ethoxy-
1,2-dihydroquinone
(relatively hydrophobic)

1,3-Dicyclohexylcarbodiimide
(relatively hydrophobic)

1-ethyl-3(3-dimethylaminopropyl)-
carbodiimide
(relatively hydrophobic)

FIGURE 5. A comparison of some reagents used for the modification of carboxyl groups in proteins.

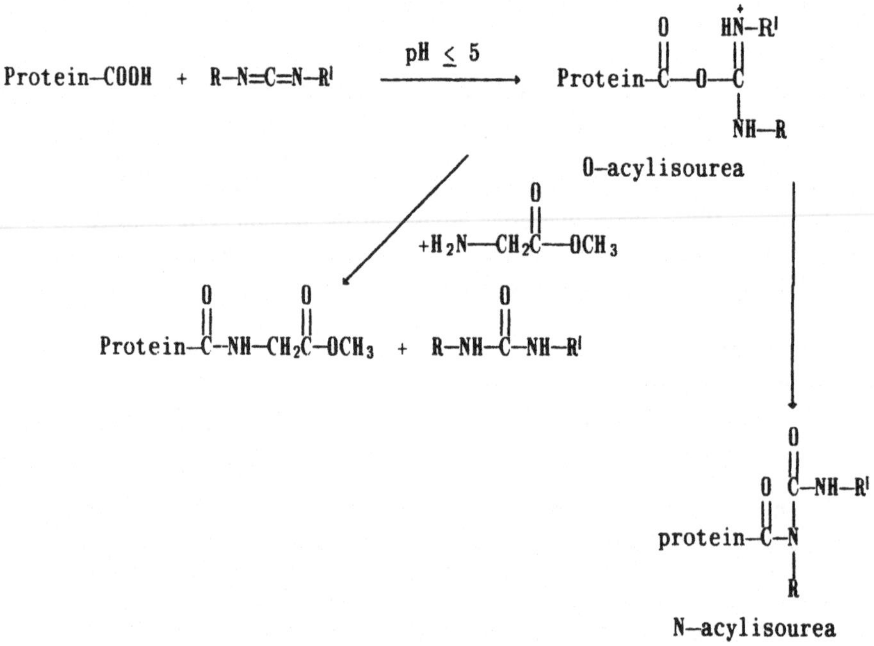

$$Protein-COOH + R-N=C=N-R^{I} \xrightarrow{pH \leq 5}$$

O-acylisourea

$+H_2N-CH_2C-OCH_3$

Protein-C--NH-CH$_2$C-OCH$_3$ + R-NH-C-NH-R^I

N-acylisourea

FIGURE 6. The reaction of carbodiimide with protein carboxyl groups.

thylsulfonic acid) has proved extremely useful.[22] It should be noted that ammonium ions can be used as the attacking nucleophile to generate asparaginyl and glutaminyl residues from "exposed" carboxyl groups. The modification was accomplished in 5.5 M NH$_4$Cl at pH 4.75 for 3 h at 25°C. Under these conditions, approximately 11 of the 15 free carboxyl groups in chymotrypsinogen were converted to the corresponding amide.[23] 1,2-Diamino-ethane or diaminomethane can be coupled to aspartic acid residues to produce a trypsin-

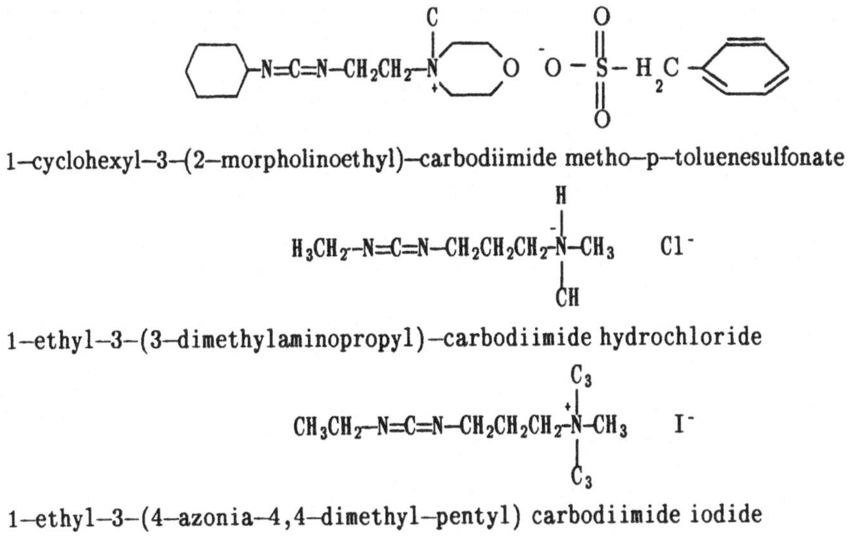

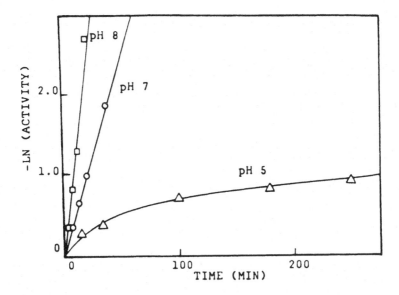

1–cyclohexyl–3–(2–morpholinoethyl)–carbodiimide metho–p–toluenesulfonate

1–ethyl–3–(3–dimethylaminopropyl)–carbodiimide hydrochloride

1–ethyl–3–(4–azonia–4,4–dimethyl–pentyl) carbodiimide iodide

FIGURE 7. Some examples of water-soluble carbodiimides.

FIGURE 8. The effect of pH on the inactivation of α-chymotrypsin by 1-cyclohexyl-3-[2-morpholinyl-(4)-ethyl]carbodiimide metho-p-toluenesulfonate (CMC). The experiments were performed in 0.1 M KCl with α-chymotrypsin (0.1 mg/ml) and 10 mM CMC at 25°C. pH was maintained with a pH stat. (From Banks, T. E., Blossey, B. F., and Schafer, J. A., *J. Biol. Chem.*, 244, 6323, 1969. With permission.)

sensitive bond.[24] Another example of using this chemistry to introduce a new functional group into a protein is provided by the work of Lin et al.[25] This procedure is outlined in Figure 9. The first step involves the water-soluble carbodiimide-mediated coupling of cystamine to protein carboxyl groups. Reduction of the coupled cystamine with dithiothreitol results in 2-aminothiol functional groups bound to protein carboxyl groups. Examples of the use of this approach are given in Table 2.

In addition to the information presented in Table 2, certain examples of carbodiimide-mediated modification should be discussed in greater detail. The inactivation of yeast

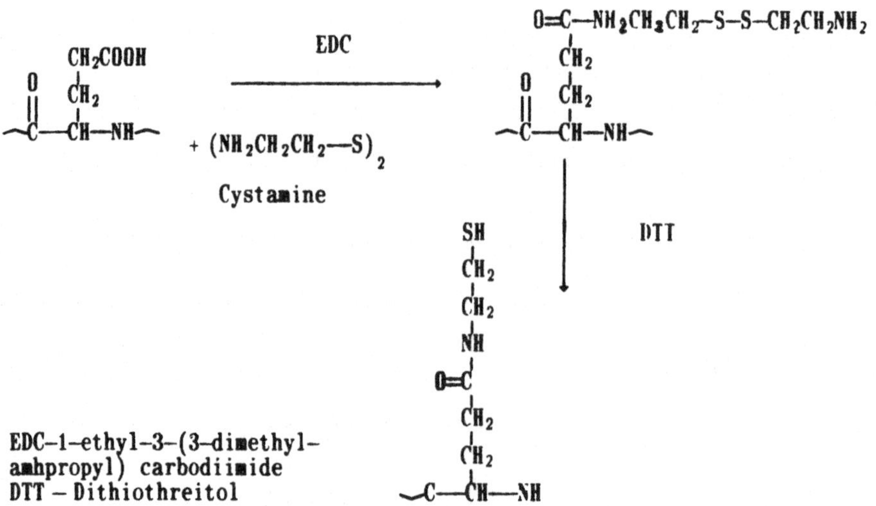

FIGURE 9.   Introduction of a sulfydryl function (2-aminoethanethiol) via isopeptide linkage mediated by a water-soluble carbodiimide.

hexokinase[26] by reaction with 1-cyclohexyl-3-(2-morpholinoethyl) carbodiimide metho-*p*-toluenesulfonate is shown in Figure 10. These experiments should be compared to those shown in Figure 11 with the same reagent in the presence of nitrotyrosine ethyl ester. The use of the nitrotyrosine derivative as the attacking nucleophile allowed the introduction of a "reporter group" onto the glutamyl residue modified in this study. The use of the nitrotyrosyl derivative also permitted the facile determination of the extent of modification (in 0.1 *M* NaOH), thus the nitrotyrosyl derivative had A_{max} at 430 nm ($\epsilon = 4.6 \times 10^{-3} M^{-1}$ cm^{-1}). Studies on the use of this carbodiimide in the modification of phosphorylase b have been reported.[27] Figure 12 shows the reaction of rabbit muscle phosphorylase with 1-cyclohexyl-3-(2-morpholinyl-(4)-ethyl) carbodiimide metho-*p*-toluenesulfonate (CMC) in the absence of added nucleophile while Figure 13 shows the effect of added nucleophiles on the rate of inactivation.

There are several observations on the use of 1-ethyl-3-(3-dimethylaminopropyl)-carbodiimide (EDC). Figure 14 compares the rate of inactivation of yeast enolase[28] with this reagent and several other carbodimides. An exogenous nucleophile was not used in these experiments. Note that 1-ethyl-3-(4-azonia-4,4-dimethylpentyl)-carbodiimide iodide (EAC) appears to be far more effective than the other two carbodiimides under these reaction conditions. In the absence of added nucleophile, the carbodiimide-activated protein carboxyl group may rearrange (Figure 15) to form a substituted *O*-acylurea as described by Borders and co-workers for the modification of thrombin by various water-soluble carbodiimides.[29,30] The selective modification of a single aspartyl residue at the active site of lysozyme (Asp-101)[31] was accomplished by the use of a low molar excess (five- to tenfold) of carbodiimide. A variety of attacking nucleophiles were used in this study (the modification reactions were performed at pH 5.0 maintained with HCl during the reaction). Of particular interest is the success achieved in the separation of the products of the reaction by ion-exchange chromatography as shown in Figure 16 and Figure 17. The modification of pancreatic phospholipase A$_2$ (Figure 18) provides a particularly useful example of the effect of pH on carbodiimide-mediated modification. Note that the inactivation is much more rapid at pH 3.5 than at pH 5.5.

Another possible reaction occurring with a water-soluble carbodiimide and a protein in the absence of added nucleophile is zero-length cross-linking via isopeptide bond formation as described in Chapter 15. This reaction is somewhat favored by participation of an

Table 2
THE MODIFICATION OF CARBOXYL GROUPS IN PROTEINS

Protein	Reaction conditions	Carbodiimide	Molar excess	Nucleophile	Carboxyl groups modified	Other functional groups modified	Ref.
Lysozyme	pH 4.75, 25°C, pH stat,[a] 0.1 M carbodiimide	N-benzyl-N'-3-[b] dimethylamino-propylcarbodiimide	140	1.0 M glycine methyl ester	2.1/11 (5 min) 4.7/11 (60 min) 8.1/11 (5—6 h)	— — —	1
Lysozyme			140	0.1 M nitro-tyrosine ethyl ester	1.4/11[c]	—	1
Trypsin			250	1.0 M glycine methyl ester	4.6/11 (5 min) 8.8/11 (60 min) 12.5/11 (5—6 h)[d]	— — —	1
Chymotrypsin			250	1.0 M glycine methyl ester	6.2/17 (5 min) 11.8/17 (60 min) 15.5/17 (5—6 h)	— — —	1
Trypsinogen	pH 4.5, 25°C	1-ethyl-3-[e] (3-dimethylamino-propyl) carbodiimide	25	1.0 M glycine[f] ethyl ester	—	—	2
Chymo-trypsinogen	pH 4.0, 25°C, pH stat pH 6.0, 25°C, pH stat pH 8.0, 25°C, pH stat	EDC		1.0 M glycine ethyl ester	13/14[g] 10/14 3/14	— — —	3 3 3
Chymotrypsin	pH 4.75, 25°C, pH stat	EDC		1.0 M glycine methyl ester	12.7[h] 15.6[i] 10.6 13.5[i]	—	4 4
Lysozyme	pH 4.75, 25°C, pH stat	BDC		0.25 M amino-methanesulfonic acid	8.5—9.5[j]	—	5
Lysozyme				1.0 M glycine methyl ester	6.5—7.5[j]	—	5
Trypsin	pH 4.75, 25°C, pH stat	EDC		1.0 M glycinamide	7.9[k] 1.7[k]	3—5 Tyr[l]	6

Table 2 (continued)
THE MODIFICATION OF CARBOXYL GROUPS IN PROTEINS

Protein	Reaction conditions	Carbodiimide	Molar excess	Nucleophile	Carboxyl groups modified	Other functional groups modified	Ref.
Albumin	pH 4.75	EDC	—	Glycine methyl ester or L-argininamide	1[m]	—	7
Chymotrypsin	pH 4.0[n]	EDC	—	Glycine ethyl ester	15/15	—	8
Papain	pH 4.75, 25°C	EDC	300—1200	Glycine ethyl ester	6/14	6—10 Tyr,[o] active site cysteinyl residue	9
Yeast hexokinase	0.1 M phosphate, pH 6.0, 20°C[p]	1-cyclohexyl-3-(2-morpholino-ethyl) carbodiimide metho-p-toluenesulfonate[q]	500—3000	Nitrotyrosine[r] ethyl ester	1	Cysteinyl (2)	10
Phosphorylase[b]	pH 5.1, 25°C	CMC	—	Glycine[s] ethyl ester	3[t]	—	11
α-Mannosidase	pH 4.2, 0.1 M MES, 1.0 M NaCl	SDC	2000	Glycine[g] ethyl ester	8/	—	12
Yeast enolase	0.050 M MES, 1 mM MgCl₂, 0.01 mM EDTA, pH 6.1	EDC, CMC[u]	2000	—	—	—[v]	13
3-Phosphoglycerate kinase	0.1 M phosphate, pH 6.1, 17°C	CMC	2000	Nitrotyrosine[v] ethyl ester	1	—	14
cAMP-dependent protein kinase	pH 6.5, 0.050 M MES, 23°C	EDC	—	Glycine ethyl ester	1.7[w]	—[x]	15
Human Fc fragment	pH 4.75	EDC	—	Glycine ethyl ester	25	—[y]	16

Pancreatic phospholipase A_2	0.25 M cacodylate, pH 5.5	EDC	—	Semicarbazide	13/15[z]	—[aa]	17
Spinach plastocyanin	pH 3.5	EDC	—	Semicarbazide	14/15[z]	—[aa]	17
	pH 6.0, 23°C borate	EDC	—	Ethylenediamine	4.3/16	—	18
Mitochondrial F_1-ATPase	0.05 M triethanolamine H_2SO_4, pH 7.0	Dicyclohexyl-carbodiimide [bb]	6	—	2[cc]	—	19
Mitochondrial trans-hydrogenase	1 mM Tricine, pH 7.0 with 0.1 M choline chloride and 2% MeOH	DCC	—	—	—	—[dd]	20
Lysozyme	pH 5.0	EDC	3.5[ee]	Ethylenediamine, ethanolamine, 4-(5)-(aminomethyl) imidazole, histamine, D-glucosamine, methylamine [ff]	1	—	21
Restriction endonuclease Eco R_1	0.1 M triethanolamine pH 7.0, 2.0 M KCl 20°C	CMC	—	—	—	—	22
Thylakoid membrane proteins	pH 7.5 (HEPES)	DDC	—	Glycine ethyl ester	—	—	23
		EDC	—	Glycine ethyl ester	—	—	

[a] It is generally necessary to add dilute HCl (0.2 M) during the course of the reaction to maintain the pH at 4.75.

[b] BCD.

[c] Reaction time not given.

[d] Excess may result from autolysis of trypsin preparations which would create "new" free carboxyl groups.

[e] EDC.

[f] Reactions are generally terminated by dilution into cold sodium acetate (1.0 M, pH 3.5—5.5).

[g] Determined by incorporation of $[^{14}C]$ glycine ethyl ester.

[h] 1-H reaction terminated with 1.0 M acetate, pH 4.75.

[i] In 7.5 M urea.

[j] Note the interesting difference in extent of modification which is dependent upon nucleophile used. There is also an interesting difference in the time course of modification.

Table 2 (continued)
THE MODIFICATION OF CARBOXYL GROUPS IN PROTEINS

k   In the presence and absence of the competitive inhibitor, benzamidine.

l   Tyrosyl residues regenerated in 0.5 *M* hydroxylamine, pH 7.1 with no effect on the EDC/glycinamide changes in catalytic activity.

m   Complete modification of the carboxyl groups was achieved in 6.0 *M* guanidine with either L-argininamide or glycine methyl ester. After reduction and carboxymethylation, approximately 20% of the carboxyl groups are unreactive with either nucleophile. There is a further decrease in modification with the reduced and cyanoethylated derivative.

n   Reaction at pH 4.0 results in apparent quantitative modification of carboxyl groups.

o   Tyrosine modification is acid-stable but reversed in 0.5 *M* hydroxylamine, pH 7.0, 5 h, 25°C. "Activated" papain irreversibly modified at active site cysteinyl residue (Cys-25) by EDC while mercuripapain is not.

p   Optimal inactivation occurred at pH 5.5—6.0 with marked decrease in extent of inactivation at more alkaline pH.

q   CMC.

r   Isolated peptide containing modified glutamic acid residue using affinity chromatography with antinitrotyrosyl γ-globulin.

s   Inactivation not dependent upon addition of nucleophile but rate is greatly enhanced.

t   Determined by incorporation of [14C] from [Metho-14C] CMC. Also, determined from the extent of incorporation of *N*-(2,4-dinitrophenyl)-ethylene diamine (spectrophotometry); ε = 15,000 M^{-1} cm^{-1}. It was determined that the modification of one carboxyl group is critical for potential catalytic function.

u   These investigators also used 1-ethyl-(4-azonia-4,4-dimethylpentyl)-carbodiimide (1-ethyl-3-(3-dimethylaminopropyl)-carbodiimide). This reagent was more effective than either EDC or CMC (least active) in the inactivation of the enzyme under these conditions.

v   Reaction at cysteine and tyrosine excluded by amino acid analysis after acid hydrolysis.

w   Determined γ-glu-gly after proteolysis with trypsin (2X), pronase, carboxypeptidases A and B, and leucine aminopeptidase.

x   Direct determination not performed. Reaction at pH 8.0 (carbodiimide is more specific for phenolic hydroxyl at alkaline pH) did not result in loss of catalytic activity.

y   Tyrosine modification excluded by amino acid analysis after acid hydrolysis.

z   Radiolabeled semicarbazide (synthesized from [14C] cyanate) incorporation.

aa   Tyrosine modification did occur. Tyrosine regenerated with neutral hydroxylamine. These investigators stressed the need to keep hydroxylamine exposure as brief as possible to avoid side reactions such as peptide bond cleavage or deamidation.

bb   DCC.

cc   From incorporation of [14C] carbodiimide.

dd   Interchain cross-linking of transhydrogenase dimer occurred under these conditions.

ee   Obtained specific modification of Asp-101 by using low molar excess of carbodiimide. Extent of modification somewhat independent of amine (nucleophile) used. These investigators speculate that increased specificity is a reflection of binding of carbodiimide to substrate binding site close to Asp-101. These investigators did purify reaction products to obtain selectively modified protein derivatives.

ff   Rate and extent of inactivation not changed by the addition of glycine ethyl ester.

References for Table 2

1. Hoare, D. G. and Koshland, D. E., Jr., A procedure for the selective modification of carboxyl groups in proteins, *J. Am. Chem. Soc.*, 88, 2057, 1966.

2. Radhakrishnan, T. M., Walsh, K. A., and Neurath, H., Relief by modification of carboxylate groups of the calcium requirement for the activation of trypsinogen, *J. Am. Chem. Soc.*, 89, 3059, 1967.

3. Abita, J. P., Maroux, S., Delaage, M., and Lazdunski, M., The reactivity of carboxyl groups in chymotrypsinogen, *FEBS Lett.*, 4, 203, 1969.

4. Carraway, K. L., Spoerl, P., and Koshland, D. E., Jr., Carboxyl group modification in chymotrypsin and chymotrypsinogen, *J. Mol. Biol.*, 42, 133, 1969.

5. Lin, T.-Y. and Koshland, D. E., Jr., Carboxyl group modification and the activity of lysozyme, *J. Biol. Chem.*, 244, 505, 1969.

6. Eyl, A. W., Jr. and Inagami, T., Identification of essential carboxyl groups in the specific binding site of bovine trypsin by chemical modification, *J. Biol. Chem.*, 246, 738, 1971.

7. Frater, R., Reactivity of carboxyl groups in modified proteins, *FEBS Lett.*, 12, 186, 1971.

8. Johnson, P. E., Stewart, J. A., and Allen, K. G. D., Specificity of α-chymotrypsin with exposed carboxyl groups blocked, *J. Biol. Chem.*, 251, 2353, 1976.

9. Perfetti, R. B., Anderson, C. D., and Hall, P. L., The chemical modification of papain with 1-ethyl-3(3-dimethylaminopropyl) carbodiimide, *Biochemistry*, 15, 1735, 1976.

10. Pho, D. B., Roustan, C., Tot, A. N. T., and Pradel, L.-A., Evidence for an essential glutamyl residue in yeast hexokinase, *Biochemistry*, 16, 4533, 1977.

11. Ariki, M. and Fukui, T., Modification of rabbit muscle phosphorylase b by a water-soluble carbodiimide, *J. Biochem. (Tokyo)*, 83, 183, 1978.

12. Paus, E., Reaction of α-mannosidase from *Phaseolus vulgaris* with group-specific reagents. Essential carboxyl groups, *Biochim. Biophys. Acta*, 526, 507, 1978.

13. George, A. L., Jr. and Borders, C. L., Jr., Essential carboxyl residues in yeast enolase, *Biochem. Biophys. Res. Commun.*, 87, 59, 1979.

14. Desvages, G., Roustan, C., Fattoum, A., and Pradel, L.-A., Structural studies on yeast 3-phosphoglycerate kinase. Identification by immunoaffinity chromatography of one glutamyl residue essential for 3-phosphoglycerate kinase activity. Its location in the primary structure, *Eur. J. Biochem.*, 105, 259, 1980.

15. Matsuo, M., Huang, C.-H., and Huang, L. C., Modification and identification of glutamate residues at the arginine recognition site in the catalytic subunit of adenosine 3':5'-cyclic monophosphate-dependent protein kinase of rabbit skeletal muscle, *Biochem. J.*, 187, 371, 1980.

16. Vivanco-Martinez, F., Bragado, R., Albar, J. P., Juarez, C., and Ortiz-Masllorens, F., Chemical modification of carboxyl groups in human Fcγ fragment: structural role and effect on the complement fixation, *Mol. Immunol.*, 17, 327, 1980.

17. Fleer, E. A. M., Verheij, H. M., and de Haas, G. H., Modification of carboxylate groups in bovine pancreatic phospholipase A₂. Identification of aspartate-49 as Ca²⁺-binding ligand, *Eur. J. Biochem.*, 113, 283, 1981.

18. Burkey, K. O. and Gross, E. L., Effect of carboxyl group modification on redox properties and electron donation capability of spinach plastocyanin, *Biochemistry*, 20, 5495, 1981.

19. Pennington, R. M. and Fisher, R. R., Dicyclohexylcarbodiimide modification of bovine heart mitochondrial transhydrogenase, *J. Biol. Chem.*, 256, 8963, 1981.

20. Esch, F. S., Böhlen, P., Otsuka, A. S., Yoshida, M., and Allison, W. S., Inactivation of the bovine mitochondrial F₁-ATPase with dicyclohexyl [¹⁴C] carbodiimide leads to the modification of a specific glutamic acid residue in the β-subunit, *J. Biol. Chem.*, 256, 9084, 1981.

21. Yamada, H., Imoto, T., Fujita, K., Okazaki, K., and Motomura, M., Selective modification of aspartic acid-101 in lysozyme by carbodiimide reaction, *Biochemistry*, 20, 4836, 1981.

22. Woodhead, J. L. and Malcolms, D. B., The essential carboxyl group in restriction endonuclease Eco RI, *Eur. J. Biochem.*, 120, 125, 1981.

23. Laszlo, J. A., Millner, P. A., and Dilley, R. A., Light-dependent chemical modification of thylakoid membrane proteins with carboxyl-directed reagents, *Arch. Biochem. Biophys.*, 215, 571, 1982.

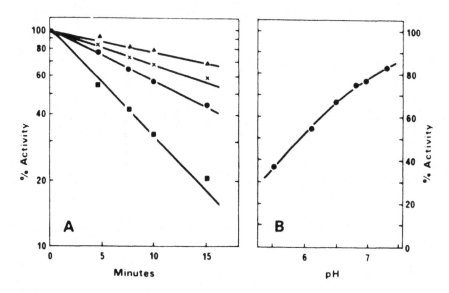

FIGURE 10. Inactivation of hexokinase by 1-cyclohexyl-3-[2-morpholinyl-(4)-ethyl]carbodiimide metho-*p*-toluenesulfonate (CMC). Panel A shows the effect of CMC concentration with 36 μ*M* enzyme in 0.01 *M* phosphate buffer, pH 6.0, at 20°C. The CMC concentration was (▲) 0.015 *M*, (x) 0.03 *M*, (●) 0.05 *M*, and (■) 0.10 *M*. Panel B shows the effect of pH (phosphate buffers) on the reaction with 0.05 *M* CMC (10-min reaction time). (From Pho, D. B., Roustan, C., Tot, A.N.T., and Pradel, L.–A., *Biochemistry*, 16, 4533, 1977. With permission.)

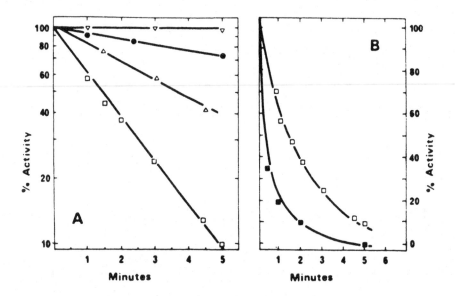

FIGURE 11. The effect of 1-cyclohexyl-3-[2-morpholinyl-(4)-ethyl]carbodiimide metho-*p*-toluenesulfonate (CMC) and nitrotyrosine ethyl ester (NTEE) on hexokinase activity. The concentration of enzyme was 36 μ*M* in 0.01 *M* phosphate buffer, pH 6.0. Panel A: (▽), 0.03 *M* NTEE alone; (●), 0.05 *M* CMC alone; (□), 0.05 *M* CMC + 0.03 *M* NTEE; and (△), 0.025 *M* glucose + 0.005 *M* ADP-Mg + 0.05 *M* CMC + 0.03 *M* NTEE. Panel B: with different concentrations of CMC; (□) 0.05 *M* CMC + 0.03 *M* NTEE and (■) 0.1 *M* CMC + 0.03 *M* NTEE. (From Pho, D. B., Roustan, C., Tot, A.N.T., and Pradel, L.–A., *Biochemistry*, 16, 4533, 1977. With permission.)

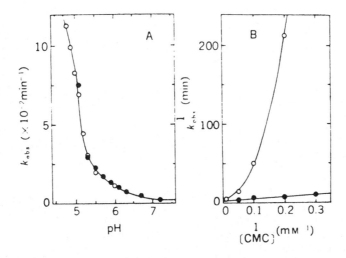

FIGURE 12.   The inactivation of phosphorylase with 1-cyclohexyl-3-[2-morpholinyl-(4)-ethyl]carbodiimide metho-*p*-toluenesulfonate (CMC). Panel A shows the pH dependence of the observed pseudo-first-order rate constant (k_{obs}) for the inactivation of phosphorylase by 20 m*M* CMC. The plot was obtained from two separate experiments, each represented by ○ and ●. Panel B shows a double reciprocal plot of k_{obs} vs. the concentration of CMC in the presence (●) and absence (○) of 50 m*M* glycine ethyl ester. (From Ariki, M. and Fukui, T., *J. Biochem.*, 83, 183, 1978. With permission.)

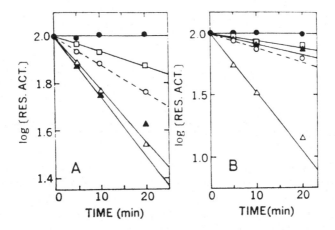

FIGURE 13.   The inactivation of phosphorylase with 1-cyclohexyl-3-[2-morpholinyl-(4)-ethyl]carbodiimide metho-*p*-toluenesulfonate (CMC) in the presence of various nucleophiles. Panel A shows the effect of various amines on the inactivation rate of phosphorylase b with 10 m*M* CMC. (●), No reagent; (○), CMC alone; (△), CMC + 50 m*M* glycine ethyl ester; (□), CMC + 50 m*M* 2-amino-2-deoxyglucose; and (▲), CMC + 50 m*M* glucosyl amine. Panel B shows the effect of amino analogs of glucose on the inactivation rate of phosphorylase b with 20 m*M* CMC. (●), No reagent added; (○), CMC alone; (△), CMC + 50 m*M* glycine ethyl ester; (▲) CMC + 50 m*M* 3-amino-3-deoxyglucose; and (□), CMC + 50 m*M* 6-amino-6-deoxyglucose. (From Ariki, M. and Fukui, T., *J. Biochem.*, 83, 183, 1978. With permission.)

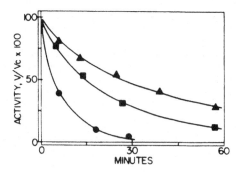

FIGURE 14. The inactivation of yeast enolase by various carbodiimides. Enolase (1 μM) was modified by 20 mM carbodiimide in 50 mM MES, 1 mM MgCl$_2$, 0.01 mM EDTA, pH 6.1, at 25°C. The carbodiimides used were (●) 1-ethyl-3-(4-azonia-4,4-dimethylpentyl)-carbodiimide iodide, (■) 1-ethyl-3-(3-dimethylaminopropyl)-carbodiimide, and (▲) 1-cyclohexyl-2-[3-morpholinyl-(4)-ethyl]-carbodiimide metho-*p*-toluenesulfonate. (From George, A. L., Jr. and Borders, C. L., Jr., *Biochem. Biophys. Res. Commun.*, 87, 59, 1979. With permission.)

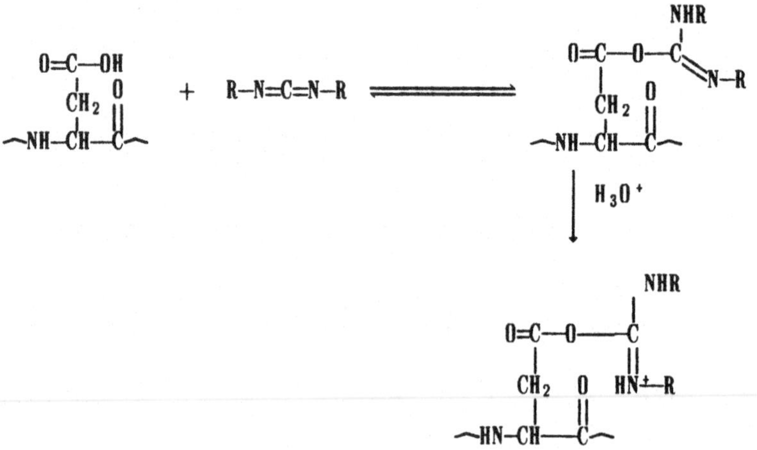

FIGURE 15.   Reaction of a protein carboxyl group with a carbodiimide in the absence of nucleophile.

unprotonated lysine residue and, hence, proceeds somewhat more rapidly at pH values greater than that generally used for protein modification with carbodiimide reagents. In work with cytochrome b$_5$ and NADH cytochrome b$_5$ reductase,[33] the cross-linking reaction was performed at pH 8.5 (5 mM sodium borate) with the proteins bound to dimyristolylphosphatidyl choline vesicles while pH 6.8 (20 mM MOPS) was used for the coupling of calmodulin and myosin light-chain kinase.[34]

Gilles et al.[35] have recently reported studies on the stability of water-soluble carbodiimides in aqueous solution. Carbodiimide concentration was measured spectrophotometrically by reaction with dimethylbarbituric acid. In 50 mM MES buffer/25°C, 1-ethyl-3-(3-dimethyl-aminopropyl)carbodiimide (EDC) has a t$_{1/2}$ of 37 h (pH 7.0), 20 h (pH 6.0), and 3.9 h (pH 5.0). The addition of 10 mM inorganic phosphate decreases the t$_{1/2}$ to 3.7 h at pH 7.0 while 100 mM glycine methyl ester decreases the t$_{1/2}$ to 15.83 (also at pH 7.0). The addition of 100 mM hydroxylamine at pH 7.0 decreases the t$_{1/2}$ to 0.39 h. 1-Ethyl-3-(4-azonia-4,4-dimethylethylpentyl) carbodiimide is approximately one order of magnitude less stable under the same reaction conditions. An effect of phosphate buffers on the modification of phosphorylase by EDC was reported by Takagi et al.[36] The inactivation reaction proceeded effectively in N,N,N',N'-tetramethylethylenediamine buffer at pH 6.2 but very poorly in the

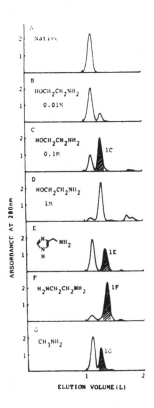

FIGURE 16. Ion-exchange chromatography of the product obtained from the reaction of egg-white lysozyme with various amines in the presence of 1-ethyl-3-[3-(dimethylamino)propyl]-carbodiimide hydrochloride. The modifications were performed at ambient temperature at pH 5.0 (maintained by the addition of HCl). The modified proteins were dialyzed exhaustively against water and then analyzed by ion-exchange chromatography on a 1 × 65 cm Bio-Rex 70 column using a linear gradient from 0.02 M borate, pH 10.0 to 0.02 M borate-0.15 M NaCl, pH 10.0. A, native lysozyme; B, reaction with 0.01 M ethanolamine; C, reaction with 0.1 M ethanolamine; D, reaction with 1 M ethanolamine; E, reaction with 4(5)-(aminomethyl)imidazole; and G, reaction with methylamine. (From Yamada, H., et al., *Biochemistry*, 20, 4836, 1981. With permission.)

presence of glycerophosphate buffer or with phosphate buffer. These results were interpreted as reflecting a specific interaction between phosphate compounds and phosphorylase.

There is additional evidence supporting the influence of solvent conditions on carbodiimide-mediated modification of proteins. Deen et al.[37] demonstrated that the use of an *N*-methylimidazole buffer for EDC-mediated coupling of peptides to carrier proteins markedly reduced the incidence of neodeterminants strictly related to coupling chemistry (in this system, such neodeterminants likely arise as *O*-acylureas).

The above observation that the majority of studies on the chemical modification of carboxyl groups utilize the carbodiimide-mediated reaction(s) is not intended to indicate that there are not other approaches to the modification of aspartyl and glutamyl residues in proteins. Indeed, there are examples of carboxyl group modification with reagents expected to react far more effectively with other nucleophiles. An example of this is the reaction of iodoacetamide with ribonuclease T₁ to form the glycolic acid derivative of the glutamic acid residue as elegantly shown by Takahashi and co-workers.[38] Another example is the modification of a specific carboxyl group in pepsin by *p*-bromophenacyl bromide[39] (the use of *p*-bromophenacyl bromide in the specific modification of proteins is not uncommon but is generally associated with the modification of cysteine, histidine, or methionine). In the study of pepsin, optimal inactivation (approximately 12-fold molar excess of reagent, 3 h, 25°C) was obtained in the pH range of 1.5 to 4.0 with a rapid decrease in the extent of inactivation at pH 4.5

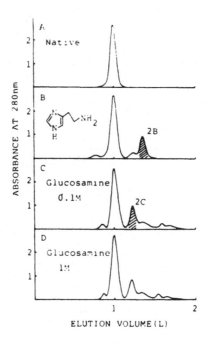

FIGURE 17. Ion-exchange chromatography of the product of the reaction of egg white lysozyme with various amines in the presence of 1-ethyl-3-[3-(dimethylamino)propyl]-carbodiimide hydrocholoride. The reactions were performed as described under Figure 16 and subjected to chromatographic analysis on a 1 × 65 cm column of Bio-Rex 70 using a linear gradient from 0.1 M phosphate, pH 7.0, to 0.4 M phosphate, pH 7.0. A, native lysozyme; B, reaction with histamine; C, reaction with 0.1 M D-glucosamine; and D, reaction with 1 M D-glucosamine.

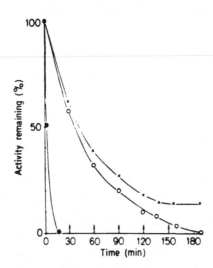

FIGURE 18. Modification of carboxylate groups in bovine pancreatic phospholipase A_2. Shown is the loss of enzyme activity vs. reaction time. Protein (5 mg/ml) was dissolved in 1 M semicarbazide. At the indicated time intervals (arrows), 5 mg 1-ethyl-3-(N,N-dimethyl)amino-propyl carbodiimide was added. (●), reaction at pH 3.5 (semicarbizide-HCl buffer) and (○), reaction at pH 5.5 (0.25 M cacodylate buffer); both reactions without Ca^{2+}. (x) Reaction at pH 5.5 in the presence of Ca^{2+} ions. The reaction was started by the addition of carbodiimide to 0.1 M. (From Fleer, E.A.M., Verheij, H. M., and de Haas, *Eur. J. Biochem.*, 113, 283, 1981. With permission.)

and above (the effect of pH greater than 5.5 to 6.0 on the modification of pepsin cannot be studied because of irreversible denaturation of pepsin at pH 6.0 and above). In studies with a 10% molar excess of p-bromophenacyl bromide at pH 2.8, 37°C, 3 h, complete inactivation of the enzyme was obtained concomitant with the incorporation of 0.93 mol of reagent/mol of pepsin (assessed by bromide analysis). Attempts to reactivate the modified enzyme with a potent nucleophile such as hydroxylamine were unsuccessful but reactivation could be obtained with sulfhydryl-containing reagents (i.e., β-mercaptoethanol, 2,3-dimercaptopropanol, thiophenol). It has been subsequently established that reaction occurs at the β-carboxy group of an aspartic acid residue (formation of 2-p-bromophenyl-1-ethyl-2-one β-aspartate).[40] These investigators noted that reduction of enzyme under somewhat harsh conditions (LiBH$_4$ in tetrahydrofuran) resulted in the formation of homoserine.

Active-site directed reactions with reactive epoxy functional groups have proved useful in several studies of the role of carboxyl groups in proteins. Tang and co-workers have used 1,2-epoxy-3-(p-nitrophenoxy) propane for the modification of catalytically important carboxyl groups in pepsin.[41,42] Active-site directed inactivation of lysozyme with an epoxy function (2′,3′-epoxypropyl β-glycoside of di-(N-acetyl-D-glucosamine)) which reacts with the β-carboxyl group of aspartic acid has been described.[43,44]

REFERENCES

1. **Wilcox, P. E.**, Esterification, *Meth. Enzymol.*, 11, 605, 1967.
2. **Wilcox, P. E.**, Esterification, *Meth. Enzymol.*, 25, 596, 1972.
3. **Rajagopalan, T. G., Stein, W. H., and Moore, S.**, The inactivation of pepsin by diazoacetylnorleucine methyl ester, *J. Biol. Chem.*, 241, 4295, 1966.
4. **Lundblad, R. L. and Stein, W. H.**, On the reaction of diazoacetyl compounds with pepsin, *J. Biol. Chem.*, 244, 154, 1969.
5. **Stein, W. H.**, Chemical studies on purified pepsin, in *Structure-Function Relationships of Proteolytic Enzymes*, Desnuelle, P., Neurath, H., and Ottesen, M., Eds., Munksgard, Copenhagen, 1970, 253.
6. **Leary, R. and Shaw, E.**, Inactivation of cathepsin B$_1$ by diazomethyl ketones, *Biochem. Biophys. Res. Commun.*, 79, 926, 1977.
7. **Widmer, F. and Viswanatha, T.**, Possible side-reactions with diazocarbonyl dipeptide esters as protein modifying reagents, *Carlsberg Res. Commun.*, 45, 149, 1980.
8. **Parsons, S. M., Jao, L., Dahlquist, F. W., Borders, C. L., Jr., Groff, T., Racs, J., and Raftery, M. A.**, The nature of amino acid side chains which are critical for the activity of lysozyme, *Biochemistry*, 8, 700, 1969.
9. **Parsons, S. M. and Raftery, M. A.**, The identification of aspartic acid residue 52 as being critical to lysozyme activity, *Biochemistry*, 8, 4199, 1969.
10. **Paterson, A. K. and Knowles, J. R.**, The number of catalytically essential carboxyl groups in pepsin. Modification of the enzyme by trimethyloxonium fluoroborate, *Eur. J. Biochem.*, 31, 510, 1972.
11. **Woodward, R. B., Olofson, R. A., and Mayer, H.**, A new synthesis of peptides, *J. Am. Chem. Soc.*, 83, 1010, 1961.
12. **Woodward, R. B. and Olofson, R. A.**, The reaction of isoxazolium salts with nucleophiles, *Tetrahedron*, Suppl. 7, 415, 1966.
13. **Bodlaender, P., Feinstein, G., and Shaw, E.**, The use of isoxazolium salts for carboxyl group modification in proteins. Trypsin, *Biochemistry*, 8, 4941, 1969.
14. **Saini, M. S. and Van Etten, R. L.**, An essential carboxylic acid group in human prostate acid phosphatase, *Biochim. Biophys. Acta*, 568, 370, 1979.
15. **Arana, J. L. and Vallejos, R. H.**, Two different types of essential carboxyl groups in chloroplast coupling factor, *FEBS Lett.*, 123, 103, 1981.
16. **Dinur, D., Kantrowitz, E. R., and Hajdu, J.**, Reaction of Woodward's Reagent K with pancreatic porcine phospholipase A$_2$: modification of an essential carboxylate residue, *Biochem. Biophys. Res. Commun.*, 100, 785, 1981.
17. **Kooistra, C. and Sluyterman, L. A. A.**, Isosteric and non-isosteric modification of carboxyl groups of papain, *Biochim. Biophys. Acta*, 997, 115, 1989.

18. **Hoare, D. G. and Koshland, D. E., Jr.,** A procedure for the selective modification of carboxyl groups in proteins, *J. Am. Chem. Soc.,* 88, 2057, 1966.

19. **Banks, T. E., Blossey, B. K., and Shafer, J. A.,** Inactivation of α-chymotrypsin by a water-soluble carbodiimide, *J. Biol. Chem.,* 244, 6323, 1969.

20. **Perfetti, R. B., Anderson, C. D., and Hall, P. L.,** The chemical modification of papain with 1-ethyl-3(3-dimethylaminopropyl) carbodiimide, *Biochemistry,* 15, 1735, 1976.

21. **Carraway, K. L. and Koshland, D. E., Jr.,** Reaction of tyrosine residues in proteins with carbodiimide reagents, *Biochim. Biophys. Acta,* 160, 272, 1968.

22. **Carraway, K. L. and Koshland, D. E., Jr.,** Carbodiimide modification of proteins, *Meth. Enzymol.,* 25, 616, 1972.

23. **Lewis, S. D. and Shafer, J. A.,** Conversion of exposed aspartyl and glutamyl residues in proteins to asparaginyl and glutaminyl residues, *Biochim. Biophys. Acta,* 303, 284, 1973.

24. **Wang, T.-T. and Young, N. M.,** Modification of aspartic acid residues to induce trypsin cleavage, *Anal. Biochem.,* 91, 696, 1978.

25. **Lin, C., Mihal, K. A., and Krueger, R. J.,** Introduction of sulfydryl groups into proteins at carboxyl sites, *Biochim. Biophys. Acta,* 1038, 382, 1990.

26. **Pho, D. B., Roustan, C., Tot, A. N. T., and Pradel, L.-A.,** Evidence for an essential glutamyl residue in yeast hexokinase, *Biochemistry,* 16, 4533, 1977.

27. **Ariki, M. and Fukui, T.,** Modification of rabbit muscle phosphorylase b by a water-soluble carbodiimide, *J. Biochem.,* 83, 183, 1978.

28. **George, A. L., Jr. and Borders, C. L., Jr.,** Essential carboxyl residues in yeast enolase, *Biochem. Biophys. Res. Commun.,* 87, 59, 1979.

29. **Chan, V. W. F., Jorgensen, A. M., and Borders, C. L., Jr.,** Inactivation of bovine thrombin by water-soluble carbodiimides: the essential carboxyl group has a pK_a of 5.51, *Biochem. Biophys. Res. Commun.,* 151, 709, 1988.

30. **Borders, C. L., Jr., Chan, V. W. F., Miner, L. A., and Weerasuriya, Y. M.,** Inactivation of human thrombin by water-soluble carbodiimides: the essential carboxyl has a pK_a of 5.6 and is one other than Asp-189, *FEBS Lett.,* 255, 365, 1989.

31. **Yamada, H., Imoto, T., Fujita, K., Okazaki, K., and Motomura, M.,** Selective modification of aspartic acid-101 in lysozyme by carbodiimide reaction, *Biochemistry,* 20, 4836, 1981.

32. **Fleer, E. A. M., Verheij, H. M., and de Haas,** Modification of carboxylate groups in bovine pancreatic phospholipase A_2. Identification of aspartate-49 as Ca^{2+}-binding ligand, *Eur. J. Biochem.,* 113, 283, 1981.

33. **Hackett, C. S. and Strittmatter, P.,** Covalent cross-linking of the active sites of vesicle-bound cytochrome b_5 and NADH-cytochrome b_5 reductase, *J. Biol. Chem.,* 259, 3275, 1984.

34. **Yamamoto, K., Sekine, T., and Sutoh, K.,** The sites on calmodulin cross-linked to myosin light chain kinase and troponin I with water-soluble carbodiimide, *J. Biochem.,* 104, 251, 1988.

35. **Giles, M. A., Hudson, A. Q., and Borders, C. L., Jr.,** Stability of water-soluble carbodiimides in aqueous solution, *Anal. Biochem.,* 184, 244, 1990.

36. **Takagi, S., Kobayashi, M., and Matsuda, K.,** Modification of essential carboxyl group in rabbit muscle phosphorylase by water-soluble carbodiimide, *J. Biochem. (Tokyo),* 105, 933, 1989.

37. **Deen, C., Claassen, E., Cerritse, K., Zegers, N. D., and Boersma, W. J. A.,** A novel carbodiimide coupling method for synthetic peptides. Enhanced anti-peptide antibody response, *J. Immunol. Meth.,* 129, 119, 1990.

38. **Takahaski, K., Stein, W. H., and Moore, S.,** The identification of a glutamic acid residue as part of the active site of ribonuclease T_1, *J. Biol. Chem.,* 242, 4682, 1967.

39. **Erlanger, B. F., Vratsanos, S. M., Wassermann, M., and Cooper, A. G.,** Specific and reversible inactivation of pepsin, *J. Biol. Chem.,* 240, PC3447, 1965.

40. **Gross, E. and Morell, J. L.,** Evidence for an active carboxyl group in pepsin, *J. Biol. Chem.,* 241, 3638, 1966.

41. **Tang, J.,** Specific and irreversible inactivation of pepsin by substrate-like epoxides, *J. Biol. Chem.,* 246, 4510, 1971.

42. **Chen, K. C. S. and Tang, J.,** Amino acid sequence around the epoxide-reactive residues in pepsin, *J. Biol. Chem.,* 247, 2566, 1972.

43. **Eshdat, Y., McKelvy, J. F., and Sharon, N.,** Identification of aspartic acid 52 as the point of attachment of an affinity label in hen egg white lysozyme, *J. Biol. Chem.,* 248, 5892, 1973.

44. **Eshdat, Y., Dunn, A., and Sharon, N.,** Chemical conversion of aspartic acid 52, a catalytic residue in hen egg white lysozyme, to homoserine, *Proc. Natl. Acad. Sci. U.S.A.,* 71, 1658, 1974.

Chapter 15

THE CHEMICAL CROSS-LINKING OF PEPTIDE CHAINS

The formation of either intramolecular or intermolecular covalent cross-links between amino acid residues in proteins is proving to be an extremely valuable tool in biochemistry with particular use in the study of protein-protein interactions. Naturally occurring inter- and intramolecular cross-links are commonly found in proteins, the most common being the disulfide bond. Other examples exist including the transglutaminase-catalyzed formation of a peptide bond between the γ-carboxyl groups of glutamic acid and the ε-amino groups of lysine.[1,2] There are also the extremely complex cross-links found in collagen.[3,4]

In addition to the study of protein-protein interactions, intramolecular cross-linking has been of value in increasing protein stability[5-7] as well as stabilizing erythrocyte structure.[8] Cross-linking between a biologically active protein and a carrier protein has been advocated for therapeutic purposes[9] although this approach will likely be supplanted by the preparation of chimeric proteins. Covalent cross-linking with the reagents described in this chapter have been used to complex peptides to carrier proteins such as hemocyanin or tetanus toxin for the preparation of antipeptide antibodies.[10] Care must be exercised in the screening of antibodies resulting from the use of peptide-carrier conjugates not only for cross-reactivity with the carrier protein but also for antibodies directly to coupling groups used in such procedures.[11]

Zero-length cross-linking[12] is a procedure which joins peptide chains via existing functional groups such that a "spacer" group is not utilized. Examples include the covalent linkage of proteins to nucleic acids, the formation of 3,3'-dityrosine mediated by tetranitromethane (see Chapter 13) and isopeptide bond formation. Isopeptide bond formation (Figure 1) mediated by carbodiimide[13,14] (see Chapter 14) has been the most extensively used approach. This technique has been applied to the cross-linking of heavy meromyosin and F-actin[15,16] and components of the *A. vinelandii* nitrogenase complex.[17] A more recent modification of this technique[18] involves a two-step procedure where one protein is first incubated with a water-soluble carbodiimide and *N*-hydroxysuccinimide resulting in the formation of an *N*-oxysuccinimide ester. The second step involves condensation with lysine residues in the second component of the reaction.

An interesting pair of reagents (Figure 2) which cross-link proteins by consecutive Michael reactions have been described.[18a] These investigators made the point that since the cross-linkage reaction is driven by consecutive Michael additions, eventually the most thermo-dynamically stable cross-link will be established, which can be subsequently stabilized by reduction of the nitro function with sodium dithionite. These investigators explored the reaction of pancreatic ribonuclease with 2-(*p*-nitrophenyl) allyl-4-nitro-3-carboxyphenyl sulfide (twofold molar excess with respect to ribonuclease in 0.1 *M* sodium phosphate, pH 10.5 at 37°C, 36 h, cross-link stabilized by sodium dithionite fivefold molar excess). No reaction occurred at pH 8.0. Analysis of the reaction mixture showed 61% monomer, 21% dimer, 10% trimer, and a trace of tetramer. The monomer fraction was characterized; the predominant cross-links occurred between lysine-7 and lysine-37 and between lysine-31 and lysine-41.

Care must be taken in the size analysis of intramolecularly linked species in any denaturing medium (i.e., sodium dodecylsulfate, guanidine hydrochloride, etc.) since, unless the cross-linking reagent is cleaved by reduction, the intramolecularly cross-linked protein will not denature properly and will probably give falsely low molecular weight results.[19,20]

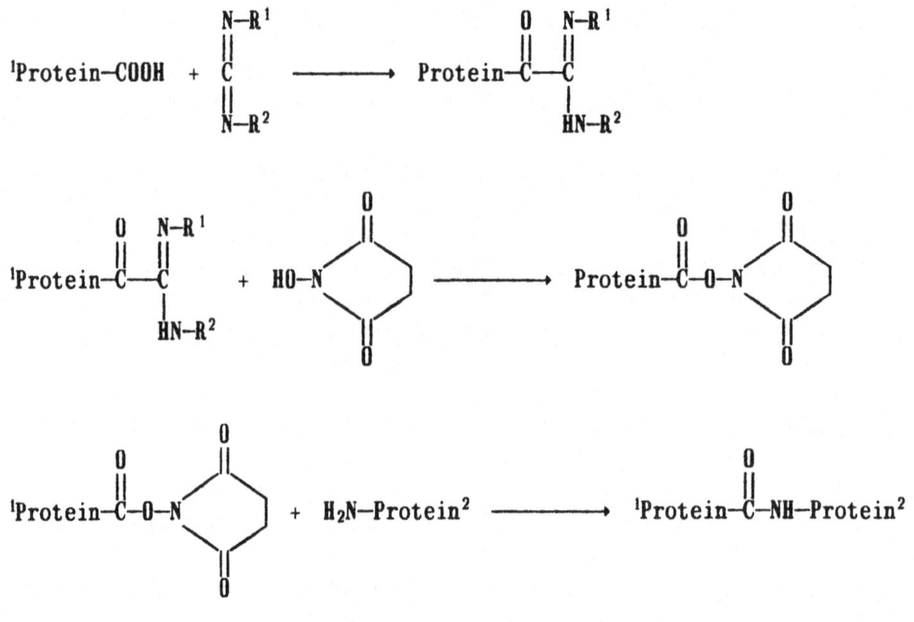

FIGURE 1. A scheme for zero-length cross-linking using a two-step process as described in Reference 18.

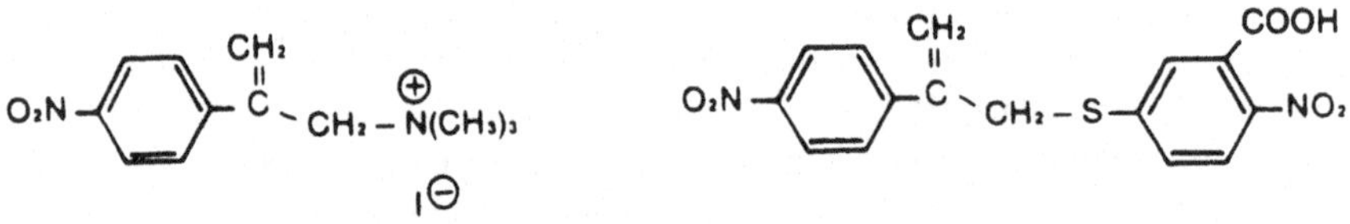

FIGURE 2. The structure of 2-(*p*-nitrophenyl)-allyltrimethylammonium iodide (on the left) and the structure of 2-(*p*-nitrophenyl)-allyl-4-nitro-3-carboxyphenyl sulfide (on the right).

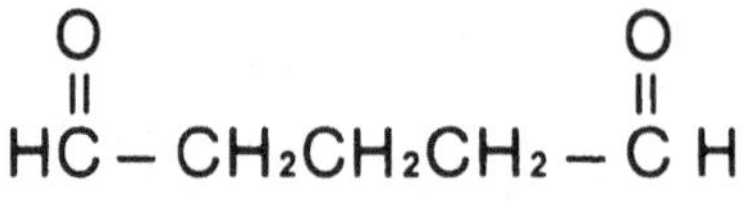

FIGURE 3. The structure of glutaraldehyde.

Intramolecular cross-linking can be enhanced by the following reaction conditions:

1. Low protein concentration (<0.1 mg/ml)
2. High net charge on protein
3. High ratio of protein reactive sites to reagent concentration

The remainder of our consideration will involve intermolecular cross-linking, which includes the cross-linking of identical protomers to form homopolymers (e.g., cross-linkage of identical subunits in an oligomeric protein).[21,22] Cross-linkage to form heteropolymers includes studies on protein-protein interactions (this could result in homopolymers in self-associating systems),[23,24] studies on multienzyme complexes,[25-27] and protein-ligand interactions with cell membrane receptors.[28-33]

The following discussion will focus on the various reagents which have been used for intermolecular protein cross-linking studies.

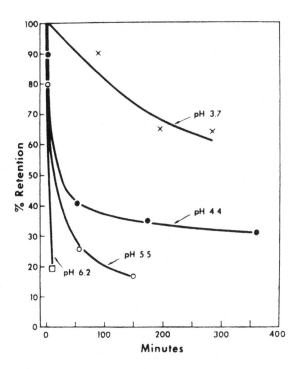

FIGURE 4. The effect of pH on the inactivation of α-chymotrypsin by glutaraldehyde. Reaction mixtures were 2.3% in glutaraldehyde and 0.2% in α-chymotrypsin at 0°C. For pH values of 3.7, 4.4, and 5.5, 0.14 N acetate was employed as buffer. The buffer for pH 6.2 was 0.034 M phosphate. (From Jansen, E. F., Tomimatsu, Y., and Olson, A. C., *Arch. Biochem. Biophys.*, 144, 394, 1971. With permission.)

Glutaraldehyde (Figure 3) should cross-link proteins with the formation of α,ω-Schiff bases, which should be a readily reversible process in the absence of reduction of the Schiff bases with a reducing agent such as sodium borohydride or sodium cyanoborohydride. This is not the case, as summarized by Richards and Knowles.[34] These investigators noted that the reaction of proteins with glutaraldehyde was essentially irreversible even without reduction and that, in the absence of reduction, there was loss of lysine on amino acid analysis following acid hydrolysis. These investigators proposed the formation of a complex reagent resulting from aldol condensation of glutaraldehyde which would then react with the protein. Studies have presented an alternative structure for glutaraldehyde.[35] It seems clear that the chemistry of the reaction of glutaraldehyde is complex. In recent years, the use of glutaraldehyde has received considerable attention in the study of the properties of protein crystals in solution.[36-40] The rationale in these studies has been to show that the properties of a protein in crystalline form are similar to those for the protein in solution.[40] Although glutaraldehyde has a fair degree of specificity for the ε-amino group of lysine, reaction has also occurred with other nucleophilic functional groups in proteins such as the sulfhydryl group of cysteine, the imidazole ring of histidine, and the phenolic hydroxyl group of tyrosine.[41]

The reaction of glutaraldehyde with proteins proceeds quite rapidly at alkaline pH as demonstrated by early studies[42] on reaction with chymotrypsin (Figure 4).

Studies[43] have utilized glutaraldehyde to measure the rate of reconstitution of porcine muscle lactic dehydrogenase. This enzyme is composed of four subunits (Figure 5) and this study demonstrated that the formation of tetramers from a denatured enzyme preparation parallels the recovery of enzymatic activity (Figure 6).

Manning and co-workers have examined the related chemistry of protein cross-linking

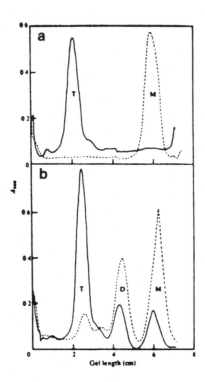

FIGURE 5.   Polyacrylamide gel electrophoresis of cross-linked porcine muscle lactic dehydrogenase (LDH) in the presence of sodium dodecyl sulfate (SDS). Cross-linking by a 2-min incubation in 0.2 *M* phosphate, 5 m*M* EDTA with 0.3 to 0.4 m*M* glutaraldehyde at 20°C was stopped by addition of 15 to 25 µ*M* SDS. Unreacted bifunctional reagent was inactivated by 3 to 4 m*M* hydrazine. The solutions were heated for 10 min (100°C) and subsequently stored for 2 h at 20°C. The protein solutions were concentrated by 24-h dialysis vs. 20% polyethylene glycol prior to electrophoresis on 5% polyacrylamide gels in the presence of SDS. The gels were stained with Coomassie blue R 250 and then scanned at 560 nm. Correlation of the bands to the tetrameric (T), dimeric (D), and monomeric (M) fractions of LDH was achieved by calibration with proteins of defined molecular weight. (a), cross-linking of native tetramers (solid line) and SDS-denatured monomers (dashed line); monomer concentration 81 n*M*. (b), Cross-linking of reactivating LDH after acid dissociation at pH 2.3. Reactivation at 20°C by dilution at pH 7.6. The final concentration of monomer was 343 nm. The dashed line indicates cross-linking after 210 s while the solid line indicates 1 h of reactivation and reassociation. (From Hermann, R., Rudolph, R., and Jaenicke, R., *Nature (London)*, 277, 243, 1979. With permission.)

using glycoaldehyde.[44] Acharya and co-workers[45] have examined the cross-linking of proteins with glyceraldehyde in some detail. A scheme for the chemistry of this reaction is shown in Figure 7. These studies provide some insight into the cross-linking of proteins with other carbohydrate-like compounds.[46]

Homobifunctional imidoesters (Figure 8) were introduced by Singer and co-workers.[47] These reagents have the advantage that the reaction with the protein results in charge preservation of the lysine residue modified. This class of reagents is highly specific for primary amines in the following reactions as shown in Figures 9 and 10. Aspects of the chemistry of this reaction are discussed further in Chapter 10. Buffer effects on the reaction have not been extensively investigated except to specify that the use of potential competing nucleophiles (e.g., Tris, imidazole) should be avoided. Most studies have used 0.02 to 0.1 *M* triethanolamine in the range of pH 8.0 to 9.0. It has been suggested that the amidation reaction is enhanced by the presence of triethanolamine in studies on the reaction of methyl-4-mercaptobutyrimidate.[31] The greatest use of these reagents has been in the study of protomer organization of oligomeric proteins and self-association systems.

The early studies of Davies and Stark with dimethyl suberimidate[21] showed that analysis of the reaction products reveals a set of species with molecular weights equal to integral

Relative peak area (%)
Relative reactivation (%)
100
40
20
0
10
20
30
40
50
Time (min)

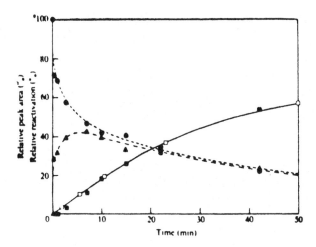

FIGURE 6. Determination of the kinetics of reassociation of porcine muscle lactic dehydrogenase by cross-linking. The experimental conditions are described in the caption to Figure 5. Reassociation (20°C) at 170 n*M* monomer concentration was analyzed by withdrawing portions from the reactivation mixture at defined times and fixation of the association products by cross-linking with glutaraldehyde. Percentage of monomers (●), dimers (▲), and tetramers (■) is defined by the respective peak areas relative to their total amount. Reactivation (□), as determined by enzymatic assay, was calculated relative to the final extent of reactivation (75% after 6 days). (From Hermann, R., Rudolph, R., and Jaenicke, R., *Nature (London)*, 277, 243, 1979. With permission.)

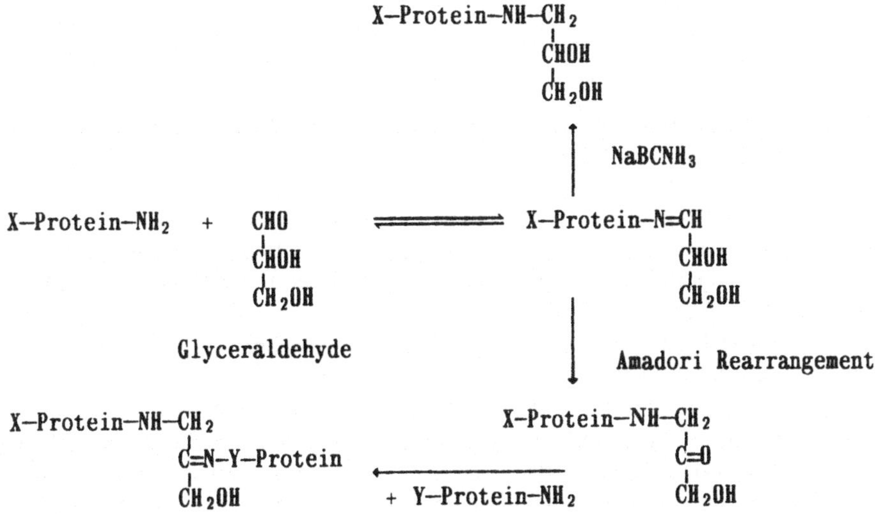

X–Protein–NH–CH2
CHOH
CH2OH
NaBCNH3
X–Protein–NH2
+
CHO
CHOH
CH2OH
Glyceraldehyde
X–Protein–N=CH
CHOH
CH2OH
Amadori Rearrangement
X–Protein–NH–CH2
C=N–Y–Protein
CH2OH
+ Y–Protein–NH2
X–Protein–NH–CH2
C=O
CH2OH

FIGURE 7. A scheme for the cross-linking of proteins using glyceraldehyde as described in Reference 45.

multiples of the protomer molecular weight. For oligomers composed of identical protomers, the number of products is equivalent to the number of protomers in the oligomer. These investigators also noted that reaction at a lower protein concentration can be used to distinguish cross-linking within an oligomer from cross-linking between two or more oligomers. Studies on leucine aminopeptidase from bovine lens[22] also provided a sound basis for the use of bifunctional imidoesters as a probe of the quaternary structure of proteins.

In this study it was emphasized that it is essential to know the effect of reaction with monofunctional reagents on biological activity before considering the effect of cross-linking on biological activity.[48] In addition, the work of Sinha and Brew[49] is worth further examination. These investigators developed a useful procedure employing the prior trace-labeling

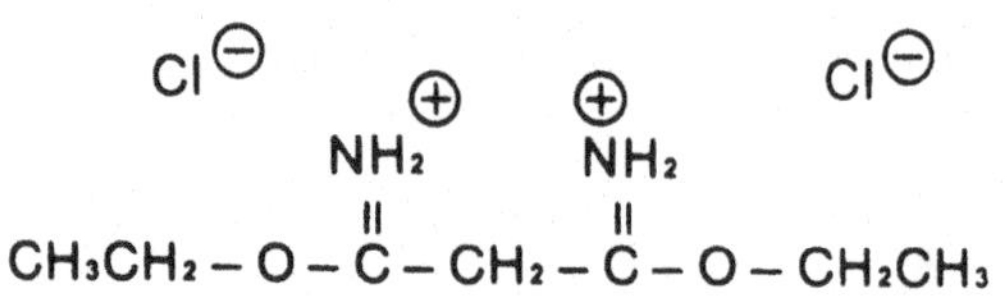

$$Cl^{\ominus} \quad \overset{\oplus}{NH_2} \quad \overset{\oplus}{NH_2} \quad Cl^{\ominus}$$
$$CH_3CH_2 - O - \overset{\overset{\displaystyle \|}{NH_2}}{\underset{}{C}} - CH_2 - \overset{\overset{\displaystyle \|}{NH_2}}{\underset{}{C}} - O - CH_2CH_3$$

FIGURE 8.   The structure of a homobifunctional imidoester.

$$2P - NH_2 + CH_3CH_2 - O - \overset{\overset{\displaystyle \|}{NH_2}}{\underset{}{C}} - CH_2 - \overset{\overset{\displaystyle \|}{NH_2}}{\underset{}{C}} - O - CH_2CH_3 \longrightarrow P - NH - \overset{\overset{\displaystyle \|}{NH_2}}{\underset{}{C}} - CH_2 - \overset{\overset{\displaystyle \|}{NH_2}}{\underset{}{C}} - NH - P$$

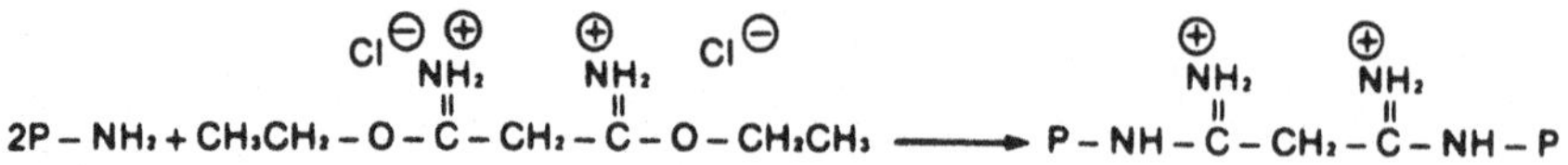

FIGURE 9.   The reaction of a homobifunctional imidoester with the primary amino groups in a protein resulting in covalent cross-linking.

$$P - NH_2 + CH_3CH_2 - O - \overset{\|}{C} - CH_2 - \overset{\|}{C} - O - CH_2CH_3 \longrightarrow P - NH - \overset{\|}{C} - CH_2 - \overset{\|}{C} - O - CH_2CH_3$$

$$P - NH - \overset{\|}{C} - CH_2 - \overset{O}{\overset{\|}{C}} - O - CH_2CH_3$$

$$+$$

$$NH_4^{\oplus} + H_2O + CH_3CH_2OH$$

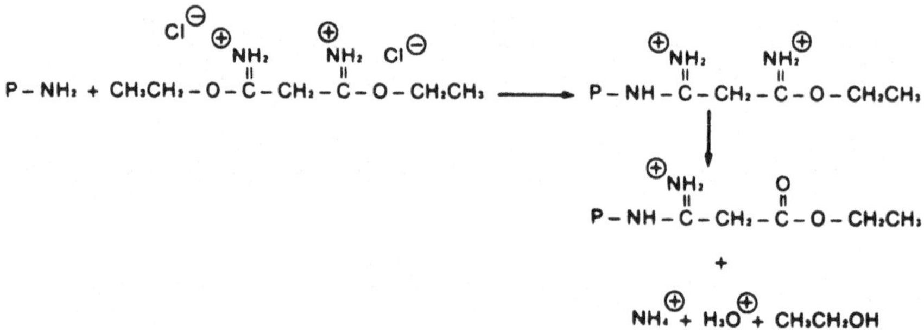

FIGURE 10.   The reaction of a homobifunctional imidoester with the primary amino groups in a protein not resulting in covalent cross-linking.

of the protein with acetic anhydride. Since reaction with acetic anhydride and imidoester is mutually exclusive, fragmentation and subsequent determination of specific radioactivity at specific lysine residues allows the identification of the site(s) of reaction with bifunctional imidoesters.

Diimidates have been used to study the glycogen phosphorylase system. Reagents of different length were used to study intermolecular and intramolecular interaction of phosphorylase b.[50] Figure 11 illustrates the effect of AMP on the cross-linkage pattern of phosphorylase b. In panel A, C_d can be viewed as a measure of association between individual dimers of phosphorylase b. Panel B is a plot of reagent (cross-linkage reagent) length vs. r_k which is a measure of total cross-link formation (inter and intra). Subsequent studies[51] from the same laboratory extended these observations to phosphorylase a and a hybrid phosphorylase ab (Figure 12), permitting the development of a model (Figure 13) of the various structural states of this highly regulated enzyme.

Disuccinimidyl ester derivatives have also seen considerable use. bis-(Sulfosuccinimidyl)suberate has been used to assess the dimerization of EGF receptors in Triton X-100 extracts of A431 cells. The introduction of a cross-linking reagent that could be subsequently cleaved, 3,3'-dithiobis(succinimidylpropionate)[53] has proved to be of considerable use in the study of proteins.[54-62] This reagent provides for the reversible formation of cross-links according to Figure 14.

The use of bifunctional maleimides is of considerable value in cross-linking between sulfhydryl groups. A particularly useful study in this area is the work of Heilmann and Holzner[63] in which the synthesis and use of a number of bifunctional maleimides for the elucidation of the structure of tryptophan synthetase is reported (Figure 15). One of the more useful derivatives is bis-*N*-maleimido-1,8-octane (Figure 16).

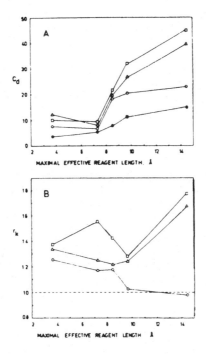

FIGURE 11. Structural changes in glycogen phosphorylase b as revealed by cross-linking with a homologous series of bifunctional imidates. Shown is the effect of AMP on the cross-link parameters (C_d, the percentage amount of protein found in the trimer and tetramer bands, C_d = (trimer + tetramer)/total × 100; r_k, the rate-constant ratio of cross-linking, $r_k = k_L/k_O$ where k_L and k_O are the apparent first-order rate constants of the disappearance of the monomeric band (as detected by gel electrophoresis) in the presence and absence of a given ligand). The cross-linking was performed in 0.2 M triethanolamine, pH 8.0. The reaction was started by the addition of the diimidoesters and allowed to proceed for 60 min at 30°C. The reaction was terminated by lowering the pH to 7.0 and the distribution of reaction products assessed by polyacrylamide gel electrophoresis in the presence of sodium dodecyl sulfate. The gels were stained with Coomassie Blue (the cross-linking did not change the staining properties of the protein). Panel A: C_d as a function of maximum effective reagent length (the maximal effective reagent lengths for malonic, adipic, pimelic, suberic, and dodecanedioic diimidates are 3.7, 7.3, 8.5, 9.7, and 14.5 A, respectively). (●), without AMP; (○), 0.1 mM AMP; (△), 0.3 mM AMP; and (□), 1.0 mM AMP. The points without AMP are the mean of at least four independent experiments. The lines connecting the points have no physical meaning; they only serve for better visualization. Panel B: r_k as a function of reagent length at various AMP concentrations. The symbols and number of experiments are the same as in panel A. (From Hajdu, J., Dombradi, V., Bot, G., and Friedrich, P., *Biochemistry*, 18, 4037, 1979. With permission.)

A cleavable bifunctional dimaleimide has been recently reported.[64] The synthesis of the reagent, maleimidomethyl-3-maleimido propionate (Figure 17), is reported as is the use of the reagent to probe spatial relationships in the erythrocyte membrane. *p*-Phenylenedimaleimide (Figure 18) has been used to cross-link subunits of transducin and cGMP phosphodiesterase complexes in bovine rod photoreceptors.[65]

Continued interest has been shown in the use of heterobifunctional reagents for crosslinking of proteins. Of particular interest has been the use of photoactivatable derivatives. An example of this type of derivative is methyl-3-[*p*-azidophenyl)dithio] propioimidate[28] (Figure 19). In these experiments, epidermal growth factor was reacted in the dark at pH 8.5 (0.1 M triethanolamine, 0.2 M NaCl, pH 8.5) for reaction of the imido ester formation with lysine. This reaction is terminated by the addition of ammonium acetate. Photoactivation in the presence of mouse 3T3 cells resulted in the specific labeling of a cell surface protein. It is noted that this reagent can be cleaved by reduction, permitting isolation of such a cell surface protein free of ligand.

The synthesis of *N*-(4-azidocarbonyl-3-hydroxyphenyl)-maleimide has been reported.[66] This reagent has been used to cross-link subunits of porcine heart lactate dehydrogenase via reaction between a cysteine residue and a lysine residue.

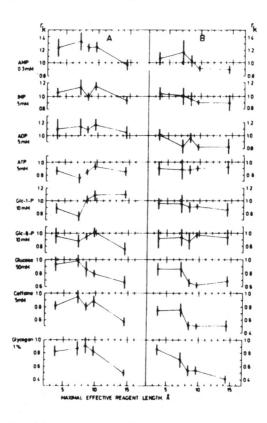

FIGURE 12.   Structural changes in glycogen phosphorylase as revealed by cross-linking with bifunctional diimidates. Shown is the effect of ligands on the r_k cross-link parameter (defined in legend to Figure 11). Panel A represents studies performed with phosphorylase ab and panel B represents studies performed with phosphorylase a. The experimental conditions are described in Figure 11 except that the cross-linking was carried out at 18°C in the experiments described in panel B. The abscissa is discontinuous. The mean ± standard deviation of three independent experiments is shown. (From Dombradi, V., Hajdu, J., Bot, G., and Friedrich, P., *Biochemistry*, 19, 2295, 1980. With permission.)

A series of homo- and heterobifunctional reagents which form acid-labile cross-links in proteins have been reported.[67] These are shown in Figure 20. The ability to be cleaved by mild acid (pH 5.0) is based on the presence of ortho ester, acetal, and ketal functional groups. Another heterobifunctional reagent which forms an acid-labile link is based on the lability of the reaction product between citraconic anhydride and lysine.[68]

The use of monofunctional and bifunctional membrane-permeant and membrane-impermeant maleimides is covered in more detail in the chapter on the chemical modification of cysteine (Chapter 6).

The use of 4-nitrophenyl esters for cross-linking and affinity labeling has been proposed.[69]

The synthesis of 4-(6-formyl-3-azidophenoxy) butyrimidate (Figure 21) has been reported.[70] The imido function can react with the amino groups on a protein (0.1 M sodium borate, pH 8.6). Cross-linking can occur either with nitrene formation from the azido functional group upon irradiation or via reductive alkylation utilizing the aldehyde formation. In either instance, radiolabel can be introduced with sodium borotritiide (NaB[^{3}T]$_4$) with conversion of the free aldehyde to an alcohol or by reducing the Schiff base formed during reductive alkylation. Sulfosuccinimidyl-2-(*p*-azidosalicylamido)-1,3-dithiopropionate has been used to identify the receptor for phytohemaglutinin in mononuclear cells.[71]

A related approach involves the use of *p*-nitrophenyl-3-diazopyruvate (Figure 22).[72] This reagent reacts with amines to form the corresponding pyruvamide derivatives. Upon

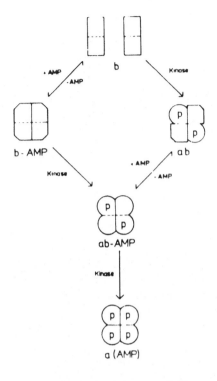

FIGURE 13. Structural changes in glycogen phosphorylase as revealed by cross-linking with bifunctional diimidates. Shown are the structural states detectable by cross-linking in rabbit muscle phosphorylase. Letters a, b, and ab denote the respective forms of phosphorylase. Square, truncated square, and circular protomer symbols indicated by the dotted line denote allosterically competent subunit contact m. "Kinase" means the incorporation of phosphate (P) at Ser-14 by phosphorylase kinase. (From Dombradi, V., Hajdu, J., Bot, G., and Freidrich, P., *Biochemistry*, 19, 2295, 1980. With permission.)

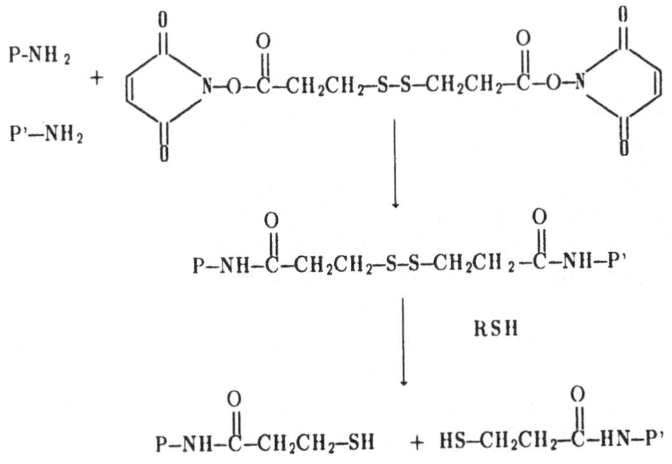

FIGURE 14. The structure of 3,3′-dithiobis(succinimidylpropionate) and the formation of reversible cross-links in proteins via coupling with primary amino groups.

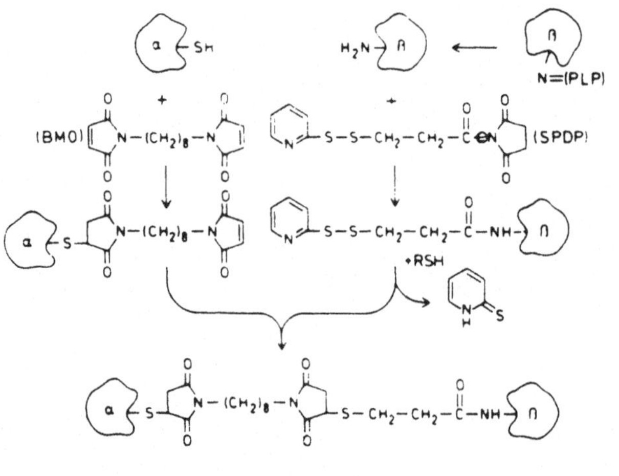

FIGURE 15. The use of bifunctional maleimides to determine the solution structure of tryptophan synthetase. Shown is a scheme for the reactions leading to covalent cross-linking of α and β subunits. β Signifies one subunit within the β_2 dimer after modification by methyl acetimidate of the bulk of the NH_2 groups accessible in the holo enzyme; (PLP) is the pyridoxal phosphate group covalently bound to β by Schiff base formation. (BMO) is bis-*N*-maleimideo-1,8-octane; (SPDP) is *N*-succinimidyl-3-(2-pyridyldithio) propionate. (From Heilmann, H. D. and Holzner, M., *Biochem. Biophys. Res. Commun.*, 99, 1146, 1981. With permission.)

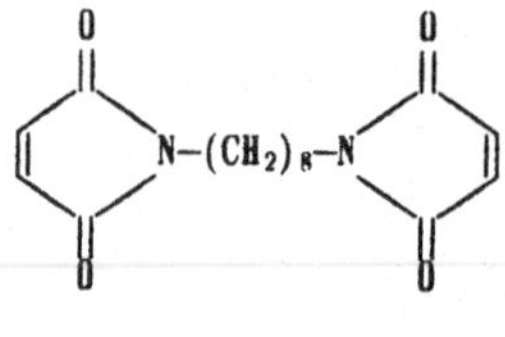

FIGURE 16.   The structure of bis-*N*-maleimido-1,8-octane.

photolysis at 300 nm, a ketene amide is formed which is highly reactive with nucleophiles to produce malonic acid derivatives.

Chong and Hodges[73,74] have reported studies of a complex bifunctional affinity reagent, *N*-(4-azidobenzoylglycyl)-5-(2-thiopyridyl)-cysteine (AGTC) (Figure 23). Figure 24 describes the effect of photolysis (350 nm) and reduction (dithiothreitol) on the spectral properties of the reagent. Figure 25 describes strategy in the use of this reagent.

One of the uses of cross-linking reagents such as those described above is the characterization of the interactions(s) between biologically active peptides and proteins and cell surface receptors. An excellent example of this approach is provided by the work of Ji and co-workers.[29,75] Some reagents developed for this purpose[76] are shown in Figure 26.

bis-Pyridoxal polyphosphates (Figure 27) have been described by Benesch and Kwong[77] as a class of specific intramolecular cross-linking agents for hemoglobin. While specifically designed for hemoglobin, this reagent would likely be useful for other site-specific cross-link reagents. In another study on hemoglobin, Hosmane and Bertha[78] describe the use of 2,2'-sulfonylbis[3-methoxy-(E,E')-2-propenitrile (Figure 28) as a cross-linking reagent. Lee et al.[79] described an interesting heterobifunctional reagent (Figure 29) designed for coupling glycopeptides to proteins.

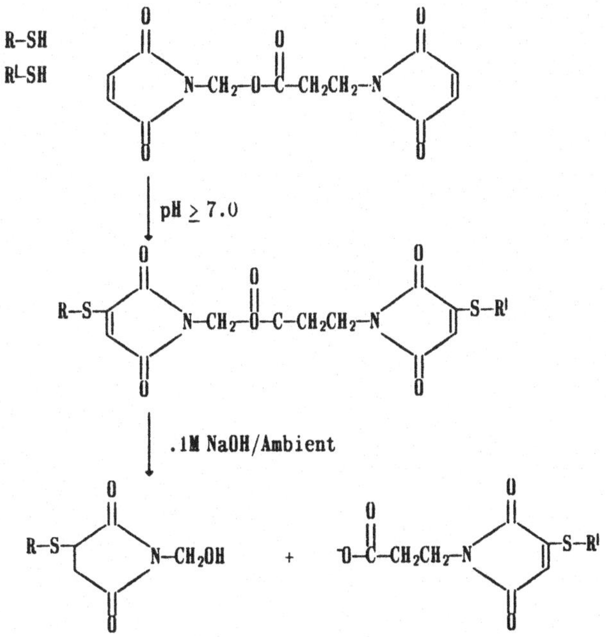

FIGURE 17. The structure of maleimidomethyl-3-maleimido propionate, the reaction of this reagent with protein sulfhydryl groups and the subsequent cleavage of this cross-link with base.

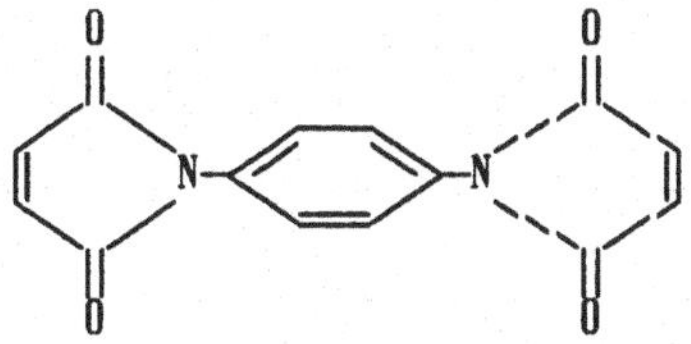

N,N' –1,4–Phenylene dimaleimide

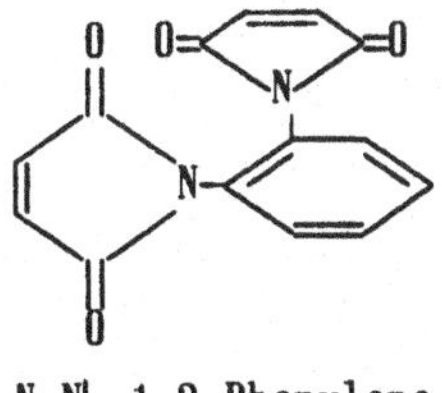

N,N' –1,2–Phenylene dimaleimide

FIGURE 18. The structures of two phenylene dimaleimides.

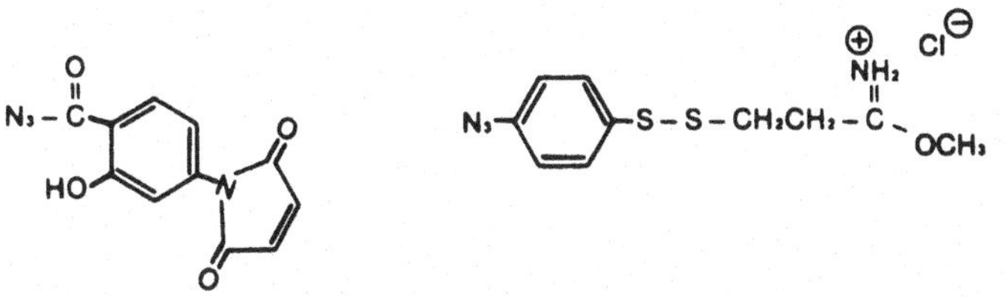

FIGURE 19. The structure of N-(4-azidocarbonyl-3-hydroxyphenyl)maleimide (on the left) and methyl-3-(p-azidophenyl)dithiopropioimidate (on the right).

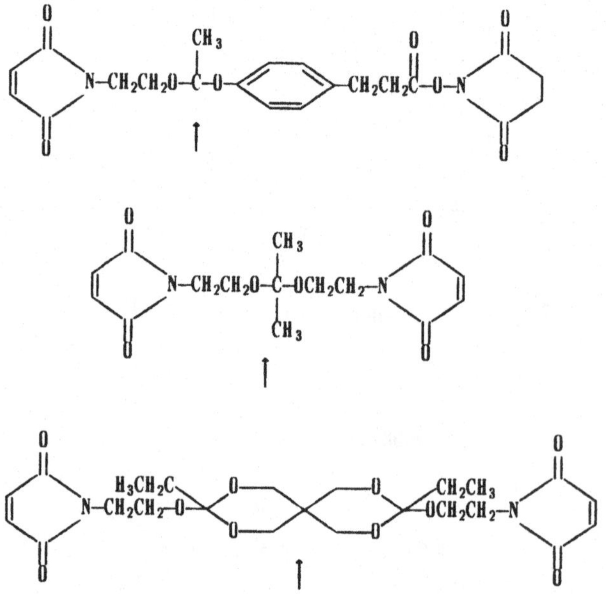

FIGURE 20. The structures of some acid-labile cross-linking reagents as described in Reference 68. I, a heterobifunctional acetal cross-linking agent; II, a maleimido ketal cross-linking agent; and III, an *ortho* ester cross-linking agent.

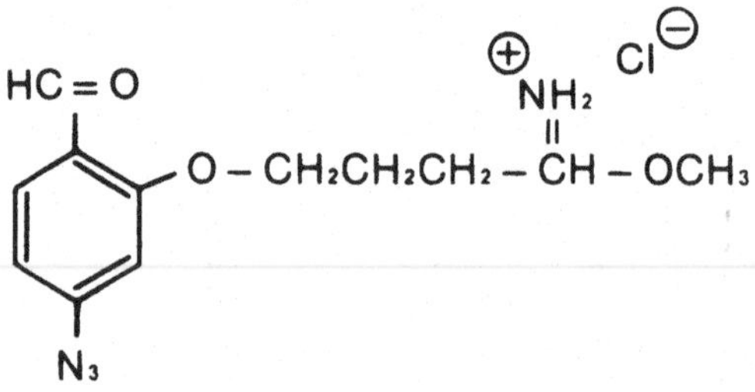

FIGURE 21. The structure of 4-(6-formyl-3-azidophenoxy)butyrimidate.

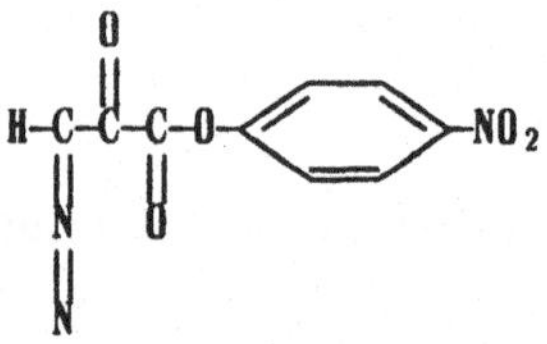

FIGURE 22. The structure of *p*-nitrophenyl-3-diazopyruvate.

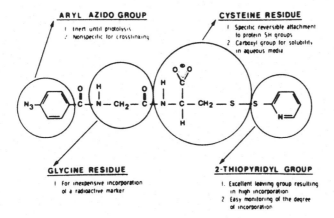

FIGURE 23. The design of a heterobifunctional cross-linking reagent for the study of biological interactions between proteins. Shown is the rationale for the design of *N*-(4-azidobenzoylglycyl)-*S*-(2-thiopyridyl)-cysteine (AGTC). (From Chong, P.C.S. and Hodges, R. S., *J. Biol. Chem.*, 256, 5064, 1981. With permission.)

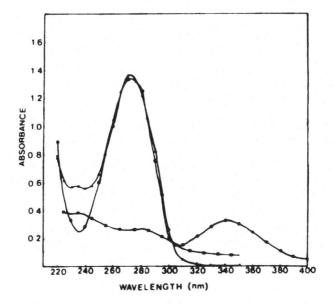

FIGURE 24. The effect of photolysis and dithiothreitol on the UV absorption spectrum of the heterobifunctional photoaffinity probe AGTC (see Figure 23). The spectrum of AGTC (50 μM) in 50 mM Tris-HCl, 0.1 M KCl buffer, pH 7.5, before (▲——▲) and after either irradiation at 350 nm at 32°C for 30 min (■——■) or treatment with 25 mM dithiothreitol for 20 min (●——●). (From Chong, P.C.S. and Hodges, R. S., *J. Biol. Chem.*, 256, 5064, 1981. With permission.)

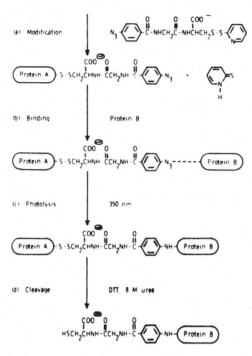

FIGURE 25. The use of a heterobifunctional cross-linking reagent for the study of the biological interactions between proteins. Shown is a scheme for the radiolabeling of a binding site on one protein which is in the vicinity of a SH group on another protein. The SH groups are modified with the heterobifunctional photoaffinity probe N-(4-azidobenzoyl[2-^{3}H]glycyl)-S-(2-thiopyridyl)cysteine. a, the introduction of the arylazide structure into a thioprotein A by thiol-disulfide interchange; b, noncovalent binding of modified protein A to protein B; c, covalent cross-linking of the proteins by photolysis of the arylazide moiety; and d, the cleavage of the disulfide bridge linking the two proteins by dithiothreitol, thus completing the transfer of radiolabel from protein A to protein B. (From Chong, P.C.S. and Hodges, R. S., *J. Biol. Chem.*, 256, 5071, 1981. With permission.)

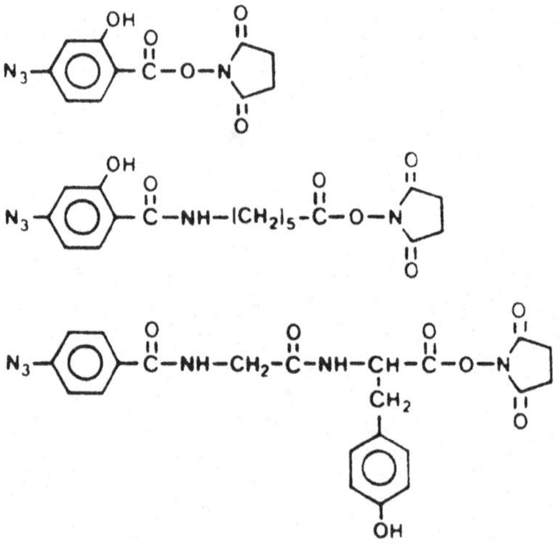

NHS-ASA

NHS-ASC

NHS-ABGT

FIGURE 26. Structures of some cross-linking reagents which have proved useful in the study of the interaction of peptide hormones with cell surface receptors. Shown is NHS-ASA, the N-hydroxysuccinimide ester of 4-azido-salicylic acid; NHS-ABGT, the N-hydroxysuccinimide ester of 4-azidoben-zoylglycyltyrosine; and HNS-ASC, the N-hydroxysuccinimide ester of N-(4-azidosalicyl)-6-aminocaproic acid. (From Ji, T. H. and Ji, I., *Anal. Biochem.*, 121, 286, 1982. With permission.)

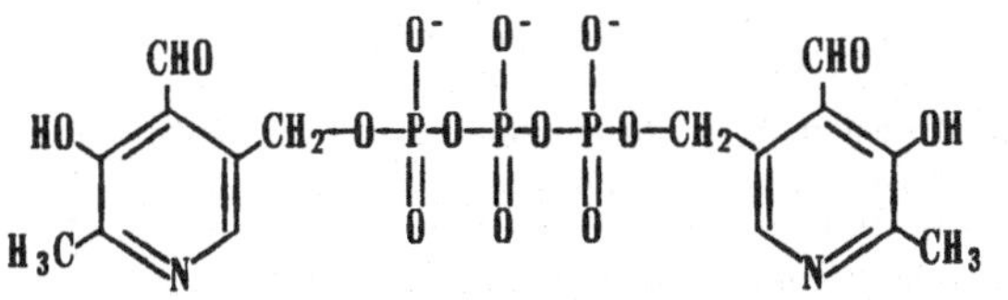

FIGURE 27. The structure of a bis-pyridoxal polyphosphate.

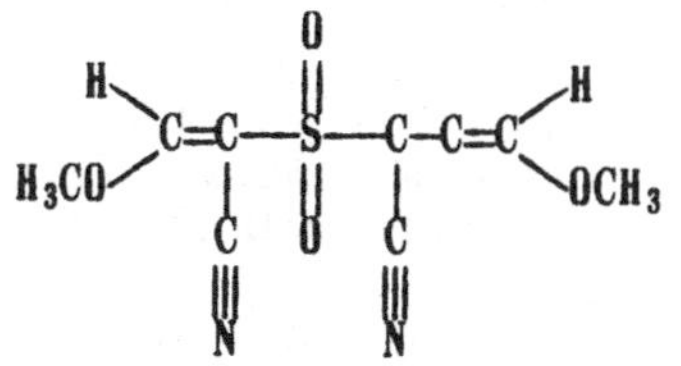

FIGURE 28. The structure of 2,2'-sulfonyl[3-methoxy-E,E']-propenenitrile.

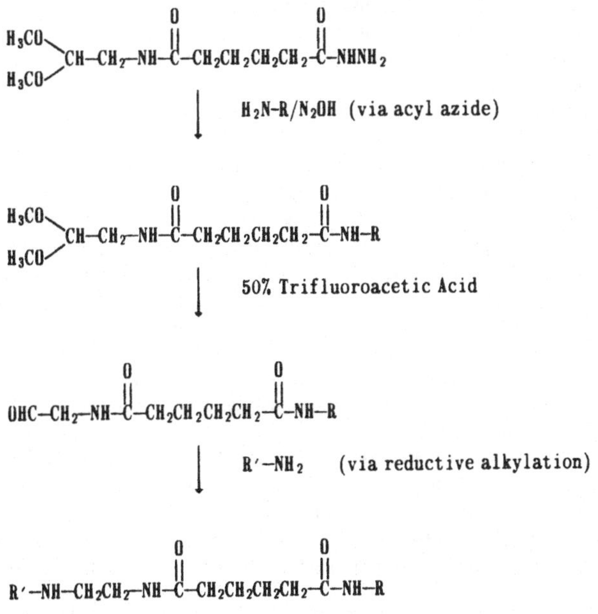

H₂N-R/N₂OH (via acyl azide)

50% Trifluoroacetic Acid

R'-NH₂ (via reductive alkylation)

FIGURE 29. A scheme for cross-linking a peptide to a protein after Reference 80.

REFERENCES

1. **Iwanij, V.,** The use of liver transglutaminase for protein labeling, *Eur. J. Biochem.,* 80, 359, 1977.
2. **Folk, J. E. and Finlayson, J. S.,** The ε-(γ-glutamyl) lysine crosslink and the catalytic rate of transglutaminases, *Adv. Protein Chem.,* 31, 1, 1977.
3. **Traub, W. and Piez, K. A.,** The chemistry and structure of collagen, *Adv. Protein Chem.,* 25, 243, 1971.
4. **Bornstein, P. and Sage, H.,** Structurally distinct collagen types, *Annu. Rev. Biochem.,* 49, 957, 1980.
5. **Shami, E. Y., Rothstein, A., and Ramjeesingh, M.,** Stabilization of biologically active proteins, *Trends Biotechnol.,* 7, 186, 1989.

6. **Shaked, Z. and Wolfe, S.,** Stabilization of pyranose 2-oxidase and catalase by chemical modification, *Meth. Enzymol.,* 137, 599, 1988.

7. **Martinek, K. and Torchilin, V. P.,** Stabilization of enzymes by intramolecular cross-linking using bifunctional reagents, *Meth. Enzymol.,* 137, 615, 1988.

8. **Bellelli, A., Benedetti, P. L., Coletta, M., Ippoliti, R., and Brunori, M.,** Human erythrocytes cross-linked with glutaraldehyde general properties and significance as a blood substitute, *Biochem. Biophys. Res. Commun.,* 156, 970, 1988.

9. **Poznansky, M. J.,** Soluble enzyme-albumin conjugates: new possibilities for enzyme replacement therapy, *Meth. Enzymol.,* 137, 566, 1988.

10. **Peeters, J. M., Hazendonk, T. G., Beuvery, E. C., and Tesser, G. I.,** Comparison of four bifunctional reagents for coupling peptides to proteins and the effect of the three moieties on the immunogenicity of the conjugates, *J. Immunol. Meth.,* 120, 133, 1989.

11. **Edwards, R. J., Singleton, A. M., Boobis, A. R., and Davis, D. S.,** Cross-reaction of antibodies to coupling groups used in the production of anti-peptide antibodies, *J. Immunol. Meth.,* 117, 215, 1989.

12. **Kunkel, G. R., Mehrabian, M., and Martinson, H. G.,** Contact-site cross-linking agents, *Mol. Cell. Biochem.,* 34, 3, 1981.

13. **Sheehan, J. C. and Hlavka, J. J.,** The use of water-soluble and basic carbodiimides in peptide synthesis, *J. Org. Chem.,* 21, 439, 1956.

14. **Sheehan, J. C. and Hlavka, J. J.,** The cross-linking of gelatin using a water-soluble carbodiimide, *J. Am. Chem. Soc.,* 79, 4528, 1957.

15. **Onishi, H., Maita, T., Matsuda, G., and Fujiwara, K.,** Evidence for the association between two myosin heads in rigor acto-smooth muscle heavy meromyosin, *Biochemistry,* 28, 1898, 1989.

16. **Onishi, H., Maita, T., Matsuda, G., and Fujiwara, K.,** Carbodiimide-catalyzed cross-linking sites in the heads of gizzard heavy meromyosin attached to F-actin, *Biochemistry,* 28, 1905, 1989.

17. **Willing, A. and Howard, J. B.,** Cross-linking site in *Azotobacter vinelandii* complex, *J. Biol. Chem.,* 265, 6596, 1990.

18. **Grabarek, Z. and Gergely, J.,** Zero-length cross-linking procedure with the use of active esters, *Anal. Biochem.,* 185, 131, 1990.

18a. **Mitra, S. and Lawton, R. G.,** Reagents for the cross-linking of proteins by equilibrium transfer alkylation, *J. Am. Chem. Soc.,* 101, 3097, 1979.

19. **Ruoho, A., Bartlett, P. A., Dutton, A., and Singer, S. J.,** A disulfide-bridge bifunctional imidoester as a reversible cross-linking reagent, *Biochem. Biophys. Res. Commun.,* 63, 417, 1975.

20. **Steele, J. C. H., Jr. and Nielson, T. B.,** Evidence of cross-linked polypeptides in SDS gel electrophoresis, *Anal. Biochem.,* 84, 218, 1978.

21. **Davies, G. E. and Stark, G. R.,** Use of dimethyl suberimidate, a cross-linking reagent, in studying the subunit structure of oligomeric proteins, *Proc. Natl. Acad. Sci. U.S.A.,* 66, 651, 1970.

22. **Carpenter, F. H. and Harrington, K. T.,** Intermolecular cross-linking of monomeric proteins and cross-linking of oligomeric proteins as a probe of quaternary structure. Application to leucine aminopeptidase (bovine lens), *J. Biol. Chem.,* 247, 5580, 1972.

23. **Tarvers, R. C., Noyes, C. M., Roberts, H. R., and Lundblad, R. L.,** Influence of metal ions on prothrombin self-association. Demonstration of dimer formation by intermolecular cross-linking with dithiobis(succinimidyl propionate), *J. Biol. Chem.,* 257, 10708, 1982.

24. **Lewis, R. V., Roberts, M. F., Dennis, E. A., and Allison, W. S.,** Photoactivated heterobifunctional cross-linking reagents which demonstrate the aggregation state of phospholipase A₂, *Biochemistry,* 16, 5650, 1977.

25. **DeAbreu, R. A., DeVries, J., DeKok, A., and Veeger, C.,** Cross-linking studies with the pyruvate dehydrogenase complexes from *Azotobacter vinelandii* and *Escherichia coli, Eur. J. Biochem.,* 97, 379, 1979.

26. **Monneron, A. and d'Alayer, J.,** Effects of cross-linking agents on adenylate cyclase regulation, *FEBS Lett.,* 109, 75, 1980.

27. **Baskin, L. S. and Yang, C. S.,** Cross-linking studies of cytochrome P-450 and reduced nicotinamide adenine dinucleotide phosphate-cytochrome P-450 reductase, *Biochemistry,* 19, 2260, 1980.

28. **Das, M., Miyakawa, T., Fox, C. F., Pruss, R. M., Aharonov, A., and Herschman, H. R.,** Specific radiolabeling of a cell surface receptor for epidermal growth factor, *Proc. Natl. Acad. Sci. U.S.A.,* 74, 2790, 1977.

29. **Ji, T. H.,** A novel approach to the identification of surface receptors. The use of photosensitive heterobifunctional cross-linking reagent, *J. Biol. Chem.,* 252, 1566, 1977.

30. **Pilch, P. R. and Czech, M. P.,** Interaction of cross-linking agents with the insulin effector system of isolated fat cells. Covalent linkage of ¹²⁵I-insulin to a plasma membrane receptor protein of 140,000 daltons, *J. Biol. Chem.,* 254, 3375, 1979.

31. **Birnbaumer, M. F., Schrader, W. T., and O'Malley, B. W.,** Chemical cross-linking of chick oviduct progesterone-receptor subunits by using a reversible bifunctional cross-linking agent, *Biochem. J.,* 181, 201, 1979.

32. **Kasuga, M., Van Obberghen, E., Nissley, S. P., and Rechler, M. M.,** Demonstration of two subtypes of insulin-like growth factor receptors by affinity cross-linking, *J. Biol. Chem.*, 256, 5305, 1981.

33. **Rebois, R. V., Omedeo-Sale, F., Brady, R. O., and Fishman, P. H.,** Covalent cross-linking of human chorionic gonadotropin to its receptor in rat testes, *Proc. Natl. Acad. Sci. U.S.A.*, 78, 2086, 1981.

34. **Richards, F. M. and Knowles, J. R.,** Glutaraldehyde as a protein cross-linking reagent, *J. Mol. Biol.*, 37, 231, 1968.

35. **Monsan, P., Puzo, G., and Mazarguil, H.,** Etude du mecánisme d'établissement des liaisons glutaraldéhyde-protéins, *Biochimie*, 57, 1281, 1975.

36. **Quiocho, F. A. and Richards, F. M.,** Intermolecular cross-linking of a protein in the crystalline state: carboxypeptidase A, *Proc. Natl. Acad. Sci. U.S.A.*, 52, 833, 1964.

37. **Wong, C., Lee, T. J., Lee, T. Y., Lu, T. H., and Hung, C. S.,** Intermolecular cross-linking of a protein crystal - acid protease from *Endothia parasitica* — in 2.7 *M* ammonium sulfate solution, *Biochem. Biophys. Res. Commun.*, 80, 886, 1978.

38. **Spillburg, C. A., Bethune, J. L., and Vallee, B. L.,** Kinetic properties of crystalline enzymes. Carboxypeptidase A, *Biochemistry*, 16, 1142, 1977.

39. **Wong, C., Lee, T. J., Lee, T. Y., Lu, T. H., and Hung, C. S.,** The structure of acid protease from *Endothia parasitica* in cross-linked form at 3.5 Å resolution, *Biochem. Biophys. Res. Commun.*, 80, 891, 1978.

40. **Tüchsen, E., Hvidt, A., and Ottesen, M.,** Enzymes immobilized as crystals. Hydrogen isotope exchange of crystalline lysozyme, *Biochimie*, 62, 563, 1980.

41. **Habeeb, A. F. S. A. and Hiramoto, R.,** Reaction of proteins with glutaraldehyde, *Arch. Biochem. Biophys.*, 126, 16, 1968.

42. **Jansen, E. F., Tomimatsu, Y., and Olson, A. C.,** Cross-linking of α-chymotrypsin and other proteins by reaction with glutaraldehyde, *Arch. Biochem. Biophys.*, 144, 394, 1971.

43. **Hermann, R., Rudolph, R., and Jaenicke, R.,** Kinetics of *in vitro* reconstitution of oligomeric enzymes by cross-linking, *Nature (London)*, 277, 243, 1979.

44. **Manning, L. R. and Manning, J. M.,** Influence of ligation state and concentration of hemoglobin A on its cross-linking by glycolaldehyde: functional properties of cross-linked, carboxymethylated hemoglobin, *Biochemistry*, 27, 6640, 1988.

45. **Acharya, A. S., Cho, Y. J., and Manjula, B. N.,** Cross-linking of proteins by aldotriose: reaction of the carbonyl function of the keto amines generated in situ with amino groups, *Biochemistry*, 27, 4522, 1988.

46. **Harding, J. J.,** Nonenzymatic covalent posttranslational modification of proteins *in vivo*, *Adv. Enzymol.*, 37, 247, 1985.

47. **Dutton, A., Adams, M., and Singer, S. J.,** Bifunctional imidoesters as cross-linking reagents, *Biochem. Biophys. Res. Commun.*, 23, 730, 1966.

48. **Monneron, A. and d'Alayer, J.,** Effects of imido-esters on membrane-bound adenylate cyclase, *FEBS Lett.*, 122, 241, 1980.

49. **Sinha, S. K. and Brew, K.,** A label selection procedure for determining the location of protein-protein interaction sites by cross-linking with bisimidoesters. Application to lactose synthase, *J. Biol. Chem.*, 256, 4193, 1981.

50. **Hajdu, J., Dombradi, V., Bot, G., and Friedrich, P.,** Structural changes in glycogen phosphorylase as revealed by cross-linking with bifunctional diimidates: phosphorylase b, *Biochemistry*, 18, 4037, 1979.

51. **Dombradi, V., Hajdu, J., Bot, G., and Friedrich, P.,** Structural changes in glycogen phosphorylase as revealed by cross-linking with bifunctional diimidates. Phospho-dephospho hybrid and phosphorylase a, *Biochemistry*, 19, 2295, 1980.

53. **Lomant, A. J. and Fairbanks, G.,** Chemical probes of extended biological structures: synthesis and properties of the cleavable protein cross-linking reagent [^{35}S] dithiobis(succinimidyl propionate), *J. Mol. Biol.*, 104, 243, 1976.

54. **Tarvers, R. C., Noyes, C. M., Roberts, H. R., and Lundblad, R. L.,** Influence of metal ions on prothrombin self-association. Demonstration of dimer formation by intermolecular cross-linking with dithiobis(succinimidylpropionate), *J. Biol. Chem.*, 257, 10708, 1982.

55. **Tarvers, R. C., Roberts, H. R., and Lundblad, R. L.,** Self-association of bovine prothrombin fragment 1 in the presence of metal ions. Use of a covalent cross-linking agent to study the reaction, *J. Biol. Chem.*, 259, 1944, 1984.

56. **Tarvers, R. C., Noyes, C. M., Tarvers, J. K., and Lundblad, R. L.,** Mechanism of the calcium dependent self-association of bovine prothrombin. Use of a covalent cross-linking reagent to study the reaction, *J. Biol. Chem.*, 261, 4855, 1986.

57. **Tarvers, R. C., Roberts, H. R., Straight, D. L., Featherstone, G. L., and Lundblad, R. L.,** Homo- and heterodimer formation with prothrombin and prothrombin fragment 1 in the presence of calcium ions, *Arch. Biochem. Biophys.*, 257, 439, 1987.

58. **Hantula, J. and Bamford, D. H.,** Chemical cross-linking of bacteriophage 6 nucleocapsid proteins, *Virology,* 165, 482, 1988.

59. **Cornell, R.,** Chemical cross-linking reveals a dimeric structure for CTP: phosphocholine cytidylyltransferase, *J. Biol. Chem.,* 264, 9077, 1989.

60. **Wiland, E., Siemieniako, B., and Trzeciak, W. H.,** Binding of low mobility group protein from rat liver chromatin with histones studied by chemical cross-linking, *Biochem. Biophys. Res. Commun.,* 166, 11, 1990.

61. **D'Souza, S. E., Ginsberg, M. H., Lam, S. C.-T., and Plow, E. F.,** Chemical cross-linking of the arginyl-glycyl-aspartic acid peptides to an adhesion receptor on platelets, *J. Biol. Chem.,* 263, 3943, 1988.

62. **Rexin, M., Busch, W., and Gehring, U.,** Chemical cross-linking of heteromeric glucocorticoid receptors, *Biochemistry,* 27, 5593, 1988.

63. **Heilmann, H. D. and Holzner, M.,** The spatial organization of the active sites of the bifunctional oligomeric enzyme tryptophan synthetase: cross-linking by a novel method, *Biochem. Biophys. Res. Commun.,* 99, 1146, 1981.

64. **Sato, S. and Nakao, M.,** Cross-linking of intact erythrocyte membrane with a newly synthesized cleavable bifunctional reagent, *J. Biochem.,* 90, 1177, 1981.

65. **Fanger, B. O., Stephens, J. E., and Staros, J. V.,** High-yield trapping of EGF-induced receptor dimers by chemical cross-linking, *FASEB J.,* 3, 71, 1989.

66. **Kolkenbrock, H., Kiltz, H.-H., and Trommer, W. E.,** Stepwise cross-linking of pig heart lactate dehydrogenase by a heterobifunctional reagent, *Biochem. Biophys. Acta,* 535, 216, 1978.

67. **Srinivasachar, K. and Neville, D. M., Jr.,** New protein cross-linking reagents that are cleaved by mild acid, *Biochemistry,* 28, 2501, 1989.

68. **Blattler, W. A., Kuenzi, B. S., Lambert, J. M., and Senter, P. D.,** New heterobifunctional protein cross-linking reagent that forms an acid-labile link, *Biochemistry,* 24, 1517, 1985.

69. **Jelenc, P. C., Cantor, C. R., and Simon, S. R.,** High yield photoreagents for protein cross-linking and affinity labeling, *Proc. Natl. Acad. Sci. U.S.A.,* 75, 3564, 1978.

70. **Maassen, J. A.,** Cross-linking of ribosomal proteins by 4-(6-formyl-3-azidophenoxy) butyrimidate. A heterobifunctional cleavable cross-linker, *Biochemistry,* 18, 1288, 1979.

71. **Shephard, E. G., de Beer, F. C., von Holt, C., and Hapgood, J. P.,** The use of S-sulfosuccinimidyl-2-(p-azidosalicylamido)-1,3'-dithiopropionate as a cross-linking reagent to identify cell surface receptors, *Anal. Biochem.,* 168, 306, 1988.

72. **Goodfellow, V. S., Settineri, M., and Lawton, R. G.,** p-Nitrophenyl 3-diazopyruvate and diazopyruvamides, a new family of photoactivatable cross-linking bioprobes, *Biochemistry,* 28, 6346, 1989.

73. **Chong, P. C. S. and Hodges, R. S.,** A new heterobifunctional cross-linking reagent for the study of biological interactions between proteins. I. Design, synthesis and characterization, *J. Biol. Chem.,* 256, 5064, 1981.

74. **Chong, P. C. S. and Hodges, R. S.,** A new heterobifunctional cross-linking reagent for the study of biological interactions between proteins. II. Application to the troponin C-troponin I interaction, *J. Biol. Chem.,* 256, 5071, 1981.

75. **Ji, I., Yoo, B. Y., Kaltenbach, C., and Ji, T. H.,** Structure of the lutropin receptor on granulosa cells. Photoaffinity labeling with the α-subunit in human choriogonadotropin, *J. Biol. Chem.,* 256, 10853, 1981.

76. **Ji, T. H. and Ji, I.,** Macromolecular photoaffinity labeling with radioactive photoactivable heterobifunctional reagents, *Anal. Biochem.,* 121, 286, 1982.

77. **Benesch, R. E. and Kwong, S.,** Bis-pyridoxal polyphosphates: a new class of specific intramolecular crosslinking agents for hemoglobin, *Biochem. Biophys. Res. Commun.,* 156, 9, 1988.

78. **Hosmane, R. S. and Bertha, C. M.,** A versatile, highly reactive, cross-linking reagent: 2,2'-sulfonylbis[3-methoxy-(E,E)-2-propenenitrile], *Biochem. Biophys. Res. Commun.,* 166, 567, 1990.

79. **Lee, R. T., Wong, T.-C., Lee, R., Yue, L., and Lee, Y. C.,** Efficient coupling of glycopeptides to proteins with a heterobifunctional reagent, *Biochemistry,* 28, 1856, 1989.

Chapter 16

AFFINITY LABELING

The use of biological affinity to label amino acid residues at enzyme active sites, allosteric binding sites, substrate binding sites, and other types of binding sites on proteins (such as the sites of binding of fatty acids and various other compounds to albumin) has proved to be a powerful tool in the study of the relationship between structure and function in proteins. This has been an area of extensive study and it is not possible to discuss all investigations. The reader is directed to reviews[1-6] covering various aspects of affinity labeling. In particular, the reader is directed toward the review by Plapp.[4]

The concept of affinity labeling can be said to have been first advanced by Singer and co-workers.[7] The early work was expanded by the studies of Baker[8] which covered the early years of this area of investigation. It is, however, fair to suggest that studies of Shaw and co-workers on the labeling of the active-site histidine residues with peptide chloromethylketones[9-11] really initiated serious study in this area. Details of these studies are presented below.

Affinity labeling is a technique for the specific modification of an amino acid residue in a protein which involves both the binding of the reagent (affinity label) on the basis of biological specificity and subsequent modification of an amino acid residue through the formation of a covalent bond. There are therefore at least two separate and distinct steps in the process of affinity labeling regardless of whether one is concerned with modification of an enzyme catalytic site or a binding site on a protein not involved in catalysis: the process of specific (selective) binding and the process of covalent bond formation.

It therefore follows that the process of affinity labeling should show saturation kinetics such as that shown for the reaction of human placental 17β-estradiol dehydrogenase/20α-hydroxysteroid dehydrogenase[12] with 5'-p-fluorosulfonyl adenosine (Figure 1). The kinetics of modification can be demonstrated as:

$$P + AL \underset{k_2}{\overset{k_1}{\rightleftharpoons}} P \cdot AL \overset{k_3}{\longrightarrow} P - AL \qquad (1)$$

$$K_{AL} = \frac{[P][AL]}{[P \cdot AL]}; \qquad k_{observed} = \frac{k_3[AL]}{K_{AL} + [AL]} \qquad (2)$$

$$\frac{1}{k_{observed}} = \frac{K_{AL}}{k_3[AL]} + \frac{1}{k_3} \qquad (3)$$

where P is the protein (not necessarily an enzyme), AL is the affinity label, P·AL is the noncovalent complex, and P−AL is the covalently bonded product of the reaction. This approach has been adapted from Powers and co-workers[13] and implies that when reagent (AL) concentration is much greater than protein concentration that decrease of P + P·AL in the reaction mixture will follow pseudo-first-order kinetics at a fixed value of AL. The observed reaction rate ($k_{observed}$) is not constant with changes in the concentration of affinity label. However, as noted by these investigators, $k_{observed}$/[AL] remains constant over a substantial concentration range for peptide chloromethyl ketones and α-chymotrypsin (Table 1).[13] This is explained by $k_{AL} \gg$ [AL] such that:

$$\frac{k_{observed}}{[AL]} = \frac{k_3}{K_{AL}} \qquad (4)$$

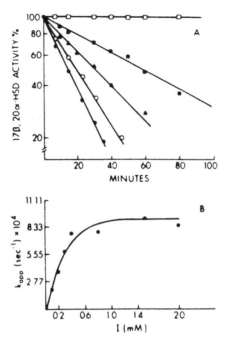

FIGURE 1.   Saturation kinetics in the reaction of 5′-[*p*-(fluorosulfonyl)benzoyl]adenosine with 17β-estradiol/20α-hydroxysteroid dehydrogenase. Shown is the inactivation of the 17β-estradiol dehydrogenase and 20α-hydroxy-steroid dehydrogenase activities by various concentrations of 5′-[*p*-(fluorosulfonyl)benzoyl]adenosine. In panel A the enzyme (2 μ*M*) in 6 ml 0.01 *M* potassium phosphate, pH 7.0, containing 5 m*M* EDTA and 20% (v/v) glycerol was incubated at 25°C with inactivator [final concentrations (■) 100 μ*M*; (▲) 200 μ*M*; (○) 300 μ*M*, and (●) 400 μ*M*] in 0.12 ml of ethylene glycol. Identical control incubations contained adenosine. At the indicated times, portions were removed and assayed for both 17β and 20α activities. The percentage of enzyme activity is a logarithmic scale along the ordinate. For simplification of the graphic presentation, the single points represent the mean of duplicate assays for both activities. In panel B the data from panel A as well as inactivation studies using saturating concentrations of inactivator (500 to 2000 μ*M*) were used to calculate the k_{app} (0.693/$t_{1/2}$) and to construct the plot demonstrating saturation kinetics. (From Tobias, B. and Strickler, R. C., *Biochemistry*, 20, 5546, 1981. With permission.)

Table 1
REACTION OF PEPTIDE
CHLOROMETHYL KETONES
WITH α-CHYMOTRYPSIN[10]

Inhibitor	$k_{observed}/[AL]$
N-Formyl-PheCH$_2$Cl	0.05
N-Acetyl-PheCH$_2$Cl	0.15
N-Tosyl-PheCH$_2$Cl	0.12
N-Acetyl-GlyPheCH$_2$Cl	0.13
N-Acetyl-AlaPheCH$_2$Cl	0.11
N-Acetyl-LeuPheCH$_2$Cl	0.32
N-Cb$_3$-GlyGlyPheCH$_2$Cl	0.32
N-Boc-AlaGlyPheCH$_2$Cl	0.33
N-Acetyl-AlaGlyPheCH$_2$Cl	0.88
N-Boc-GlyLeuPheCH$_2$Cl	1.29

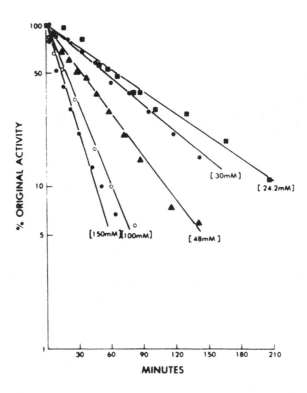

FIGURE 2. Loss of creatine kinase activity upon incubation with
epoxycreatine (*N*-(2,3-epoxypropyl)-*N*–amidinoglycine). Conditions were as follows: creatine kinase (1 mg/ml) in 10 m*M* HEPES,
pH 7.5, at 0°C. The epoxycreatine concentrations are noted on the
figure. (From Marletta, M. A. and Kenyon, G. L., *J. Biol. Chem.*,
254, 1879, 1979. With permission.)

The reader is referred to Powers and co-workers,[13,14] Wold,[15] and Plapp[3] for a more extensive consideration of the kinetics of interaction of affinity labels with proteins.

There are at least three major considerations which must be satisfied in order to justify identification of a compound as a true affinity label. First, the reaction must show a rate saturation effect as one increases inhibitor (affinity label) concentration (Figure 1). Secondly, substrate, competitive inhibitor, or ligand must protect against modification and inactivation. Finally, the reaction must demonstrate stoichiometry with respect to sites modified/functional subunit. The modification of creatine kinase by *N*-(2,3-epoxypropyl)-*N*-amidinoglycine[16] provides an excellent example of these considerations. Figure 2 shows the time course for the loss of activity by creatine kinase upon reaction with the epoxycreatine derivative in 0.010 *M* HEPES, pH 7.5 (0°C) at several concentrations of reagent. When the t$^{1/2}$ (inactivation half-time) is plotted vs. the reciprocal of inhibitor concentration a straight line is obtained[17] with the y intercept equal to T$^{1/2}$ (minimum inactivation half-time). Such a graph for the data obtained from the experiments described in Figure 2 is shown in Figure 3. The minimum inactivation half-time obtained from this analysis is 4.2 min corresponding to a pseudo-first-order rate constant of 2.8×10^{-3} s^{-1}. A value for K_{INACT} (concentration of inhibitor giving half-maximal inactivation rate) is obtained either from the slope of the line or the negative of the reciprocal of the intercept on the X axis and, in these experiments, is 355 m*M*. The stoichiometry for this reaction is presented in Figure 4 and is consistent with the incorporation of 1 mol of reagent per mole of enzyme subunit. In the presence of epoxycreatine, there is an increase in amounts of ADP generated based on comparison with a control experiment in the absence of epoxycreatine suggesting that epoxycreatine is phosphorylated by the

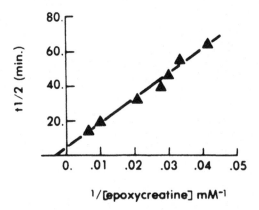

FIGURE 3. The half-time of inactivation of creatine kinase as a function of the reciprocal of the epoxycreatine concentration. The half-times of inactivation were obtained from Figure 2. (From Marletta, M. A. and Kenyon, G. L., *J. Biol. Chem.*, 254, 1879, 1979. With permission.)

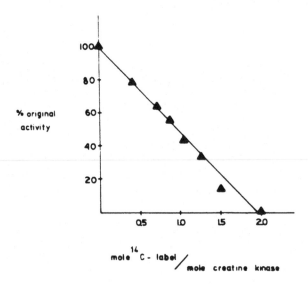

FIGURE 4. Stoichiometry for the inactivation of creatine kinase by epoxycreatine. Shown is the loss of creatine kinase activity upon incorporation of [^{14}C]epoxycreatine. Conditions were as follows: creatine kinase (17 mg/ml, 209 μM) and epoxycreatine (39 mM) in 10 mM HEPES, pH 7.5 at 0°C. (From Marletta, M. A. and Kenyon, G. L., *J. Biol. Chem.*, 254, 1879, 1979. With permission.)

enzyme. This indicates that epoxycreatine does interact with the active site of the enzyme. Further support for this interaction is shown in Figure 5 where the Mg^{2+}-ADP-creatine complex does protect the enzyme from inactivation.

There is almost an infinite variety of compounds which can be used as affinity labels. First are derivatives which form relatively stable analogs/homologs of enzyme intermediates. Examples of this class include diisopropylphosphorofluoridate,[18] peptide aldehydes,[19] and compounds such as *p*-nitrophenyl-*p'*-guanidinobenzoate which serve as "active-site titrants"

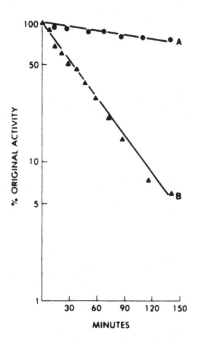

FIGURE 5. The ability of substrate to protect creatine kinase from inactivation by the active-site-directed reagent, N-(2,3-epoxypropyl)-N-amidinoglycine (epoxycreatine). Shown is protection from inactivation by the MgADP·NO$_3$ creatine complex. Conditions were as follows: (A) creatine kinase (1.0 mg/ml), epoxycreatine (48 mM), ADP (8 mM), magnesium acetate (8 mM), NaNO$_3$ (8 mM), and creatine (40 mM) in 10 mM HEPES, pH 7.5 at 0°C; (B) the same except ADP, magnesium acetate, NaNO$_3$, and creatine were all deleted. (From Marletta, M. A. and Kenyon, G. L., *J. Biol. Chem.*, 254, 1879, 1979. With permission.)

of serine proteases.[20-22] Second are the so-called K$_s$ reagents, which are isosteric with respect to substrate or ligands and possess a relatively unreactive functional group such as a sulfonyl fluoride[23] (Figure 6) or a halomethyl ketone derivative such as L-1-tosylamido-2-phenylethyl chloromethyl ketone (TPCK),[9] bromoacetylcholine,[24] and 1-chloro-2-oxo-hexanol-6-phosphate.[25] With this type of reagent, the functional group (i.e., sulfonyl halide, α-keto alkylhalide) is comparatively unreactive and reaction with a nucleophile (i.e., lysine, cysteine, histidine) is accomplished by enhanced local reagent concentration caused by specific binding. In another type of modification, the reactive species is generated after binding of the reagent to the protein. Photoaffinity reagents, which will be discussed in greater detail below, have been the most extensively studied reagents in this category. The most popular reagent class within this group are aryl azides which, upon irradiation with ultraviolet light, will generate short-lived, highly reactive nitrenes. Examples of aryl azides include 4-fluoro-3-nitrophenyl azide which has been used to modify trypsin and chymotrypsin,[26] N-4-azido-2-nitrophenyl-aminobutyryl ADP which has been used to modify adeninine nucleotide binding sites on proteins,[27] 8-azidoadenosine 3′,5′-monophosphate[28] which has been used to identify a 3′,5′-cyclic AMP receptor, and 3-azido-2,7-naphthalene disulfonate[29] (Figure 7) which has been used as a hydrophilic surface probe.

Suicide inhibitors of enzymes[30,31] can be considered a class of affinity labeling reagents.[4] In general, however, these reagents are used more frequently as probes of enzyme mechanisms rather than for the site-specific modification of proteins. Some recent elegant examples of this approach include the studies on isocoumarin derivatives by Powers and co-workers[32] and substituted benzoxazinones by Abeles and co-workers.[33] In the former study,[32] 3,4-dichloroisocoumarin was found to be an effective inhibitor of serine proteases such as human leukocyte elastase and chymotrypsin but had no effect on a related sulfydryl protease such as papain. Isocoumarin alone had no effect and the 3-chloroisocoumarin was much less

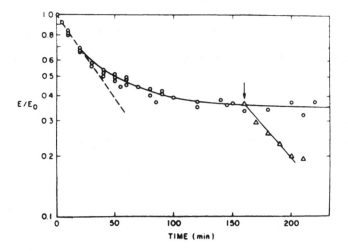

FIGURE 6. The inactivation of yeast pyruvate kinase by 5'-*p*-fluorosulfonylbenzoyl adenosine (5'-*p*-FSO$_2$BzAdo). Pyruvate kinase (0.22 to 0.49 mg/ml) was incubated with 1.1 m*M* 5'-*p*-FSO$_2$BzAdo (○ —— ○) at 25°C in 20 m*M* potassium barbital buffer, pH 8.6, containing 200 m*M* KCl, 0.5 m*M* EDTA, and 4.4% dimethylformamide. At the indicated times, a portion of the reaction mixture was withdrawn and assayed for enzymatic activity. After 160 min of reaction with the reagent, an additional 2 μl of 51 m*M* 5'-*p*-FSO$_2$BzAdo in dimethylformamide was added to 100 μl of the reaction mixture (△ —— △) and 2 μl of dimethylformamide to 100 μl of the control. (From Likos, J. J., Hess, B., and Colman, R. F., *J. Biol. Chem.*, 255, 9388, 1980. With permission.)

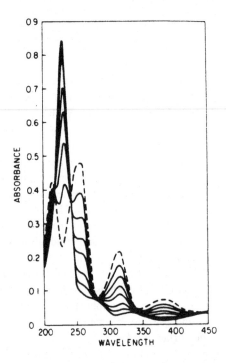

FIGURE 7. Change in the UV absorption spectrum of 3-azido-2,7-naphthalene disulfonate (ANDS) upon irradiation. Shown are the flashed spectra of 30 μ*M* ANDS in 10 m*M* sodium phosphate, pH 7.0, at 25°C. The dashed line is the spectrum of the ANDS before flash. Each solid line represents a 15-s exposure to a 366-nm hand-held UV light. The λmax of ANDS shifts from 260 nm to 233 nm during irradiation. (From Moreland, R. B. and Dockler, M. E., *Anal. Biochem.*, 103, 26, 1980. With permission.)

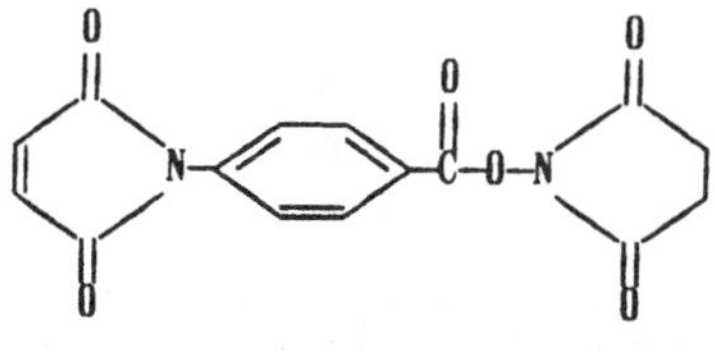

FIGURE 8. The structure of maleimido-*N*-hydroxysuccinimide.

effective. In the latter study, the catalysis-dependent inactivation of chymotrypsin with the formation of an ortho-substituted benzoyl-chymotrypsin. This inactive derivative slowly reactivates with the release of benzoyleneurea.

Irrespective of mechanism, the process of affinity labeling is conceptually a markedly different process from the "serendipitous" modification of a uniquely reactive residue at the active site of an enzyme[34-39] (see Reference 1 for a more detailed discussion of this concept).

The past six years have seen a continued use of affinity labeling to explore structure-function relationships in enzymes and other biologically active proteins.[40-57] There has, however, been only a limited increase in our understanding of the chemistry of such reactions and it is the author's sense that the majority of this effort has been directed towards photoaffinity labeling (see below).

In the area of non-photoaffinity-based reagents, the majority of the new work has been directed toward the development of more complex reagents based on the interaction between peptides and/or proteins and cell surface receptors or other examples of higher-order biochemical organization. Many of these have been based on either homobifunctional[58] or heterobifunctional[59,60] reagents such as those described in the chapter on cross-linking (Chapter 15). An example is the use of maleimido-*N*-hydroxysuccinimide (Figure 8) to prepare a derivative of choleocystokinin to label binding proteins on rat pancreatic plasma membranes.[60,61] Another example is the preparation of derivatives of calmodulin.[62]

Since the effectiveness of an affinity label is dictated largely by binding, the greater the quality of structural information in the probe, the greater the effectivenss.

An excellent example of the use of increasing structural information in the quality of the inhibition (inactivation) is the work on chymotrypsin initiated by Schoellmann and Shaw[9] and extended during the subsequent decade by Powers and co-workers. The initial studies used L-1-tosylamido-2-phenylethyl chloromethyl ketone.[9] Reaction of L-1-tosylamido-2-phenylethyl chloromethyl ketone (TosPheCH$_2$Cl) with chymotrypsin is dependent upon the structure of the native enzyme; chymotrypsin previously exposed to 8.0 *M* urea does not react with reagent. This incidentally is an excellent test for specificity of affinity labeling; reaction should not occur with denatured enzyme. The D-isomer of TosPheCH$_2$Cl does not react with the active-site histidine.[63] These investigators also reported that modification of the methionine residue at the active site (Met-192) occurred, but this reaction is apparently nonspecific and stereochemistry of the modifying reagent did not have any apparent role. The methionine residue in question was modified by iodoacetate but not with the affinity label. Morihara and Oka[64] examined the reaction of chymotrypsin with a closely related compound, carbobenzoxy-L-phenylalanine chloromethyl ketone (CBZPheCH$_2$Cl). CBZPheCH$_2$Cl reacted effectively with the active-site histidine of chymotrypsin; a greater than tenfold decrease in the observed first-order rate constant was seen if the complexity of the reagent was increased to carbobenzoxy-glycyl-L-phenylalanyl chloromethyl ketone. However if the complexity of the reagent was increased to carbobenzoxy-L-alanyl-glycyl-L-phenylalanine chloromethyl ketone, an approximate sevenfold increase in reaction rate was observed (Figure 9). It is of interest that CBZGlyPheCH$_2$Cl was approximately 8 times more

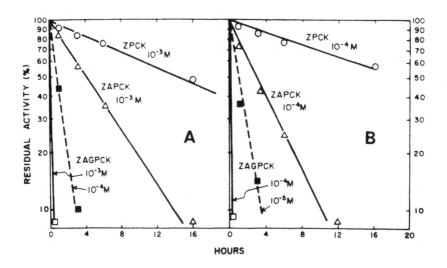

FIGURE 9.   The inactivation of subtilisin BPN′ by peptide chloromethyl ketone derivatives. The derivatives are: ZPCK, carbobenzoxy-L-phenylalanine chloromethyl ketone; ZAPCK, carbobenzoxy-L-phenylalanyl chloromethyl ketone; ZAGPCK, carbobenzoxy-L-alanyl-glycyl-L-phenylalanine chloromethyl ketone. Shown is the loss of esterase activity on incubation of the enzyme in 0.05 M Tris-HCl, pH 7.0, containing 0.001 M CaCl$_2$ and either 25% (panel A) or 10% (panel B) dioxane at 40°C. The enzyme concentration was 5 μM and inhibitor concentrations were as indicated in the figure. (From Morihara, K. and Oka, T., *Arch. Biochem. Biophys.*, 138, 526, 1970. With permission.)

effective than CBZPheCH$_2$Cl with subtilisin BPN′ at pH 7.0 (0.05 M Tris, 0.001 M CaCl$_2$, 10% dioxane) while CBZAlaGlyPheCH$_2$Cl was greater than 200 times more effective. Thus, affinity labels need not show the same order of effectiveness with different enzymes of similar specificity. Powers and co-workers have also pursued a systematic analysis of the reaction of peptide chloromethyl ketones with various serine proteases. Most noteworthy for present consideration is the study of the reaction of peptide chloromethyl ketones with chymotrypsin.[13] The results of a study of this influence of increasing structural quality of the inhibitor on the rate of inactivation of α-chymotrypsin is presented in Table 1. These observations when combined with an elegant application of crystallographic analysis[65,66] (see Figures 10, 11, and 12) provide considerable information regarding secondary substrate binding sites. The concept of greatest importance in considering this information is that the greater the specificity information (quality) built into an affinity label, the greater the significance of the study of the reaction of the compound with the protein (enzyme) under investigation. D-ProPheArgCH$_2$Cl has been prepared as a specific inactivator of thrombin.[67,68] Subsequent crystallographic studies[69] have shown that the specificity of this inhibitor is largely generated through hydrophobic interactions from a "cage" formed by tryptophanyl residues at the substrate binding site.

The reaction of peptide chloromethyl ketones with sulfhydryl proteases has been investigated.[70,71] Despite the presence of a histidine residue at the active site of these enzymes, reaction occurs at the active-site sulfhydryl group. Comparison of the rates of reaction of TosLysCH$_2$Cl with free cysteine and with papain demonstrated that reaction with the enzyme occurs approximately 10^6 times more rapidly. Rate enhancement of this order of magnitude is seen on occasion with putative affinity labels. While not necessarily as dramatic as this, differences should be seen in comparing either the rates of reaction of affinity label with model compound and protein (as seen above with papain) or the rates of reaction of affinity label and its functional group with protein. In studies on the affinity labeling of rat muscle hexokinase type II,[72] Connolly and Trayer observed that bromoacetic acid inactivated the

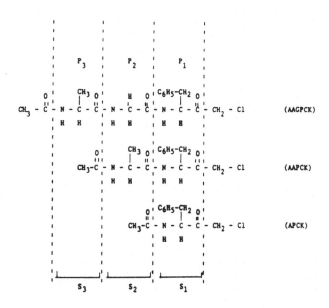

FIGURE 10. Schematic diagram of the inhibitors, acetyl-L-alanyl-glycyl-L-phenylalanine chloromethyl ketone (AAGPCK), acetyl-L-alanyl-L-phenylalanine chloromethyl ketone (AAPCK) and acetyl-L-phenylalanine chloromethyl ketone (APCK) and their interactions with the binding site on chymotrypsin according to the notation of Schechter and Berger. (From Segal, D. M. et al., *Cold Spring Harbor Symp. Quant. Biol.*, 36, 85, 1971.

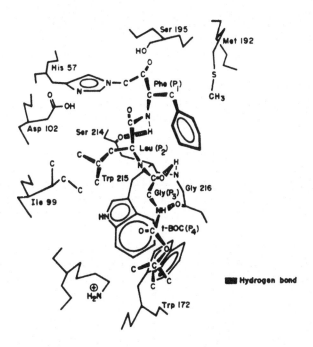

FIGURE 11. A schematic drawing of the inhibitor moiety, Boc-Gly-Leu-PheCH$_2$Cl, bound to chymotrypsin A$_\alpha$. Only the portion of the enzyme which can interact with the inhibitor is shown. (From Kurachi, K., Powers, J. C., and Wilcox, P. E., *Biochemistry*, 12, 771, 1973. With permission.)

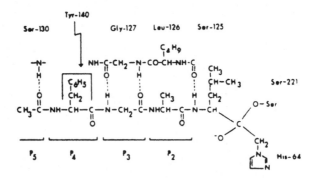

FIGURE 12.   A schematic representation of the inhibitor moiety, Ac-Phe-Gly-Ala-LeuCH$_2$ bound to the active site of subtilisin BPN′. The probable interactions are based on crystallographic studies of subtilisin inhibited with other chloromethyl ketones. (From Powers, J.C., Lively, M.O., III, and Tippett, J.T., *Biochim. Biophys. Acta*, 480, 246, 1977. With permission.)

enzyme at one fifth the rate of the affinity label, *N*-bromoacetyl-2-amino-2-deoxy-D-glu-copyranose. The difference in rate is likely larger than this since it could not be determined that the two reagents were acting at the same site(s). The differences in the reaction of peptide chloromethyl ketones with serine proteases and sulfhydryl proteases have been considered in some detail by Brocklehurst and Malthouse.[73]

As described above, α-keto-halo compounds can modify histidyl and/or cysteinyl residues at the active site. Further versatility in the reaction of this class of derivative was shown by the work of Hass and Neurath[74,75] on the affinity labeling of bovine carboxypeptidase A (Figures 13 and 14). Here the affinity label, *N*-bromoacetyl-*N*-methyl-L-phenylalanine, reacts with the active-site carboxylic acid (Glu-270) with the formation of a glycolic acid derivative. Modification of an active-site carboxyl group with an α-keto-halo compound also occurs with an affinity label described by Rasnick and Powers[76] (Figure 15). The active-site-directed inhibitor used, *N*-chloroacetyl-*N*-hydroxyleucine methyl ester, is novel in that a substantial portion of the "affinity" is provided by interaction with the zinc atom at the active site (see Figure 16).[77] Replacement of the P′ amide hydroxyl with a hydrogen obviates the majority of the quality of this inhibitor.

Photoaffinity labeling has emerged as an extremely active area of research. Reagents based on photoactivation have a distinct advantage in that the reactive species, generally a nitrene or carbene, will modify a wide variety of chemical bonds in a protein including insertion into a carbon-carbon bond. Thus, one is not limited by the presence of specific functional groups at the site of interest. In addition, the reactive species can be generated at the site at the convenience of the investigator. The reader is directed to a number of general works on photochemistry[78-84] and, in particular to reviews by Bayley and Knowles[85] and Bayley[86] for a detailed consideration of the chemistry involved in these reactions.

The affinity reagents using in the photoaffinity labeling for proteins are composed of two distinct moieties: one, an affinity component which possesses characteristics complementary to the binding site being studied and a second moiety which can generate either a nitrene (an aromatic azide) or a carbene (an aliphatic carbonyldiazo compound or a diazarine). A particularly good example, 8-azido adenosine triphosphate, is shown in Figure 17. This compound has been extensively used to modified nucleotide binding sites in proteins.[87,88] The specificity is provided by the adenosine triphosphate moiety while the reactive group is a nitrene derived from photolysis of the aromatic azide function. A fluorescent derivative related to 8-azido adenosine triphosphate, 8-azido-2′-*O*-dansyl adenosine triphosphate (Figure 18) has been synthesized.[89]

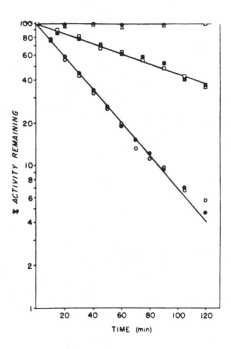

FIGURE 13. Affinity labeling of bovine carboxypeptidase A_γ^{Leu} (CPA_γ^{Leu}) by N-bromoacetyl-N-methyl-L-phenylalanine (BAMP). Shown is the loss of peptidase and esterase activities of CPA_γ^{Leu} as a function of time during incubation with L-BAMP, D-BAMP, and bromoacetate. CPA_γ^{leu} (0.1 mg/ml) was treated with 1 mM L-BAMP, 10 mM D-BAMP, or 10 mM bromoacetate in a solution containing 1 N NaCl, 0.05 M Tris-chloride (pH 7.5). The esterase (L-BAMP (●); D-BAMP (■); bromoacetate (▲)) and peptidase (L-BAMP (○) D-BAMP (□); bromoacetate (△)) activities of the enzyme were monitored as a function of time. (From Hass, G. M. and Neurath, H., *Biochemistry*, 10, 3535, 1971. With permission.)

The variety of photoactivated reagents is limited only by the imagination of the investigator. The criteria for a suitable photoaffinity reagent are discussed in detail elsewhere[85,86] and will only be summarized here. First, the synthesis of the precursor azide, diazo compound, or diazirine should be reasonable and a stable product obtained which can be stored until use. The precursor must be stable under the solution conditions to be used in the photolysis reaction. For example, a reducing environment should be avoided with aryl azides as such a compound can be reduced by dithiothreitol to the corresponding amine.[91] Other possibilities with thiol groups include the oxidation of cysteine to cystine during photolysis of an aromatic azide, such as that observed with cytosolic phosphoenolpyruvate carboxykinase and 8-azidoguanosine 5′-triphosphate.[92] The active species, either a nitrene or a carbene, must be generated under conditions where the absorption characteristics of the biologic system under study does not present difficulties. An excitation wavelength less than 300 nm should be avoided when working with either proteins or nucleic acids. Photolysis properties of the precursor can be altered by changing the chemistry of the reagent. This is illustrated by the examples in Figure 19 (adapted from Reference 86). The parent compound, phenyl azide (I) absorbs at 250 nm. Changing the chemistry of the ring by addition of a carboxylate function increases the wavelength of maximum absorption to 280. Placement of even strongly electron-withdrawing component, a nitro function, further increases the absorption maximum to approximately 330 nm. The photolysis process should be efficient in that the precursor has a high extinction coefficient with generation of the active species with a reasonably high quantum yield. Finally, the reactive species should have a short lifetime (highly reactive species).

The actual conditions for photolysis vary with the protein and affinity label. The two

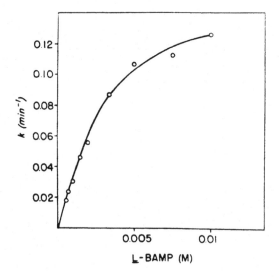

FIGURE 14. Psuedo-first-order rate constant, k, for the inactivation of CPA$_\gamma^{Leu}$ as a function of L-BAMP concentration at pH 7.5. Incubation mixtures contained 0.1 mg/ml of CPA$_\gamma^{Leu}$ in 1 *N* NaCl, 0.05 *M* Tris-chloride (pH 7.5), including different amounts of L-BAMP. Esterase activity was monitored as a function of time at each concentration of L-BAMP and pseudo-first-order rate constants were calculated from the following equation:

$$\ln \left(\frac{E_1}{E_2} \right) = k(T_2 - T_1)$$

(From Hass, G. M. and Neurath, H., *Biochemistry*, 10, 3535, 1971. With permission.)

IRREVERSIBLE INHIBITION OF THERMOLYSIN

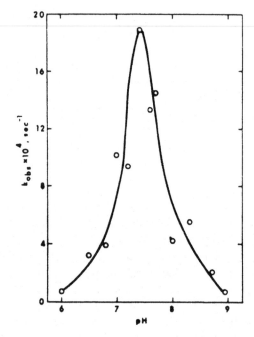

FIGURE 15. pH Dependence of the inactivation of thermolysin by *N*-chloroacetyl-DL-*N*-hydroxyleucine methyl ester (ClCH$_2$CO-DL-(N-OH)Leu-OCH$_3$). The concentration of the enzyme was 4.2 μ*M* and the concentration of the inhibitor was 2.3 m*M*. The buffers used were: PIPES (pH 6.0), HEPES (pH 6.50 to 7.70), and Tris (pH 8.00 to 8.95); all were 0.1 *M* and contained 0.01 *M* CaCl$_2$. (From Rasnik, D. and Powers, J. C., *Biochemistry*, 17, 4363, 1978. With permission.)

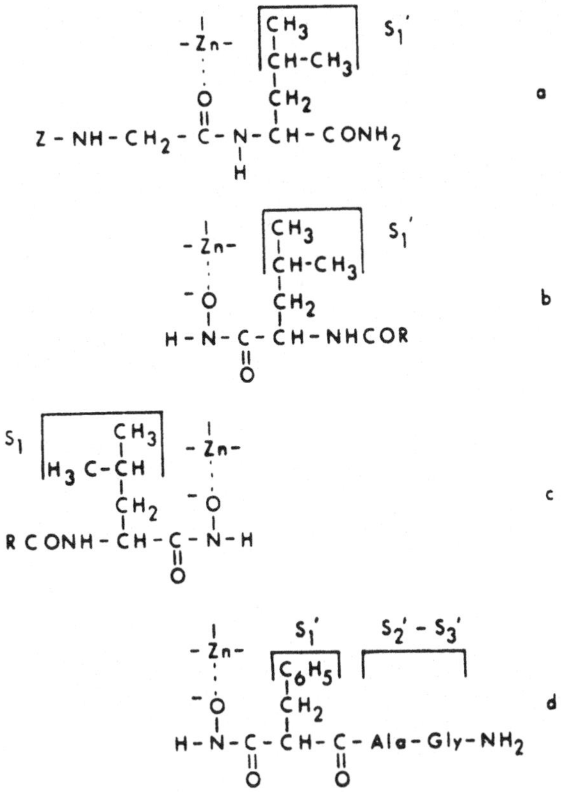

FIGURE 16. Peptide hydroxamic acids as inhibitors of thermo-lysin. Shown are schematic drawings demonstrating the binding of a substrate (a) to the active site of thermolysin and possible binding modes for hydroxamic acid inhibitors (b-d). (From Nishino, N. and Powers, J. C., *Biochemistry,* 17, 2846, 1978. With permission.)

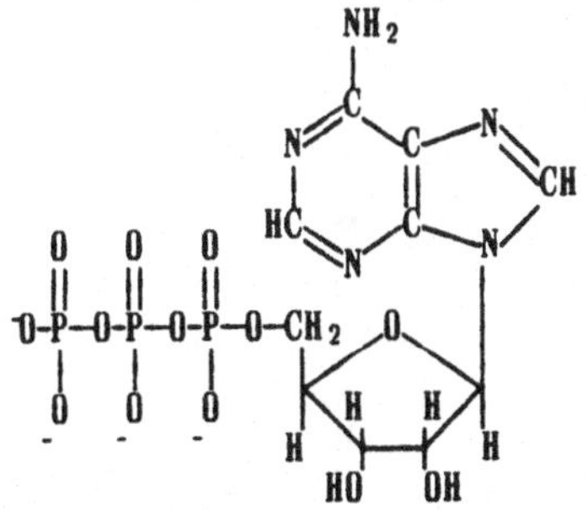

FIGURE 17. The structure of 8-azido adenosine triphosphate.

general reviews cited above[85,86] contain extensive detail regarding solvent/temperature selection and irradiation conditions (including lamp selection).

Several photoaffinity reagents have been designed to probe membrane structure and affinity use based on reagent hydrophobicity. 3-(Trifluoromethyl)-3-(*m*-iodophenyl)diazirine (Figure 20) was developed to selectively modify intrinsic membrane proteins.[93,94] More recently this reagent has been used to label ''hydrophobic'' regions of proteins interacting with lipid vesicles.[95,96] Radiolabeled (^{125}I) reagent has been used to monitor the extent of modification

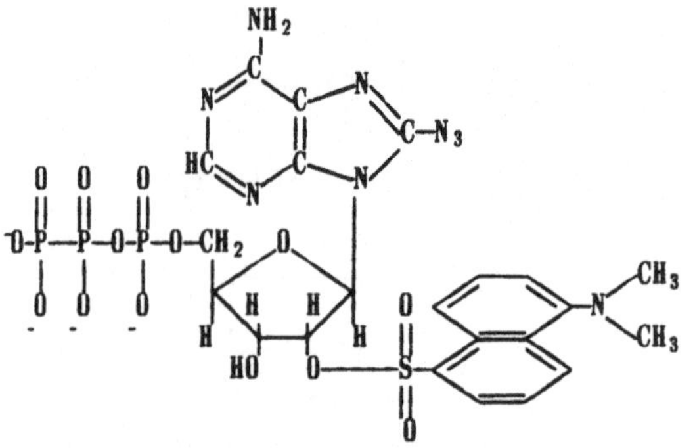

FIGURE 18. The structure of 8-azido-2'-*O*-dansyl adenosine triphosphate.

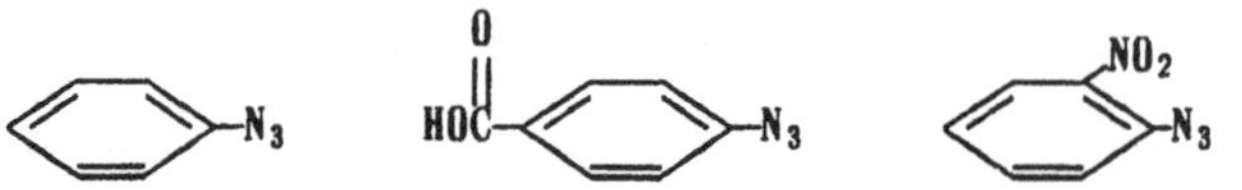

FIGURE 19. The structure of phenyl azide (I) and two derivatives with electron-withdrawing substituents. *p*-Azidobenzoic acid (II) and 2-nitrophenyl azide (III) have excitation maximum at higher wavelengths than the parent compound (see text).

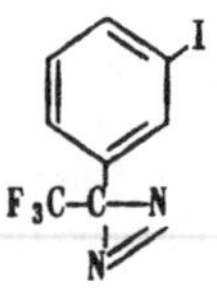

FIGURE 20. The structure of 2-(trifluoromethyl)-3-(*m*-iodophenyl)diazirine.

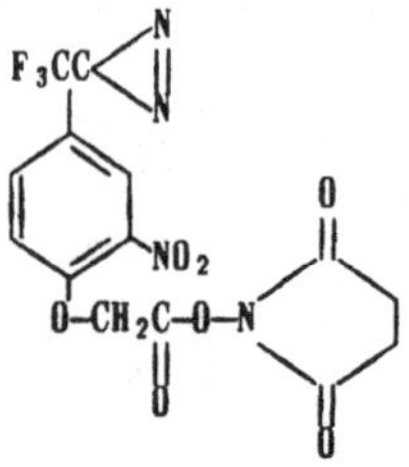

FIGURE 21. The structure of [[2-nitro-4-(trifluoromethyl-3H-diazirin-3-yl)]phenoxy]acetyl-*N*-hydroxysuccinimide.

in these studies. A chromogenic derivative of 3-(trifluoromethyl)-3-(*m*-iodophenyl)diazirine (Figure 21) has recently been synthesized[97] which can also be used as a cross-linking agent via the *N*-hydroxysuccinimide ester function. A peptide-bound derivative, 2-[3-(trifluoromethyl-3H-diazirin-3-yl)phenoxy]acetyl-*S*-methyloxycarbonyl-sulfonyl-L-cysteinyl-D-valine has been used to label isopenicillin *N*-synthetase using laser photolysis.[98]

Diazofluorene and the related 9-diazofluorene-2-butyric acid (Figure 22) are other useful

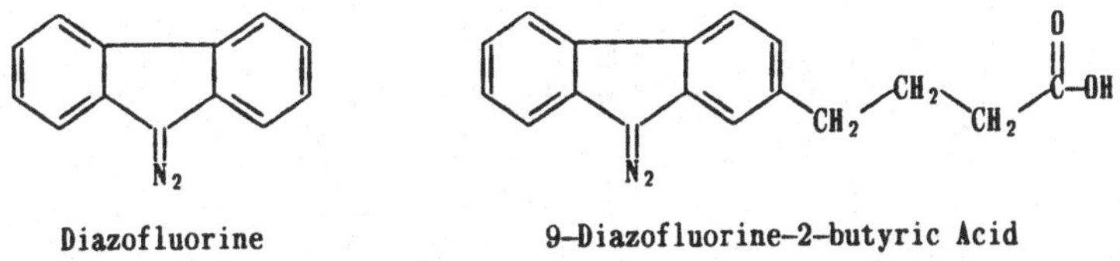

Diazofluorine   9-Diazofluorine-2-butyric Acid

FIGURE 22.   The structures of 2-diazofluorene and 9-diazofluorene-2-butyric acid.

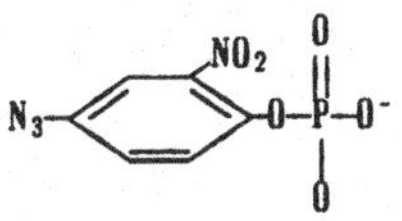

FIGURE 23.   The structure of 4-azido-2-nitrophenyl phosphate.

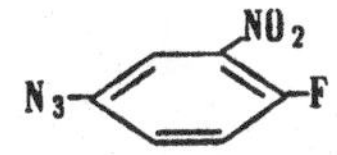

FIGURE 24.   The structure of 4-fluoro-3-nitrophenyl azide.

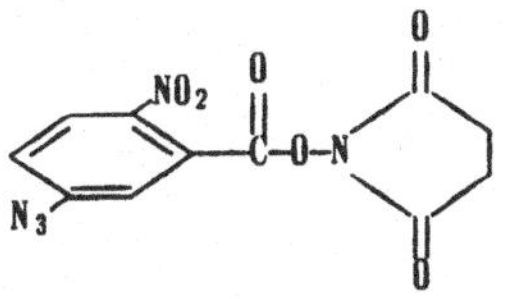

FIGURE 25.   The structure of N-(5-azido-2-nitrobenzoyl)-N-oxysuccinimide.

hydrophobic probes.[99,100] The latter derivative can be used to label membrane components at different depths within the membrane by varying the length of the alkyl carboxylic acid side chain.

4-Azido-2-nitrophenylphosphate (Figure 23) is a photoaffinity reagent for labeling phosphate-binding sites in proteins[101,102] which has recently been used to label residues at the phosphate-binding site of mitochondrial ATPase.[103]

More complex peptide photoaffinity reagents have been developed by incorporating modified amino acids capable of generating an activated species. Examples include 6-nitrotryptophan in choleocystokinin,[104] N-ε-azidobenzolysine in oxytocin[105] (biotinyl and fluorescent derivatives were also prepared using the same synthetic strategy), and p-azidophenylalanine in vasotocin.[106] Another related approach involves the incorporation of p-benzoyl-L-phenylalanine into a peptide substrate for cAMP-dependent protein kinase[107] and 3-(4'-benzoylphenyl)propionyl-phenylalanyl transfer RNA.[108]

Another approach to the preparation of a complex photoaffinity label is the use of heterobifunctional cross-linking reagents (see Chapter 15) where one of the functional groups possesses the capability of generating a nitrene or carbene on photolysis. One of the early examples of this type of reagent is 4-fluro-3-nitrophenyl azide (Figure 24).[109] This reagent has been recently used to prepare a photoaffinity derivative of parathyroid hormone.[110] A related reagent, N-(5-azido-2-nitrobenzoyl)-N-oxysuccinimide (Figure 25) has been used to prepare a photoaffinity label based on atrial naturetic factor,[111] insulin-like growth factor,[112]

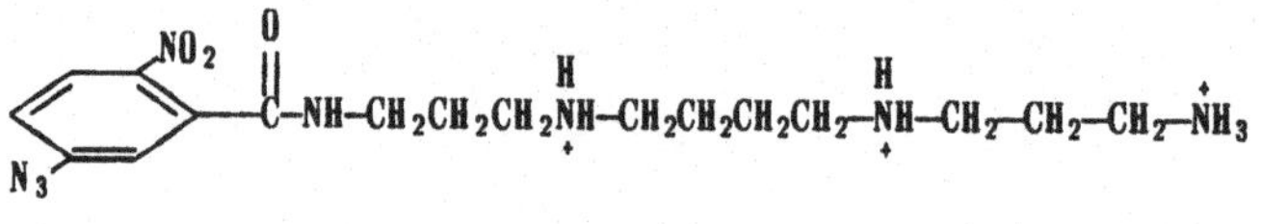

FIGURE 26.   The structure of azidonitrobenzoyl-spermine.

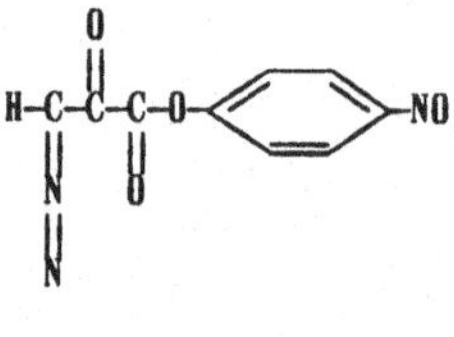

FIGURE 27.   The structure of *p*-nitrophenyl-3-diazopyruvate.

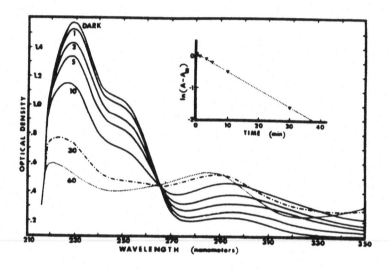

FIGURE 28.   The effect of photolysis on the UV absorption spectra of *m*-azidobenzamidine. The concentration of *m*-azidobenzamidine was 0.187 m*M*. Solid line for 0 (dark), 1, 3, 5, and 10 min of photolysis (performed with a model 457 Micropulser, Xenon Corp., equipped with a Zenon flash lamp, N-725C-WC; energy was delivered at a rate of 14 pulses per second utilizing a 6-kV potential on the lamp, located 2.5 cm from the sample; samples were contained in Pyrex Petri dishes, 1.5 × 5.0 cm, fitted with 5.0-cm diameter polystyrene Falcon Petri dish covers to act as filters; this configuration provided efficient thermal equilibration in addition to a very sharp filter cutoff of wavelengths below 295 nm; the entire lamp housing and sample compartment were maintained at 5 to 7°C (by enclosure in a small refrigerator). Dashed and dotted lines represent 30 and 60 min, respectively. Photolysis rate (inset) is $k_m = 7.4 \pm 0.9 \times 10^{-5}$ per pulse. The solvent was 0.1 *M* succinate, pH 6.2. (From DeTraglia, M. C., Brand, J. S., and Tometsko, A. M., *J. Biol. Chem.*, 253, 1846, 1978. With permission.)

tubulin,[113] and spermine[114] (Figure 26). *p*-Nitrophenyl-3-diazopyruvate (Figure 27)[115] has been used to prepare a photoaffinity derivative of calmodulin.[116]

Photoaffinity labels have become extremely popular. These reagents are essentially unreactive until exposed to light, whereupon the active species is generated (i.e., a nitrene is formed from an azide) which then reacts instantaneously with a variety of groups. Particular attention must be paid to photolysis rate and solvent conditions. As noted by DeTraglia and co-workers,[90] characterization of the rate(s) of photolysis vs. wavelength of irradiation provides useful information to control photoaffinity labeling (see Figures 28 and 29). Another potential problem in the use of aryl azides is the ease of reduction to the corresponding amine with a mild reducing agent such as dithiothreitol.[91] Selected examples of affinity labels are given in Table 2.

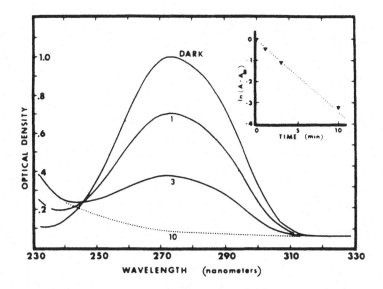

FIGURE 29. The effect of photolysis on the UV absorption spectrum of *p*-azidobenzamidine. The experiments were performed as described under Figure 23 with 0.181 m*M* *p*-azidobenzamidine. Solid lines for 0 (dark), 1, and 3 min of photolysis while the dashed line represents 10 min. Photolysis rate (inset) is $k_p = 4.2 \pm 0.5 \times 10^{-4}$ per pulse. (From DeTraglia, M. C., Brand, J. S., and Tometsko, A. M., *J. Biol. Chem.*, 253, 1846, 1978. With permission.)

Table 2
SELECTED EXAMPLES OF AFFINITY LABELS

Compound	Substrate or Ligand[a]	Enzyme	Residue modified[b]	Ref.
Tosylphenylalanine chloromethyl ketone (TPCK, Tos-PheCH₂Cl) L-1-tosylamido-2-phenylethyl chloromethyl ketone	Tosylphenylalanine methyl ester	Chymotrypsin	His / His	1 / 2
Tosyllysyl chloromethyl ketone (TLCK; TosLysCH₂Cl) 1-chloro-3-tosylamido-7-amino-2-heptanone	Tosyl lysine methyl ester	Trypsin	His	3
	Adenosine 5′-phosphate	Adenylosuccinate lyase		4

Table 2 (continued)
SELECTED EXAMPLES OF AFFINITY LABELS

Compound	Substrate or Ligand[a]	Enzyme	Residue modified[b]	Ref.
N-Bromoacetyl-N-methyl-L-phenylalanine	N-Acetyl-L-phenylalanine ester	Carboxypeptidase	Glu	5,6
p-Amidinophenacyl bromide	Benzamidine	Trypsin		7
p-Guanidinophenacyl bromide	Benzamidine	Trypsin	Ser	7
m-[O-(2-chloro-5-fluorosulfonyl[c] phenylureido) phenoxybutoxy] benzamidine	Benzamidine	Trypsin Thrombin		8,9 10
DL-α-Bromo-β-(5-imidazoyl)-propionic acid	Imidazole[f]	Horse liver alcohol dehydrogenase, yeast alcohol dehydrogenase	Cys	11
p-Azidobenzamidine	Benzamidine	Trypsin		12
m-Azidobenzamidine	Benzamidine	Trypsin		13
Iodoacetyldiethylstilbestrol	Glutamate		Cys	14

Table 2 (continued)
SELECTED EXAMPLES OF AFFINITY LABELS

Compound	Substrate or Ligand[a]	Enzyme	Residue modified[b]	Ref.

ClCH₂ — C — N — CH — C — OCH₃ (structure)

| 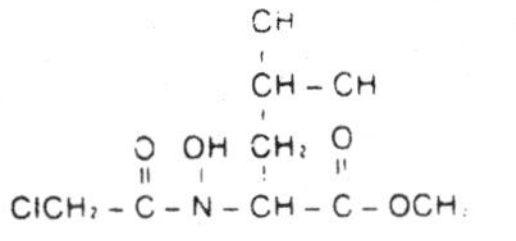 | Metal affinity | Thermolysin | Glu | 15 |

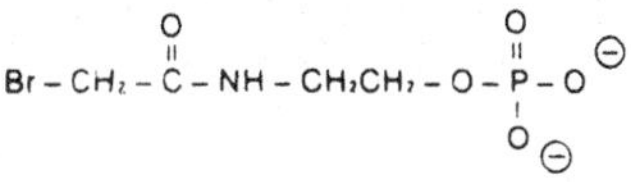

Br – CH₂ – C – NH – CH₂CH₂ – O – P – O (structure)

Bromoacetylcholine

| | Acetylcholine | Acetylcholine receptor | Cys | 16 |

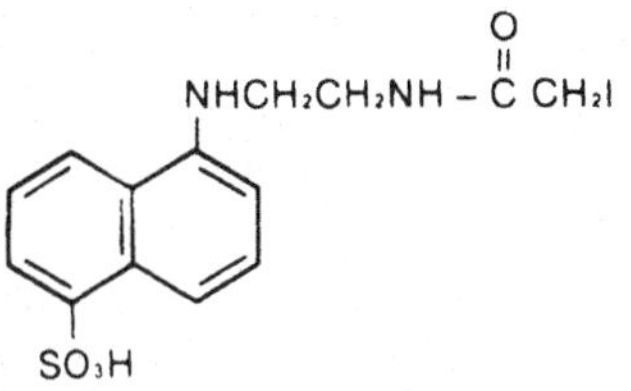

NHCH₂CH₂NH – C CH₂I (structure) SO₃H

N-(Iodoacetylamino-ethyl)-5-naphthylamine-1-sulfonic acid

| | | Phosphoenolpyruvate carboxykinase | Cys | 17 |

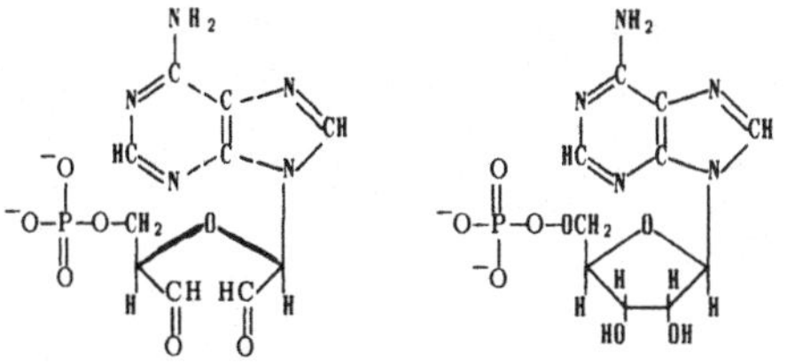

AMP Dialdehyde structures

AMP Dialdehyde (adenosine-5'-monophosphate-2',3'-dialdehyde)

| | Adenosine-5'-phosphate | Fructose 1,6-bisphosphatase | Lys[d] | 18 |

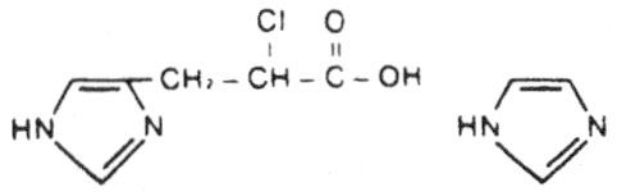

2-Chloro-3-(5-imidazodyl) propionic acid structure

2-Chloro-3-(5-imidazodyl) propionic acid

| | Metal affinity | Horse liver alcohol dehydrogenase, yeast alcohol dehydrogenase | | 19 |

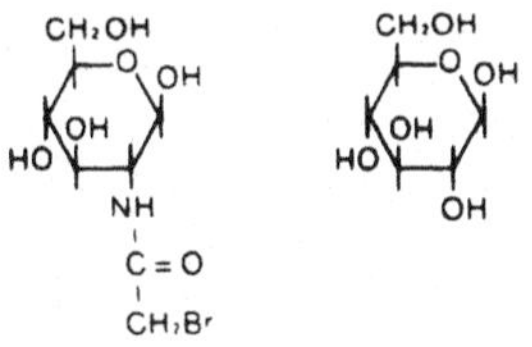

N-Bromoacetylglucosamine structures

N-Bromoacetylglucosamine

| | Glucose | Rat muscle hexokinase II | Cys | 20 |

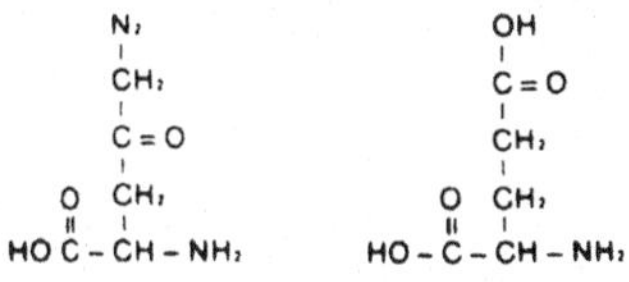

6-Diazo-5-oxo-D-norleucine structures

6-Diazo-5-oxo-D-norleucine

| | D-Glutamate | γ-Glutamyl transpeptidase | | 21 |

Table 2 (continued)
SELECTED EXAMPLES OF AFFINITY LABELS

Compound	Substrate or Ligand[a]	Enzyme	Residue modified[b]	Ref.
N-4-Azido 2-nitrophenyl-γ-aminobutyryl-adenosine diphosphate	Adenine nucleotides	F1-ATPase		22,23
5-[^{125}I]-iodonaphthyl-1-azide	"Hydrophobic" probe	Cytochrome c oxidase		24
5-(4-Azido-2-nitrophenyl)-[^{35}S]-thiophenol	"Hydrophobic" probe	Cytochrome c oxidase		24
N-(2,3-Epoxypropyl)-*N*-amidinoglycine	Creatine	Creatine kinase	Carbo	25
4-(3-Bromoacetylpyridinio)-butyldiphosphoadenosine	NAD	Horse liver alcohol dehydrogenase	Cys	26
		Yeast alcohol dehydrogenase	Cys	26
		Bacillus stearothermophilus alcohol dehydrogenase	Cys	27

Table 2 (continued)
SELECTED EXAMPLES OF AFFINITY LABELS

Compound	Substrate or Ligand[a]	Enzyme	Residue modified[b]	Ref.
CH₃, CH₃ (structure) ⊕N₂ ⊖F p-Dimethylaminobenzene dia-zonium fluoride[c]		Acetylcholine esterase		28
(structure) 5'-p-Fluorosulfonyl-benzoyl adenosine	Adenosine-5'-phosphate	Yeast pyruvate kinase	Tyr[i] Lys	29
(structure) 4-Nitrophenyl-α-D-galactopyranoside[f]	β-Galactoside	Lac carrier protein		30
(structure) Azidofluorescein diacetate				31
(structure) 17β-Hydroxy-4,6-androsta-dien-3-one[h] (Δ⁶-testosterone)	17-β-Hydroxy-5-androstan-3-one	**Androgen binding proteins**		32
(structure) 3-Azido-2',7-naphthalene disulfonate	Hydrophilic surface probe			33

Table 2 (continued)
SELECTED EXAMPLES OF AFFINITY LABELS

Compound	Substrate or Ligand[a]	Enzyme	Residue modified[b]	Ref.
2-(2-Nitro-4-azidophenyl) aminoethyl 16-doxyl-stearate (1,14 Nap)		Ca²⁺ ATPase in sarcoplasmic reticulum		34
Adenosine triphosphate-γ-*p*-azidoanilide	Adenosine triphosphate	Arginine kinase	Cys	35
Bromopyruvate		Flavocytochrome b₂	Cys	36
Bromoacetyl derivative of pleuromutilin	Tiamulin (pleuromutilin)	Ribosome		38
5'-*p*-Fluorosulfonyl-benzoyl adenosine	NADH	17 β-Estradiol dehydrogenase		
5'-*p*-Fluorosulfonyl-benzoyl guanosine	Guanosine nucleotide	Phosphoenolpyruvate carboxykinase		39
1,2-di-*O*-hexylglycero-3-(ethyldiazomalonamido-ethyl phosphate)	Phosphatidyl-ethanolamine	Phospholipase A₂	Val	40

Table 2 (continued)
SELECTED EXAMPLES OF AFFINITY LABELS

Compound	Substrate or Ligand[a]	Enzyme	Residue modified[b]	Ref.

| 5-*p*-Fluorosulfonyl-benzoyl-1-*N*⁶-ethenoadenosine | Nucleotide | Pyruvate kinase | Cys | 41 |

| *N*-Bromoacetyl-L-Thyroxine | Thyroxine | Thyroxine-binding globulin | Met | 42 |

| (RS)-3-bromo-2-ketoglutarate | α-Ketoglutarate | Isocitrate dehydrogenase | | 43 |

| 5'-*p*-Fluorosulfonyl-benzoyl-adenosine | Adenosine-5'-phosphate | Cyclic GMP-dependent protein kinase | — | 44 |

| Iodoazidobenzyl-pindolol[¹] (±)-1-(indol-4-yloxy)-3-[1-(*p*-azido-*m*-iodophenyl)-2-isobutylamine]-2-propanol | β-Adrenergic agonists | β-Adrenergic receptors | — | 45 |

| 2-Azido-4-ethylamine-6-iso-propylamine-5-triazine (azido-triazine) | Atrazine | Chloroplast membranes | — | 46 |

Table 2 (continued)
SELECTED EXAMPLES OF AFFINITY LABELS

Compound	Substrate or Ligand[a]	Enzyme	Residue modified[b]	Ref.
[³H]-3'-O-(4-[N-4-azido-2-ni-trophenyl] amino butyryl-adenosine-5'-diphosphate ([³H]-NAP₄-ADP)	Adenosine diphosphate	Adenosine-5-triphosphatase	—	47
[³H]-3'-O-(4-[N-(4-azido-2-ni-trophenyl) amino] butyryl adenosine triphosphate ([³H]NAP₄-ATP)	Adenosine triphosphate	Adenosine-5-triphosphatase	—	47
3-Azido-9[(4-diethylamino)-1-methyl-butylamine]-7-methoxyacridine	Quinacrine[ᵏ]	Acridine dye binding sites		48
1-Chloro-2-oxohexanol-6-phosphate	Glucose-6-phosphate	Phosphoglucose isomerase		49
8-Azidoguanosine-5'-triphosphate	Guanosine-5-triphosphate	Guanosine-5-triphosphatase		50

Table 2 (continued)
SELECTED EXAMPLES OF AFFINITY LABELS

    Model for affinity label.
ᵇ   From amino acid analysis unless otherwise indicated.
ᶜ   Affinity based on metal chelating ability.
ᵈ   Stabilization required (reduction of Schiff base).
ᵉ   Photoaffinity labeling by using energy transfer from tryptophanyl residue.
ᶠ   Two different sites modified in enzyme.
ᵍ   Photoaffinity label. Photolysis with a mercury arc lamp (100 W, type AH-4) with a Corning 0-54 filter to eliminate light below 300 nm)
ʰ   Subject to photoexcitation at 345 nm (n → π* transition) resulting in formation of reactive species.
ⁱ   Small extent of modification at Lys, Tyr, and His.
ʲ   Iodohydroxybenzylpindolol, a related compound, was demonstrated to have a k_D with duck erythrocyte membranes of 0.22 nM.
ᵏ   3-Chloro-9-[(4-(dimethylamino)-1-methylbutyl)amino]-7-methoxyacridine; an antimalarial agent and flavin antagonist.

References for Table 2

1. **Schoellman, G. and Shaw, E.,** Direct evidence for the presence of histidine in the active center of chymotrypsin, *Biochemistry,* 2, 252, 1963.
2. **Morihara, K. and Oka, T.,** Subtilisin BPN': inactivation by chloromethyl ketone derivatives of peptide substrates, *Arch. Biochem. Biophys.,* 138, 526, 1970.
3. **Shaw, E., Mares-Guia, M., and Cohen, W.,** Evidence for an active-center histidine in trypsin through the use of a specific reagent, 1-chloro-3-tosylamido-7-amino-2-heptanone, the chloromethyl ketone derived from Nα-tosyl-L-lysine, *Biochemistry,* 4, 2219, 1965.
4. **Hampton, A. and Harper, P. J.,** The potential of carboxylic-phosphoric mixed anhydrides as specific reagents for enzymic binding sites for alkyl phosphates. Inactivation of an enzyme by an anhydride isosteric with adenosine 5'-phosphate, *Arch. Biochem. Biophys.,* 143, 340, 1971.
5. **Hass, G. M. and Neurath, H.,** Affinity labeling of bovine carboxypeptidase A,ᴸᵉᵘ by N-bromoacetyl-N-methyl-L-phenylalanine. I. Kinetics of inactivation, *Biochemistry,* 10, 3535, 1971.
6. **Hass, G. M. and Neurath, H.,** Affinity labeling of bovine carboxypeptidase A,ᴸᵉᵘ by N-bromoacetyl-N-methyl-L-phenylalanine. II. Sites of modification, *Biochemistry,* 10, 3541, 1971.
7. **Schroeder, D. D. and Shaw, E.,** Active-site-directed phenacyl halides inhibitory to trypsin, *Arch. Biochem. Biophys.,* 142, 340, 1971.
8. **Bing, D. H., Andrews, J. M., and Cory, M.,** Affinity labeling of thrombin and other serine proteases with an extended reagent, in *Chemistry and Biology of Thrombin,* Lundblad, R. L., Fenton, J. W., and Mann, K. G., Eds., Ann Arbor Science, Ann Arbor, Mich., 1977, 159.
9. **Bing, D. H., Cory, M., and Fenton, J. W., II,** Exo-site affinity labeling of human thrombins. Similar labeling on the A chain and B chain/fragments of clotting α– and non-clotting γ/β–thrombins, *J. Biol. Chem.,* 252, 8027, 1977.
10. **Bing, D. H., Cory, M., and Doll, M.,** The inactivation of human C1 by benzamidine and pyridinium sulfonyl fluorides, *J. Immunol.,* 113, 584, 1974.
11. **Dahl, K. H. and McKinley-McKee, J. S.,** Affinity labelling of alcohol dehydrogenases. Chemical modification of the horse liver and the yeast enzymes with α-bromo-β-(5-imidazolyl)-propionic acid and 1,3-dibromoacetone, *Eur. J. Biochem.,* 81, 223, 1977.
12. **DeTraglia, M. C., Brand, J. S., and Tometsko, A. M.,** Characterization of azidobenzamidines as photoaffinity labels for trypsin, *J. Biol. Chem.,* 253, 1846, 1978.
13. **Tometsko, A. M. and Turula, J.,** Inactivation of trypsin and chymotrypsin with a photosensitive probe, *Int. J. Peptide Protein Res.,* 8, 331, 1976.
14. **Michel, F., Pons, M., Descomps, B., and Crastes de Paulet, A.,** Affinity labelling of the estrogen binding site of glutamate dehydrogenase with iodoacetyldiethylstilbestrol. Selective alkylation of cysteine-8ᵘ, *Eur. J. Biochem.,* 84, 267, 1978.
15. **Rasnick, D. and Powers, J. C.,** Active-site directed irreversible inhibition of thermolysin, *Biochemistry,* 17, 4363, 1978.
16. **Damle, V. N., McLaughlin, M., and Karlin, A.,** Bromoacetylcholine as an affinity label of the acetylcholine receptor from *Torpedo californica, Biochem. Biophys. Res. Commun.,* 84, 845, 1978.
17. **Silverstein, R., Rawitch, A. B., and Grainger, D. A.,** Affinity labelling of phosphoenolpyruvate carboxykinase with 1,5-I-AEDANS, *Biochem. Biophys. Res. Commun.,* 87, 911, 1979.
18. **Maccioni, R. B., Hubert, E., and Slebe, J. C.,** Selective modification of fructose 1,6-bisphosphatase by periodate-oxidized AMP, *FEBS Lett.,* 102, 29, 1979.

References for Table 2 (continued)

19. **Dahl, K. H., McKinley-McKee, J. S., Beyerman, H. C., and Noordam, A.,** Metal-directed affinity labelling. Inactivation and inhibition studies of two zinc alcohol dehydrogenases with twelve imidazole derivatives, *FEBS Lett.,* 99, 308, 1979.

20. **Connolly, B. A. and Trayer, I. P.,** Affinity labelling of rat muscle hexokinase type II by a glucose-derived alkylating agent, *Eur. J. Biochem.,* 93, 375, 1979.

21. **Inoue, M., Horiuchi, S., and Marino, Y.,** Affinity labelling of rat kidney γ-glutamyl transpeptidase by 6-diazo-5-oxo-D-norleucine, *Eur. J. Biochem.,* 99, 169, 1979.

22. **Lunardi, J., Lauquin, G. J. M., and Vignais, P. V.,** Interaction of azidonitrophenylaminobutyryl-ADP, a photoaffinity ADP analog with mitochondrial adenosine triphosphatase. Identification of the labeled subunits, *FEBS Lett.,* 80, 317, 1977.

23. **Lunardi, J. and Vignais, P. V.,** Adenine nucleotide binding sites in chemically modified F1-ATPase. Inhibitory effect of 4-chloro-7-nitrobenzofurazan on photolabeling by arylazido nucleotides, *FEBS Lett.,* 102, 23, 1979.

24. **Cerletti, N. and Schatz, G.,** Cytochrome c oxidase from baker's yeast. Photolabeling of subunits exposed to the lipid bilayer, *J. Biol. Chem.,* 254, 7746, 1979.

25. **Marletta, M. A. and Kenyon, G. L.,** Affinity labelling of creatine kinase by N-(2,3-epoxypropyl)-N-amidinoglycine, *J. Biol. Chem.,* 254, 1879, 1979.

26. **Woenckhaus, C., Jeck, R., and Jörnvall, H.,** Affinity labelling of yeast and liver alcohol dehydrogenases with the NAD analogue, 4-(3-bromoacetylpyridinio)butyldiphosphoadenosine, *Eur. J. Biochem.,* 93, 65, 1979.

27. **Jeck, R., Woenckhaus, C., Harris, J. I., and Runswick, M. J.,** Identification of the amino acid residue modified in *Bacillus stearothermophilus* alcohol dehydrogenase by the NAD⁺ analogue 4-(3-bromoacetyl-pyridinio) butyldiphosphoadenosine, *Eur. J. Biochem.,* 93, 57, 1979.

28. **Godner, M. P. and Hirth, C. G.,** Specific photolabeling induced by energy transfer: application to irreversible inhibition of acetylcholinesterase, *Proc. Natl. Acad. Sci. U.S.A.,* 77, 6439, 1980.

29. **Likos, J. J., Hess, B., and Colman, R. F.,** Affinity labelling of the active site of yeast pyruvate kinase by 5'-p-fluorosulfonylbenzoyl adenosine, *J. Biol. Chem.,* 255, 9388, 1980.

30. **Kaczorowski, G. J., LeBlanc, G., and Kaback, H. R.,** Specific labelling of the *lac* carrier protein in membrane vesicles of *Escherichia coli* by a photoaffinity reagent, *Proc. Natl. Acad. Sci. U.S.A.,* 77, 6319, 1980.

31. **Rotman, A. and Heldman, J.,** Azidofluorescein diacetate — a novel intracellular photolabelling reagent, *FEBS Lett.,* 122, 215, 1980.

32. **Taylor, C. A., Jr., Smith, H. E., and Danzo, B. J.,** Photoaffinity labelling of rat androgen binding protein, *Proc. Natl. Acad. Sci. U.S.A.,* 77, 234, 1980.

33. **Moreland, R. B. and Dockter, M. E.,** Preparation and characterization of 3-azido-2,7-naphthalene disulfonate: a photolabile fluorescent precursor useful as a hydrophilic surface probe, *Analyt. Biochem.,* 103, 26, 1980.

34. **Fellmann, P., Andersen, J., Devaux, P. F., le Maire, M., and Bienvenue, A.,** Photoaffinity spin-labelling of the Ca²⁺ ATPase in sarcoplasmic reticulum: evidence for oligomeric structure, *Biochem. Biophys. Res. Commun.,* 95, 289, 1980.

35. **Vandest, P., Labbe, J. -P., and Kassab, R.,** Photoaffinity labelling of arginine kinase and creatine kinase with a γ-P-substituted arylazido analogue of ATP, *Eur. J. Biochem.,* 104, 433, 1980.

36. **Alliel, P. M., Mulet, C., and Lederer, F.,** Bromopyruvate as an affinity label for baker's yeast flavo-cytochrome b₂. Stoichiometry of incorporation and localization on the peptide chain, *Eur. J. Biochem.,* 105, 343, 1980.

37. **Högenauer, G., Egger, H., Ruf, C., and Stumper, B.,** Affinity labelling of *Escherichia coli* ribosomes with a covalently binding derivative of the antibiotic pleuromutilin, *Biochemistry,* 20, 546, 1981.

38. **Tobias, B. and Strickler, R. C.,** Affinity labelling of human placental 17β-estradiol dehydrogenase and 20α-hydroxysteroid dehydrogenase with 5'-[p-(fluorosulfonyl) benzoyl] adenosine, *Biochemistry,* 20, 5546, 1981.

39. **Jadus, M., Hanson, R. W., and Colman, R. F.,** Inactivation of phospoenolpyruvate carboxykinase by the guanosine nucleotide analogue, 5'-p-fluorosulfonylbenzoyl guanosine, *Biochem. Biophys. Res. Commun.,* 101, 884, 1981.

40. **Huang, K.-S. and Law, J. H.,** Photoaffinity labelling of *Crotalus atrox* phospholipase A₂ by a substrate analogue, *Biochemistry,* 20, 181, 1981.

41. **Likos, J. J. and Colman, R. F.,** Affinity labelling of rabbit muscle pyruvate kinase by a new fluorescent nucleotide alkylating agent 5-[p-(fluorosulfonyl)benzoyl]-1,N⁶-ethenoadenosine, *Biochemistry,* 20, 491, 1981.

42. **Erard, F., Cheng, S.-Y., and Robbins, J.,** Affinity labelling of human serum thyroxine-binding globulin with N-bromoacetyl-L-thyroxine: identification of the labelled amino acid residues, *Arch. Biochem. Biophys.,* 206, 15, 1981.

References for Table 2 (continued)

43. **Hartman, F. C.**, Interaction of isocitrate dehydrogenase with *(RS)*-3-bromo-2-ketoglutarate. A potential affinity label for α-ketoglutarate binding sites, *Biochemistry*, 20, 894, 1981.
44. **Hixson, C. S. and Krebs, E. G.**, Affinity labelling of the ATP binding site of bovine lung cyclic GMP-dependent protein kinase with 5'-*p*-fluorosulfonylbenzoyladenosine, *J. Biol. Chem.*, 256, 1122, 1981.
45. **Rashidbaigi, A. and Ruoho, A. E.**, Iodoazidobenzylpindolol, a photoaffinity probe for the β-adrenergic receptor, *Proc. Natl. Acad. Sci. U.S.A.*, 78, 1609, 1981.
46. **Pfister, K., Steinback, K. E., Gardner, G., and Arntzen, C. J.**, Photoaffinity labelling of an herbicide receptor protein in chloroplast membranes, *Proc. Natl. Acad. Sci. U.S.A.*, 78, 981, 1981.
47. **Lunardi, J., Satre, M., and Vignais, P. V.**, Exploration of adenosine-5'-diphosphate-adenosine 5'-triphosphate binding sites of *Escherichia coli* adenosine-5'-triphosphatase with arylazido adenine nucleotides, *Biochemistry*, 20, 473, 1981.
48. **Mueller, D. M., Hudson, R. A., and Lee, C.-P.**, Azide photoaffinity analogues for acridine dye binding sites, *J. Am. Chem. oc.*, 103, 1860, 1981.
49. **Schnackerz, K. D., Chirgwin, J. M., and Noltmann, E. A.**, Synthesis of 1-chloro-2-oxohexanol 6-phosphate, a covalent active-site reagent for phosphoglucose isomerase, *Biochemistry*, 20, 1756, 1981.
50. **Takemoto, D. J., Haley, B. E., Hansen, J., Pinkett, O., and Takemoto, L. J.**, GTPase from rod outer segments: characterization by photoaffinity labelling and tryptic peptide mapping, *Biochem. Biophys. Res. Commun.*, 102, 341, 1981.

REFERENCES

1. **Shaw, E.**, Selective chemical modification of proteins, *Physiol. Rev.*, 50, 244, 1970.
2. **Jakoby, W. B. and Wilchek, M., Eds.**, *Affinity Labeling, Methods in Enzymology*, Vol. 46, Academic Press, New York, 1977.
3. **Seiler, N., Jung, M. J., and Koch-Weser, J., Eds.**, *Enzyme-Activated Irreversible Inhibitors*, Elsevier/North-Holland, Amsterdam, 1978.
4. **Plapp, B. V.**, Application of affinity labeling for studying structure and function of enzymes, *Meth. Enzymol.*, 87, 469, 1982.
5. **Bazaes, S.**, Affinity labels as probes of the active site of enzymes. The use of dialdehyde derivatives of nucleotides, in *Chemical Modification of Enzymes: Active Site Studies*, Eyzaguirre, J., Ed., Ellis Norwood, Chichester, 1987, 35.
6. **Shaw, E.**, Cysteinyl proteinases and their selective inactivation, *Adv. Enzymol.*, 63, 271, 1990.
7. **Wofsy, L., Metzger, H., and Singer, S. J.**, Affinity labeling — a general method for labeling the active sites of antibody and enzyme molecules, *Biochemistry*, 1, 1031, 1962.
8. **Baker, B. R.**, *Design of Active-Site-Directed Irreversible Enzyme Inhibitors*, John Wiley & Sons, New York, 1967.
9. **Schoellmann, G. and Shaw, E.**, Direct evidence for the presence of histidine in the active center of chymotrypsin, *Biochemistry*, 2, 252, 1963.
10. **Mares-Guia, M. and Shaw, E.**, Studies on the active center of trypsin. The binding of amidines and guanidines as models of the substrate side chain, *J. Biol. Chem.*, 240, 1579, 1965.
11. **Shaw, E., Mares-Guia, M., and Cohen, W.**, Evidence for an active-center histidine in trypsin through the use of a specific reagent, 1-chloro-3-tosylamido-7-amino-2-heptanone, the chloromethyl ketone derived from Nα-tosyl-L-lysine, *Biochemistry*, 4, 2219, 1965.
12. **Tobias, B. and Strickler, R. C.**, Affinity labeling of human placental 17β-estradiol dehydrogenase and 20α-hydroxysteroid dehydrogenase with 5'-[*p*-(fluorosulfonyl)benzoyl] adenosine, *Biochemistry*, 20, 5546, 1981.
13. **Kurachi, K., Powers, J. C., and Wilcox, P. E.**, Kinetics of the reaction of chymotrypsin Aα with peptide chloromethyl ketones in relation to its subsite specificity, *Biochemistry*, 12, 771, 1973.
14. **Powers, J. C., Lively, M. O., III, and Tippett, J. T.**, Inhibition of subtilisin BPN' with peptide chloromethyl ketones, *Biochim. Biophys. Acta*, 480, 246, 1977.
15. **Wold, F.**, Affinity labeling — an overview, *Meth. Enzymol.*, 46, 3, 1977.
16. **Marletta, M. A. and Kenyon, G. L.**, Affinity labeling of creatine kinase by *N*-(2,3-epoxypropyl)-*N*-amidinoglycine, *J. Biol. Chem.*, 254, 1879, 1979.
17. **Meloche, H. P.**, Bromopyruvate inactivation of 2-keto-3-deoxy-6-phosphogluconic aldolase. I. Kinetic evidence for active site specificity, *Biochemistry*, 6, 2273, 1967.

18. **Main, A. R.**, Affinity and phosphorylation constants for the inhibition of esterases by organophosphates, *Science*, 144, 992, 1964.

19. **Brayer, G. D., Delbaere, L. T. J., James, M. N. G., Bauer, C.-A., and Thompson, R. C.**, Crystallographic and kinetic investigations of the covalent complex formed by a specific tetrapeptide aldehyde and the serine protease from *Streptomyces griseus*, *Proc. Natl. Acad. Sci. U.S.A.*, 76, 96, 1979.

20. **Kezdy, F. J., Lorand, L., and Miller, K. D.**, Titration of active centers in thrombin solutions. Standardization of the enzyme, *Biochemistry*, 4, 2302, 1965.

21. **Chase, T., Jr. and Shaw, E.**, Comparison of the esterase activities of trypsin, plasmin, and thrombin on guanidinobenzoate esters. Titration of the enzymes, *Biochemistry*, 8, 2212, 1969.

22. **Livingston, D. C., Brocklehurst, J. R., Cannon, J. F., Leytus, S. P., Wehrly, J. A., Peltz, S. W., Peltz, G. A., and Mangel, W. F.**, Synthesis and characterization of a new fluorogenic active-site titrant of serine proteases, *Biochemistry*, 20, 4298, 1981.

23. **Likos, J. J., Hess, B., and Colman, R. F.**, Affinity labeling of the active site of yeast pyruvate kinase by 5'-*p*-fluorosulfonylbenzoyl adenosine, *J. Biol. Chem.*, 255, 9388, 1980.

24. **Damle, V. N., McLaughlin, M., and Karlin, A.**, Bromoacetylcholine as an affinity label of the acetylcholine receptor from *Torpedo californica*, *Biochem. Biophys. Res. Commun.*, 84, 845, 1978.

25. **Schnackerz, K. D., Chirgwin, J. M., and Noltmann, E. A.**, Synthesis of 1-chloro-2-oxohexanol 6-phosphate, a covalent active-site reagent for phosphoglucose isomerase, *Biochemistry*, 20, 1756, 1981.

26. **Tometsko, A. M. and Turula, J.**, Inactivation of trypsin and chymotrypsin with a photosensitive probe, *Int. J. Peptide Protein Res.*, 8, 331, 1976.

27. **Lunardi, J. and Vignais, P. V.**, Adenine nucleotide binding sites in chemically modified F_1-ATPase. Inhibitory effect of 4-chloro-7-nitrobenzofurazan on photolabeling by arylazido nucleotides, *FEBS Lett.*, 102, 23, 1979.

28. **Aiba, H. and Krakow, J. S.**, Photoaffinity labeling of the adenosine cyclic 3',5'-monophosphate receptor protein of *Escherichia coli* with 8-azidoadenosine 3,5'-monophosphate, *Biochemistry*, 19, 1857, 1980.

29. **Moreland, R. B. and Dockler, M. E.**, Preparation and characterization of 3-azido-2,7-naphthalene disulfonate: a photolabile fluorescent precursor useful as a hydrophilic surface probe, *Anal. Biochem.*, 103, 26, 1980.

30. **Abeles, R. H. and Maycock, A. L.**, Suicide enzyme inhibitors, *Acc. Chem. Res.*, 9, 313, 1976.

31. **Walsh, C.**, Recent developments in suicide substrates and other active site-directed inactivating agents of specific target enzymes, *Horizons Biochem. Biophys.*, 3, 36, 1977.

32. **Harper, J. W., Hemmi, K., and Powers, J. C.**, Reaction of serine proteases with substituted isocoumarins: discovery of 3,4-dichloroisocoumarin, a new general mechanism based serine protease inhibitor, *Biochemistry*, 24, 1831, 1985.

33. **Hedstrom, L., Moorman, A. R., Dobbs, J., and Abeles, R. H.**, Suicide inactivation of chymotrypsin of benzoxazinones, *Biochemistry*, 23, 1753, 1984.

34. **Light, A.**, The reaction of iodoacetate and bromoacetate with papain, *Biochem. Biophys. Res. Commun.*, 17, 781, 1964.

35. **Shaw, D. C., Stein, W. H., and Moore, S.**, Inactivation of chymotrypsin by cyanate, *J. Biol. Chem.*, 239, PC671, 1964.

36. **Heinrikson, R. L., Stein, W. H., Crestfield, A. M., and Moore, S.**, The reactivities of the histidine residues at the active site of ribonuclease toward halo acids of different structures, *J. Biol. Chem.*, 240, 2921, 1965.

37. **Fruchter, R. G. and Crestfield, A. M.**, The specific alkylation by iodoacetamide of histidine-12 in the active site of ribonuclease, *J. Biol. Chem.*, 242, 5807, 1967.

38. **Lin, M. C., Stein, W. H., and Moore, S.**, Further studies on the alkylation of the histidine residues at the active site of pancreatic ribonuclease, *J. Biol. Chem.*, 243, 6167, 1968.

39. **Holbrook, J. J. and Ingram, V. A.**, Ionic properties of an essential histidine residue in pig heart lactate dehydrogenase, *Biochem. J.*, 131, 729, 1973.

40. **Rao, R., Cunningham, D., Cross, R. L., and Senior, A. E.**, Pyridoxal 5'-phosphate-5'-adenosine binds at a single site on isolated alpha-subunit from Escherichia coli F1-ATPase and specifically reacts with lysine 201, *J. Biol. Chem.*, 263, 5640, 1988.

41. **Tamura, J. K., LaDine, J. R., and Cross, R. L.**, The adenine nucleotide binding site on yeast hexokinase PII. Affinity labeling of Lys-111 by pyridoxal 5'-diphospho-5'-adenosine, *J. Biol. Chem.*, 263, 7907, 1988.

42. **Slepneva, I. A. and Weiner, L. M.**, Affinity modification of NADPH-cytochrome P-450 reductase, *Biochem. Biophys. Res. Commun.*, 155, 1026, 1988.

43. **Van Berkel, W. J. H., Müller, F., Jekel, P. A., Weijer, W. J., Schreuder, H. A., and Wierenga, R. K.**, Chemical modification of tyrosine-38 in *p*-hydroxybenzoate hydroxylase from *Pseudomonas fluorescens* by 5'-*p*-fluorosulfonylbenzoyladenosine: a probe for the elucidation of the NADPH binding site? Involvement in catalysis, assignment in sequence and fitting to the tertiary structure, *Eur. J. Biochem.*, 176, 449, 1988.

44. **Ohmi, N., Hoshino, M., Tagaya, M., Fukui, T., Kawakita, M., and Hattori, S.,** Affinity labeling of *ras* oncogene product p21 with guanosine diphospho- and triphosphopyridoxals, *J. Biol. Chem.,* 263, 14261, 1988.

45. **Dominici, P., Scholz, G., Kwok, F., and Churchich, J. E.,** Affinity labeling of pyridoxal kinase with adenosine polyphosphopyridoxal, *J. Biol. Chem.,* 263, 14712, 1988.

46. **Saavedra, C., Araneda, S., and Cardemil, E.,** Affinity labeling of *Saccharomyces cerevisiae* phosphoenolpyruvate carboxykinase with the 2′,3′-dialdehyde derivative of ATP, *Arch. Biochem. Biophys.,* 267, 38, 1988.

47. **King, M. M., Shell, D. J., and Kwiatkowski, A. P.,** Affinity labeling of the ATP-binding site of type II calmodulin-dependent protein kinase by 5′-*p*-fluorosulfonylbenzoyl adenosine, *Arch. Biochem. Biophys.,* 267, 467, 1988.

48. **Vaz, A. D. N. and Schoellmann, G.,** Affinity labeling of bovine opsin by trans-retinoyl chloromethane, *Biochem. Biophys. Res. Commun.,* 160, 942, 1989.

49. **Tritsch, D., Eiler-Samama, B., Svircevic, J., Albrecht, A.-M., Branlant, G., and Biellmann, J.-F.,** 4-Chloroacetylpyridine adenine dinucleotide — a highly reactive and chromophoric affinity label of glyceraldehyde-3-phosphate dehydrogenase from sturgeon, *Eur. J. Biochem.,* 181, 215, 1989.

50. **Tian, W.-X., Wang, Y., and Hsu, R. Y.,** Affinity labeling of chicken liver fatty acid synthase with chloroacetyl-CoA and bromopyruvate, *Biochim. Biophys. Acta,* 998, 310, 1989.

51. **Slepneva, I. A. and Weiner, L. M.,** Affinity modification of microsomal flavoproteins by NAD(P) 2′,3′-dialdehydes, *Biochem. Biophys. Res. Commun.,* 164, 758, 1989.

52. **Wu, J. C., Lin, J., Chuan, H., and Wang, J. H.,** Determination of the roles of active sites in F_1-ATPase by controlled affinity labeling, *Biochemistry,* 28, 8905, 1989.

53. **Grant, P. G., DeCamp, D. L., Bailey, J. M., Colman, R. W., and Colman, R. F.,** Three new potential cAMP affinity labels. Inactivation of human platelet low K_m cAMP phosphodiesterase by 8-[(4-bromo-2,3-dioxobutyl)thio]adenosine 3′,5′-cyclic monophosphate, *Biochemistry,* 29, 887, 1990.

54. **Rabinkov, A. G. and Amontov, S. V.,** Affinity labelling of rat liver acetyl-CoA carboxylase by a 2′,3′-dialdehyde derivative of ATP, *Biochim. Biophys. Acta,* 1037, 216, 1990.

55. **Tasayco J., M. L. and Prestwich, G. D.,** A specific affinity reagent to distinguish aldehyde dehydrogenases and oxidases. Enzymes catalyzing aldehyde oxidation in an adult moth, *J. Biol. Chem.,* 265, 3094, 1990.

56. **LaCasse, E. C., Howell, G. M., and Lefebvre, Y. A.,** Microsomal dexamethasone binding sites identified by affinity labelling, *J. Steroid Biochem.,* 35, 47, 1990.

57. **Bateman, R. C., Jr., Kim, Y.-A., Slaughter, C., and Hersh, L. B.,** N-Bromoacetyl-D-leucylglycine. An affinity label for neutral endopeptidase 24.11, *J. Biol. Chem.,* 265, 8365, 1990.

58. **Herzig, M. C. S. and Weigel, P. H.,** Synthesis and characterization of N-hydroxysuccinimide ester chemical affinity derivatives of asialoorosomucoid that covalently cross-link to galactosyl receptors on isolated rat hepatocytes, *Biochemistry,* 28, 600, 1989.

59. **Cooperman, B. S.,** Affinity labeling of ribosomes, *Meth. Enzymol.,* 164, 341, 1988.

60. **Madison, L. D., Rosenzweig, S. A., and Jamieson, J. D.,** Use of the heterobifunctional cross-linker *m*-maleimidobenzoyl-N-hydroxy-succinimide ester to affinity label choleocystokinin binding proteins on rat pancreatic plasma membranes, *J. Biol. Chem.,* 259, 14818, 1984.

61. **Klueppelberg, U. G., Powers, S. P., and Miller, L. J.,** Protease peptide mapping of affinity labeled rat pancreatic choleocystokinin-binding proteins, *Biochemistry,* 28, 7124, 1989.

62. **Vale, M. G. P.,** Affinity labeling of calmodulin-binding proteins in skeletal muscle sarcoplasmic reticulum, *J. Biol. Chem.,* 263, 12872, 1988.

63. **Stevenson, K. J. and Smillie, L. B.,** The inhibition of chymotrypsins A_4 and B with chloromethyl ketone reagents, *Can. J. Biochem.,* 46, 1357, 1968.

64. **Morihara, K. and Oka, T.,** Subtilisin BPN′: inactivation by chloromethyl ketone derivatives of peptide substrates, *Arch. Biochem. Biophys.,* 138, 526, 1970.

65. **Segal, D. M., Cohen, G. H., Davies, D. R., Powers, J. C., and Wilcox, P. E.,** The stereochemistry of substrate binding to chymotrypsin $A_γ$, in *Cold Spring Harbor Symp. Quant. Biol.,* 36, 85, 1971.

66. **Segal, D. M., Powers, J. C., Cohen, G. H., Davies, D. R., and Wilcox, P. E.,** Substrate binding site in bovine chymotrypsin $A_γ$. A crystallographic study using peptide chloromethyl ketones as site-specific inhibitors, *Biochemistry,* 10, 3728, 1971.

67. **Kettner, C. and Shaw, E.,** D-Phe-Pro-ArgCH₂Cl-A selective affinity label for thrombin, *Thromb. Res.,* 14, 969, 1979.

68. **Kettner, C. and Shaw, E.,** Inactivation of trypsin-like enzymes with peptides of arginine chloromethyl ketone, *Meth. Enzymol.,* 80, 826, 1981.

69. **Bode, W., Mayr, I., Baumann, Y., Huber, R., Stone, S. R., and Hofsteenge, J.,** The refined 1.9 Å crystal structure of human alpha-thrombin: interaction with D-Phe-Pro-Arg-chloromethyl ketone and significance of the Tyr-Pro-Pro-Trp insertion sequence, *EMBO J.,* 8, 3467, 1989.

70. **Stein, M. J. and Liener, I. E.,** Inhibition of ficin by the chloromethyl ketone derivatives of N-tosyl-L-lysine and N-tosyl-L-phenylalanine, *Biochem. Biophys. Res. Commun.,* 26, 376, 1967.

71. **Tsai, I.-H. and Bender, M. L.**, Conformation of the active site of thiolsubtilisin: reaction with specific chloromethyl ketones and arylacryloylimidazoles, *Biochemistry*, 18, 3764, 1979.

72. **Connolly, B. A. and Trayer, I. P.**, Affinity labelling of rat-muscle hexokinase type II by a glucose-derived alkylating agent, *Eur. J. Biochem.*, 93, 375, 1979.

73. **Brocklehurst, K. and Malthouse, J. P. G.**, Mechanism of the reaction of papain with substrate-derived diazomethyl ketones. Implications for the difference in site specificity of halomethyl ketones for serine proteinases and cysteine proteinases and for stereoelectronic requirements in the papain catalytic mechanism, *Biochem. J.*, 175, 761, 1978.

74. **Hass, G. M. and Neurath, H.**, Affinity labeling of bovine carboxypeptidase A_γ^{Leu} by *N*-bromoacetyl-*N*-methyl-L-phenylalanine. I. Kinetics of inactivation, *Biochemistry*, 10, 3535, 1971.

75. **Hass, G. M. and Neurath, H.**, Affinity labeling of bovine carboxypeptidase A_γ^{Leu} by *N*-bromoacetyl-*N*-methyl-L-phenylalanine. II. Sites of modification, *Biochemistry*, 10, 3541, 1971.

76. **Rasnick, D. and Powers, J. C.**, Active-site directed irreversible inhibition of thermolysin, *Biochemistry*, 17, 4363, 1978.

77. **Nishino, N. and Powers, J. C.**, Peptide hydroxamic acids as inhibitors of thermolysin, *Biochemistry*, 17, 2846, 1978.

78. **Wagner, R. P.**, *Principles and Applications of Photochemistry*, Oxford University Press, Oxford, 1988.

79. **Kalyanasundarum, K.**, *Photochemistry in Microheterogeneous System*, Academic Press, Orlando, FL, 1982.

80. **Horspol, W. M.**, *Aspects of Organic Photochemistry*, Academic Press, London, 1976.

81. **Wells, C. H. J.**, *Introduction to Molecular Photochemistry*, Chapman and Hall, London, 1972.

82. **Coxon, J. M. and Holton, B.**, *Organic Photochemistry*, Cambridge University Press, Cambride, 1972.

83. **Roberts, R., Ouellette, R. P., Muradoz, M. M., Cozzens, R. F., and Cheriemisinoff, P. N.**, *Applications of Photochemistry*, Technamic Publishing, Lancaster, PA, 1984.

84. **Jackson, W. M. and Harvey, A. B., Eds.**, *Lasers as Reactants and Probes in Chemistry*, Howard University Press, Washington, D.C., 1985.

85. **Bayley, H. and Knowles, J. R.**, Photoaffinity labeling, *Meth. Enzymol.*, 46, 69, 1977.

86. **Bayley, H.**, Photogenerated reagents in biochemistry and molecular biology, in *Laboratory Techniques in Biochemistry and Molecular Biology*, Work, T. W. and Burden, B. H., Eds., Elsevier, 1983.

87. **Haley, B. E. and Hoffman, J. F.**, Interactions of a photoaffinity ATP analogue with calcium-stimulated adenosine triphosphatases of human red cell membranes, *Proc. Natl. Acad. Sci. U.S.A.*, 71, 3367, 1974.

88. **Potter, R. L. and Haley, B. E.**, Photoaffinity labeling of nucleotide binding sites with 8-azidopurine analogues: techniques and applications, *Meth. Enzymol.*, 41, 613, 1983.

89. **Chuan, H., Lin, J., and Wang, J. H.**, 8-Azido-2′-*O*-dansyl-ATP. A fluorescent photoaffinity reagent for ATP-binding proteins and its application to adenylate kinase, *J. Biol. Chem.*, 264, 7981, 1989.

90. **DeTraglia, M. C., Brand, J. S., and Tometsko, A. M.**, Characterization of azidobenzamidines as photoaffinity labels for trypsin, *J. Biol. Chem.*, 253, 1846, 1978.

91. **Staros, J. V., Bayley, H., Standring, D. N., and Knowles, J. R.**, Reduction of aryl azides by thiols: implications for the use of photoaffinity reagents, *Biochem. Biophys. Res. Commun.*, 80, 568, 1978.

92. **Lewis, C. T., Haley, B. E., and Carlson, G. M.**, Formation of an intramolecular cystine disulfide during the reaction of 8-azidoguanosine 5′-triphosphate with cytosolic phosphoenolpyruvate carboxykinase (GTP) causes inactivation without photolabeling, *Biochemistry*, 28, 9248, 1989.

93. **Brunner, J. and Semenza, G.**, Selective labeling of the hydrophobic core of membranes with 3-(trifluoromethyl)-3-(*m*-[^{125}I]iodophenyl)diazirine, a carbene-generating reagent, *Biochemistry*, 20, 7174, 1981.

94. **Hoppe, J., Brunner, J., and Jorgensen, B. R.**, Structure of the membrane-embedded F_0 part of F_1F_0 ATP synthase from *Escherichia coli* as inferred from labeling with 3-(trifluormethyl)-3-(*m*-[^{125}I]iodophenyl)diazirine, *Biochemistry*, 23, 5610, 1984.

95. **Krieg, U. C., Isaacs, B. S., Yemui, S. S., Esmon, C. T., Bayley, H., and Johnson, A. E.**, Interaction of blood coagulation factor Va with phospholipid vesicles examined by using lipophilic photoreagents, *Biochemistry*, 26, 103, 1987.

96. **Kim, J. and Kim, H.**, Interaction of alpha-lactalbumin with phospholipid vesicles as studied by photoactivated hydrophobic labeling, *Biochim. Biophys. Acta*, 983, 1, 1989.

97. **Hatanaka, Y., Yoshida, E., Nakayama, H., and Kanaoka, Y.**, Chromogenic diazirine: a new spectrophotometric approach for photoaffinity labeling, *Bioorganic Chem.*, 17, 482, 1989.

98. **Baldwin, J. E., Coates, J. B., Halpern, J. B., Moloney, M. G., and Pratt, A. J.**, Photoaffinity labelling of isopenicillin N synthetase by laser-flash photolysis, *Biochem. J.*, 261, 197, 1989.

99. **Pradhan, D. and Lala, A. K.**, Photochemical labeling of membrane hydrophobic core of human erythrocytes using a new photoactivable reagent 3[^{3}H]Diazofluorene, *J. Biol. Chem.*, 262, 8242, 1987.

100. **Lala, A. K., Dixit, R. R., and Koppaka, V.**, Depth-dependent photolabelling of membrane hydrophobic core with 9-diazofluorene-2-butyric acid, *Biochim. Biophys. Acta*, 978, 333, 1989.

101. **Lauquin, G., Pougeois, R., and Vignais, P. V.**, 4-Azido-2-nitrophenyl phosphate, a new photoaffinity derivative of inorganic phosphate. Study of its interaction with the inorganic phosphate binding site of beef heart mitochondrial adenosine triphosphatase, *Biochemistry*, 19, 4620, 1980.

102. **Tommasino, M., Prezioso, G., and Palmieri, F.**, Photoaffinity labeling of the mitochondrial phosphate carrier by 4-azido-2-nitrophenyl phosphate, *Biochim. Biophys. Acta*, 890, 39, 1987.

103. **Garin, J., Michel, L., Dupuis, A., Issartel, J.-P., Lunardi, J., Hoppe, J., and Vignais, P.**, Photo-labeling of the phosphate binding site of mitochondril F_1-ATPase by [^{32}P]azidonitrophenyl phosphate. Identification of the photolabeled amino acid residues, *Biochemistry*, 28, 1442, 1989.

104. **Klueppelberg, U. G., Gaisano, H. Y., Powers, S. P., and Miller, L. J.**, Use of a nitrotryptophan-containing peptide for photoaffinity labeling the pancreatic cholecystokinin receptor, *Biochemistry*, 28, 3468, 1989.

105. **Buku, A., Yamin, N., and Gazis, D.**, Fluorescent, photoaffinity, and biotinyl analogs of oxytocin, *Peptides*, 9, 783, 1988.

106. **Buku, A., Gazis, D., and Eggena, P.**, Photoaffinity, biotinyl, and iodo analogues as probes for vasotocin receptors, *J. Med. Chem.*, 32, 2432, 1989.

107. **Miller, W. T. and Kaiser, E. T.**, Probing the peptide binding site of the cAMP-dependent protein kinase by using a peptide-based photoaffinity label, *Proc. Natl. Acad. Sci. U.S.A.*, 85, 5429, 1988.

108. **Kuechler, E., Steiner, G., and Barta, A.**, Photoaffinity labeling of peptidyltransferase, *Meth. Enzymol.*, 164, 361, 1988.

109. **Fleet, G. W. J., Knowles, J. R., and Porter, R. R.**, The antibody binding site. Labelling of a specific antibody against the photo-precursor of an aryl nitrene, *Biochem. J.*, 128, 499, 1972.

110. **Shigeno, C., Hiraki, Y., Keutmann, H. T., Stern, A. M., Potts, J. T., Jr., and Segre, G. V.**, Preparation of a photoreactive analog of parathyroid hormone [Nle^6, Lys(N-ε-4-azido-2-nitrophenyl)^{13}, Nle^{18}, Tyr^{34}] bovine parathyroid hormone-(1-34)NH$_2$, a selective, high-affinity ligand for characterization of parathyroid hormone receptors, *Anal. Biochem.*, 179, 268, 1989.

111. **Ricard, B., Fourquet, P., Massacrier, A., and Couraud, F.**, Photoaffinity labeling of ANF receptor in cultured brain neurons, *Biochem. Biophys. Res. Commun.*, 152, 1031, 1988.

112. **Furlanetto, R. W.**, Metabolism of photoaffinity-labeled insulin-like growth factor-I receptors by human cells *in vitro*, *Endocrinology*, 126, 1334, 1990.

113. **Balczon, R. D. and Brinkley, B. R.**, Synthesis of azidotubulin: a photoaffinity label for tubulin-binding proteins, *Biochemistry*, 28, 8490, 1989.

114. **Morgan, J. E., Calkins, C. C., and Matthews, H. R.**, Discovery and mapping of discrete binding sites on nucleosome core particles for a photoaffinity derivative of spermine, *Biochemistry*, 28, 5095, 1989.

115. **Goodfellow, V. S., Settineri, M., and Lawton, R. G.**, p-Nitrophenyl 3-diazopyruvate and diazopyruvamides, a new family of photoactivatable cross-linking bioprobes, *Biochemistry*, 28, 6346, 1989.

116. **Harrison, J. K., Lawton, R. G., and Gnegy, M. E.**, Development of a novel photoreactive calmodulin derivative: cross-linking of purified adenylate cyclase from bovine brain, *Biochemistry*, 28, 6023, 1989.

INDEX

A

Acetic acid, 9, 49—50
Acetic anhydride, 132, 291—292
Acetol, 150
Acetone, 145
Acetonitrile, 31
2-Acetoxy-5-nitrobenzyl bromide, 231
Acetylation, 132
Acetylcholine receptor, 69
N-Acetyl-3-dansylaminotyrosine ethyl ester, 261
Acetylhydroxamate, 244
N-Acetylimidazole, 242—245
N-Acetyl-3-nitrotyrosine, 11, 251—253, 260—261
N-Acetyltryptophan ethyl ester (ATEE), 215, 217
N-Acetyltyrosine, 247—248
N-Acetyltyrosine ethyl ester, 215, 218—219
Acid phosphatase, 200, 211, 267, 269
Acid proteinase, 268
Acidification, 11, 14—15, 37
Acylation, 131—132
Acyl-CoA:cholesterol acyltransferase, 118
Adenyl cyclase, 200, 209
Adenylate cyclase, 139—140
ADP, 307—308
ADP-glucose synthetase, 7
Affinity labeling, 305—331
  characteristics, 307
  examples of, 321—328
  kinetics, 305—306
  types, 308—309, 311
Albumin, 80, 82, 153, 155—156
Alcohol dehydrogenase, 62, 140—141
Alcohol oxidase, 119—120, 125
Aldehyde reductase, 198, 203
Aldolase, 141, 145
Alkalinity, 174—175
Alkyl halides, 62, see also Individual entries
Alkylation, 99—100, 102
Amadori rearrangement, 158—159
Amines, 146, 290, 292
D-Amino acid oxidase, 109
D-Amino acid transaminase, 74, 77
Amino acids
  α-amino acids, 189—190
  analysis, 21—26
  sequence determination
    COOH-terminal degradation, 45
    direct Edman degradation 39—45
    indirect Edman degradation, 37—39
α-Amino acids, 189—190
α-Amino groups, 176, 185
ε-Amino groups, 109, 163
4-Aminosulfonyl-7-fluoro-2,1,3-benzoxadiazole, 86, 88
5-Amino-1H-tetrazole, diazotized, 240—241

Ammonium ions, 162—163, 272
α-Amylase, 220—222
β-Amylase, 62
Anion transport, 69—70
Anticoagulant activity, placental, 105
Apolipoprotein, 12—13, 17—18
Apo-serine hydroxylmethyltransferase, 145
Arachin, 134
Arginine, 173—211
  2,3-butanedione reactions, 188—198
  1,2-cyclohexanedione reactions, 195, 197, 200, 205, 211
  phenylglyoxal reactions, 173, 176—188, 196—197
Arsanilic acid, diazotized, 239—240
Aryl halides, 309
Asparaginase, 241
Asparaginyl-glycyl residues, 54
Aspartate aminotransferase, 255
Aspartate transcarbamylase, 1—2, 260
Aspartic acid, 272—273
ATEE, see N-Acetyltryptophan ethyl ester
ATPase
  2,3-butanedione reaction, 200, 209
  photoaffinity labeling, 319
  pyridoxal-5'-phosphate reaction, 145—146
8-Azido adenosine triphosphate, 314, 317
m-Azidobenzamidine, 320—321
N-(4-Azidobenzoylglycyl)-5-(2-thiopyridyl)-cysteine, 296, 299—300
N-(4-Azidocarbonyl-3-hydroxyphenyl)maleimide, 297
8-Azido-2'-O-dansyl adenosine triphosphate, 314, 318
3-Azido-2,7-naphthalene disulfonate, 309, 311
N-(5-Azido-2-nitrobenzoyl)-N-oxysuccinimide, 319
Azidonitrobenzoyl-spermine, 320
4-Azido-2-nitrophenyl phosphate, 319
Azocarboxypeptidase, 241

B

N-Benzylmaleimide, 68—69
Bicarbonate buffers, see Buffers
Bimanes, 69—70
Biological activity
  N-bromosuccinimide-tryptophan reaction, 216
  changes and chemical modification, 2—3
  histidine loss, 105—107
Biotin, 54—55, 63—64, 164—165
Biotin-EDTA, 54—55
Blood coagulation factors, 12, 16—17, 30
BNPS-Skatole, 53
Borate, 187—189
Boulton-Hunter reagent, 163
Bovine serum albumin, 18, 97

Bromoacetate, 100
N-Bromoacetyl-N-methyl-L-phenylalanine,
     314—316
2-Bromoethane sulfonate, 86
2-Bromoethanol, 62—63
p-Bromophenacyl bromide, 106, 283, 285
N-Bromosuccinimide
     N-acetyltryptophan ethyl ester reaction, 215,
          217—218
     N-acetyltyrosine ethyl ester reaction, 215,
          218—219
     α-amylase reaction, 220—222
     asparaginase reaction, 241
     dihydrofolate reductase reaction, 216, 219—220
     DNase reaction, 216, 218
     galactose oxidase reaction, 218—220
     glucoamylase reaction, 221—222
     lactose repressor reaction, 222—223
     oxidation by, 99
     peptide cleavage, 52—53
     protein modification, 224—225
     transcarboxylase reaction, 223
     tryptophan reaction, 215—216
     xylanase reaction, 223
Bronsted acids and bases, 8
Buffers
     arginine modifications, 178, 186—188
     2,3-butanedione arginine modification, 200, 208
     carbodiimide-carboxyl group reaction, 282—283
     glutamate carboxylase-phenylglyoxal reaction,
          197—198, 202—203
     high-performance liquid chromatography, 31
     homobifunctional imidoester cross-linking, 290
2,3-Butanedione
     arginine modification, 173
     adenyl cyclase reaction, 200, 209
     aldehyde reductase reaction, 198, 203
     arginine reactions, 188—191
     ATPase reaction, 200, 209
     energy-dependent transhydrogenase, 196—197,
          199
     fatty acid synthetase reaction, 198, 204
     isocitrate dehydrogenase reaction, 199—200, 207
     photophosphorylation, 196, 198
     pyridoxamine-5'-phosphate oxidase modification,
          7
     saccharopine dehydrogenase, 200, 210
     stearyl-CoA desaturase reaction, 200, 208

C

Calcitonin, 132
Calmodulin, cleavage of, 54—55
Camphorquinone-10-sulfonic acid, 175—176
Carbamylation, 137—140
Carbene, 314, 319
Carbobenzoxy-L-phenylalanine chloromethyl ketone,
     311
Carbodiimide, water-soluble, 271—277, 282
Carbonyl compounds, 150
2-Carboxy-4,6-dinitrochlorobenzene, 129—131

Carboxyl group, see also Individual entries
     carbodiimide modification, 271—285
     diazo compounds and, 267—271
     isoteric modification, 271
     isoxazolium salt modification, 267, 269—271
Carboxyl terminals, 45
Carboxymethylation, 105—106, 108
Carboxypeptidase, nitrated, 11
Carboxypeptidase A
     N-acetylimidazole reaction, 244
     affinity labeling, 314—316
     2,3-butanedione reaction, 189
     diazonium salt modification, 240—241
     p-hydroxymercuribenzoate reaction, 81, 83
Cell surface protein, cross-linking, 293, 296, 300
Chain elongation factor Tu, 105
Chalcone isomerase, 81
CHD, see 1,2-Cyclohexanedione
Chemical modification, site specific, 1—18
Chemical mutations, 4
Chloramine T
     iodination by, 242
     methionine oxidation, 99—100
     UV spectra, 101—102
Chloroacetamide, 60—62
Chloroacetic acid
     cysteine modification, 59—60
     papain modification, 60—62
N-Chloroacetyl-N-hydroxyleucine methyl ester, 314,
     316—317
2-Chloromercuri-4-nitrophenol, 66, 81, 83—84
4-Chloro-7-nitrobenzofurazan, see 4-Chloro-7-nitro-
     benzo-2-oxa-1,3-diazole
4-Chloro-7-nitrobenzo-2-oxa-1,3-diazole, 83,
     85—88
7-Chloro-4-nitrobenzo-2-oxa-1,3-diazole, 242—243
1-p-Chlorophenyl-4,4-dimethyl-5-diethylamino-1-
     penten-3-one hydrobromide, 87, 89
Chloroplasts, 162
N-Chlorosuccinimide, 53, 99, 223
Choline acetyltransferase, 199, 206
Chromium ion, 22
Chymotrypsin, 311—313, see also α-Chymotrypsin
α-Chymotrypsin
     affinity labeling, 306
     1-cyclohexyl-3-(2-morpholinyl-(4)-
          ethyl)carbodiimide metho-p-toluenesulfonate
          reaction, 271, 273
     diazonium salt modification, 239—241
     glutaraldehyde reaction, 289
Chymotrypsinogen, 134, 230
Chymotrypsinogen A, 239
Citraconic anhydride, 134—136
Citrate synthase, 73—76
Cleland's reagent, see Dithiothreitol
Cobalt ion, 155—156
Competitive inhibition
     microenvironment changes, 10—12
     nitrocarboxypeptidase, 253—255
     nuclease, 254, 259
     thermolysis, 111—112, 120—121

Competitive labeling, 109, 132, 134
Copper ions, 267
Creatine kinase
  affinity labeling, 307—309
  2-nitro-5-thiocyanobenzoic acid reaction, 70—71
Cross-linking
  acid-labile agents, 294, 298
  bifunctional agents, 292, 295—297, 299
  cell surface, 296, 300
  covalent, tetranitromethane, 250—251
  heterobifunctional agents, 293—294, 298—299,
    301, 319—320
  intermolecular, 288, 296, 299
  reagents, 288
  zero length, 274, 282, 287—288
Crystals, protein, 288
Cyanate, 83, 85, 137—139
Cyanation, 109
Cyanide, 52, see also Potassium cyanide
S-Cyanocysteine, 51—52, 72
Cyanogen bromide, 32, 49—51, 109
Cyanopropyl columns, 31
Cyanuric fluoride, 242—243
S-Cyanylation reactions, 71—73
1,2-Cyclohexanedione
  acid phosphatase reaction, 200, 211
  ADP-glucose synthetase modification, 7
  aldehyde reductase reaction, 198, 203
  arginine modification, 173, 189, 195—197
1-Cyclohexyl-3-(2-morpholinyl-(4)-
    ethyl)carbodiimide metho-p-toluenesulfonate
  α-chymotrypsin reaction, 271, 273
  enolase reaction, 274, 281
  hexokinase reaction, 274, 280
  phosphorylase reaction, 274, 281
Cysteine, 314
  active site modification, 4
  4-chloro-7-nitrobenzo-2-oxa-1,3-diazole reaction
    with, 85
  methyl-2-pyridyl disulfide NMR spectrum, 80
  modification, 59—89, see also Sulfhydryl groups
  residues
    cleavage at, 51—52
    pKa values, 59, 61
    tetranitromethane modification, 249—250
    structure of, bound, 60
Cystine, 52, 95—97
Cytochrome, 134
Cytochrome b$_5$, 111, 241
Cytochrome c
  2-carboxy-4,6-dinitrochlorobenzene reaction, 131
  formylation, 226
  iodination of, 241
  peptide cleavage, 53
  tetranitromethane reaction, 255
Cytochrome P-450, 131

D

DABITC (Dimethylaminoazobenzene-4'-isothio-
  cyanate), 40

Dabsyl chloride, 23—24
Dansyl aziridine, 87, 89
Dansyl chloride
  D-amino acid oxidase reaction, 109
  fluorescent probes, 12—13, 17—18
  lysine modification, 129
  peptide degradation, 38—39
Dansyl-Edman degradation, 38—39
Deoxyribonuclease
  N-bromosuccinimide reaction, 216, 218
  methyl picolinimidate reaction, 140, 143
  p-nitrobenzenesulfonyl fluoride reaction, 262
  potassium cyanate reaction, 142
  2,4,6-trinitrobenzenesulfonic acid reaction, 140,
    144
Deoxyribonuclease A, 138—139, 141
Deoxythymidine 3',5'-diphosphate, 254, 259
Derivatization
  post-column, 23
  pre-column, 21, 24, 26
Dextran maleimide, 69
Di-(N-acetyl-D-glucosamine, epoxy function, 285
Diagonal method, for cysteine peptide identification,
  65—66
Diaminomethane, 272—273
Diazoacetyl compounds, 268
Diazoacetyl-norleucine methyl ester, 267
Diazofluorene, 319
9-Diazofluorene-2-butyric acid, 319
Diazomethane, 267
Diazonium salts, 239—241
Diazonium-1H-tetrazole, 241
p-Diazophenylphosphate, 240
5'-(4-Diazophenyl phosphoryl)uridine 2'(3')-phos-
  phate, 240
Dicarboxylic acid anhydride, 243
Dichlorisocoumarin, 309
Dielectric constant, protein, 8—9
Diethylpyrocarbonate
  acyl-CoA:cholesterol acyltransferase reaction, 118
  alcohol oxidase reaction, 119—120, 125
  dihydrofolate reductase reaction, 120, 125—126
  histidine modification, 6—8, 110
  lactate dehydrogenase reaction, 119, 124
  pyridoxamine-5'phosphate oxidase reaction, 5,
    112, 121—123
  ribulose-bisphosphate carboxylase reaction, 119,
    124
  thermolysis reaction, 111—112, 118—121
Dihydrofolate reductase
  N-bromosuccinimide reaction, 216, 219—220
  diethylpyrocarbonate reaction, 120, 125—126
Diimidates, 292—293
Diisopropylphosphorofluoridate
  affinity label, 308
  trypsin conformation, 10, 12—13
4-4'-Diisothiocyanstilbene 2,2'-disulfonic acid,
  69—70
Diketene, 136
Dimethyl suberimidate, 139—140, 290
Dimethyl sulfoxide, 23

Dimethylamine borane, 155, 157—158
Dimethylaminoazobenzene-4'-isothiocyanate/phenyl-
     isothiocyanate, 40
1-Dimethylaminonaphthalene-5-sulfonyl chloride,
     see Dansyl chloride
N-(3-dimethyl aminopropyl)-N-ethyl carbodiimide
     HCl, 9—10
1,5-Dimethyl-1,5-diazaundecamethylene poly-
     methobromide (Polybrene), 41—42
Dimethyl(2-hydroxy-5-nitrobenzyl) sulfonium bro-
     mide, 230
2,4-Dinitrofluorobenzene
     luciferase reaction, 131—133
     peptide cleavage, 51—52
2,4-Dinitrophenyl cysteinyl disulfide, 80, 82
2,4-Dinitrophenylsulfenyl chloride, 234—235
N,N'-1,2-Diphenylenedimaleimide, 68—69
6,6-Diselenobis(3-nitrobenzoic acid), 74, 76
Dissociation, of acids, 9
Disuccinimidyl esters, 292
2,2'-Dithiobis(S-nitropyridine), 74
3,3'-Dithiobis(succinimidylpropionate), 292, 295
5,5'-Dithiobis(2-nitrobenzoic acid)
     creatine kinase reaction, 71
     cysteinyl residue reaction, 72—74
     2-keto-4-hydroxyglutarate aldolase reaction,
          248—249
     structure, 74
4,4'-Dithiodipyridine, 74, 76
Dithioerythritol, 96
2,2'-Dithiopyridine, 82
Dithiothreitol, 96, 273, 296, 299
Di(trimethylsilylethyl)trimesic acid, 134—135,
     243—244
DNase, see Deoxyribonuclease
Dodecylphosphocholine, 260, 262
DTNB, see 5,5'-Dithiobis(2-nitrobenzoic acid)
Dynein adenosine triphosphatase, 162

E

Edman degradation
     direct
          automated, 41—42
          dimethylaminoazobenzene-4'-isothiocyanate
               identification methods, 43—45
          manual, 39—40
          spinning-cup sequenator, 40—42
     indirect, 37—39
Elastase, 132
Electroblotting, 51
Electrolytic protein reduction, 97
Ellman's reagent, see 5,5'-Dithiobis(2-nitrobenzoic
     acid)
Elution systems, 29—30
Enolase, 274, 282
Eosin isothiocyanate, 131
Eosin-5-maleimide, 67—68
Epoxycreatine, 307—309
1,2-Epoxy-3-(p-nitrophenoxy) propane, 285
Epsilon toxin, 223, 225

Erythropoietin, 163—164
ESR, 13—15
Esterase, 13
17β-Estradiol dehydrogenase, 305—306
Ethoxyformic anhydride, see Diethylpyrocarbonate
Ethyl acetimidate, 139
1-Ethyl-3-(4-azonia-4,4-dimethylpentyl)-carbodi-
     imide iodide, 274, 282
1-Ethyl-3-(3-dimethylaminopropyl)-carbodiimide,
     274, 282
Ethyleneimine, 86, 89, 100
N-Ethylmaleimide, 63, 65—67
N-Ethyl-5-phenylisoxazolium-3'-sulfate, 267,
     269—270
Ethylthiofluoroacetate, 134

F

Fatty acid synthetase, 198, 204
FDNB, see 2,4-Dinitrofluorobenzene
Fluorescamines, 23
Fluorescein isothiocyanate, 131
Fluorescence
     arginine-9,10-phenanthrenequinone reaction,
          176—178
     peptide detection, 31
     probes
          4-chloro-7-nitrobenzo-2-oxa-1,3-diazole as, 83
          cysteine modification, 66—68
          N-methyl-2-anilino-6-napthalenesulfonyl chlo-
               ride as, 131
          protein structure, 12, 16—18
1-Fluoro-2,4-dinitrobenzene, 109
Fluorogenic reagents, 23, 86, 88
4-Fluoro-3-nitrophenyl azide, 319
5'-p-Fluorosulfonyl adenosine, 305—306
Formaldehyde, 155, 157
Formic acid, 49, 226—227
Formylation, 225—227
4-(6-Formyl-3-azidophenoxy)butyrimidate, 294, 298

G

Galactose oxidase, 218—220
β-Galactosidase, 62
Gas-liquid solid-phase sequenator, 42
Gas-phase hydrolysis, 23
Gel filtration, 250—251
Glucoamylase, 221—222
Glucocorticoid receptor, hepatic, 145—146
D-Glucose, 159
Glutamate carboxylase, 197, 202
Glutamate dehydrogenase, 161
Glutamine synthetase, 139
Glutaraldehyde, 288—291
Glutathione, 81
Glutathione maleimide, 69
Glutathione reductase, 162
Glyceraldehyde, 158—159
Glycinamide, 9—10
Glycoaldehyde, 150, 290—291

Glycopeptides, 296, 301
Glyoxal, 174
Glyoxylate, 164—165
Gradient elution, vs. isocratic, 43
Guanidation, 163—164
Guanylate cyclase, 78
Guanyl-3,5-dimethyl pyrazole, 163—164

H

Haloacetates, 59, see also Individual entries
α-Haloacids
    cysteine modification, see Individual entries
    histidine residues and, 105—107
α-Haloamines, cysteine modification, see Individual
        entries
Hemoglobin
    cross-linking, 296, 301
    cyanate reactions, 137—140
    monosaccharide reactions, 159—160
    tryptic peptide mapping, 30
Heptafluorobutyric acid (HFBA), 41
Hexadecylphosphocholine, 260—261
Hexokinase
    affinity labeling, 312—313
    1-cyclohexyl-3-(2-morpholinyl-(4)-
        ethyl)carbodiimide metho-p-toluenesulfonate
        reaction, 274, 280
    phenylglyoxal reaction, 197, 200
    pyridoxal-5'-diphospho-5'adenosine reaction, 148
HFBA, see Heptafluorobutyric acid
High-performance liquid chromatography (HPLC)
    amino acid analysis, 23—24, 26
    Edman degradation products, 43
    peptide analysis, 4
    reverse-phase, 29—34
Histidine residues, 109—126
    active site modification, 7—8
    cyanation, 109
    diethylpyrocarbonate and, 110—126
    methylation, 107
Histidinol dehydrogenase, 147—148
Homocitrulline, 138—139, 141
Homoserine lactone, 49—50
HPLC, see High-performance liquid chromatogra-
        phy
Human serum albumin, 260
Hydrazine, 176
Hydrochloric acid-trifluoracetic acid, 22—23
Hydrogen binding, 9
Hydrogen peroxide, 99, 215
Hydrolysis
    amino acid analysis, 22
    diethylpyrocarbonate, 111
    Edman degradation products, 45
    homocitrulline, 138—139, 141
Hydrophobicity, 68—69, 136
Hydroxide, 161—162
Hydroxylamine
    arginine modification, 196
    decarboxylation, 110

peptide cleavage, 54
    tyrosine modification, 244, 247
p-Hydroxymercuribenzoate, 80—81, 83
2-Hydroxy-5-nitrobenzyl alcohol, 228—229
2-Hydroxy-5-nitrobenzyl bromide
    chymotrypsinogen reaction, 230
    laccase reaction, 229—230
    protein modification, 232
    structure, 231
    tryptophan reaction, 227—228
p-Hydroxyphenylglyoxal, 187—188
20α-Hydroxysteroid dehydrogenase, 305—306
N-Hydroxysuccinimide, 163—165

I

Imidoesters
    covalent cross-linking, 139—140
    homobifunctional, 290—294
Indole, 22
Initiation factor, 147
Insulin, 96, 242
Iodate, 96
Iodination, 241—242
Iodine, 241—242
Iodine, radiolabeled, 317—318
Iodine monochloride, 242
Iodoacetamide, 62, 105—106, 283
5-Iodoacetamido-fluorescein, 63—64
4-(2-iodoacetamido)-TEMPO, 63—64
Iodoacetate
    biotin probe, 63—64
    cysteine modification, 59, 61
    histidine modification, 105—106, 108
    methionine modification, 99—102
Iodoacetic acid, 129
5-[2-((Iodoacetyl)amino)ethyl]naphthalene-1-sulfonic
        acid, 63—64
o-Iodosobenzoic acid, 54
Ion exchange chromatography, 21, 274, 283—284
Isocitrate dehydrogenase, 199—200, 207
Isocratic elution, 29
Isopenicillin N-synthetase, 318
Isopeptide bond, 287—288
Isoteric modification, 271
Isothiocyanate, 45
Isoxazolium salts, 267, 269—270

K

α-Keto-halo compounds, 314—316
2-Keto-4-hydroxyglutarate aldolase, 248—250
K$_s$ agents, 309

L

Labeling, competitive (trace), see Competitive label-
        ing
Laccase, 229—230

Lactate dehydrogenase
  active site histidine of, 119, 124
  cross-linking, 293
  glutaraldehyde cross-linking in, 288—289, 291
  pyridoxal-5'-phosphate reaction, 146, 148
Lactose, 158—159
Lactose repressor, 66—67, 222—223
Lewis acids and bases, 8
Luciferase, 131—134
Lysine, 129—165
  citraconic anhydride modification, 134—136
  competitive labeling, 132, 134
  guanidation, 163—164
  methyl acetimidate reaction, 139, 143
  as nucleophile, 129
  pyridoxal phosphate modificaiton, 141—148
  reductive alkylation, 150, 152
  structure, 130
  succinic anhydride modification of, 134
Lysolecithin, 251—252
Lysozyme
  N-bromosuccinimide reaction, 222
  HPLC separation, 31—32
  2-nitrophenylsulfenyl chloride reaction, 233—234
  sodium borohydride reaction, 150, 153
  thiol reactions, 95

M

Maleimides, 69
  bifunctional cross-linking, 6, 292, 296—297
  cysteine probes, 66—68
Maleimido-*N*-hydroxysuccinimide, 311
Maleimidomethyl-3-maleimido propionate, 293, 297
6,4-Maleimido-2,2,6,6-tetramethylpiperidine-1-oxyl, 67
Malic anhydride, 132
Malic enzyme, 118
Membrane, 162, 317—318
β-Mercaptoethanol, 85—87, 103
2-Mercapto-5-nitrobenzoic acid, 71—73
Mercurials, organic, UV spectra, 82—88, see also
    Individual entries
Mercuric chloride, 81
Metal ions, 22
Methanesulfates, 61
Methanesulfonic acid, 22
Methionine
  chloramine T oxidation, 100—102
  cyangogen bromide peptide cleavage, 49—51
  reversible modification, 103
  structure, 99—100
Methionine sulfoxide, 99, 102
Methyl acetimidate, 139, 143
Methyl acetyl phosphate, 148, 152
N-Methyl-2-anilino-6-napthalenesulfonyl chloride, 131
Methyl-3-(*p*-azidophenyl)dithiopropioimidate, 293, 297
Methyl cellosolve, 23
Methylene blue, 105

Methylglyoxal, 187—188, 198, 203
O-Methylisourea
  amino group reactions, 140
  cysteine reaction, 83, 85
  protein guanidation, 163—164
Methylmaleic anhydride, see Citraconic anhydride
N-Methylmercaptoacetimide, 99
Methyl methanethiosulfonate, 59—60, 131—132
Methyl *p*-nitrobenzenesulfonate, 107, 109
Methyl 3-nitro-2-pyridyl disulfide, 78—79
Methyl picolinimidate, 139—141, 143
Methyl-2-pyridyl disulfide, 79—80
Michael reactions, 287—288
Microenvironment polarity, 9
Microwaves, 23
Mixed disulfide, 76, 78, see also Individual entries
Mobile phase, high-performance liquid chromatogra-
    phy, 29
Modification, reversal
  biological activity, 5—7
  tyrosine, 244, 247
  tryptophan, 226—227
Monellin, 149
Monobromobimane, 70
Monobromotrimethylammonium bimane, 70
Monosaccharides, 158, 160—161
Mutagenesis, site-specific, 4—5
Myoglobin, 32, 109
Myosin, 131, 197, 201

N

NAD(P)H:quinone reductase, 162, 262
Nbf-Cl, see 4-Chloro-7-nitrobenzo-2-oxa-1,3-diazole
NBSF, see *p*-Nitrobenzenesulfonyl fluoride
NH$_2$ terminal, 38—39
Nickel ion, 155—156
Ninhydrin
  amino acid analysis, 23—25
  arginine reaction, 173, 175
  ribonuclease reaction, 173—174
Nitration, of tyrosyl residues, 251—253
Nitrene, 314, 319
Nitroazocarboxypeptidase, 241
p-Nitrobenzenesulfonyl fluoride, 262
Nitrocarboxypeptidase, 251—252
Nitroformate, 247—248
p-Nitrophenol acetate, 231
2-(*p*-Nitrophenyl)-allyl-4-nitro-3-carboxyphenyl sul-
    fide, 287—288
2-(*p*-Nitrophenyl)allyltrimethylammonium iodide,
    287—288
p-Nitrophenyl-3-diazopyruvate, 294—295, 298, 320
p-Nitrophenylglyoxal, 187—188
p-Nitrophenyl-*p*'-guanidinobenzoate, 308
2-Nitrophenylsulfenyl chloride, 231, 233
o-Nitrophenylsulfenyl chloride, see 2-Nitrophenyl-
    sulfenyl chloride
3-Nitro-2-pyridone, 78—79
2-Nitro-5-thiocyanobenzoic acid, 70—72

[[2-Nitro-4-(trifluoromethyl-3H-diazirin-3-yl)]phenoxy]acetyl-*N*-hydroxysuccinimide, 318

Nitrotyrosine ethyl ester, 274, 280

3-Nitrotyrosine, 255, 259

Notexin, 231

NTCB, see 2-Nitro-5-(thiocyanato)benzoic acid

Nuclease, streptococcal, 253—255

Nucleophiles, dissociation constants, 8

Nucleophilic centers, proteins, 8, 129

Nucleoproteins, 136

O

Ornithine transcarbamylase, 81, 83—84

Ovomucoid, 153, 155, 157—158

Oxidative cleavage, 54

Oxyhemoglobin S, 137—138, 158—159

P

Packing, high-performance liquid chromatography, 29, 31

Papain

    carbodiimide reaction, 271

    haloacetate modification, 60—62

    methyl-2-pyridyl disulfide reaction, 81

Partial acid hydrolysis, 49

Pepsin, 4, 267, 283, 285

Pepsinogen, 11, 14—15

Peptide chloromethyl ketones, 306, 311—312, 314

Peptide bonds, chemical cleavage, 49—55, see also specific compounds

Peptide chains, cross-linking, see Cross-linking

Peptides

    mapping methods, 29—34

    subtractive degradation, 38—39

Peptidyltransferase, 108—109

Permeability, 69—70

Peroxidase, 242

pH effects

    acetyltyrosine-tetranitromethane reaction, 247

    N-bromosuccinimide-glucoamylase reaction, 221—222

    carbodiimide carboxyl group reactions, 274, 284

    disulfide bond cleavage, 97

    N-ethylmaleimide-cysteine reaction, 65

    luciferase-fluorodinitrobenzene reaction, 131, 133

    lysine deacylation, 136

    methyl-2-pyridyl disulfide UV spectrum, 78—79

    papain modification, 60—62

    photooxidation, 105

    reductive methylation, 153—154

    spin-labeled pepsinogen, 15

    thymidylate synthetase inactivation, 198, 205

    tyrosine modification, 253—254

9,10-Phenanthrenequinone, 176—178

Phenyl azide, 315, 318

o-Phenylenediamine, 176

Phenylenedimaleimides, 293, 297

Phenylglyoxal

aldehyde reductase reaction, 198, 203

arginine modification, 173, 176, 178—188

energy-dependent transhydrogenase, 196—197, 199

fatty acid synthetase reaction, 198, 204

glutamate carboxylase, 197, 202

hexokinase reaction, 197, 200

methodology, 176—177

myosin reaction, 197, 201

photophosphorylation, 196, 198

thymidylate synthetase reaction, 198—199, 205

transketolase modification, 6

Phenylhydrazine, 158—159

Phenylisothiocyanate (PITC)

    Edman degradation, 37—40

    pre-column derivatization, 23—24, 26

β-Phenylpropionate, 13, 253—254

Phosphate, 31

Phosphate-acetonitrile eluent, 30

Phosphoenolpyruvate carboxylase, 129, 131

Phosphofructokinase, 72—73

Phosphoglucomutase, 242

Phosphoglycerate kinase, 52

Phospholipase, 260—261

Phospholipase A_2

    p-bromophenacyl bromide reaction, 106—107

    carbodiimide reaction, 274, 284

    carboxyl group modification, 269, 271

    tetranitromethane reaction, 250—252

Phospholipase C, 200, 210

Phospholipid, 12, 16—17

N-(Phosphonyl)-*n*-hexylmaleimide, 70

Phosphoric acid, 31

Phosphorothioate, 95—96

Phosphorylase, 274, 281

Phosphorylase b, 292—295

Photoaffinity labels, 309, 311, 314—315

Photolysis

    cross-linking agents, 296, 299

    photoaffinity labeling, 315, 317, 320—321

Photooxidation, 105, 107—108

Photophosphorylation, 196, 198

o-Phthalaldehyde, 23

PITC, see Phenylisothiocyanate

pKa values, nucleophiles, 8—9

Polar probes, 69—70

Polarity gradient, 8—9

Polyacrylamide gel, 51

Polybrene, 41—42

Polymerization, 250—252

Polypeptides, separation, 31

Polyvinyldifluoride (PVDF) membranes, 51

Potassium chloride, 73—74

Potassium cyanate

    chalcone isomerase reactivation, 81

    deoxyribonuclease I reaction, 142

    ribulose-bisphosphate carboxylase reaction, 139

    reductive alkylation, 155—156

Pre-column derivatization, see Derivatization, pre-column

Primary structure analysis, proteins, 9—10

Proenzyme, 11, 15
Progesterone receptor, 145
Proteinase, 59—60
PTH amino acids
    high-performance liquid chromatography identification, 43
    hydrolysis, 45
    spinning-cup sequenator, 41—42
    thin-layer chromatography, 43—44
N-(Pyrenyl)maleimide, 67—68
Pyridoxal, 145
bis-Pyridoxal phosphates, 296, 301
Pyridoxal-5'-diphospho-5'adenosine, 148, 151
Pyridoxal-5'-phosphate, 141, 144—151
Pyridoxamine, 145
Pyridoxamine phosphate oxidase, 5
P,ridoxamine-5'-phosphate oxidase, 7, 112, 121—123
Pyridylethylation, 62
2-(2'-pyridylmercapto)-mercuri-4-nitrophenol, 84
Pyruvate kinase, 311

Q

Quadrol sequenator program, 41—42

R

Reagents, see also Individual entries
    cross-linking studies, 288—301
    hydrophobilic vs. hydrophilic, 70
    reaction patterns, 1—2
    spin-labeled, 10—11
Reducing agents, 99, 102
Reductive alkylation, 148, 150, 152, 155
Reductive methylation, 148—149, 153—155, 157—158
Reporter groups
    2-chloromercuri-4-nitrophenol as, 81, 83
    2-hydroxy-5-nitrobenzyl bromide as, 228—229
    3-nitrotyrosine as, 255, 259
    nitrotyrosine ethyl ester and, 274
    microenvironment changes, 10—12
Reverse-phase high-performance liquid chromatography, see High-performance liquid chromatography, reverse-phase
Rhodanese, 72
Ribonuclease, see also Ribonuclease A; Ribonuclese T
    p-diazophenylphosphate reaction, 240
    lactose reaction, 158—159
    2-(p-nitrophenyl)-allyl-4-nitro-3-carboxyphenyl sulfide cross-linking, 287
    phosphorothioate in study of, 95
    4-sulfonyl-2-nitrofluorobenzene reaction, 129—130
Ribonuclease A
    cleavage, 86—87
    phenylglyoxal reaction, 176, 179, 185
Ribonuclease T, 175, 283
Ribosomes, 105—106

Ribulose-bisphosphate carboxylase, 119, 124, 139, 145
Robot chemists, see Spinning-cup sequenator
Rose bengal, 105, 107

S

Saccharopine dehydrogenase
    2,3-butanedione reaction, 200, 210
    pyridoxal-5'-phosphate reaction, 146, 149—151
Sakaguchi reaction, 176
Salt, 74
Secretin, 109
Selenium analogs, 76, 78
Selenocysteine, 65—66
6-Seleno-3-nitrobenzoate, 74, 76
Sequenators, 40—42
Sequence determination, amino acids, see Amino acids, sequence determination
Serine protease, 230—231
Sickle cell hemoglobin, see Oxyhemoglobin S
Silica, 29
Silica gel, 44
Site-specific mutagenesis, 69—70, 162
S_N1 mechanism, 8
S_N2 mechanism, 8, 59
Sodium borohydride
    reduction, 146, 150, 152—153, 155
    structure, 157
Sodium cyanoborohydride
    monosaccharide-protein reactions, 158—160
    reduction, 149—150, 152—153
Sodium periodate, 99
Sodium sulfite, 97
Sodium tetrathionate, 59—60
Solid-phase sequenator, 42
Spin-labeled reagents, 10—11, 15
Spinning-cup sequenator, 40—42
Stationary phase, 29
Stearyl-CoA desaturase, 200, 208
Stoichiometry, of modification, 1
Stopped-flow kinetics, 220—222
Subtilisin, 4, 311—312, 314
Subtractive degradation, 38—39
Succinate dehydrogenase, 67—68
Succinic anhydride, 134
N-Succinimidyl-3(4-hydroxyphenyl)propionate. 163
Succinyl-CoA:3 ketoacid coenzyme A transferase, 72—73
Sugars, 158, 160—161
Suicide inhibitors, 309, 311
Sulfanic acid, diazotized, 242
Sulfenylation, 231, 234
Sulfhydryl (sulfydryl) groups, 59—89, see also specific reagents used
    of cysteine, 59, 62
    localization using membrane permeability, 69—70
    tetranitromethane, 247—248, 250
Sulfhydryl oxidase, 95
Sulfonium salts, 100—101, 230

2,2'-Sulfonylbis(3-methoxy-E,E')-2-propenitrile, 296, 301

Sulfonyl fluoride, 309, 311

4-Sulfonyl-2-nitrofluorobenzene, 129—130

Supports, reverse-phase, 29—31

Surface polarity, 9

T

Taipoxin, 106

Taurine transporter, human placental, 262

Temperative, reductive methylation, 154—155

Tetranitromethane
    apolipoprotein C-III modification, 13, 17
    aspartate transcarbamylase reaction, 260
    free/buried tyrosyl residues, 255
    human serum albumin reaction, 261
    2-keto-4-hydroxyglutarate aldolase reaction, 248—250
    phospholipase A$_2$ reaction, 250—252
    tyrosine modification, 247, 256—257

Thermolysin, 314, 316—317

Thermolysis
    carboxylic acid anhydride reaction, 136—137
    diethylpyrocarbonate reaction, 111—112, 118—121

Thin-layer chromatography, 43—44

Thiol groups, 87—88, 242—243

Thiol-subtilisin, subtilisin modification, 4

'Thiol-trypsin (Trypsin S195C), 5

Thiolysis, 231, 234—235

Thiomethylation, 119, 124

5-Thio-2-nitrobenzoate, 74—75

2-Thiopyridone, 79—80

Thioredoxin, 62—63

Thrombin, 3, 139

Thymidylate synthetase, 198—199, 205

TNB, see 5-Thio-2-nitrobenzoate

Tosyl acid, 22

L-1-Tosylamido-2-phenylethyl chloromethyl ketone, 311

Trace labeling, see Competitive labeling

Transcarboxylase, 223

Transhydrogenase, energy-dependent, 196—197, 199

Transketolase, 6

Trialklyoxonium fluoroborate salts, 268—269

2,4,6-Tribromo-4-methyl-cyclohexadione, 53—54

Trifluoroacetic acid, 49

2,2,2-Trifluoroethylamine, 145, 147

2-(Trifluoromethyl)-3-(m-iodophenyl)diazirine, 317—318

Trifluoroperazine-EDTA, 54—55

Trimesylation, 243—244

Trimethylamine borane, 155, 157—158

Trimethyloxonium fluroborate, 4

Trinitrobenzenesulfonic acid
    amino group reactions, 160—161

    ammonium reaction, 162—163
    deoxyribonuclease reaction, 140, 144
    hydroxide reaction, 161—162

Tri-n-butylphosphine, 97

Trypsin
    carboxy group modification, 267, 270
    dansyl chloride reaction, 129
    reductive methylation, 148—149
    spin-label derivatives and microenvironment of, 10, 12—13
    tryptophan formylation, 226—227

β-Trypsin, 9—10

Trypsin S195C, 5

Trypsinogen, 95

Tryptic digest, 30—34

Tryptophan, 215—235
    N-bromosuccinimide reaction, see N-Bromosuccinimide
    formylation, 225—227
    2-hydroxy-5-nitrobenzyl bromide reaction, 227—228
    recovery, 22
    residue cleavage, 52—54
    structure, 216

Tryptophan synthetase, 292, 296

Tryptophanase, 99

Tsou plots, applications, 3—6

Tyrosine, 1
    N-acetylimidazole and, 243—247
    diazonium salts and, 239—241
    iodination of, 241—242
    tetranitromethane and, 247—261

Tyrosyl residues, "free" vs. "buried", 255

U

Ultrasphere-ODS, 30, 44

Urea, 137, 223

Urokinase, 95

V

VydacTP column, 30—31

W

Woodward's reagent K, see N-Ethyl-5-phenylisoxazolium-3'-sulfate

X

Xylanase, 223

D-Xylose isomerase, 111

Z

Zero-length cross-linking, see Cross-linking, zero length

Zorbax TMS column, 30